AF145426

Psychiatry after Kraepelin

George Ikkos · Thomas Becker

Editors

Psychiatry after Kraepelin

Ambition Images Practices 1926-2026

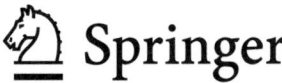 Springer

Editors
George Ikkos
Department of Liaison Psychiatry
Royal National Orthopaedic Hospital
Stanmore, UK

Thomas Becker
Department of Psychiatry and
Psychotherapy
University of Leipzig Medical Center
Leipzig, Sachsen, Germany

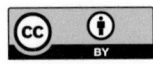

ISBN 978-3-032-09474-2   ISBN 978-3-032-09475-9   (eBook)
https://doi.org/10.1007/978-3-032-09475-9

This work was supported by Professor Burns.

© The Editor(s) (if applicable) and The Author(s) 2026. This book is an open access publication.

Open Access This book is licensed under the terms of the Creative Commons Attribution 4.0 International License (http://creativecommons.org/licenses/by/4.0/), which permits use, sharing, adaptation, distribution and reproduction in any medium or format, as long as you give appropriate credit to the original author(s) and the source, provide a link to the Creative Commons license and indicate if changes were made.
The images or other third party material in this book are included in the book's Creative Commons license, unless indicated otherwise in a credit line to the material. If material is not included in the book's Creative Commons license and your intended use is not permitted by statutory regulation or exceeds the permitted use, you will need to obtain permission directly from the copyright holder.
The use of general descriptive names, registered names, trademarks, service marks, etc. in this publication does not imply, even in the absence of a specific statement, that such names are exempt from the relevant protective laws and regulations and therefore free for general use.
The publisher, the authors and the editors are safe to assume that the advice and information in this book are believed to be true and accurate at the date of publication. Neither the publisher nor the authors or the editors give a warranty, expressed or implied, with respect to the material contained herein or for any errors or omissions that may have been made. The publisher remains neutral with regard to jurisdictional claims in published maps and institutional affiliations.

This Springer imprint is published by the registered company Springer Nature Switzerland AG
The registered company address is: Gewerbestrasse 11, 6330 Cham, Switzerland

If disposing of this product, please recycle the paper.

Foreword: Emil Kraepelin and His Legacy

Kraepelin dominated psychiatry in his own day and continues to dominate it today. His contributions to descriptive psychiatry, classification, psychopathology, experimental psychiatry and psychology, epidemiology, genetics, transcultural psychiatry, and forensics were pioneering, seminal, and remain as influential now as during his lifetime.

My purpose in this foreword is to provide a quick summary of Kraepelin's contributions to psychiatry and why they still matter from a North American perspective, though not narrowly so. I will paint a "warts and all" portrait—highlighting the highs, but not cloaking the harms of his career. Although Kraepelin advanced psychiatry in many useful and innovative directions, his narrow biological reductionism has been a heavy anchor on the field. And there is no way to avoid the fact that Kraepelin's noxious social positions added pseudoscientific fuel to the Nazi fires. But these two serious flaws do not reduce the grandeur of Kraepelin's other contributions or their enduring relevance. Anyone who wants to really understand psychiatry has to know Kraepelin.

Establishing Psychiatry Within Medicine

Psychiatry is, relatively speaking, a young specialty. Beginning with Hippocrates twenty-five hundred years ago and until Philippe Pinel (1745–1826) in the early 1800s, the major advances in psychiatry were made by generalist doctors who spent most of their time treating and describing patients with diverse medical illnesses. The one notable exception was medieval Islamic medicine, which was first to create the specialty of psychiatry a thousand years before it was recreated in Enlightenment Europe [1].

Psychiatry became a profession when it did for the same reason in both places— the establishment of asylums that specialized in caring for the mentally ill. The doctors placed in charge of asylums became the first psychiatrists. It was thus no accident that the term "psychiatry" was coined by Johann Reil (1759–1818) in 1808—just after Pinel had freed mental patients from their chains and treated them as people. The term "Psychiatry" was based on a great choice of root words, combining the ancient Greek words for "soul" (psyche) (ψυχή) and "doctor" (ἰατρός or ἰατήρ).

Ironically, no sooner had psychiatry become a medical specialty than it began a steady drift away from medicine. The heads of the usually geographically remote asylums were isolated from each other, from other doctors, and from medical schools. By the middle of the nineteenth century, they had acquired the weird new name "Alienist"—a shortened form of the French "*medecin alieniste*," a doctor who treats the "*aliene*" (literally meaning "foreign," but in usage applied to the mentally ill). Medicine was making extraordinary scientific advances, and it appeared that psychiatry would be left out and that "alienists" would serve a mostly administrative function running asylums. Kraepelin helped to bury the term "alienist" by restoring psychiatry's place in medicine.

In fact, it may be that Kraepelin's most enduring contribution was his insistence that psychiatry develop as a legitimate specialty, closely integrated with the rest of medicine. His core belief was that mental disorders are caused by brain malfunctioning in the same way as medical diseases are caused by malfunctions of other organs. He was an epistemological "realist" who believed he was describing "natural disease entities" in psychiatry equivalent to the diseases in the rest of medicine. Kraepelin applied to psychiatry the same kind of research tools that were transforming medicine: detailed, objective, and systematic clinical observation; application of the experimental method; neuropathological examination; and clinical/pathological correlation. By virtue of his prestigious professorial positions at several of the top German universities, he was also to embed psychiatry able within the mainstream of academia. His remarkably influential textbook left an indelible mark on how psychiatry has been taught in medical schools and hospitals.

Kraepelin the Great Classifier

The history of psychiatric classification is long in years and rich in contributors. But no one before Kraepelin, or since, has ever been a more determined systematizer and classifier. The order he imposed on the seeming chaos of psychiatric presentations was so compelling that it helped to develop psychiatry as a clinical science and still remains embedded in our current official nomenclatures.

Hippocrates provided the first classification in western psychiatry—including conditions we would call depression, mania, paranoia, and phobia. Galen described four temperaments (sanguinary, phlegmatic, melancholic, and choleric) which he associated with the four humors (blood, phlegm, black, and yellow bile) and suggested that imbalances predisposed to medical and psychiatric illness. Medieval Islamic psychiatry created an expanded classification that included mania, melancholia, reactive depression, delusions, and hallucinations. There was little further progress until the burst of psychiatric classifications during the eighteenth century, stimulated by Carl Linnaeus' (1707–1778) comprehensive organization of all then known plant and animal life. The two most popular psychiatric classifications, offered by Boissier de Sauvages (1706–1767) and William Cullen (1710–1709), comprised long lists of individual symptoms.

Thomas Sydenham (1624–1629) had previously taken a giant step in the classification of medical diseases late in the seventeenth century, but it was not picked up by psychiatry until early in the nineteenth century. He proposed that individual symptoms were the wrong unit for classification. It would be more productive to classify based on syndromes (clusters of symptoms that appear frequently together and help to predict course and prognosis). Pinel, Jean-Étienne Dominique Esquirol (1772–1840), Karl Ludwig Kahlbaum (1828–1899), Ewald Hecker (1843–1909), and others applied Sydenham's syndromal approach to classification in psychiatry. The value of the syndromal approach in psychiatry was first established by the rapid progress it facilitated in understanding "general paresis of the insane" (syphilis). The new paradigm was that describing a cluster of characteristic symptoms and determining their distinct course would eventually lead to discovering underlying causation (e.g., the *Treponema pallidum* bacterium in the case of general paresis). Kraepelin hoped and expected that the path from description to explanation which worked so well in unraveling general paresis would eventually work equally well in understanding the other psychiatric syndromes that he was so carefully describing. This optimism made great sense at the time, but turned out to be false hope—the major psychiatric syndromes have eluded causal explanation because their presumed causes are so numerous, so interacting, and so complicated.

The rest of this piece will describe the many specific ways Kraepelin contributed to psychiatric classification, but the main point here is that the whole of his influence was much greater than the sum of its parts. Kraepelin provided a compelling framework for describing psychiatric syndromes that is as modern as DSM-5 (the American Psychiatric Association Diagnostic and Statistical Manual, fifth edition) and ICD-11 (the World Health Organization's International Classification of Diseases, eleventh edition). It does not detract from his achievement that his descriptive/classificatory model has so far yielded so little in the way of causal explanations for psychiatric disorders [2].

Kraepelin the Great Observer and Describer

I was lucky enough during several visits to the Munich Hospital, where Kraepelin worked to review the cards he used to notate patient contacts. They are written neatly and compactly, with separate sections devoted to presenting symptoms, onset, course, and personal history—each done in different colored inks. I have no precise idea how many patients Kraepelin evaluated and documented in this meticulous and well-ordered way—but it must have been thousands. Using multi-colored cards was Kraepelin's best available method of storing and aggregating data across patients regarding which symptoms tended to cluster together into syndromes and what was the most typical onset and course of each syndrome. Having myself lived in the pre-computer era, I can fully appreciate just how tedious and painstaking this effort was to sort the clinical chaos of psychiatric symptoms into neat little research piles.

Kraepelin's passion for detail surely derived from his personality, but also reflects how high seemed the stakes. A century ago, there was good reason to believe that careful classification in any field could lead to explanatory gold. Linnaeus' descriptive classification of plants and animals led to Darwin's evolutionary explanations. Dmitri Ivanovich Mendeleev's (1834–1907) descriptive "Periodic Table" of elements led to atomic theory and the prediction of new elements. Description of medical diseases led to a revolutionary understanding of their causes and exciting discoveries of new treatments. Kraepelin's devotion to psychiatric classification made great sense, given his plausible hope it would facilitate the search for underlying causes.

Though enthusiasm for descriptive psychiatry waned after Kraepelin's death because no biological markers or causal mechanisms were discovered, his descriptive approach and passion for classification made a great comeback in the 1970s during the preparation of DSM-III. Neuroscience had advanced dramatically with the availability of powerful new research tools—brain imaging, genetics, and molecular biology. There was renewed hope that a reliable diagnostic system would yield brilliant insights into causal pathogenesis mechanisms. Fifty years later, the results have been disappointing. We still lack biological markers, and we still lack causal understanding.

Kraepelin would have had a partial understanding of this failure. He was skilled enough as a clinician to appreciate that patient presentations do not sort neatly. He knew there were no pathognomonic symptoms to pin down a diagnosis; that the symptoms characterizing any disorder are heterogeneous; and that the boundary between disorders is inherently fuzzy. Kraepelin also knew that complexity would be a great obstacle in making the leap from description to causal explanation—but he never lost faith that the gap could be bridged. What Kraepelin could not possibly know was just how ridiculously complicated the brain is and just how elusive its secrets are. There was no low-hanging fruit during Kraepelin's lifetime, and there is no low-hanging fruit during ours [3].

Kraepelin's Textbook

Textbooks usually summarize a field; rarely do they determine its future course, and never do they still have great influence 140 years after publication. Kraepelin's *A Textbook: Foundations of Psychiatry and Neuroscience* was a unique exception. Early in his career, a publisher asked Kraepelin to write a textbook of psychiatry. He agreed to do the project only for its financial, not its possible intellectual or professional, rewards. But the textbook took on a remarkable life of its own, soon to become much more than a textbook.

First published in 1883, during the next forty-four years it went through nine editions (the last one published posthumously in 1927) and evolved from a single slim book into four fat volumes. Like the DSM's (the American Psychiatric Association's five succeeding editions of its Diagnostic and Statistical Manual), the length of Kraepelin's text had increased by tenfold from first to last editions, expanding the number of mental disorders, and the detail with which each was covered.

The Table of Contents of Kraepelin's textbooks became the source of his classification and the first explication of the crucial distinction between manic depressive disorder and dementia praecox. Every subsequent classification system has since followed what started as a simple textbook—it forms the skeleton upon which DSM-5 is built. How ironic then that Kraepelin's greatest and most defining contribution to psychiatry was inspired by the most mundane of motivations—his need to make a little extra money.

Influence on Psychiatric Research

Kraepelin had hoped to have a career doing laboratory research and particularly enjoyed his experiences as the first medical doctor to work with Wilhelm Wundt (1832–1920), the father of experimental psychology. But this was not to be his fate—when Wundt could not fund a permanent place for him, Kraepelin had to leave the lab and make his living in clinical medicine. However, research always remained his first love, and he never let his administrative and educational duties interfere with it. Kraepelin was a thorough-going empiricist who rejected subjectivity and fancy theorizing, instead always promoting the virtues of systematic observation and experiment.

A strong case could be made that research was Kraepelin's greatest legacy to psychiatry. His lasting impact did not result from any particular finding, but rather from how he wove research into the fabric of psychiatry's clinical practice and education. In 1912, he began planning for a research institute devoted exclusively to psychiatry. He succeeded in doing so in 1917, in the midst of World War I—one of the first anywhere in the world. From its modest start with just a few rooms and a few investigators and aided by grants from the Rockefeller Foundation, Kraepelin's brainchild grew to become one of the leading centers in the world for psychiatric research. Renamed "The Max Planck Institute of Psychiatry," it has furthered its founder's interest in every aspect of psychiatry and embodies his insistence on rigor and excellence.

Distinguishing Dementia Praecox Versus Manic Depressive Disorder

Kraepelin's most important contribution to psychiatric classification was distinguishing "dementia praecox" (today's "schizophrenia") from "manic depressive disorder" (today's bipolar disorder). The mood disorder side of this was easy. Kraepelin just had to synthesize a long and well-traveled tradition—Hippocrates was first to describe manic-depressive patients twenty-five hundred years ago, and many others have since provided clear descriptions of melancholia, mania, and the switches that occur from one to the other.

But "dementia praecox" was then (and still remains) a much more elusive, heterogenous, and fuzzy construct lacking a long history and clear definition. Several nineteenth-century psychiatrists (Bénédict Augustin Morel (1809–1873), Thomas Clouston (1840–1915), Kahlbaum, and Hecker) had described psychotic disorders that shared an early onset and chronic course—but the symptom patterns they described were a confusing hodgepodge. Kraepelin's achievement was to integrate the diversity of presentations under one rubric (which he labeled dementia praecox) and to treat the previously independent symptom patterns as nine different subtypes of one unified disorder.

Kraepelin was aware (as many of his followers subsequently were not) that there is no pathognomonic symptom for dementia praecox and that its boundaries were inherently fuzzy. This is precisely why he put such great reliance on the more clearly distinguishing features of early onset, chronic course, and progressive deterioration. There was (and is) great clinical value in discriminating "dementia praecox" from "manic depression." This differential diagnosis often helps predict proper treatment, likely course, prognostic probabilities, and family transmission.

But the more we learn about schizophrenia and bipolar disorder, the less distinct they seem. On paper, their criteria seem worlds apart, but in the real world, patients often present with hybrid, overlapping symptoms at a fuzzy boundary. This eventually necessitated the inclusion of a fudge-factor diagnosis, "schizoaffective disorder." Course is also not always a clearly distinguishing feature—some patients with severe mood disorders have a chronic course and deteriorating outcome; some patients with schizophrenia do quite well. Medication is not a useful "diagnostic dissection tool"—antipsychotics are not at all specific, working well for both conditions. And it even turns out that the same polygenic risk factors are associated with both schizophrenia and mood disorder. Kraepelin's hope that carefully distinguishing the clinical characteristics of different mental disorders would lead to a better understanding that their distinct pathogenesis was plausible and appealing in his time—but has so far failed to deliver in ours.

Kraepelin's construct, dementia praecox (today's schizophrenia), also created new problems as it was solving old ones. Using chronic and deteriorating course as a defining requirement resulted in therapeutic nihilism and neglect of the fact that an appreciable percentage of patients have a stable course or even improve. Moreover, Kraepelin's biological determinism neglected the important role of psychosocial factors in triggering onset and exacerbations and in providing treatment. Dementia praecox was always a flawed and poorly named construct, but after more than a century of debate and intense research, we have not come up with anything much better, either in definition or in name [4].

Rescuing Alzheimer's Disease from Obscurity

Had Emil Kraepelin been pushier and Alois Alzheimer (1864–1915) more shy, what we now call "Alzheimer's disease" (the only eponymous label left in DSM) would instead have been "Kraepelin's disease." In 1903, Kraepelin (then Professor of

Clinical Psychiatry at the University of Munich) recruited Alzheimer to join him so that they could collaborate on dementia research. There was a natural division of skills and labor between the two: Kraepelin was the clinical classifier; Alzheimer the neuropathologist. They also had complementary personalities: Kraepelin was ambitious and public; Alzheimer shy and retiring.

Auguste Deter (1850–1906) was the first "Alzheimer's disease" patient. At age 51, she suffered a sudden and severe deterioration of memory accompanied by confusion; inability to perform household tasks; chronic insomnia; aggressive outbursts; jealousy regarding her husband having affairs; and the belief that neighbors and strangers intended to kill her. Alzheimer followed Deter as a patient for several years before her death, performed the autopsy, and conducted postmortem neuropathological studies. The results were amazing—he was able to identify distinctive plaques and neurofibrillary tangles in the brain histology.

Kraepelin was delighted and immediately saw the great significance of the discovery. He encouraged the reluctant Alzheimer to present his findings in a paper titled "A Peculiar Severe Disease Process of the Cerebral Cortex" to 88 participants at the 37th Meeting of South-West German Psychiatrists, held in Tubingen on November 3, 1906. Alzheimer's presentation turned out to be a dud—no questions were asked, no comments made. He was a poor speaker, but the audience may have been indifferent because the next talk was on "compulsive masturbation," a much hotter research topic at the time. There was also little interest when Alzheimer accumulated several more cases and published two papers describing the clinical course and brain findings of presenile dementia.

But Kraepelin knew that Alzheimer was on to something very big. It was a basic tenet of Kraepelin's belief and teaching that there is a specific brain lesion responsible for each mental disorder. He realized that Alzheimer had discovered a biological marker and potential cause of presenile dementia, which could now be distinguished from natural aging and from the many other forms of dementia caused by various medical and neurological illnesses. He gave a prominent place to Alzheimer's neuropathological discovery in the eighth edition of his textbook, published in 1910, and generously named presenile dementia "Alzheimer's disease." Inclusion in Kraepelin's textbook put Alzheimer's disease on the map, guaranteed its inclusion in all later classifications, and made it the subject of intense research ever since.

Including Psychopathic Personality Within Psychiatry

Kraepelin can be credited, or blamed, for the fact that "antisocial personality" is considered a mental disorder—rather than just simple bad or criminal behavior. He held the strong belief that recidivist criminal activity must indicate the presence of mental illness. Starting with the 1904 revision, his textbook added a new section devoted to "psychopathic personalities," including several specific subtypes. The powerful and enduring influence of Kraepelin's textbook resulted in the (somewhat mindless) inclusion of antisocial behavior as a psychiatric diagnosis in all subsequent systems of psychiatric classification.

Kraepelin was much influenced by the theories of the criminologist, Cesare Lombroso (1835–1909). Both argued that some people are "born criminals," suffering from a "moral defect" due to hereditary degeneration and brain pathology—a "lack or weakness of those sentiments which counter the ruthless satisfaction of egotism." Kraepelin's logic followed the seemingly plausible chain of logic—if crimes are committed because of brain disease, criminals have reduced responsibility for their acts; they should be treated, not just punished; and psychiatrists should have considerable influence in determining the length of their sentence and what occurs in prison settings.

Kraepelin's proposed extension of psychiatry into the courtroom and correctional system was once promising and popular—but it has not worked out very well. There is no effective psychiatric treatment for Antisocial behavior, and psychiatry's involvement in adversarial court proceedings has resulted in opposing expert opinions that create much heat and little light. Kraepelin's biological reductionism also blinded him to the obvious fact that criminal behavior is not just inborn and biologically determined, but also heavily influenced by parents, peers, and economic and environmental circumstances. Kraepelin's blurring of the distinction between "bad vs mad" also resulted in two unfortunate unintended consequences. First, it casts stigma on the mentally ill—the vast majority of whom are well-meaning, well-behaved, and deserve better than to be lumped with bad actors. Second, including a category of bad behavior within the psychiatric classification has provided an excuse for the bad actors—"my illness made me do it."

As Chair of the DSM-IV Task Force, I argued that "antisocial personality disorder" should be eliminated from the manual on the grounds that it describes a bad person, not mental illness; that there is no treatment for it; and that it plays no meaningful role in psychiatric practice. But Kraepelin's influence was much stronger than mine and, to my chagrin, "antisocial personality disorder" continues to be considered a mental disorder in DSM-5 [5].

Kraepelin and Psychopharmacology

Kraepelin was a pioneer in the then newly emerging field of psychopharmacology. He hoped it would provide a window into how best to sort mental illnesses; to understand their causes; and to develop better and more specific treatments. Kraepelin was the first to do experiments on the effects of drugs on psychological test performance. He studied the impacts of alcohol, morphine, chloroform, chloral hydrate, coffee, and tea. In clinical work, his medication of choice was potassium bromide to promote sleep and calm agitated patients.

By the 1950s, especially in the United States, Kraepelin's influence on psychiatry had waned with the growing popularity of psychoanalysis as a model and psychotherapy as a treatment. But Kraepelin's star rose again in subsequent decades with the exploding development of powerful new psychiatric medications (lithium, antipsychotics, antidepressants, and benzodiazepines) and research tools (brain imaging, genetics, molecular biology). By 1980, biological psychiatry was dominating psychiatry, and Kraepelin was again king [6].

Influence on Later Official Classifications

The evolving chapter headings in the successive editions of Kraepelin's textbook became the template of all subsequent psychiatric classifications. The first detailed official system in the United States, the 1918 "Statistical Manual for the Use of Institutions for the Insane," described 21 disorders, of which 19 were psychotic. Unlike previous systems which were based on individual symptoms, these were described with syndromal complexity and sometimes with causal inference [7].

Responding to the needs of soldiers during World War II, the US Army developed an expanded psychiatric classification that combined the (largely inpatient) psychotic disorders described by Kraepelin with newly included (largely outpatient) psychoneurotic and personality disorders, mostly described by Sigmund Freud (1856–1939) and his followers. After the war, the US Veterans Administration expanded the Army classification even further to account for outpatient problems. In 1949, the sixth edition of the "International Classification of Diseases" for the first timed added a special section for mental disorders, again heavily influenced by Kraepelin's descriptions of psychotic disorders and Freud's descriptions of neurotic disorders.

DSM I, published in 1950 by the American Psychiatric Association, reflected three main influences—Kraepelin's psychotic disorders; Freud's psychoneurotic disorders; and Adolph Meyer's (1866–1950) view that mental disorders are at least partly a reaction to life stresses and circumstances. A slightly modified DSM II was published in 1968. DSM-I and DSM-II had very brief, impressionistic descriptions of mental disorders that were almost completely unreliable and largely ignored.

The DSM-III's "Neo-Kraepelinian" Gang

Most of the people who worked on DSM-III described themselves proudly and triumphantly as "Neo-Kraepelinians." They were like Kraepelin in their desire to return psychiatry to a more scientific and strictly biological discipline. They shared Kraepelin's (still unrealized) hope and expectation that a clear, reliable classification of mental disorders would soon promote an understanding of their biological precursors. They believed that the new psychotropic drugs (which then seemed to have specific indications) provided confirmation of Kraepelin's syndromes. They were like Kraepelin in their passionate preoccupation with descriptive psychiatry—the delineation of syndromes and attempts to distinguish boundaries between them. Like Kraepelin, they sought to provide psychiatry with a common language for clinical communication, education, and research. And, finally, they cherished Kraepelin's empiricism and worshiped "reliability" as the highest goal of the diagnostic system.

The Neo-Kraepelinians also rechanneled some of Kraepelin's less useful tendencies. They reproduced his naive realism, that the syndromes they concocted in committee meetings would somehow necessarily reflect the inherent nature of things and represent the best or only way to construct a psychiatric classification. They equally adhered to Kraepelin's biological reductionism, neglecting the crucial role psychological and social factors have in describing, understanding, and treating mental disorders. Like Kraepelin, the Neo-Kraepelinians were also aggressively anti-Freudian and felt it their mission to eliminate what they regarded as Freudian contaminants from the pure gold of scientific biological psychiatry. This sometimes led to silly over-reach. After fierce controversy, the Neo-Kraepelinians successfully removed the term "neurosis" from the DSM system. Their eagerness to do this was based on the false belief that the term was of Freudian origin, when in fact it was first coined in 1769 by William Cullen and had been in continuous use ever since by psychiatrists all around the world, many of whom either opposed Freud or never heard of him.

I was the token clinician among the DSM-III Neo-Kraepelinians (most of whom saw patients only as part of research studies or not at all). Their lack of everyday clinical experience allowed them to see a clarity in criteria building that I knew did not at all reflect the heterogeneity, fuzzy boundaries, and comorbidity of real-world patients. I was also given the thankless and impossible task of liaison to representatives of psychodynamic, family, and group therapy associations, all of whom were rightly concerned that DSM-III would have a detrimental impact on psychotherapy. I could provide no reassurance. The Neo-Kraepelinians, like Kraepelin, were strongly biased toward biological treatment and either hostile or indifferent toward psychotherapy.

It turned out, however, that I was far more Kraepelinian than the Neo-Kraepelinians on one issue—the proper definition of schizophrenia. They recklessly abandoned Kraepelin's requirement that schizophrenia have a chronic course and instead shifted the definition to emphasize Kurt Schneider's (1887–1967) "First Rank" symptoms (i.e., thought echo, insertion, withdrawal, or broadcasting; delusions of control, influence, or passivity; hallucinatory voices conducting a running commentary or discussing the patient; and bizarre delusions). There was a laudable motivation, in switching away from a longitudinal course and toward cross-sectional evaluation of symptoms, the now not so Neo-Kraepelinians were hoping to facilitate earlier diagnosis and more timely treatment. But there is a big problem with Schneider's "First Rank" symptoms: they are not really first rank because they are not specific to schizophrenia and don't predict its typically chronic course. Reliance on first rank symptoms leads to massive overdiagnosis of schizophrenia, causing great overuse of harmful medicines, avoidable demoralization, and needless stigma. Kraepelin understood something the Neo-Kraepelinians did not: there are no pathognomonic symptoms for schizophrenia or other mental disorders, and there are fuzzy boundaries between them. It turns out that on this issue I was right to stick with Kraepelin; the Neo-Kraepelians were wrong to abandon him.

Transcultural Psychiatry

Kraepelin made early systematic contributions to transcultural psychiatry. As a frequent and adventurous traveler (often accompanying his brother Karl, a prominent botanist, on collecting trips to exotic places), he began the systematic study of whether and how psychopathology presents itself differently in different cultures. This research began in 1904 with patients in an Indonesian psychiatric hospital. Kraepelin compared the symptom presentations and course of 100 European, 100 indigenous, and 25 Chinese patients. He next planned to organize a comparative study of the rates and presentations of psychiatric disorders in seven European countries, but this had to be canceled because of World War I. Kraepelin's last study, shortly before his death, compared American Indian, Afro-American, and Latin American patients hospitalized in the United States, Mexico, and Cuba. Numerous transcultural studies conducted since reveal that the rates of the different mental disorders are not radically different around the world but that cultural factors do have a significant influence on symptom presentation and course [8].

Comparing Kraepelin and Freud

Despite striking parallels in their lives and work, Kraepelin and Freud never once met or corresponded and rarely referenced each other. The two pioneers of modern psychiatry were born in the same year, just 3 months and 300 miles apart. Both trained in neuroanatomy and were heavily influenced by Charles Darwin's (1809–1882) then startling evolutionary theories. Both studied with Jean-Martin Charcot (1825–1893) in Paris. Both were forced to leave laboratory science for clinical work in order to make a living. Both were great observers and elegant writers. They shared the same professional interest in describing and explaining psychiatric symptoms. During the prime of their careers, Kraepelin and Freud lived and worked in cities, Munich and Vienna, that were only 250 miles apart (but interestingly, neither ever bothered to visit the other, although both were great travelers). They even looked enough alike as young men to be mistaken for brothers.

Kraepelin and Freud also shared the same critical flaw—they were both bad epistemologists. Kraepelin was a biological reductionist and naive realist who believed he was carving nature at its joints. He assumed that he was describing and classifying actual diseases that would eventually be explained by brain pathology, rather than just sorting symptoms into very heterogeneous syndromes with very fuzzy boundaries and ridiculously complex and interacting causes. Freud's bio/psych/social model of mental illness was much more rounded and accurate in describing the complexity of human behavior and mental illness. But he was equally epistemologically naive in assuming that psychoanalysis was a useful research tool to uncover the complex pathogenesis of mental disorders.

But here the many surprising congruences between Kraepelin and Freud stop. Both shaped modern psychiatry, but took it in very different, and sometimes opposing, directions. Kraepelin worked almost exclusively in hospital settings with inpatients suffering from the most severe psychiatric disorders. Except for six months of training in psychiatry, Freud worked exclusively with much better-functioning outpatients. Kraepelin was an esteemed professor who had risen quickly within the highly competitive German academic system. Freud was a defiant outsider, much better known to the general public, but often reviled within mainstream academic circles. Kraepelin focused on describing psychiatric presentations, classifying them into distinct syndromes, and carefully tracing their course and outcome. Freud was much more interested in explaining the origin of symptoms than in describing them (although he was an excellent describer and has had a profound, if largely unrecognized, influence on DSM-V).

Kraepelin and Freud never competed directly, but their followers certainly did. Their ideas and methods have had inverse periods of popularity. Kraepelin's follows a U-curve; his work dominated psychiatry at the turn of the twentieth century, was then largely eclipsed by Freud (especially in the United States) during its middle, and has again become dominant during the last 50 years. Freud's influence was at its height when Kraepelin's was lowest and has since steadily declined with the current Neo-Kraepelinian revival. Freud was greatly overrated during his own time, but is greatly underrated in ours.

The Good, Bad, and Ugly of Kraepelin's Social Legacy

Once he attained fame and influence, Kraepelin increasingly spoke out on social and political issues. Some of his influence was beneficial, but much of it was horribly misguided and fed directly into Nazi dogma and the Holocaust.

On the positive side, Kraepelin was often a voice for the voiceless, advocating strongly for better care and treatment of the severely ill and against their neglect and criminalization. His causes then are still our causes now. He spoke out against the barbarous treatment that was prevalent in the psychiatric asylums of the time and fought against imprisoning, rather than treating, the mentally ill. His focus on the innate biological origins of mental disorders reduced the personal blame and stigma that was then, and is now, attached to having psychiatric problems. He also crusaded against capital punishment [8, 9].

But many of Kraepelin's social positions were inhumane and dangerous. His enthusiastic support of the then thriving eugenics movement had the tragic unintended consequence of legitimizing Nazi atrocities. He was a Social Darwinist, arguing that the welfare state (more advanced in Germany than in any other developed country) would necessarily interfere with the competitive workings of natural selection and cause an increase in mental illness, addiction, and criminality. He also supported the then popular idea that careful family history taking could predict which people were at risk for passing bad genes on to future generations and that they should be discouraged from having children as a way of protecting the genetic integrity of the German people. Most chillingly, he singled out Jews as being particularly vulnerable to nervous and mental disorders. Similarly, Kraepelin's dangerous views on homosexuality were widely held at the time but gained added currency by being espoused from his position of scientific authority. Unlike Freud, he considered homosexuality to be a vice, not a biological predisposition, and attributed it to degeneration and excessive masturbation. His prescriptive solution—"educational discipline"—was transformed by the Nazis into brutal treatment and extermination [10].

Kraepelin was not himself a member of the Nazi party, and he died seven years before it came into power. But he was a member of another nationalist party that promoted authoritarian rule, extreme patriotism, and aggressive nationalism. It is unknowable how Kraepelin would have felt and reacted to Nazi atrocities had he lived long enough to experience them. His passionate opposition to the death penalty suggests he would have felt disgusted and ashamed. And it may be considered by some unfair for us to retrospectively blame Kraepelin for holding views on eugenics, race, and sexuality that, though by no means universal, were then widespread among psychiatrists and the general public (not just in Germany but throughout Europe and most passionately in the United States). And even more unfair to blame him for the Nazi atrocities that began after his death. The Nazis would most certainly have been Nazis had Kraepelin never existed or if his views were opposite to what they were. Nor could Kraepelin have anticipated the horrors perpetrated by his students—the prominent Nazi psychiatrists Robert Gaupp (1870–1953), Paul Nitsche (1876–1948), and Ernst Rüdin (1874–1952), who were responsible for the "euthanasia" programs that killed tens of thousands of the mentally ill. But I think we must accept that Kraepelin the great psychiatrist and humanitarian was also Kraepelin the promulgator of horrible social views that greased the Nazi slope to cold-blooded murder on a scale never before experienced by humanity [10, 11].

Conclusion: Emil Kraepelin and This Book

This book marks the hundredth anniversary of Kraepelin's death and explores ways his work remains influential. There are many hundreds of psychiatrists who have been famous and powerful in their own times who are completely forgotten in ours. What is different about Kraepelin? Why does his work still matter so much?

Certainly, it was not creativity. Kraepelin's two biggest innovations (connecting syndromes to course and distinguishing what we call schizophrenia from bipolar disorder) were not particularly novel and instead were built on work done by many others prior to him and within his lifetime. What distinguished Kraepelin was his ability as a systematizer—no one before or since has been better at describing patients so clearly *and* classifying them so well into categories based on symptom correlations and course. It also helped spread his influence widely that Kraepelin presided through eight revisions of the most influential textbook ever written (perhaps in any field) and that he chaired one of the most prestigious psychiatry departments in the world. He was extremely good at what he did, and he did a lot.

But there is also another factor responsible for Kraepelin's continuing influence that says less about his greatness and more about the slowness of advances in psychiatry. In no other medical specialty would this much reference be made to bygone leaders who accomplished no more than furthering the description of syndromes. The action now in medicine has moved rapidly from description to explanation via a precise understanding of the genetics and molecular biology of various diseases. The fact that such great leaps forward have not occurred in psychiatry is not for any want of trying—tens of billions of dollars have been spent in a so far mostly failed effort to understand the fundamental causes of psychiatric disorders. And thousands of brilliant minds have spent decades of their careers on the hot pursuit. We have learned a great deal about the brain in the past 50 years, using remarkably powerful gene, molecular biology, and imaging tools. It has been a great intellectual adventure. But this has not provided biomarkers of mental disorder, or understanding of pathogenesis, or radical improvements in treatment. Sad to say, part of Kraepelin's long lingering name and influence results from the fact that psychiatry has a much steeper mountain to climb than most of medicine, has progressed much more slowly, and is still mostly stuck at Kraepelin's descriptive level.

The brain is by far the most complex thing in the known universe (though artificial intelligence is rapidly catching up). Three pounds of squiggly tissue contains 86 billion neutrons connected to each other by several hundred trillion synapses. The choreography that allows 20,000 genes to create a functioning brain is weirdly complicated in itself and gets even more awe-inspiring when you consider the great influence environment has on gene expression and neuron connectivity. It is hard enough to understand what goes wrong to produce malfunctions in relatively simple tissues like breast and liver; it is orders of magnitude harder to decipher the brain.

Kraepelin's role in psychiatry will diminish, only if and when we get a clearer and deeper knowledge of what causes the psychiatric problems he was describing and attempting to classify. It is the notable merit of this book that it squares up both to the grandeur and harm of his legacy. Its chapters trace in detail the origins and evolution of some of their key aspects. But it also looks beyond Kraepelin's influence both in terms of spread of geographical practice and across time. And it gives due attention to alternative methodologies and approaches, including what has been perhaps the single most positive development since his time, namely the service user perspective.

The view that the greatness of a scientist should be measured not by the years she or he advanced their field but by how many years they have held it back, has been attributed to Danish physicist Niels Bohr (1885–1962). Kraepelin's most important contribution has been to secure psychiatry's position in medicine, but it is clear now that the continuing espousal of his perspective will hold it back both within the profession and beyond. Contributors to this volume show us that there have always been other ways of doing things and offer strong hints about how they may be done differently in the future.

Acknowledgment

Most of what I know about Kraepelin, I learned from Professor Hanns Hippius, who succeeded him as Medical Director (1971–1994) of the Department of Psychiatry and Psychotherapy at the Ludwig Maximilian University in Munich and edited the fascinating "Emil Kraepelin Memoirs." Hans was a great teacher, clinician, researcher, mentor, and friend [12].

Department of Psychiatry and Behavioral Science   Allen Frances
Duke University School of Medicine
Durham, UK

Suggested Readings

1. Pormann P, Savage-Smith E. The clinico-diagnostic perspective in psychopathology. Physicians and Society, Ch. 3 in Medieval Islamic Medicine, Edinburgh UPBerrios GE: Hist Psychiatry. 2007;18(70 part 2):231–3.
2. Kraepelin E. Patterns of mental disorder, Ch.1: In Themes and variations in European Psychiatry, Hirsch SR, Shepherd M, editors. University Press of Virginia; 1974.
3. Hippius H, Neundörfer G. The discovery of Alzheimer's disease. Dialogues Clin Neuroscience. 2003;5(1):101–108. https://pmc.ncbi.nlm.nih.gov/articles/PMC3181715/.
4. Jablenski A. The diagnostic concept of schizophrenia: its history, evolution, and future prospects. Dialogues Clin Neurosci. 2010;12(3):271–87. https://pmc.ncbi.nlm.nih.gov/articles/PMC3181977/.
5. Hoff P. Emil Kraepelin and forensic psychiatry. Int J Law Psychiatry. 1998. https://pubmed.ncbi.nlm.nih.gov/9870176/.
6. Müller U. The origin of pharmacopsychology: Emil Kraepelin's experiments in Leipzig, Dorpat and Heidelberg (1882-1892). Psychopharmacology. 2006. https://pubmed.ncbi.nlm.nih.gov/16378216/.
7. Statistical Manual for the Use of Institutions for the Insane. 1918. https://openlibrary.org/works/OL1201453W/Statistical_manual_for_the_use_of_institutions_for_the_insane
8. Steinberg H. Emil Kraepelin's ideas on transcultural psychiatry. Aust Psychiatry. 2015;23(5). https://journals.sagepub.com/doi/abs/10.1177/1039856215590253?download=true&journalCode=apya
9. Jilek WG. Emil Kraepelin and comparative sociocultural psychiatry. European Arch Psychiatry Clin Neuroscience. 1995. https://pubmed.ncbi.nlm.nih.gov/7578286/#:~:text=One%20year%20before%20his%20unexpected,E%20Kraepelin
10. Mildenberger F. Kraepelin and the 'urnings': male homosexuality in psychiatricdiscourse. Hist Psychiatry. 2007;18:321–35.
11. Shepherd M. Two faces of Emil Kraepelin. Br J Psychiatry 1995,167:174–183, "Emil Kraepelin Memoirs" (Hippius H, Peters G, Ploog G, editors), Springer-Verlag, Heidelberg; 1987.

Introduction: Psychiatry After Kraepelin and Beyond

The historian is a prophet looking backwards. (Friedrich Schlegel, *Atheneum Fragments* [1])

We need history, but our need for it differs from that of the jaded idlers in the garden of knowledge. (Friedrich Nietzsche, *On the Advantages and Disadvantages of History for Life* [2])

It may be that continuity is mere semblance. But then precisely the persistence of the semblance of persistence provides it with continuity. (Walter Benjamin, *The Arcades Project* [3])

The year 2026 marks 100 years since the death of Emil Kraepelin (15 February 1856–7 October 1926) and only a little over 125 years since he first used the term "dementia praecox" to label the syndrome he had first described in 1899 and which later, following Bleuler, came to be called schizophrenia [4]. He wrote beautifully, was thoroughly committed to the scientific method, was systematic in his observations and meticulous in his record keeping, and developed a formidable clinical and research department and professional legacy. Arguably, the nine editions of his *Handbook of Psychiatry* and his original descriptions of schizophrenia and manic depression (manisch-depressives Irresein, now bipolar disorder) have provided the most consistent backbone for research and clinical practice in psychiatry since his time. However, both his observations and formulations have been repeatedly challenged and his views on degeneration and eugenics have continued causing concern ever since.

Our Intentions

The present volume attempts neither a comprehensive record nor assessment of Kraepelin, nor of psychiatry. On the occasion of the centenary of his death, however, it hopes to bear on both. And, with respect to psychiatry as a field, it aims to note developments beyond Kraepelin, those that would have pleased him, others that might have surprised him, and yet others that might have shocked him. It is important to emphasise, however, that though inspired by the centenary of Kraepelin, this book is neither about him, nor against him. The enduring influence of his work and resonance of his concerns have acted as a catalyst, but it would be wrong to examine 100 years of psychiatry simply through the lens of Kraepelin. In some ways psychiatry has moved so far beyond him that this would be too restrictive. A most important example here is the increasing voice of the service user movement and the need for co-creation and co-production of recovery and mental health [5]. Therefore, our intention has been to create a montage occasioned by Kraepelin's centenary which is in dialectic tension with it.

Today's contested geopolitics, with threats and imperial wars under other names, might have been familiar to Kraepelin. However, including in psychiatry, we are an eternity away from his time. Developments in science, technology, society, and culture have transformed the world, much as the nineteenth century had transformed itself compared to the previous one. No doubt, this will tempt or persuade many to think that it would be best to forget him, just focus on today's promises. In contrast, we expect that those who read these lines will want to learn the lessons arising from the dismal gap between Kraepelin's confident expectations and what followed [6], including reality now [7]. And we would argue that it is this gap which keeps presenting itself and the opportunity to reflect on it that can also be part of Kraepelin's legacy and a foundation for a better future. And, also, that it is by reflecting not only on the texts of our montage but also on the spaces between them that the reader may benefit most.

The Book

In putting together our montage, we have thought along two axes. One is that of Kraepelin's take on psychopathology, biology, culture, and experience. The other, psychiatry's ambitions, public image and actual practices. The outcome has been a six-part volume as follows:

Part A "Emil Kraepelin" aims to meet Kraepelin in his times and bring him directly face to face with today's psychiatry. Emil Kraepelin remains a towering and contested figure in the history of psychiatry, not only for the systems he proposed but for the questions he left unresolved. His legacy is visible in the way modern psychiatry still grapples with how best to classify, understand, and treat mental disorders. While he helped shape a more systematic and observational approach to diagnosis, critics—both then and now—have challenged the limits of this method, arguing that it overlooks the depth and nuance of subjective experience. These chapters revisit these enduring tensions, showing how Kraepelin's work sparked important debates about the relationship between biology, lived experience, and meaning in psychiatry. Rather than treating him as simply a founder or a figure of the past, the authors use his work as a lens through which to examine the ongoing struggle to develop a psychiatry that does justice to both scientific insight and human complexity.

Part B "After Darwin: Biology in the Evolution of Psychiatry" examines complex key issues relating to Darwin's legacy in psychiatry, some of them mediated by Kraepelin initially, yet others beyond him. This is not simply about biology but about biology, psychiatry, and society more broadly. Some of Kraepelin's early biological assumptions, particularly his endorsement of degeneration theory and eugenic thinking, reflected broader scientific and societal biases shared by some in his time and later definitely proved both scientifically flawed and ethically catastrophic. In contrast, contemporary genetics and neuroscience take a more nuanced view of human variation. Rather than supporting rigid categories or deterministic views of inheritance, modern research emphasises how genetic risk factors for mental health conditions are probabilistic, often overlapping across diagnoses, and shaped by interactions with the environment. This means that traits linked to vulnerability in one context may contribute to strengths in another. Similarly, neuroimaging studies reveal patterns of brain structure and function that can be associated with certain mental health conditions, but these findings are typically dimensional rather than categorical—illustrating gradients rather than clear-cut boundaries between health and illness. Together, these advances challenge older dichotomies and support more flexible, person-centred understandings of mental health.

Part C "Psychiatric Diagnosis: Concepts and Challenges" examines relevant developments in relation to psychiatric diagnosis both from more narrowly empirical positive scientific and more socially critical points of view. His own late doubts notwithstanding, Kraepelin's early and determined insistence on discrete diagnostic entities and his distinction between schizophrenia and manic depression are perhaps his most enduring legacies in psychiatry and its lasting controversies.

Understanding psychiatric diagnosis requires attention not only to biological or clinical indicators but also to the overlapping and often ambiguous nature of human psychological suffering. Symptoms associated with certain diagnoses—such as emotional volatility, social withdrawal, or unusual perception—can arise from diverse origins including infection, substance use, trauma, or developmental variation. Rather than fitting individuals neatly into rigid categories, it may be more useful to view mental distress along spectrums that reflect the full range of human neurobiological and experiential diversity. Concepts like neurodiversity invite us to rethink difference not as disorder but as variation—and highlight how traits that may challenge social norms can also contribute to focus, innovation, or creativity, particularly when individuals are adequately supported in environments that value inclusion.

The use of diagnostic labels has not only shaped clinical practice but has also carried profound social consequences, especially when tied to political ideologies or systems of control. History offers stark examples of how psychiatric categories were weaponised, most horrifically under Nazi rule, when individuals deemed mentally unfit were subjected to sterilisation, institutionalisation, or even extermination. In response to such abuses, some postwar movements within psychiatry have aimed to humanise care, drawing inspiration from philosophical, psychoanalytic, and sociological traditions to create more participatory and respectful therapeutic environments. More recently, a grassroots intellectual movement known as Mad Studies has emerged, led by individuals with lived experience. Challenging traditional power structures in psychiatry, this movement advocates for recognition of survivor perspectives and promotes alternative ways of teaching, researching, and understanding mental health across academic and clinical settings.

Part D "Image, Imagination and Experience" looks at brain imaging, but also at the imagination, and images emerging directly from the experience of psychiatry or philosophical reflection on it. The discovery and widespread use of Computerised Axial Tomography (CAT) in the 1970s has had a profound methodological impact on psychiatric research. Yet, the importance of other images and imagination require attention of their own. The chapters highlight the need for psychiatry to balance scientific insight with a deeper appreciation of lived experience and subjective meaning. While advances in neuroscience offer valuable perspectives on how trauma and adversity shape brain function, they cannot replace the complexity of personal narratives. The importance of approaching concepts such as the self not as fixed scientific objects but as evolving constructs shaped by both biology and experience is highlighted. Attention is drawn to the contributions of thinkers who foreground the richness of individual perception and the existential dimensions of mental distress. Through personal testimonies and reflective accounts, the chapters invite a rethinking of how experience—particularly in distressing circumstances—can inform and enrich both clinical understanding and human connection in mental health care.

Part E "Mental Health Services: Reality and Ambition" looks at the history and ambitions of psychiatry with respect to theories of psychiatry and the practical development of mental health services. Both in relation to and beyond Kraepelin, it surveys a range of countries and regions across the world during the twentieth century. The chapters explore how psychiatric ideas evolved and were adapted across various geopolitical and cultural contexts throughout this period. They examine the imprint of colonial legacies, authoritarian regimes, and Cold War tensions on psychiatric practices and theories. They highlight how local responses were shaped by broader ideological and historical forces. Case studies include postcolonial mental health strategies, the politicisation of psychiatry in totalitarian states, and the philosophical underpinnings of reform movements in both Western Europe and Latin America. Together they illustrate a dynamic interplay between global influences and local conditions in the transformation of mental health care.

Part F "Psychiatry and Mental Health Services Today and Tomorrow" looks at psychiatry's future from the perspectives of psychiatric research, peer support, clinical treatment and services, and justice and vocation. The authors detail how psychiatry is being reimagined in the light of both scientific advancements and shifting societal expectations. They reflect on the role of neuroscience and translational research in shaping future directions and a growing recognition of the value of lived experience in care delivery. Innovative approaches to understanding psychosis challenge the clinical utility of the diagnostic label of schizophrenia, while national case studies, such as Denmark, illustrate how constructive professional and campaigning group dialogue can generate effective policy alignment to ensure political prioritisation of mental health and secure resources to drive systemic reform. The concluding reflections engage with historical, ethical, and philosophical dimensions relevant to psychiatry's future, questioning how justice, empathy, and professional purpose can be sustained in the face of evolving political, economic, and ecological pressures.

To Readers

Our authors come to psychiatry from very diverse fields and experiences. Therefore, in order to give them the opportunity to bring to this volume what they think is best about their approach, our instructions to them have been very limited. However, we have also tried to assist readers by suggesting the presence in each chapter of an abstract (online publication only), keywords (online publication only), introduction, conclusion, and five key bullet points at the end. Unavoidably, the language in a number of chapters remains highly technical. In some, we have tried to assist somewhat through lists of abbreviated terms, glossaries, and images.

We hope that readers will find this a forward-looking volume. We intend that our montage both inform about the range and subtlety of issues and stimulate new ideas and debate. With respect to the latter, where necessary, it should help to bring into sharper focus the differences of evidence, experience, and opinion and promote more dialogue and understanding. This, in turn, should help psychiatry learn from and move on decisively beyond its long twentieth century 1899–2026 [8].

George Ikkos
Thomas Becker

References

1. Schlegel F. Athenaeum Fragments, published in: German History in Documents and Images. 1798. https://germanhistorydocs.org/en/the-holy-roman-empire-1648-1815/ghdi:document-5363. December 13, 2024.
2. Nietzsche F. On the advantages and disadvantages of history for life. 1873, quoted as epigram to Thesis XII in Benjamin W. 1999. On the concept of history, in tr Zorn H. eds Eilan H, Jennings MW. 2003. p. 394.
3. Benjamin W. N19,1 in tr. Eiland H, McLaughlin E, editors. The Arcades project. Belknap Press of Harvard University Press; 1999. p. 486.
4. Emil Kraepelin Memoirs. Hippius H, Peters G, Ploog D, editors. Berlin: Springer Verlag; 1987.
5. Ikkos G, Bouras N, editors. Epilogue: Mind, state, society and 'Our psychiatric future'. In: Mind, state and society: Social history of psychiatry and mental health in Britain 1960–2010. Cambridge University Press; 2021.
6. Ikkos G, Stanghellini G, Morgan A. History, 'nowtime' (jetztzeit) and dialectical images: introduction to Walter Benjamin for psychiatry (I). Int Rev Psychiatry. 2024;36(6):585–99. https://doi.org/10.1080/09540261.2024.2359468.
7. Harrington A. The mind fixers: Psychiatry's troubled search for the biology of mental illness. 2019.
8. Ikkos G, Stanghellini G, Becker T. The precision of images: Emil Kraepelin, Walter Benjamin and a space for rethinking psychiatry. Int Rev Psychiatry. 2024;36(6):553–6. https://doi.org/10.1080/09540261.2024.2382022.

Advance Reviews

Psychiatry After Kraepelin: Ambition Images and Practices 1926-2026, edited by George Ikkos and Thomas Becker, makes a unique contribution which successfully integrates the numerous authors' perspectives on psychiatry and mental health for the contemporary world.

Each of the seven parts of the book can stand alone as a valuable, autonomous collection, offering substantial insight and knowledge. This also holds true for each of the 27 chapters, all written by leading experts from a wide range of disciplines—from psychiatry to philosophy.

Using Kraepelin's work as a common foundation, *Psychiatry After Kraepelin* offers a reflective and historically informed analysis of the current state of mental health. It presents a panoramic view of the evolution of psychiatry in relation to global social, cultural, scientific, and ideological transformations and identifies key issues that have emerged from truly paradigmatic shifts in modern life, causing profound impacts on mental health.

The editors' conception and integration of the sections and chapters reveal a holistic understanding of human subjectivity. They place psychiatry and mental health within the broader context of human experience—encompassing changes in natural and social science, technology, culture, society, and ideology. Through a strong and well-founded scientific discourse, mediated by their authors, they advocate for prioritizing mental health and call for a more human-centered way of life.

In an era characterized by individualism and fragmentation—even within our professional lives—Ikkos and Becker have created a volume that shows how science can contribute to the humanization of our world by combating the growing dehumanization we face today. In the spirit of Aristotle's concept of *politikē* (πολιτική), it embodies high political value, too.

Psychiatry After Kraepelin is a volume that should be read not only by those interested in the future of psychiatry and mental health but by all who care about the future of our world. *Professor Dimitris C. Anagnostopoulos, MD, PhD, Emeritus Professor of Child and Adolescent Psychiatry, National and Kapodistrian University of Athens, Greece, and Immediate Past President of the European Society for Child and Adolescent Psychiatry*

This compelling and accessible book charts the evolution of modern psychiatry, grounded in Kraepelin's pioneering work and its enduring influence. Bridging a long-standing gap in the literature, it offers a global, historically informed view of how mental illness has been classified, understood, and challenged over the past century. Authored by internationally renowned experts, it is essential reading for anyone interested in the scientific and historical foundations of psychiatry—and in the future direction of mental health care and clinical practice. *Professor Nick Bouras, MD, PhD, Emeritus Professor of Psychiatry, Institute of Psychiatry, Psychology and Neuroscience: King's College: London*

Emil Kraepelin's ideas and research programme have exercised an unparalleled influence in shaping psychiatry as a medical discipline in what the editors of this volume label as its "long 20th century 1899–2026". The book's sections and chapters trace his influence, as well as the impact of further developments in the medical sciences and technologies, the humanities and service user movements, and political and economic disasters and opportunities. At a time of rapid increase in demand for mental health services but also fears both of the overmedicalisation of everyday life and the excessive demedicalisation of psychiatry, this is no idle endeavour. It is essential thought leadership on issues concerning the core identity of psychiatry and the place of psychiatrists in society. *Psychiatry after Kraepelin* is an essential text for current and aspiring psychiatrists; a resource not just for the personal library but also to trigger vital discussions in clinical and educational supervision and journal clubs worldwide. *Professor Subodh Dave, FRCPsych, MMed (Clinical Education) Dean, Royal College of Psychiatrists; Professor of Psychiatry, University of Greater Manchester; Consultant Psychiatrist and Deputy Director of Undergraduate Medical Education, Derbyshire Healthcare Foundation Trust*

Marking 100 years since Emil Kraepelin's death, this remarkable volume brings together world-leading experts across disciplines—from molecular genetics and neurodiversity to philosophy and evolutionary psychiatry—to reflect on his enduring legacy. The editors have curated a compelling account of psychiatric practice, policy, and research over the past century, including critical perspectives on the realities of mental health care and the evolution of psychiatric nosology. With 27 chapters, the book offers a consistent thread tracing Kraepelin's influence while openly addressing his troubling views on eugenics and degeneration. Far more than a historical text, it raises vital questions about the future direction of psychiatry. This is an essential resource not only for psychiatrists, but for all involved in mental health—clinicians, policymakers, researchers, and patient advocates alike. With this authoritative and thought-provoking work, Professors George Ikkos and Thomas Becker have created a legacy of their own. *Professor Kevin Gournay, CBE, FMedSci, FRCPsych (Hon), PhD, CPsychol, RN, Emeritus Professor of Psychiatric Nursing: Institute of Psychiatry, Psychology and Neuroscience, King's College, London; Honorary Professor: Matilda Centre, Faculty of Medicine and Health, University of Sydney*

Eugen Bleuler's nomination of Emil Kraepelin for the Nobel Prize in 1917 serves as a poignant reminder of the challenges involved in understanding psychiatry. Bleuler likened the pursuit of knowledge in this field to climbing a glass mountain, with Kraepelin's pioneering work acting as a set of stairs cutting through the mountain by providing a scientific basis for the discipline. However, our understanding of Kraepelin's legacy and its impact on psychiatry has evolved over time, shaped by various layers of memory and influenced by social, intellectual, and philosophical contexts.

On the occasion of the centenary of Kraepelin's death, the editors of this volume have undertaken an initiative to re-examine the current state of psychiatry. They start with Kraepelin's contributions but also consider the broader historical and philosophical contexts that have shaped the field. They aim to provide a nuanced understanding of how the past influences present and future psychiatry, including the social, intellectual, and philosophical factors that have contributed to its development.

To achieve this ambitious goal, the editors have compiled a volume that showcases the benefits of interdisciplinarity. The book offers a unique perspective on the past century of psychiatry, featuring contributions from psychiatrists and authors from the arts and humanities, as well as experts from other fields, including the emerging field of mad studies. The chapters provide a postcolonial, international comparative analysis of the evolution of psychiatry, highlighting the complexities and challenges involved in understanding human behaviour, mentality, and mental health.

This volume is more than a collection of essays; it is a thoughtful, clever, and intelligently compiled handbook on the path dependencies that have shaped psychiatry. The editors' modest description of the book as a "montage" does not do justice to its significance. Rather, it is a valuable resource that offers insights into the historical and philosophical contexts that have influenced current perspectives on psychiatry, with both positive and negative effects on humanity, mental health, and public health.

Anyone interested in mental health, regardless of their professional background, will find this book to be a valuable read from start to finish. The editors' comprehensive and nuanced exploration of the evolution of psychiatry and its current state is a testament to the importance of interdisciplinary collaboration and ongoing critical reflection within the field. *Professor Dr. Heiner Fangerau, Professor and Head of the Department of History, Philosophy and Ethics of Medicine, Heinrich-Heine-Universität Düsseldorf*

This authoritative text with a stellar cast of authors provides an unparalleled exploration and analysis of the thinking underpinning one of the founders of the profession of psychiatry. It faces head-on both the brilliance of Kraepelin's thesis and its many flaws and reframes them using current evidence, placing them within a contemporary context. Whilst Kraepelin can be rightly credited with a major (possibly the prime) role in establishing psychiatry as a full medical specialty, this book highlights the richness that comes from complementary and contrary biological and psychological dimensions and the complex interplay with culture and politics. Accessible, insightful and exploratory it is a recommended read for all who share the challenging and rewarding mental health world. *Dr. Adrian James, Immediate Past President Royal College of Psychiatrists and Consultant Forensic Psychiatrist of Devon Partnership NHS Trust*

Psychiatry After Kraepelin is an outstanding contribution to the history and future of psychiatric thought. Bringing together leading experts from diverse fields, this volume offers a profound exploration of Emil Kraepelin's legacy and its impact on modern psychiatric diagnosis, treatment, and research. By bridging historical perspectives with contemporary debates, it provides invaluable insights into the evolution of psychiatric practice and its societal implications. A must-read for anyone interested in the past, present, and future of mental health care. *Prof. Dr. med. Steffi G. Riedel-Heller, MPH, Full Professor and Director of the Institute of Social Medicine, Occupational Health and Public Health (ISAP), University of Leipzig*

Acknowledgments

The editors owe a great debt of gratitude to Professor Tom Burns, Emeritus Professor of Social Psychiatry, Oxford University. First, for our mutual introduction and his encouragement for cooperation. Equally, for securing full funding for the Open Access publication of *Psychiatry after Kraepelin: Ambitions Images Practices 1926-2026*. It is doubtful that this volume would have happened but for his facilitation.

We would also like to thank Professors Allen Frances and Matthew Broome, for their foreword and afterword respectively, and all our authors for their outstanding contributions. It has been a great pleasure and learning experience to collaborate with them. A definite highlight in our now rather long careers.

George Ikkos would like to thank the Royal Society of Medicine (RSM) Psychiatry Section and the Royal College of Psychiatrists (RCPsych) History of Psychiatry (HoPSIG) and Philosophy and Psychiatry (PhilSIG) Special Interest Groups for providing fora where ideas could be shared, opinions tested, and opportunities for networking of immediate relevance to this book could emerge. He would particularly like to thank the members of the organizing committee of the conference "After Kraepelin: Ambition, Images and Practices in the History of Psychiatry 1926–2026" hosted by the RSM Psychiatry Section and held in association with HoPSIG and PhilSIG on March 6 and 7, 2025: Professor Nicol Ferrier (Vice-chair); Drs. Graham Ash, Peter Carpenter and John Mason and Professor Marius Turda (HoPSIG); Drs Anastasios Dimopoulos and Iain Smith (PhilSIG); and Drs Gordana Milavic and Jacqueline Phillips Owen and Professor Femi Oyebode (RSM Psychiatry Section). This volume represents the authors' views, not theirs.

Thomas Becker would like to thank Professor Steffi Riedel-Heller, Professor of Social and Occupational Medicine and Public Health, and Professor Georg Schomerus, Professor of Psychiatry and Psychotherapy, both at Leipzig University, for their invaluable support. He also wants to acknowledge the great support received from Sabine Heitmann at the Department of Psychiatry and Psychotherapy, Leipzig University in handling the work on this book.

Finally, we would like to thank Dr. Sylvana Freyberg, PhD, Senior Editor of Medicine Books Continental, Europe and UK; Ms. Smitha Diveshan, Production Editor (Books); and their colleagues at Springer Nature for their thorough professionalism and ready advice and support.

George Ikkos
Thomas Becker

Contents

About the Editors and Contributors

Riadh Abed qualified in medicine from Baghdad School of Medicine in 1974 and completed his training in psychiatry in the UK. He worked as a consultant psychiatrist and Hon. Senior Lecturer (University of Sheffield) in South Yorkshire for 25 years with 7 years as Medical Director of an NHS Trust. He has had a longstanding interest in the application of evolutionary theory to the understanding of mental disorder and has published numerous peer-reviewed evolutionary articles and chapters including novel theories on eating disorders, OCD, schizophrenia, and the evolutionary origins of human personality traits. He is the founding chair of the evolutionary psychiatry special interest group at the Royal College of Psychiatrists and the chair of the Section of Evolutionary Psychiatry in the World Psychiatric Association. He is also co-editor of *Evolutionary Psychiatry: Current Perspectives on Evolution and Mental Health* published jointly by the RCPsych and Cambridge University Press.

Awais Aftab is a Clinical Assistant Professor of Psychiatry at Case Western Reserve University and psychiatrist at Southwest General Medical Center in Cleveland, Ohio. His academic, educational, and public-facing work focuses on conceptual and critical issues in psychiatry. He led the interview series Conversations in Critical Psychiatry for Psychiatric Times, and a book adaptation was published in 2024 from Oxford University Press. He is a senior editor for the journal *Philosophy, Psychiatry, & Psychology*. He writes online on his Substack newsletter Psychiatry at the Margin.

Ana Antic is Professor of European history and medical humanities at the University of Copenhagen, and head of the Centre for Culture and the Mind (DNRF Centre of Excellence). She is a historian of psychiatry, and has published on the relationship between psychiatry, violence and politics, decolonisation of psychiatry, and history of psychiatry in Eastern and Southeast Europe. She has published a number of articles and two monographs: *Therapeutic Fascism: Experiencing the Violence of the Nazi New Order* (2017) and *Non-aligned Psychiatry in the Cold War* (2022).

Simon Baron-Cohen is Professor of Developmental Psychopathology and Director of Autism Research Centre, Cambridge University, and leads 12 programmes of research, all focusing on autism. Six of these are in basic research: (a)

Perception and Cognition; (b) Neuroscience; (c) Genetics and Environmentl; (d) Hormones; (e) Epidemiology; and (f) Synaesthesia. The other six programmes are in applied research: (g) Screening and Diagnosis; (h) Employment; (i) Education; (j) Criminal Justice; (k) Physical Health; and (l) Mental Health. In 2017, he gave a keynote address to the United Nations on Autism Awareness Day on the topic of Autism and Human Rights. In 2021, he received a knighthood in the New Year's Honours List for his services to autism. The Medical Research Council (MRC) awarded him with the MRC Millennium Medal 2023 in recognition of his pioneering MRC-funded research into the prenatal sex steroid theory of autism, his establishment of the ARC, and his work in the public understanding of neurodiversity.

Thomas Becker is a psychiatrist in retirement with a current affiliation at Leipzig University. Following his MD thesis work on the Italian psychiatric reform in Turin, Piedmont in Italy (1982–1983), he worked as a resident in internal medicine and neurology, trained in psychiatry and worked as senior clinician at Würzburg University (1984–1995), and was awarded a Humboldt Foundation fellowship and worked at the Section of Community Psychiatry at the (then) Institute of Psychiatry, King's College London in the UK (1995–1998). He received the Hermann Simon Award of the DGPPN (German Association for Psychiatry, Psychotherapy and Psychosomatics) in 1998. Following work as a senior clinician and the appointment to a Public Health professorial post at the Department of Psychiatry of Leipzig University (1998–2002), he was appointed chair of psychiatry and head of the Department of Psychiatry II of Ulm University at the Bezirkskrankenhaus Günzburg and held that post from 2002 to 2022. His main research focus has been in mental health services research, and his current interest is in theoretical issues relevant to social psychiatry. Following retirement at Ulm University, he was appointed Senior Professor at the Department of Psychiatry and Psychotherapy at Leipzig University in 2022. He was a member of the Executive Committee of the European Network for Mental Health Service Evaluation (ENMESH, 2001–2007) and chairman of the Section of Epidemiology and Social Psychiatry of the European Psychiatric Association (EPA, 2008–2012).

Peter Beresford is Visiting Professor at the University of East Anglia and Co-Chair of the UK user led organisation Shaping Our Lives. He is also Emeritus Professor at Brunel University London and Essex University. He identifies as a long-term user of mental health services. He is an academic and activist who has been actively involved in the development of policy, practice, and research through affiliations and strong networks with national (and international) government, research, policy, practice, and service user organisations and structures. He has been a pioneer in the development and analysis of participation and service user involvement in research and evaluation, as writer, researcher, activist, and educator. He has also played an ongoing role in the international development of participatory and emancipatory research. His areas of particular interest are disability, Mad Studies, mental health, palliative care, social work and social care, welfare reform, social work education, and participatory research. He has published widely in these fields. His latest book is *The Antidote: How People Powered Movements Can Renew Politics, Policy and Practice* (Policy Press, 2025), https://policy.bristoluniversitypress.co.uk/the-antidote.

Francesca Brencio is Teaching Fellow in Mental Health at the Institute for Mental Health at the School of Psychology at the University of Birmingham (UK) with a full-time teaching position. She is also the Director of the *PhenoLab—A Theoretical Laboratory in Phenomenology and Mental Health*, officially recognised as an organizational partner at The Collaborating Centre for Values-based Practice in Health and Social Care at the St Catherine's College at the University of Oxford (UK). She is also Executive Committee Member of *The Royal College of Psychiatrists—* Special Interest Group in Philosophy.

Francesca is a scholar in the phenomenological and Heideggerian tradition. Her scholarly contributions advance the integration of phenomenology and hermeneutics within clinical education and practice, enriching the theoretical framework for understanding lived experiences in mental health. Her investigations encompass fundamental aspects of human experience, including perceptual processes, attentional mechanisms, emotions (individual and social emotions), affective life, and the role of the body in psychopathological experiences.

Together with Prof. Matthew Broome, Director of the IMH at the University of Birmingham (UK), she co-leads *The Birmingham Network for Phenomenology and Mental Health*, funded by the University of Birmingham (UK).

Francesca published extensively in prestigious international journals, both in philosophy and psychiatry. She has authored and edited the following books: *Phenomenology, Neuroscience and Clinical Practice. Transdisciplinary Experiences* (Springer Nature, Cham 2024); *Metaphors in Action. Humanities, Medicine and the Digital World* (Springer-Nature, Cham, forthcoming, 2025); *Heidegger and Neuroscience. Ontology, Medicine and Psychoanalysis in Dialogue* (Routledge, forthcoming 2025). She is among the contributors of *The APA Handbook of Humanistic and Existential Psychology* (American Psychological Association Press, 2025), and *The Oxford Handbook of Phenomenological Psychopathology* (Oxford University Press, Oxford 2019).

She also works as Certified APPA Philosophical Counsellor.

Matthew Broome is Chair in Psychiatry and Youth Mental Health, Director of the Institute for Mental Health, and Director of The Midlands Translational Centre, Mental Health Mission at the University of Birmingham; Distinguished Research Fellow, Oxford Uehiro Centre for Practical Ethics, University of Oxford; and Visiting Professor, Suor Orsola Benicasa University of Naples. In the NHS, he is Honorary Consultant Psychiatrist to East Birmingham Early Intervention in Psychosis Team, Birmingham, and Solihull Mental Health NHS Foundation Trust.

Matthew studied Pharmacology and Medicine at the University of Birmingham and trained in psychiatry at the Maudsley Hospital, Bethlem Royal Hospital, and the National Hospital for Neurology and Neurosurgery. He has a PhD in Psychiatry from the Institute of Psychiatry, University of London and in Philosophy from the University of Warwick. He is series editor to the OUP series, International Perspectives in Philosophy and Psychiatry; was editor and deputy editor of *The British Journal of Psychiatry* from 2014 to 2023; and is currently editor for *Social Psychiatry and Psychiatric Epidemiology*. He co-edited *Risk Factors for Psychosis:*

Paradigms, Mechanisms, and Prevention (Elsevier Press, 2020), *The Oxford Handbook of Phenomenological Psychopathology* (Oxford University Press, 2019), *The AMDP System: Manual for Assessment and Documentation of Psychopathology in Psychiatry* (Hogrefe, 2017), *The Maudsley Reader in Phenomenological Psychiatry* (Cambridge University Press, 2013), and *Psychiatry as Cognitive Neuroscience: Philosophical Perspectives* (Oxford University Press, 2009).

Matthew's research interests include youth mental health, the prodromal phase of psychosis, delusion formation, mood instability, functional neuroimaging, interdisciplinary methods, mental health humanities, phenomenology, and the philosophy and ethics of psychiatry. His research is funded by the Wellcome Trust, NIH, MRC, NIHR, EU, and the Wolfson Foundation.

Martin Brüne graduated in medicine at the Westphalian Wilhelms University in Münster in 1988. He completed his neurology training in 1993, and his psychiatry training in 1995. His subsequent training included a Visiting Research Scientist fellowship at the Centre for the Mind, a joint venture of the Australian National University and University of Sydney. He is currently Professor of Psychiatry and Head of the Division of Cognitive Neuropsychiatry and Psychiatric Preventive Medicine at the LWL University-Hospital, Ruhr-University Bochum, Germany.

Dr Brüne has authored more than 300 articles and book chapters. He has also authored the *Textbook of Evolutionary Psychiatry and Psychosomatic Medicine: The Origins of Psychopathology* (2nd edn., Oxford University Press, 2016). He also edited the *Oxford Handbook of Evolutionary Medicine* (together with Prof. Wulf Schiefenhövel; Oxford University Press, 2019), as well as the book *Evolutionary Roots of Human Brain Diseases* (together with Nico Diederich, Christopher G. Goetz, and Katrin Amunts; OUP, 2024).

His current clinically oriented research projects include the analysis of social cognition and nonverbal behaviour, the behavioural performance of psychiatric populations in evolutionary game-theoretical scenarios, the effect of oxytocin on social perception and cognition in psychiatric disorders, as well as genetic and epigenetic aspects of interpersonal behaviour. He is also interested in evolutionary aspects of gut-brain-interactions, and somatic comorbid diseases in psychiatric populations.

Dr Brüne's research approach is grounded in evolutionary theory, that is, how and why cognition, emotion, and behaviour in psychiatric conditions relate to adaptive function of psychological traits. Dr Brüne's interests also include cross-species comparison and psychopathological conditions in nonhuman primates.

Dr Brüne is a member of several psychiatric and neuroscientific societies (Deutsche Gesellschaft für Psychiatrie, Psychotherapie und Nervenheilkunde (DGPPN), International Society for Human Ethology (ISHE), Gesellschaft für Anthropologie (GfA), and the International Graduate School of Neuroscience (IGSN), Ruhr-University Bochum. He also acted as a Co-PI in the ARC Centre of Excellence in Cognition and its Disorders, Belief Formation Program at the Macquarie University, Sydney, Australia.

José Miguel Caldas de Almeida is Professor of Psychiatry at Nova Medical School, Nova University of Lisbon. He was Director of the University Department of Psychiatry and Mental Health for more than 20 years and Dean of the NOVA Medical School (2007–2013). He currently serves as Chair of the Lisbon Institute of Global Mental Health and Coordinator of the "Global and Population Mental Health Group" of the Comprehensive Health Research Centre, Nova Medical School. He has been at the forefront of mental health services reform at national and global levels since the 1980s. In Portugal, he has been responsible for the creation of one of the first community-based mental health services in the country, coordinator of the National Mental Health Plan (2007–2011), and member of the group responsible for drafting the new Mental Health Act adopted in 2023. He has held several high-ranking positions on the international stage, including Head of the Mental Health Unit at the Pan American Health Organization, Regional Office of the World Health Organization for the Americas in Washington D.C. (2000–2005), Leader of the EU Joint Action for Mental Health (2013–2016), and Vice Chair of the EU Cost Action FOSTREN: Fostering and Strengthening Approaches to Reducing Coercion in European Mental Health Services (2020–2024). He collaborated with Benedetto Saraceno in the creation and coordination of the Gulbenkian Global Mental Health Platform (2011–2016) and the coordination of Master Courses on mental health policy, mental health systems, and global mental health, developed in collaboration with WHO at the Nova Medical School (since 2010). His main research focus has been in psychiatric epidemiology, mental health services research, and mental health and human rights. He has been President of the Portuguese Society of Psychiatric Epidemiology (1993–1997), Portuguese Mental Health Association (1995–2000), and Lisbon Society of Medical Sciences (2013–2017).

Giulia Cattarinussi is a postdoctoral research associate working at the Department of Psychological Medicine at the Institute of Psychiatry, Psychology and Neuroscience at King's College London. She obtained her medical degree and trained as a psychiatrist at the University of Udine (Italy). During her PhD in Neuroscience at the Department of Neuroscience at the University of Padova (Italy), she studied extensively neuroimaging abnormalities in schizophrenia and bipolar disorder. Her research focuses on neuroimaging, and cognitive and inflammatory abnormalities in affective and psychotic disorders, with a particular focus on young adults.

Paola Dazzan is Professor of Neurobiology of Psychosis, Theme Co-Lead for Psychosis and Mood Disorders at the NIHR Maudsley Biomedical Research Centre. After obtaining her medical degree, she trained as a psychiatrist at the Maudsley Hospital, became a Member of the Royal College of Psychiatrists (MRCPsych), and subsequently a Fellow. She completed her PhD at the Institute of Psychiatry, King's College London. She is internationally known for her work on the relationship between brain Magnetic Resonance Imaging (MRI) data and other biological measures such as neurodevelopmental indices, stress and inflammatory markers, reproductive hormones, and the onset and outcome of psychoses and severe mental health problems. She studies these phenomena in adolescents and young individuals in the early stages of psychosis and was first to conduct neuroimaging studies in women at risk of postpartum psychosis. More recently, she has also been focusing on the role of childhood adversities on brain development. Her work has been extensively published in high-impact papers, with more than 300 publications and recognition as 2019, 2020, 2021, 2022, and 2023 Highly Cited Researcher Awardee by Clarivate Analytics. She has received several prestigious International Awards, including the Academic of the Year Award from the Royal College of Psychiatrists, three NARSAD Investigator Awards, and an Honorary Membership of the American Psychiatric Association in recognition of her contribution to psychiatry. She also received the Guy's, King's, and St Thomas's Award for "Outstanding Contribution to Student Experience," for her work as Lead of Psychiatry teaching in the Medical School. Most recently, she has received a Senior Investigator Award from the UK National Institute of Health Research.

Lene Falgaard Eplov is a psychiatrist and head of research at Copenhagen Research Unit of Recovery, Mental Health Center Amager. Her primary research interests include clinical and personal recovery, peer support, integrated care, stigmatisation, and art in mental health services. She maintains strong connections with key researchers both in Denmark and internationally, and she collaborates actively with various stakeholders in the mental health field. This collaboration fosters impactful, cross-sectional projects that span regions and municipalities. For example, she is involved in the Individual Placement and Support (IPS) project, the Collaborative Care for Anxiety and Depression D(Collabri) project, and the "Paths to Everyday Life" (PEER) project, which is co-produced in close collaboration with the Peer Partnership Association. Driven by a deep commitment to improving the lives of individuals facing mental health challenges, she is particularly passionate about implementing evidence-based recovery interventions across Denmark.

Peter Falkai is professor and chair of the Department of Psychiatry at the Ludwig-Maximilians-University (LMU) Munich in Germany. Additionally, he is director of the Clinical Translation Department at the Max Planck Institute of Psychiatry Munich. He has a long-standing interest in understanding the pathophysiology of schizophrenia and the development of mechanistically informed innovative treatments. He is a member of a multidisciplinary research team combining clinical, neuropsychological, imaging, genetic, and post-mortem research expertise to define a pathophysiological pathway from risk factors to brain abnormalities to behavioural correlates in schizophrenia.

Nicol Ferrier is Emeritus Professor of Psychiatry at the University of Newcastle. He trained in Medicine at the University of Glasgow. After 3 years of post-graduate study in Medicine in Glasgow, he moved to Northwick Park Hospital in NW London to train in Psychiatry under the tutelage of Professor T.J. Crow and Professor E.C. Johnstone. During his time there he was in receipt of MRC and Wellcome Training Fellowships. In 1984 he moved to Newcastle as an MRC Clinical Scientist and Consultant Psychiatrist. In 1990 he was appointed to the

Chair in Psychiatry at Newcastle University, a post he held until his retirement in 2017. His research interests were in neurobiology and treatment of severe affective disorders, and he has published about 300 papers in this field. He is a past President of the British Association or Psychopharmacology and was a member of MRC and Wellcome Trust Fellowship and Grant Committees. From 2017 to 2024 he conducted a PhD in the History of Psychiatry examining mortality in Victorian asylums. He edits the RCPsych History of Psychiatry Special Interest Group's Newsletter.

Angelo Fioritti is a psychiatrist and former Director of the Department of Mental Health and Substance Abuse of AUSL Bologna (Local Health Trust). From 2015 to 2017 he was Medical Director of the same Trust. He has been President of the "Italian College of the Departments of Mental Health" (2020–2024). In addition to his clinical work at the mental health services of various health authorities in Emilia-Romagna, he has carried out research and teaching activities on the themes of psychiatric legislation, psychiatric epidemiology, mental health policy, integration between mental health and addiction services, forensic psychiatry, protection of human rights in psychiatry, and strategies to improve access to work for citizens with mental health problems. For four years (2006–2010) he was Chief Officer of Mental Health, Pathological Addictions and Health in Prisons at the Regional Council of Emilia-Romagna. He is author of over 70 international publications and more than a hundred articles in Italian journals and books.

Allen Frances is Professor Emeritus of Psychiatry and former Chair at Duke University. He was chair of the DSM IV Task Force and was instrumental in the preparation of DSM III and DSM III-R. He has written several hundred peer-reviewed papers; dozens of book chapters; a dozen books; and has received a dozen research grants. He is the author of *Saving Normal*; *Essentials of Psychiatric Diagnosis*; and *Twilight of American Sanity*.

Uta Gühne is a psychologist and research associate at the Institute of Social Medicine, Occupational Medicine and Public Health (ISAP) at the University of Leipzig. She gained clinical experience in child and adolescent psychiatry at various clinics in Germany. She wrote her doctoral thesis at the Department of Psychiatry and Psychotherapy at Leipzig University in the field of epidemiology of mental illness (2005–2006). In her habilitation thesis, she addressed topics related to the psychosocial care of people with severe mental illnesses. She is one of the authors of the treatment guideline "Psychosocial Therapies for Severe Mental Illness" of the German Association for Psychiatry, Psychotherapy and Psychosomatics. Since 2022, she has been leading the working group for guidelines and psychosocial care research at ISAP. Further research interests include implementation research and participation in guideline processes.

Lorenzo Gilardi is an independent scholar in the field of the phenomenological psychopathology of schizophrenia. He is also a student of Mathematics at Insubria University in Como. His interests span from mathematics to history, from philosophy to economics, from classics to psychiatry. In his research he has written book chapters and articles for different journals, such as *Philosophy, Psychiatry and Psychology*, *Le Cercle Hermeneutique*, *World Psychiatry*, *Psychopathology*, and *Philosophical Psychology*. Some are: Gilardi, Lorenzo & Stanghellini, Giovanni. (2021). "I Am Schizophrenic, Believe It or Not! A Dialogue about the Importance of Recognition". *Philosophy, Psychiatry, & Psychology*. 28. 1–10; Gilardi, Lorenzo & Stanghellini, Giovanni. (2021). "The Schizophrenic Person as a Moral Agent". *Philosophy, Psychiatry, & Psychology*. 28. 35–39. Fusar-Poli, Paolo & Estradé, Andrés & Stanghellini, Giovanni et al. (2022). "The lived experience of psychosis: a bottom-up review co-written by experts by experience and academics". *World Psychiatry*. Stanghellini, Giovanni & Aragona, Massimiliano & Gilardi, Lorenzo & Ritunnano, Rosa. (2022). "The person's position-taking in the shaping of schizophrenic phenomena". *Philosophical Psychology*. Tewes, C. and Stanghellini, G. "Time and Body. Phenomenological and Psychopathological Approaches," Gilardi, L., Ch. 4.1 *The Epiphany of the Body: Some Remarks on the Translation of Leib from German*, Cambridge University Press, 2021; Gennart, M. La vulnérabilitè—Approache phénoménologique, existentielle et psychopathologique, Ch. 2, Stanghellini, G. and Gilardi, L., *Préhistoire du corps—Corps symbolique et circonscription dans l'expérience de la vulnerabilité de la personne schizophréne*, Le Cercle Hermeneutique, Vrin, 2021.

Stephan Heckers studied philosophy and medicine at the Universities of Munich and Cologne in Germany. He completed clinical training in psychiatry at the Massachusetts General Hospital in Boston, MA. He was a faculty member at Harvard Medical School from 1997 until 2005 and the Director of the Schizophrenia and Bipolar Disorder Program at McLean Hospital from 2003 until 2005. He has been serving as Chair of Psychiatry and Behavioral Sciences at Vanderbilt University since 2006.

Dr Heckers studies the neural basis of schizophrenia and bipolar disorder and has explored the mechanism of memory deficits in psychotic patients. He is the recipient of several awards, including Dr Paul Janssen Schizophrenia Research Award, A.E. Bennett Award (Society of Biological Psychiatry), Paul Hoch Award (American Psychopathological Association), and Outstanding Translational Research Award (Schizophrenia International Research Society).

Dr Heckers is a member of several editorial boards and of the Scientific Council for the Brain & Behavior Research Foundation. He served as editor of *JAMA Psychiatry* from 2015 until 2017.

Chalotte Heinsvig Poulsen
holds MSc in medical science and health promotion and PhD in public health, and is a senior researcher at Copenhagen Research Unit for Recovery at Mental Health Center Amager. She is a dedicated lived experience researcher specialising in trauma-informed, peer-led recovery-oriented interventions aimed at promoting well-being and mental health. Drawing on published research into peer support effectiveness, including findings from the "Paths to everyday life" (PEER) project, and her role in founding a national network of lived experience researchers, she brings a uniquely valuable perspective to her research. Beyond her academic

pursuits, she is a passionate advocate for transforming the mental health system and communities toward a recovery-oriented approach. Her personal journey as an experienced yoga enthusiast deeply informs her understanding of holistic well-being and the power of embodied practices. She is committed to building peer relationships that challenge existing perspectives, reshape conversations, and strengthen connections within the mental health landscape. Her work is driven by a profound belief in the potential for positive social change and the importance of lived experience in shaping a more compassionate and effective mental health system.

Paul Hoff received his medical degree at the University of Mainz, Germany, in 1980, and his philosophical degree at the University of Munich, Germany, in 1988. From 1981 to 1996 he worked at the Departments of Psychiatry and Neurology at the University of Munich, where, in 1994, he was appointed university lecturer. He received his accreditation as psychiatrist and neurologist in 1989 and as psychotherapist in 1996. In 1997 he was appointed university professor of psychiatry at the Technical University of Aachen, Germany (RWTH). From June 2003 until his retirement in May 2021, he was head psychiatrist and deputy medical director of the Department of Psychiatry, Psychotherapy and Psychosomatics at the Psychiatric University Hospital in Zurich, Switzerland. Since June 2021 he has been working as an affiliated scientist at the Psychiatric University Hospital in Zurich and continues to see outpatients at the Private Hospital Hohenegg in Meilen (Canton Zurich). He has been elected chairman of the Central Ethics Committee (CEC) of the Swiss Academy of Medical Sciences (SAMS) for the periods 2021–2024 and 2025–2028.

His main areas of work are

- Psychopathology from an empirical and theoretical point of view, including descriptive approaches and epistemological issues such as concepts of illness, implications of neurosciences on psychiatry, subjectivity and objectivity in clinical medicine, medicine of the person
- Conceptual history of psychiatry with focus on Emil Kraepelin, Eugen Bleuler, Karl Jaspers, Arthur Kronfeld and their relevance for twenty-first-century psychiatry
- Ethical and juridical aspects of psychiatry, especially regarding coercive measures

George Ikkos is Consultant Liaison Psychiatrist at the Royal National Orthopaedic Hospital UK, Clinical Fellow of the International Neuropsychoanalysis Association, and Honorary Fellow of the Royal College of Psychiatrists (RCPsych). He is immediate past Chair of the RCPsych History of Psychiatry Special Interest Group (HoPSIG) and former President of the Royal Society of Medicine (RSM) Pain Medicine and Psychiatry Sections. He was Honorary Visiting Research Professor at the School of Health and Social Care London South Bank University. He has been a pioneer of service user engagement in postgraduate psychiatric education in the UK and was Medical Advisor to the Edinburgh Festival Fringe award-winning play "The Shape of Pain," directed by an expert by experience. Since 2021 he has been the Coordinating Lead of the international collaboration group "The Precision of

Images: Emil Kraepelin, Walter Benjamin and the History of Psychiatry 1926–2026". His jointly edited Ikkos, G, Bouras, N. eds. (2021) *Mind State and Society: a Social History of Psychiatry and Mental Health in Britain 1960–2010* (RCPsych and Cambridge University Press) won joint Silver Award in the Association of American Publishers PROSE Awards 2022 in the category of History of Science, Medicine and Technology (available open access https://doi.org/10.1017/9781911623793).

Sanjeev Jain is an Emeritus Professor of Psychiatry at the Department of Psychiatry, National Institute of Mental health and Neurosciences, Bangalore, India. The history of mental health services in India, from the colonial to the contemporary period, and understanding the interface between science and medicine, and social responses to mental illness in India, has been a focus of interest. Documenting the attempts to build a comprehensive healthcare system for India, within a techno-scientific framework, is still work in progress. This work also laid the foundation for the Heritage Centre, at NIMHANS, two books (*Mindscape and Landscape*; *The Psychological Impact of the Partition of India*), and several articles related to history of psychiatry; mental health policy; etc. The Wellcome Trust, UK, has supported some of this work. He also contributed to the Molecular Genetics Laboratory at the Dept. of Psychiatry at NIMHANS, which explores the genetics and genomics of psychoses, OCD, alcoholism, dementia and neurodegenerative disease, and the broader issues of the interfaces between psychopathology and biology. The work has spanned the spectrum from bedside research on disease definition and outcomes, to gene discovery and molecular biology, and stem cell biology. He has also been involved with volunteer work with both governmental and voluntary organisations (Chittadhama; the Banyan) that work with marginalised communities with mental health issues, and has been a member of the committee for drafting the Mental Health Policy document for India.

Stephen MacGregor Lawrie is a Professor of Psychiatry in Edinburgh, mainly interested in early detection and the development of interventions to enhance outcomes and possibly even prevent psychosis. He is also clinically active in a geographically sectorised general adult psychiatry service. As Head of Psychiatry from 2010 to 2020, he oversaw an expansion of Principal Investigators and Professors in Psychiatry (which was rated 3rd in the UK in REF2014 and REF2021 with Neuroscience & Psychology). He has published more than 400 papers in peer-reviewed journals, many of which have been highly cited (Web of Science h-index >75, with >20,000 citations; Google Scholar >100 and >40,000), including his contributions using structural and functional brain imaging to predict schizophrenia, to elucidate the neurobiology of schizophrenia and develop multi-centre neuroimaging capabilities, as well as to the practice of evidence-based psychiatry. He has supervised more than 30 doctoral and 30 master's level students to completion, including three now full Professors, and obtained PhD funding for another 60 or so through PsySTAR, Translational Neuroscience, and other PhD programmes. In narrow financial terms, his career PI/Co-PI grant income is >£80M. These achievements have been recognized in Fellowships of the Royal College of Psychiatrists, the

Royal College of Physicians of Edinburgh, and the Royal Society of Edinburgh. As a Beltane Public Engagement Fellow, he has made several appearances and contributions in various media to increase knowledge and reduce stigmatization of mental illness, including shows on the Edinburgh Fringe Festival. He has been profiled twice in *The Lancet* (2011 378:1911 and 2017 389:1090) and twice in *The Lancet Psychiatry* (2016 3:931 and 2018 5:e26). He has published seven books and recently co-authored with Erica Crompton *The Beginners Guide to Sanity: A Self-Help Book for People Affected by Psychosis* which was shortlisted for the People's Book prize.

Helene Cæcilie Mørck is an academic, choreographer, and expert by experience and works at the University of Southern Denmark. She is educated at the Danish National School of Performing Arts and the Victorian College of the Arts in Melbourne. She holds a BA in English from the University of Southern Denmark and an MA in Literature and Culture from the University of Birmingham. As an artist, she has worked as a choreographer in film, theatre, and contemporary dance for over 20 years and has twice been the recipient of the Danish Actors' Association Choreography Grant. She has shared her lifelong experience with schizophrenia through articles in *Schizophrenia Bulletin* and the *Journal of Psychopathology*. Her book *My Mind Is Thin Paper—A Testimony* will be published in 2025. She was recently elected to the EPA's Scientific Section of Philosophy and Psychiatry and is currently looking for funding to support her PhD proposal.

Alastair Morgan is a Senior Lecturer at the University of Manchester in the School of Health Sciences. His most recent book is *Continental Philosophy of Psychiatry. The Lure of Madness*, published with Palgrave MacMillan in 2022. More information can be found here: Alastair Morgan — Research Explorer The University of Manchester.

Merete Nordentoft is Professor of Psychiatry at the Department of Clinical Medicine, University of Copenhagen, Director of Research at CORE—Copenhagen Research Centre for Mental Health, Mental Health Services in the Capital Region, and President of the Danish Psychiatric Society (2021–2025).

The work of Merete Nordentoft's group has led to the development of several intervention programmes, most notably the creation and launch of OPUS in 1998. OPUS is an outreach, early intervention service for young people (age 18–35 years) experiencing their first episode of psychosis, with active family involvement. Today, OPUS is the standard clinical practice that has resulted in fewer and shorter hospitalisations, greater symptom remission, significantly improved user satisfaction, and a reduced risk of early death. The OPUS model has inspired similar initiatives in many countries worldwide.

Through various register-based epidemiological studies, she and her group have identified groups at the highest immediate risk of suicide. The results of these studies have played a crucial role in shaping the Danish National Plan for Suicide Prevention. To ensure assertive follow-up treatment after suicide attempts, she developed the concept of regional suicide prevention clinics, now operating with national coverage. Furthermore, her team's work has brought attention to the high risk of suicide shortly after hospital discharge, fostering targeted preventive measures.

In register-based and clinical cohort studies, she and her group have shown that children of parents with severe mental illness are at significantly higher risk of developing mental health issues themselves, failing to complete primary school, and experiencing increased clinical symptoms and adverse life events, along with reduced motor and cognitive functions. These findings have helped raise awareness about this vulnerable group at both national and international levels.

As President of the Danish Psychiatric Society, she has played a pivotal role in advocating for increased funding for psychiatric services, particularly in relation to the Danish National 10-Year Plan for Psychiatry.

Michael Owen is Professor of Psychological Medicine at Cardiff University and Chair of Trustees of Mental Health Research UK. He trained in medicine and obtained a PhD in neuroscience at Birmingham University before moving to London to train in psychiatry at the Maudsley Hospital and molecular genetics at St. Mary's Hospital Medical School. He was appointed as Senior Lecturer in Cardiff in 1990, Professor of Neuropsychiatric Genetics in 1995, and from 1998 to 2019 Professor of Psychological Medicine and Head of the Department of Psychological Medicine and Clinical Neurosciences. He was Director of the MRC Centre for Neuropsychiatric Genetics and Genomics from 2009 to 2019, and of the Cardiff University Neuroscience and Mental Health Research Institute from 2010 to 2014. He practised as a consultant psychiatrist until February 2016.

His research focuses on the genetics of psychiatric and neurodevelopmental disorders and is aimed at understanding disease mechanisms, improving diagnostic processes, and identifying new treatment opportunities.

He was President of the International Society of Psychiatric Genetics (ISPG) from 2000 to 2005 and has twice been elected to the council of the Academy of Medical Sciences. He was awarded the Stromgren Medal for psychiatric research in 2011, the Lieber Prize for schizophrenia research in 2012, the William K Warren Distinguished Investigator Award for schizophrenia research in 2013, the Lifetime Achievement Award of ISPG in 2015, and the British Neuroscience Association Award for Outstanding Contribution to Neuroscience in 2017. He was knighted for services to psychiatry and neuroscience in 2014, awarded MD (Honoris Causa) by the University of Birmingham in 2018, and Honorary Fellowship of the Royal College of Psychiatrists in 2020.

Femi Oyebode is Honorary Professor of Psychiatry, University of Birmingham. He is the author of *Sims' Symptoms in the Mind: Textbook of Descriptive Psychopathology* (4th–7th editions), *Psychopathology of Rare and Unusual Syndromes, Madness at the Theatre*, and *Mindreadings: Literature and Psychiatry*. He is Honorary Fellow of the Royal College of Psychiatrists and received the Lifetime Achievement Award of the Royal College of Psychiatrists in 2016.

Sergi Papiol is a member of the research staff of the Max Planck Institute of Psychiatry and leads the Genomics group at the Institute of Psychiatric Phenomics and Genomics (IPPG) at the LMU Munich. His research interests have focused on the role of the polygenic risk background as a modulator of the beneficial effects of therapeutic interventions in schizophrenia.

Jesús Ramírez-Bermúdez leads the Neuropsychiatry Program at the National Institute of Neurology and Neurosurgery in Mexico. His clinical research focuses on the cognitive, affective, and behavioural aspects of brain disease. He is the author of academic books on the principles of neuropsychiatry and the clinical application of brain imaging. He is also actively engaged in scientific outreach and has published several books that blend creative essay, scientific thought, and clinical narrative. He was awarded the National Literary Essay Prize by the Institute of Fine Arts in Mexico.

Lukas Roell is a postdoctoral researcher at the Max-Planck-Institute of Psychiatry and the Department of Psychiatry and Psychotherapy of the Ludwig-Maximilians-University (LMU) Munich in Germany. He employs neuroimaging to investigate mechanisms driving symptomatic changes in schizophrenia, while considering the genetic predisposition of patients.

Moritz Rossner is professor and head of the Laboratory for Molecular and Behavioral Neurobiology at the Department of Psychiatry and Psychotherapy of the Ludwig-Maximilians-University (LMU) Munich in Germany. His research covers the development and analysis of transgenic mouse and human cellular stem cell derived models for mental disorders.

Andrea Schmitt is professor and research group leader at the Ludwig-Maximilians-University Munich in Germany. She is focusing on post-mortem investigations in schizophrenia with emphasis on oligodendrocytes. Additionally, she is contributing to clinical aerobic exercise studies and biomarkers in schizophrenia and affective disorders.

Georg Schomerus born 1973, is Full Professor of Psychiatry at University of Leipzig, and Chair of the Department of Psychiatry and Psychotherapy at University of Leipzig Medical Center. His scientific work focuses on the stigma of mental illness, the stigma of substance use, help-seeking, and inequality and health-service use.

Dr Schomerus attended Medical School in Freiburg and King's College London. After earning his medical doctorate in 2002 with a thesis on Medical Ethics in Germany and Britain between 1903 and 1933, he received his postgraduate training in clinical psychiatry in Hannover and Leipzig, and worked as a consultant and Professor of Psychiatry at Greifswald University.

Dr Schomerus is leading a National long-term study on changes of stigma and mental health literacy among the general public in Germany, based on large repeated cross-sectional representative population surveys in 1990, 1993, 2001, 2011, and 2020. He is author of several books and book chapters, and more than 250 peer-reviewed scientific papers. He was awarded the 2019 Ulrike-Fritze-Lindenthal Award for his work on substance use stigma. Together with Patrick Corrigan, he is

Editor of *The Stigma of Substance Use Disorders* (Cambridge University Press, 2022).

Giovanni Stanghellini is a psychiatrist and Professor of Dynamic Psychology at Florence University and Profesor Adjuncto at "D. Portales" University (Santiago, Chile). He founded the *International Network for Philosophy and Psychiatry*, the *European Psychiatry Association (EPA) Section on Philosophy and Psychiatry*, and the *Scuola di Psicoterapia Fenomenologico-Dinamica* (Florence, Italy). He authored more than 200 Scopus papers on the structures of the lived worlds of people with schizophrenia, melancholia and so-called eating disorders, borderline, obsessive and hysteric conditions; and on the phenomenological basis of psychotherapy. Among his books in English: *Nature and Narrative* (co-edited with K.W.M. Fulford, K. Morris and J.Z. Sadler, Oxford University Press 2003), *Disembodied Spirits and Deanimated Bodies. The Psychopathology of Common Sense* (OUP 2004), *Emotions and Personhood* (with R. Rosfort, OUP 2013), *One Century of Karl Jaspers' General Psychopathology* (co-edited with T. Fuchs, OUP 2013), *Oxford Handbook of Philosophy and Psychiatry* (co-edited with K.W.M. Fulford et al., OUP 2013), *The Therapeutic Interview in Mental Health. A Values-Based and Person-Centered Approach* (with M. Mancini, Cambridge University Press, Cambridge, 2017), and *Oxford Handbook of Phenomenological Psychopathology* (co-edited with M.R. Broome et al., OUP 2019).

Holger Steinberg born in 1967, is an associate professor teaching the history of medicine at the Medical Faculty of Leipzig University. Since 1997, he has been conducting research at the Centre of the History of Psychiatry within the Department of Psychiatry at Leipzig University. His research primarily focuses on the history of psychiatry, psychotherapy, and neurology in German-speaking countries during the nineteenth and twentieth centuries.

Over the years, Steinberg has published a variety of monographs on these subjects, including a notable book on Emil Kraepelin's years in Leipzig and his lifelong correspondence with Wilhelm Wundt. Additionally, Steinberg authored a comprehensive review on the life and work of the influential nineteenth-century psychiatrist and neurologist Paul Julius Möbius. His extensive accounts on the history of psychiatry and neurology at Leipzig University have garnered significant attention.

To date, Steinberg has written 150 papers, mostly as a solo author, in indexed journals worldwide. His work covers various topics, including the history of mental and neurological syndromes, disorders, illnesses, and therapeutic approaches. Moreover, he has extensively written on Johann Christian August Heinroth, the first-ever professor of psychiatry in the Western world, and his theories from the first half of the nineteenth century. Steinberg has also explored various aspects of the history of psychiatry in East Germany (German Democratic Republic).

Paul St John-Smith is a former chair and co-founder of the Evolutionary Psychiatry Special Interest Group (EPSIG) of the Royal College of Psychiatrists. He is currently an EPSIG executive committee member and the editor of its newsletter. He is a retired adult psychiatrist who worked as an in-patient and community psychiatrist in London and Hertfordshire and as part of a substance abuse dual diagnosis service. He was formerly section head of psychotropic drug development for Roche Products UK. He is now an independent scholar and author with a degree in Natural sciences from the University of Oxford. His current academic interests are in evolution, specifically evolutionary psychiatry, the philosophy of science, psychopharmacology, evidence-based psychiatry, and substance use. He has authored numerous papers and articles as well as contributed chapters to textbooks. His most recent book was jointly edited with Riadh Abed: *Evolutionary Psychiatry: Current Perspectives on Evolution and Mental Health* (Cambridge: CUP, 2022).

Anna Toropova is an Assistant Professor of History at the University of Warwick (UK). Her research explores interchanges between the psy-disciplines and the field of cultural production during the Stalin era. She is the author of *Feeling Revolution: Cinema, Genre and the Politics of Affect under Stalin* (Oxford: OUP, 2020), and co-editor of *Technologies of Mind and Body in the Soviet Union and the Eastern Bloc* (London: Bloomsbury, 2023).

Marius Turda Fellow of the Royal Historical Society and member of the American Psychological Association, is Professor of Biomedicine and Director of the Centre for Medical Humanities at Oxford Brookes University. He is a visiting professor at the Sapienza University in Rome, having previously taught at UCL and University of Oxford, where he was also the founding director of the "Cantemir Institute". He has authored, co-authored, and edited more than 20 books on the history of eugenics, race, and racism in East-Central Europe and beyond, including Bloomsbury's *A Cultural History of Race* published in 6 volumes in 2021 (paperback 2025). His most recent publication is *In Search of the Perfect Romanian: National Specificity, Racial Degeneration and Social Selection in Modern Romania* (2024; 2nd ed. 2025; English ed. 2026). He has also curated four exhibitions on eugenics, racial anthropology, and biopolitics, most notably "We are not Alone": Legacies of Eugenics (2021–2025). His public engagement project can be found at www.confront-eugenics.org.

Stefan Weinmann is a psychiatrist and psychotherapist working as deputy medical director and head of the outpatient department at the university-affiliated Center for Integrative Psychiatry in Lübeck, Germany. He is also affiliated at University of Basel where he is teaching psychiatry. He was trained in psychiatry in different academic hospitals in Germany and Switzerland. In addition, he worked for the German government in international health projects in Latin America, Asia, and Africa. His main research interests are mental health services research, innovative care approaches, home treatment, inclusion of people with lived experience, reduction of coercion, and critical psychopharmacology.

Part I

Emil Kraepelin

This part aims to meet Kraepelin in his times and bring him directly face-to-face with today's psychiatry.

Chapter 1 refers to his early career, particularly his relationship with Wilhem Wundt, the father of experimental psychology. It describes how Kraepelin abandoned his early ambition to set the foundations of psychiatry as a medical specialty in experimental psychology. Chapter 2 describes how he worked to establish the discipline through clinical nosology, the biological sciences and 'pharmacopsychology', culminating in the establishment of the multidisciplinary *Deutsche Forschungsanstalt für Psychiatrie* (now Max Planck Institute of Psychiatry) in Munich. Chapter 3 contrasts his philosophical reductionism with the approaches of his contemporaries Karl Jaspers and Arthur Kronfeld and suggests that all three remain relevant today and that only by attending carefully to their broad range of concerns can psychiatry overcome the current obstacles in the advancement of the biopsychosocial model in research and practice.

Emil Kraepelin, Wilhelm Wundt and Leipzig University: Short-Term Stay, Long-Term Impact

1

Holger Steinberg and Georg Schomerus

1.1 On Emil Kraepelin

Emil Kraepelin (1856–1926) is regarded as one of the most influential figures in the history of international psychiatry. But Kraepelin also paved the way in other related sciences. His pharmaco-psychological experiments, for instance, which contain several methodological innovations, form a basis of modern psychopharmacology [1, 2] (eds: see Chap. 2). Against this background, it is surprising that his contributions to psychology, particularly to the psychology of work (work curve, the so-called question of 'overburdening'), are rarely acknowledged today. This is even more true of Kraepelin's research in experimental psychology. Experimental psychology as a scientific discipline was established in Leipzig by philosopher, physiologist and psychologist Wilhelm Wundt (1832–1920) and he inspired a large number of psychologists from all over the world. He also inspired Kraepelin and the two were in a lifelong friendship. The ideas that Kraepelin pursued and started working on under Wundt's guidance in Leipzig, and how much he hoped to gain from working in this field, however, are barely recognised today. Wundt believed that simple mental phenomena and simple basic mental functions are the result of the effect of external stimuli on the nervous system. He therefore researched individual basic psychological functions with the help of time measurements, reaction measurements or association tests through experiments with changing stimuli. He

H. Steinberg (✉)
Research Center for the History of Psychiatry, Department of Psychiatry, Medical Faculty of the University of Leipzig, Leipzig, Germany
e-mail: Holger.Steinberg@medizin.uni-leipzig.de

G. Schomerus
Department of Psychiatry, Medical Faculty of the University of Leipzig, Leipzig, Germany
e-mail: georg.schomerus@uni-leipzig.de

© The Author(s) 2026
G. Ikkos, T. Becker (eds.), *Psychiatry after Kraepelin*,
https://doi.org/10.1007/978-3-032-09475-9_1

worked exclusively with mentally healthy people. Kraepelin had the idea that mental illnesses are based on disturbed or altered basic mental functions. This means that mentally ill people react slower, faster or not at all to external stimuli or generally react differently. Or that mentally ill people form different associations. Kraepelin therefore wanted to introduce Wundt's experimental methods into psychiatry, experiment with mentally ill people and discover the deviating basic functions that he had assumed to be present in mental illnesses. Kraepelin assumed that certain mental illnesses were always characterised by the same deviating basic functions. In his experiments, which would ultimately yield masses of data, he would therefore have to find regularities. This would make it possible to recognise natural laws and clinical entities. However, he was unable to implement this first and early research programme. (For a general comment on Wundt's impact on Kraepelin, see [3], pp. 33–88; 4, pp. 75–251).

Consequently, we show in this chapter how Kraepelin's failures in using experimental psychology to advance the understanding of mental illness prompted him to undertake a complete, and ultimately extremely successful scientific re-orientation (on Kraepelin see: [3–5]).

1.2   On Wilhelm Wundt

In 1875, Wundt was appointed one of two professors of philosophy at Leipzig University. In this post, he adopted particular emphasis on a scientific approach, which matched perfectly the wish of the faculty [6, 7]. Four years later he established the world's first experimental psychological laboratory, which began as his very personal undertaking [8–11]. This initiative became a starting point for the establishment of psychology as a discipline in its own right and its separation from philosophy, a process whose conclusion was only to be achieved after 1945. By the second half of the 1880s, Wundt's new approach to psychology had won recognition, but what particularly promoted its dissemination was the continuing growth in interest by a new generation of psychologists, philosophers and scientists as well as, finally, medical professionals. It was they who spread Wundt's approach throughout the European continent and beyond and in particular to the Americas.

Wundt used experiments and observations to study how people perceive things around them and to understand simple mental processes. He measured these processes to uncover their basic rules. He later applied these methods to associations, which are the building blocks of more complex thoughts. However, Wundt did not believe in using these experimental methods to study higher mental processes like conscious thinking and morality [12]. He thought these should be studied through fields like sociology, ethnology, mythology, history, and religion, not through scientific measurements.

On the other hand, Kraepelin wanted to use these methods to study mentally ill individuals, hoping to find specific patterns that could help distinguish different mental illnesses from one another [13–15].

1.3   Getting in Touch: The Beginnings

Emil Kraepelin was born in the rural town of Neustrelitz. His brother Carl, eight years his senior, who was to become a renowned zoologist and botanist, was the dominant influence on him during his childhood and adolescence. They often wandered together through the Mecklenburg countryside to observe natural phenomena enjoying to classify what they discovered by the Linnéan classification system of organisms, i.e. the division of natural phenomena according to naturally occurring criteria. Thus young Emil became sensitive to the 'naturally-given' order and developed a deep interest in biogenetic but also psychological issues, when he came across Wundt's 'Lectures on the human and animal soul' (*Vorlesungen über die Menschen- und Thierseele*; [16]) in the private library of a country doctor who was a close friend of the Kraepelin family and had made a lasting impression on young Emil ([17], p. 3; [18], pp. 109, 115). Influenced particularly by the first volume of this edition (and obviously neglecting the second), young Kraepelin decided to become a doctor specialising in insane people, a career in which he assumed he could integrate his deep interest in experimental psychology into a bread-and-butter job as a doctor ([17], p. 3).

From the start, and guided by his brother, Kraepelin followed the philosophical direction of his mentor only selectively, since in his book of 1863 Wundt had already warned explicitly that the experimental approach alone could not guarantee certainty of understanding the human soul. At this stage in Wundt's life, the experimental and the sociological and psychological aspects of his work stood 'side by side almost unconnected' ([19], p. 177), probably explaining the selective approach ([3], p. 36–45) that young Kraepelin adopted.

It was natural that Kraepelin should enrol at Leipzig University in the summer semester of 1874 to study medicine, as his brother Carl had studied and undertaken work for his doctorate there and was then lecturing at a school in the city. (On Kraepelin in Leipzig, see: [4, 20]) After only three semesters he moved to Würzburg University to continue his studies—a decision he was soon to regret. After having worked through Wundt's 'Principles of Physiological Psychology' (*Grundzüge der physiologischen Psychologie*; [21]), he decided to return to Leipzig where the now 43-year-old author of this book had meanwhile been appointed professor of philosophy. Soon after his return in March 1877, he made himself known to Wundt ([17], p. 5). In a letter to his family he offered a detailed account of this first encounter stating how surprised he was that Wundt had made a 'rather natural, very business-like impression' and 'did not make any specific enquiries'. Following this initial meeting Kraepelin was able to get to know Wundt even better through eagerly attending his seminar on 'The Psychological Society' ([5], vol. III, p. 96–97). A factual description of their meeting, which his scientifically uneducated relatives could understand without difficulty, was followed by an enthusiastic and detailed account of the book by this 'giant spirit' (*Riesengeist*), as he referred to Wundt.

During the summer semester of 1877, Kraepelin not only attended this private seminar held 'early on Wednesday evening' ([22], 1877 p. 15), which was not even part of a medical student's syllabus, but also volunteered to contribute a presentation on the sensitivity to light ([17], 1983, pp. 5–6). Presumably it was his talk and his general keen interest that attracted Wundt's attention. This could explain why in a letter of March 1880 (date not entirely certain) Kraepelin asked his mentor to pen a review on his first piece of writing or, even better, a letter of recommendation, which he could use to persuade a publisher to release it as a brochure. Wundt's letter of response dated 20 March 1880 marks the beginning of a correspondence that lasted over 40 years. This exchange provides an unconventional insight into the biographies of two outstanding men of science and bears vivid witness on the one hand to the cautious formation of their friendship and understanding based on deep mutual respect and, on the other, to the difficult phase of self-discovery of both scientific psychology and modern clinical psychiatry ([18]; see also [23]).

1.4   On Someone Having a 'Favoured Inclination Towards Psychology', Yet 'Having to Stay a Psychiatrist Out of Necessity' for the Time Being

In August 1878, Kraepelin began working as an assistant at the Upper-Bavarian county asylum in Munich. He later reflected in his memoirs on the emotional toll of his work, describing how he was depressed by what he perceived as the vanity, the trivia and the untidiness of the 150 inpatients, who were, according to him, demented, whining, yelling and always at the edge of violence. The work left him anxious and sleep-deprived, and he felt scientifically dissatisfied. The 'confusing bustle' of patients, combined with the limited medical therapeutic tools of the time, led him to feel helpless in the face of mental illnesses that still lacked scientific understanding ([17], pp. 11–13).

Kraepelin's frustration grew as he questioned whether his supervisor, Bernhard von Gudden, a proponent of the brain-anatomical school, was pursuing a productive approach. Gudden focused on finding organic causes of mental illness through brain anatomical and histological findings, which Kraepelin believed was ultimately a waste of time ([17], pp. 15–17). He did not want to end up like Auguste Forel, mocked by colleagues for his repetitive brain-slicing as 'Präparätchenassistent' (eds: [brain] 'preparation assistant') ([24], p. 73). Kraepelin sought alternative ways to address the 'confusing bustle' of patients, by finding criteria by which patients could be diagnosed reliably during their lifetime rather than trying to find out what they had suffered from post mortem.

Psychiatry in the 1880s had made progress with exogenous illnesses but struggled with endogenous and psychogenic disorders. Kraepelin felt the need to identify the underlying processes of mental illness and analyse the differences between healthy individuals and the mentally ill. He turned to Wundt's research on basic psychological processes in healthy people, believing that Wundt's methods could advance psychiatry by showing how the mentally ill perceive and associate differently. Wundt's approach, which varied experimental conditions in order to establish cause-and-effect links, impressed Kraepelin and convinced him that these methods could offer valuable insights into mental illness ([21], p. 5). In fact, Kraepelin believed that by using Wundt's methods mental disorders could be classified like natural phenomena. He also assumed that each mental phenomenon, just like physical phenomena, could be traced to an external cause, an interpretation that was more absolute than Wundt's own views.

Kraepelin's dissatisfaction with his work and the conditions at the Munich asylum drove him to seek a closer relationship with Wundt. In his letter of 18 January 1881, he asked for advice on whether it was feasible to dedicate himself to psychological studies under Wundt's guidance, and whether Wundt's methods could be applied to psychiatry. He also inquired if a year in Leipzig could prepare him to apply these methods independently. Kraepelin told Wundt that once again he faced the necessity of making a fundamental decision as to which career to follow and that only against this background he dared 'once again to bother' his much respected professor 'with a request that could prove of utmost importance for my future career, namely for advice no other person except you could possibly give. [...] As I had hinted earlier, I have been thinking of following my favoured inclination of psychology and, should that be possible, dedicating myself exclusively to psychological studies under your guidance. Unfortunately though, given the current circumstances realising this idea is far from simple and for various reasons I have to consider the situation very carefully before leaving my present secure position here. As I am not a man of means and therefore have to stay a psychiatrist out of necessity, it is essential for me to know how far you think it possible to utilise the psychological studies I can do under your guidance in psychiatry. Have the psychophysical methods [...], the mastery of which one cannot acquire from books, but only by practicing them, reached such a level that one could legitimately apply them fruitfully in psychiatry? I would prefer with all my heart not to have to make this my guiding principle, yet I have already committed myself and these obligations only allow me to follow my inclinations, if these provide an opportunity of advancing my career as a physician for the insane. These are the circumstances under which I am approaching you, as the only person that can give me competent advice. Would it on the one hand be possible for me to learn to practise the modern methods of psychological research, during, let us say, a half- to one-year stay in Leipzig, to such an extent that I could apply them independently afterwards? And do you believe that these methods could be applied to psychiatry successfully?' ([18], pp. 41–42).

1.5 Wundt's Recommendation

Kraepelin's mentor replied five days later on 23 January 1881—without, however, offering certainty in response to his student's main concern. Wundt stated he did not have enough psychiatric expertise and experience to evaluate if the psychophysical experimental methods could 'ever' be 'applicable' in psychiatry, 'that is to say usable for experiments on mentally ill patients on a larger scale'. He pointed out that 'undoubtedly experiments on the insane are likely to prove *extremely* [underlined in original] difficult. If one were seeking reliable results, they would require a lot of attention, diligence and intelligence as well as, finally, a great deal of good will and the absence of deliberate deception'. However, he ended by saying that 'many things that one once deemed impossible have become a distinct possibility' and though the experimental methods themselves had without doubt their imperfections, the time Kraepelin had suggested for getting to grips with them would be sufficient. However, after careful consideration of both the research programme Kraepelin had outlined and his situation, Wundt continued: 'Considering all these points I *cannot* [underlined in original] recommend to give up your secure job for the uncertain chances your studies in experimental psychology might open to your own career in psychiatry'. Nevertheless it should be possible to pursue the one interest without forsaking the other altogether and Wundt therefore concluded: 'Would it be helpful for you to find a job at our local psychiatric hospital which is going to open under Flechsig in a few months' time and for which your work under Gudden will provide good references? It would seem to me that, given the lack of competent and hard-working young psychiatrists and particularly those who have had training in anatomy, you would have an excellent chance. Were you to write to Flechsig and refer to me by name, I should be pleased to support your application' ([18], pp. 44–45).

Wundt was clearly suggesting that Kraepelin's brain-anatomical experience, on which the young psychiatrist himself placed little worth, could be a distinct advantage. After all, Wundt was familiar enough with contemporary psychiatry to know that, equally to Gudden, Paul Flechsig (1847–1929) was a proponent of the brain-anatomical school that almost monopolised university-based psychiatry at that time. If we understand the quote from Wundt's letter correctly, he also suggested that Flechsig could be happy to employ a psychiatrist like the young Kraepelin, with practical clinical experience, for Flechsig himself had none. He had only been made associate professor of psychiatry in 1878, and designated as head of the university psychiatric hospital due to open in 1882, because no anatomical or physiological chairs were vacant as his preferred alternative ([4, 25], pp. 29–68).

Through his letter of 23 January 1881, Wundt had a lasting influence on Kraepelin's life, for in February 1882 his student did indeed become the senior assistant in Flechsig's hospital. At the same time, he was to have the chance of working in Wundt's laboratory. Yet his mentor expected Kraepelin would do so 'on the side … as much as you care and can manage' ([18], p. 51).

1.6   The Application of Psychophysical Methods on Psychiatric Objects

Wundt had been rather vague as to the chances of success in applying 'his' approach to psychiatry. Still, Kraepelin in his next letter of 27 January 1881 outlined definite plans, almost ignoring Wundt's reservations. And these plans were not only very detailed, but also extremely optimistic: 'It is clear that for the majority of mentally ill patients all methods that are not objective by nature, but require the assistance of the person being studied are completely impractical. Yet there is still a residue of patients on whom certain studies, such as the measurement of mental time and stimulus threshold, could be undertaken and are likely to come up with interesting results. First and foremost I am thinking of patients suffering from slight melancholia, mild rage and paralytics at an initial stage […]. In general I should not apply these methods to the severely mentally ill, since innumerable sources of potential error could exist. Yet it would rather seem to me that the experiments on the persons as proposed above could prove important since they could provide us with usable clues for an understanding of the so-called neuropathic disposition. This term, which plays a significant role in present-day psychiatry, is by its nature most unclear and many sided. Consequently our understanding of both the aetiology and nature of mental disorders will barely progress, unless this mysterious 'something' has been neurophysiologically precisely defined. As you can see, I am planning to develop the fruitful thought your work has inspired in me and whose importance to psychiatry I have only hinted at. I am strongly convinced that all 'predisposing' moments produce their effects by altering the mode of reaction. They can either effect all the nerves simultaneously or only those of certain, individual areas. A person with a strong hereditary predisposition, an alcoholic, a morphine addict, an epileptic, or someone convalescing from typhoid will respond differently to external stimuli than the normal, 'sthenic' person. Consequently, should it not be possible to identify differences in the reactions between these groups of individuals with the help of your psychophysical methods? I am thinking of differences in the changes of stimulus threshold or mental time under the influence of various agents (emotions, alcohol) or differences as to how soon the individual being tested gets tired or enraged (and to what degree). […] Most importantly, however, we would also gain insight into the nature and impact of hereditary degeneration, which has been hypothesised to be responsible for a great many of mental disorders, of which we, sadly, do not have a clear understanding. Yet I'd rather not continue giving free reign to my fantasy, but I do think that the ideas mentioned above will suffice to show ways in which I see chances for psychophysical methods being applied to psychiatric objects [sic! Kraepelin's original wording preserved]. Please blame the boundless optimism and the phantasm contained in my exposition on my youth. […] I am convinced that there is at least a grain of truth in what I have said. However, I cannot say whether this truth can be found already or whether it might be me who will be able to do so. Yet, I think, it is worth giving it a try and not even your rather negative reply […] has left me doubting my resolution to carry out my intentions' ([18], pp. 47–48).

1.7   Kraepelin in Leipzig

On 25 February 1882, Kraepelin took up his duties as senior assistant and deputy director at the *Irrenklinik* ('mental hospital') of Leipzig University. From the very beginning, he and his boss Flechsig clashed and Kraepelin was constantly at the edge of being fired. Several facts may explain why the two of them did not get along well. Firstly, both were very similar in being extremely stubborn, proud and wanting to be in charge. Secondly, it is well established that Kraepelin and Flechsig were rather intolerant towards different opinions and hence also scientific approaches that were different from their own views. Their antagonism may have been exacerbated by Kraepelin turning down Flechsig's admittedly rather vague offer to help him write and defend his *Habilitation* (second MD thesis necessary to be appointed professor). After all, he had not chosen to investigate and report on a brain-anatomical topic or a clinical matter, but rather on an experimental psychological subject, a pharmaco-psychological one to be precise [20].

Immediately after Flechsig had accepted him as his senior assistant, that is, still in Munich and before going to Leipzig, Kraepelin sent Wundt his quasi-application: 'As has often been the case in the past, and with your kind permission, I shall seek your advice and support in dedicating myself more and more to psychology which has always been my favoured inclination' ([18], pp. 52–53). And right away he beseeched his teacher for help: 'a kingdom for a topic'. Might he dare 'think of [...] analysing the impact of some of the most well-known nervines [eds: calming and restorative substances] [...] on the response time. Admittedly, this is not very original, but nevertheless appropriate. [...] Should you, however, have another topic up your sleeve which you deem suitable and which you would like me to explore, I should really appreciate it if you could tell me something about it, so that I can do the necessary reading here [in Munich] and thus be well prepared to start the experimental work immediately upon my arrival' ([18], p. 56).

Wundt's response reveals that, contrary to Kraepelin, he was more interested in cognitive psychology rather than the application of experimental psychological methods to psychiatry. He suggested that Kraepelin should not just investigate the changes in response time certain nervines bring about: 'it may perhaps be worthwhile observing in addition the changes of decision and will times under the influence of certain substances in order to dissect extremely complex alterations in their individual functional components employing appropriate methods of combination and elimination'. For this purpose, Wundt suggested, Kraepelin should perhaps restrict himself to one substance ([18], p. 58).

Ultimately, Kraepelin and Wundt made a deal that provided the main reason for Flechsig's constant and increasing dissatisfaction with his senior assistant. It became soon clear to him that Kraepelin simply took advantage of him as the provider of the necessary financial support to enable Kraepelin to pursue his 'pet subject' and make his experiments at Wundt's laboratory rather than at his, Flechsig's, brain-anatomical laboratory. Possibly, the head of the Leipzig department could have developed some acceptance for his situation, had Kraepelin not greatly neglected his duties at the hospital. Flechsig had been seeking: a competent and efficient assistant who would free him of his duties as a physician and enable him to dedicate himself totally to his own research interests in his brain-anatomical laboratory. Yet, this was not possible as Kraepelin's work both at Wundt's and his own experimental laboratory in Flechsig's hospital was very time-consuming. This situation was made worse by the fact that, at least at the time, Kraepelin lacked interest in the patients and the interest he did show in them was rather research-oriented, psychopathological in nature using them as subjects for his experiments ([26, 27], p. 27; [28, 29], p. 217; [30], pp. 153–160). It was only a matter of time before the work at the hospital suffered and this would consequently lead to open conflict with Flechsig. This made Flechsig dismiss Kraepelin without notice in mid-June. The sources we were able to locate in archives provide evidence that this dismissal was fully justified, given the serious failures in hygiene and other shortcomings Flechsig described.

So Kraepelin found himself in a financially difficult situation. Still, he was determined to qualify as soon as possible as *Privatdozent*, which would give him the right to teach at university and collect fees from his students. Barely 14 days after his dishonourable dismissal from Flechsig's hospital, Kraepelin handed in his application to be granted the title of *Privatdozent* for psychiatry at Leipzig University—the very clinical academic subject that Flechsig represented and who, therefore, was definitely to be included in the *Privatdozent* examinations committee. As if applying so to say with the man who had fired him just two weeks earlier were not enough, he filed a very special request on top of that. This request was to accept, instead of the 'separate postdoctoral thesis' normally required, three papers he had already published to 'assess my scientific capabilities' ([31], p. 1).

The papers Kraepelin enclosed instead of a postdoctoral thesis were 'On the Duration of Simple Psychological Processes' [*Ueber die Dauer einfacher psychischer Vorgänge*] [32], 'On the Modulation of Simple Psychological Processes by Some Medicines' [*Ueber die Einwirkung einiger medikamentöser Stoffe auf die Dauer einfacher psychischer Vorgänge*] [33] and 'On the Influence of Acute Diseases on the Development of Mental Illnesses' [*Ueber den Einfluss acuter Krankheiten auf die Entstehung von Geisteskrankheiten*] [34]. Leipzig's medical faculty had these works reviewed by Erb and Flechsig's mentor, physiologist Carl Ludwig (1816–1895). Ludwig was very critical of the two psychological studies, but thanks to an enthusiastic review of the third study by Erb, the faculty council approved Kraepelin's written works thus allowing the *Habilitation* procedure to continue. After successfully passing the oral examination, which was the second component of the Habilitation procedure, Kraepelin was awarded the title *Privatdozent* and on 20 October 1882 officially included in the teaching staff of Leipzig's medical faculty ([35], vol. 1, p. 436).

As Kraepelin could not find paid employment in Leipzig at the time, he was pleased to accept an offer from Ambrosius Abel Publishers to author a concise textbook of psychiatry, which was to appear within the renowned 'Abel's medical compendia' series ([4], p. 236; [17], p. 28). This 'Compendium der Psychiatrie' [36], published in 1883, is the first edition of his 'Textbook of Psychiatry'. By 1926, this textbook saw nine editions and from the 1890s to 1930s was the standard work in its area, the 'Bible of Psychiatry' ([37], p. 116). His 'Compendium' is cited here, since even as early as when he penned the introduction, Kraepelin was making extensive reference to his basic idea of integrating the experimental psychological approach into psychiatry. He regarded this as the silver bullet, the only way to make progress in psychiatry: 'In order to fully understand mental disorders, it is essential to break down given symptoms into their smallest components and to ascribe these elementary alterations of mental processes to pathological changes of basic mental functions in general. The clinical approach in psychiatry [i.e. clinical observation and registration of patients' symptoms, which was described as the second key principle of psychiatric research in the chapter before—H.S.] can only prove successful if it is coupled with an exact analysis of basic mental phenomena and a profound knowledge of basic mental functions established by scientifically based psychology. Without this, facing mental disorders […] will be like trying to analyse urine without the help of our chemical and physiological knowledge. It would be totally impossible to identify the real pathological components, let alone to ascribe them to a specific organic illness. Hence our uncertainty as to the nature of certain mental illnesses is mainly the result of the severe lack of an appropriate psychological approach. […] It is therefore essential not only to undertake clinical observations and record pathological symptoms, but also to analytically study them. The science that can provide us with the means to take this third path is experimental psychology'.

So here, in the introduction of his 'Compendium', written in the Easter break of 1883, experimental psychology, 'which is the necessary extension of a 'pathology of the cerebral cortex' (all quotes from [36], p. 12–14), is proposed as a complement to clinical observation. This search for complementarity between experimental method and clinical observation can be interpreted as a first forerunner of the pluridimensional approach to mental disorders Kraepelin was to apply later. Moreover, it seems to anticipate the reduced importance Kraepelin attributed to Wundt's method later on. Only two years earlier, in his letters to Wundt, Kraepelin had referred to them as the key to open up the mysterious bustle of mental illnesses. A further three years after the release of his 'Compendium', Kraepelin was to regard experimental psychiatry as one of several auxiliary disciplines in psychiatry. A transition in Kraepelin's views was taking place, a re-orientation of his scientific approach.

1.8   The Value of Experimental Psychology to Psychiatry Is Reduced

Kraepelin left Leipzig in October 1883 to work at Gudden's hospital in Munich but stayed only a few months. He then became a senior assistant at the Silesian Province Asylum in Leubus (now Lubiąż, Poland) but again had a brief tenure. His time there may have influenced his scientific concepts, possibly through contact with Karl Ludwig Kahlbaum (1828–1899) [38]. Shortly after, he moved to the Dresden Municipal Hospital as a senior consultant in wards for the mentally ill and internal medicine. These frequent changes stemmed from his desire to marry his long-time fiancée, which he believed required a stable income. However, his short stays also highlight his search for a role suited to his interests and abilities.

Despite these shifts, Kraepelin remained focused on starting his own experimental psychological studies using Wundt's methods. In contrast to the experimental, his accounts of his clinical work itself during this period are scarce (cf. [17], pp. 30–40). After his workload at Leubus eased in autumn 1884 with the appointment of two junior assistants, he resumed the experiments he had started at Gudden's clinic. Unlike Gudden, who was sceptical of Wundt's methods ([17], p. 15), Leubus director Wilhelm Alter (1843–1918) gave Kraepelin a free hand scientifically. In the rural isolation of Leubus, however, it was not easy to find test subjects. So, Kraepelin took measurements of psychological time on his recently married wife. Strikingly, no evidence suggests he carried out any experiments on Leubus's 194 patients by late 1884 [39]. Why he would bypass this opportunity remains unclear.

On 1 June 1886, Kraepelin took up his duties as newly appointed professor of psychiatry and head of the psychiatric hospital at the German-speaking University of Dorpat (present-day Tartu in Estonia, which at that time was part of the Russian Empire). His almost five years there were of decisive importance for the theoretical foundation of his clinical-empirical approach to psychiatry, just as the Heidelberg years later mark the practical realisation of this approach. Parallel to developing his new clinical-empirical approach, Kraepelin's disappointment that the experimental psychological methods could not be satisfactorily applied to mentally ill patients was growing. He was dissatisfied with the time those experiments and the efforts to minimise sources for errors took, for he could really have used this time instead to improve his ability to communicate with his foreign-speaking patients as well as to meet his obligations as both clinical and administrative head of a university department, for whose financial affairs he was fully, and solely, responsible. This work pressure was increased by the fact that his hospital was remotely situated from both the town and the other university departments so that communication, and his presenting seminars and lectures, were impeded.

Yet, despite these pressures, Kraepelin tried to continue his experimental psychological studies 'on the side, as much as I can'. Even today one can state that his activities left their mark in Dorpat, since until the present day Kraepelin is referred to as 'by far the most important experimental psychologist to have been associated with Estonia' [40]. As one of his early activities, Kraepelin founded a Psychological Society in the autumn of 1887 in order to enhance the image of both the subject and his department with the general public and within the university. As we can see from the outcome in terms of studies, Kraepelin was able to 'attract a considerable number of enthusiastic and self-sacrificing workers' ([17], p. 59). First Kraepelin was able to find room available for their tests at the Physiological Institute. From 1888, he was able to locate more rooms to establish a psychological laboratory within his psychiatric hospital.

In the same year 1888, Kraepelin reported to his mentor in Leipzig: 'Most progress has been made in investigating the influence of exercise and fatigue. For this study I had everyday processes (like reading, writing, calculating, counting etc.) analysed systematically in order to obtain standard values. These could later be used as comparative material for tests on mentally ill people, for whom the application of more exact chronometric methods would be too complicated. It seems it will be possible to work out an adaptation, an exercise and a fatigue coefficient for each of these processes and for each individual, which will reflect both the momentary state of mind and general capability'.

At the beginning, Kraepelin stuck closely to the procedures and methods that had been developed by Wundt. In the course of the experiments, however, he soon complemented these with methods he designed and developed himself ([41], p. 1249). It can be assumed that it was the clinical experience that he gathered that particularly enhanced and optimised the conditions and methodology of the experiments. As Jaroševskij ([42], p. 262) has pointed out before, this experience made Kraepelin aware of the fact that when a single experiment and, even more so, if a whole series of experiments is conducted, it is always numerous parameters that impact the experiments and their outcome, particularly when experimental subjects demonstrate significant individual variation in their responses to the experimental procedures. All this enabled Kraepelin to revise and correct the results of earlier experiments. In general, the results of the tests carried out in Dorpat were much more exact than those of the experiments carried out among others in Leipzig and through their accuracy more convincing, and of a totally new quality. This development illustrates a general trait in all of Kraepelin's work, both psychiatric and psychological: He regarded all his findings and views as provisional, results to be improved and optimised by better methods, further eliminating sources of error, and by widening the database by including more and different test subjects.

The experimental psychological and psychopharmacological studies [43, 44] published during his Dorpat years provide revealing insights into the problems that drove him and the efforts he made to solve them. Thus his essay 'On the Knowledge of Psychophysical Methods' reveals his deep dissatisfaction with the stagnation in the methodology of experimental psychology at the time. He pointed out that discussing the methods of measurements took up 'an unreasonable amount of space in the psychophysical literature', whereas progress could only be achieved by 'producing new, more thoroughly elaborated practical experience' ([45], p. 503). In the printed version of a talk given in 1890 'On Mental Functional Disorders', he even drew the discouraging conclusion that the results of tests on mental time carried out on mentally ill patients were 'nearly useless'. Moreover, a material number of methodological problems had to be overcome before the experimental approach could be applied 'successfully in the pathological field' ([46], pp. 522, 524). He concluded that unfortunately he had not been able to realise his original research programme of identifying and classifying the natural regularities that underlay psychological processes in mentally ill people, at least not to the extent originally planned ([17], p. 50; [47], p. 12).

In his 90-page overview on 'The Psychological Experiment in Psychiatry', Kraepelin drew the modest and rather depressing conclusion that 'What experimental psychology can do for us today will hardly be of material help in making the diagnosis of illnesses any easier'. Significantly it was in his 1892 study 'On Influencing Simple Mental Processes by Several Drugs' [*Ueber die Beeinflussung einfacher psychischer Vorgänge durch einige Arzneimittel*] that Kraepelin appeared to put a provisional final line under his first scientific period, which had been closely linked with experimental psychology. Although the book is dedicated 'to his dear teacher Wilhelm Wundt as a symbol of his steadfast gratitude and devotion' ([48], p. IV), we can also read here that 'other' projects and topics were becoming more important—most probably since they seemed more promising to him: 'Since my heavy workload and other pressing scientific challenges do not allow me to foresee if and when I shall be able to continue my work, I have now strived to bring to an end the present study, work on which has taken more than the 'nonum annum'.

Despite being less optimistic about the outcomes achievable with this method, experimental psychology remained a 'favoured inclination' to Kraepelin. Over time however it became more and more a secondary field of his activities, and he increasingly delegated the troublesome and time-consuming finicky work to his undergraduate and postgraduate students. This shift in attention had nothing to do with Kraepelin taking on new responsibilities as professor at Heidelberg University in April 1891, which supposedly denied him the necessary time to pursue his pet subject ([17], p. 65; [49], p. 1; see also, [50], p. 816). The real reason for this shift becomes clear from many references in the 1892 book ([48], pp. V–VI). Still Kraepelin never gave up hope that one day experimental psychology would bring results as he had hoped and so he kept providing adequate premises and funding, both while at Heidelberg and later at Munich University and also at the German Research Institute for Psychiatry, founded by him in 1917. This way Kraepelin guaranteed that experimental psychological investigations have always been an integral part of psychiatric research. Still it is a proven fact that at the time, the results of Kraepelin's experimental psychological school were not acknowledged accordingly, nor his approach adopted by others for several decades—neither in psychiatry, nor psychology (for a similar view, see: [51, 52]). It was not before the late 1970s and 1980s that experimental and pharmaco-psychological research, in the tradition of Kraepelin's investigations of the late nineteenth and first decades of the twentieth century, took off again ([2], p. 151).

Kraepelin's approach and theories can be recognised as relevant to present-day cognitive neurosciences, including clinical neuropsychology. Between 1883 and 1893 he espoused more and more a pluridimensional approach to research and thus laid the foundations for his clinical-empirical approach to psychiatry. It was through working on the fourth edition of his 'Textbook of Psychiatry' [53] that this broader and more sophisticated approach slowly emerged. His nosological classification of mental illnesses is the most significant and visible fruit of all his efforts, and herein it is his division of endogenous mental illnesses into two large groups that stands out [54]. This division, which is still basically used today, could never have been achieved by means of the experimental psychological approach alone. In this regard, Kraepelin was right to downgrade the latter approach from 'the key science' to one of several auxiliary sciences in a combined pluridimensional approach. Nevertheless, although undoubtedly Kraepelin had fruitful links with a variety of people and schools of thought, he still felt the most intense, emotional and steadfast bond with one man, namely Wilhelm Wundt. Even though his experimental psychological schooling with Wundt had not resulted in the desired breakthrough, but rather guided him to become an empirical and wide-ranging scientific researcher, he valued the bond enormously, based as it was on 'feelings of most faithful and sincere gratitude to you, to whom I owe so much in the spiritual fulfilment of my life. While it makes me very proud to be able to demonstrate to you through my actions that the seed you planted into the heart of your youthful student has grown and thrived, I am still aware of the limitations of my own capabilities. I feel strongly that my psychological achievements are only an extension of what I learnt under your guidance and in your laboratory' ([18], p. 98).

1.9 Conclusion

Although the psychological methods Kraepelin adopted from Wundt did not enable him to reach his original scientific goals to bring order to the 'confusing bustle' of manifestations of mental illness, this failure paved the way to his greatest scientific achievement, the description and classification of mental disorders based on long-term clinical observations as laid out in his comprehensive 'Textbook of Psychiatry'.

Key Points
- Kraepelin admired the experimental psychologist Wilhelm Wundt from the beginning of his career, which led to his decision to return from Munich to Leipzig in 1882 to study under Wundt.
- Despite scepticism voiced by Wundt, Kraepelin set out to use Wundt's experimental methods to bring order to the 'confusing bustle' of manifestations of mental illness.
- During his work in Leubus and Dorpat, Kraepelin continued improving on experimental psychological methods, but grew more and more frustrated with its failure to enable the identification of specific mental disorders.
- This failure led him to adopt a pluridimensional approach to psychiatry, leading to his clinical-empirical scientific agenda and ultimately his greatest achievement, the description and classification of mental disorders based primarily on long-term clinical observations.
- Even though his experimental psychological schooling with Wundt had not resulted in the desired breakthrough, but rather guided him to become an empirical and wide-ranging scientific researcher, he considered Wundt a key scientific inspiration throughout his life.

References

1. Müller U, Fletcher PC, Steinberg H. The origin of pharmacopsychology: Emil Kraepelin's experiments in Leipzig, Dorpat and Heidelberg (1882–1892). Psychopharmacology. 2006;184:131–8.
2. Steinberg H, Müller U. Emil Kraepelin 1822/83 in Leipzig und seine frühen pharmakopsychologischen Arbeiten im Licht der aktuellen Forschung. In: Angermeyer MC, Steinberg H, editors. 200 Jahre Psychiatrie an der Universität Leipzig. Personen und Konzepte. Heidelberg: Springer; 2005. p. 121–54.
3. Hoff P. Emil Kraepelin und die Psychiatrie als klinische Wissenschaft. Berlin/Heidelberg: Springer; 1994.
4. Steinberg H. Kraepelin in Leipzig. Eine Begegnung von Psychiatrie und Psychologie. Bonn: Psychiatrie-Verlag; 2001.
5. Weber MM, Holsboer F, Hoff P, Ploog D, Hippius H. Edition Emil Kraepelin (5 vols.). München: Belleville; 2000–2005.
6. Wundt W. Erlebtes und Erkanntes. Stuttgart: Kröner; 1920.
7. Der SH. Psychologe und Philosoph Wilhelm Wundt und eine Widmung seines Schülers Emil Kraepelin. Nervenarzt. 2001;72:884.

8. Sächsisches Hauptstaatsarchiv Dresden. Bestand: 10281/322. Ministerium für Volksbildung, Universität Leipzig. Das Psychologische Institut.
9. Universitätsarchiv Leipzig. Bestand: Rentamtsakten. 979. Akten über das Seminar für experimentelle Psychologie ... 1882–1943.
10. Wundt W. Das Institut für experimentelle Psychologie. In: Festschrift zur Feier des 500 Jährigen Bestehens der Universität Leipzig, vol. 4, Part 1. Leipzig: Hirzel; 1909. p. 118–33.
11. Fensch D. Zur Rolle Wilhelm Wundts bei der Institutionalisierung der Psychologie. In: Gesellschaft für Psychologie der DDR, editor. Psychologiehistorische Manuskripte. Berlin: w/o publisher; 1977. p. 60–6.
12. Jüttemann G. Wilhelm Wundts anderes Erbe. Ein Missverständnis löst sich auf. Göttingen: Vandenhoeck & Ruprecht; 2006.
13. de Freitas AS. Wie aktuell ist Wilhelm Wundts Stellung zum Leib-Seele-Problem? Schriftenreihe der Deutschen Gesellschaft für Geschichte der Nervenheilkunde. 2006;12:199–208.
14. Rieber R, Robinson D. Wilhelm Wundt in history. New York: Kluwer Academic; 2001.
15. Bringmann W, Tweney R. Wundt studies. Toronto: Hogrefe; 1980.
16. Wundt W. Vorlesungen über die Menschen- und Thierseele. (2 vols). Leipzig: Voß; 1863.
17. Kraepelin E. In: Hippius H, Peters G, Ploog D, editors. Lebenserinnerungen. Berlin: Springer; 1983.
18. Steinberg H. Der Briefwechsel zwischen Wilhelm Wundt und Emil Kraepelin. Zeugnis einer jahrzehntelangen Freundschaft. Bern: Huber; 2002.
19. Hehlmann W. Geschichte der Psychologie. 2nd ed. Stuttgart: Kröner; 1967.
20. Steinberg H. Emil Kraepelin in Leipzig: Wie einer Entlassung eine Habilitation folgen kann – Eine Quellenstudie. In: Steinberg H, editor. Leipziger Psychiatriegeschichtliche Vorlesungen. Leipzig: Evangelische Verlagsanstalt; 2005. p. 75–102.
21. Wundt W. Grundzüge der physiologischen Psychologie. Leipzig: Engelmann; 1874.
22. Verzeichniss der im Sommer (bzw. Winter)-Halbjahre 18XX auf der Universität Leipzig zu haltenden Vorlesungen. Leipzig: Edelmann; respective years.
23. Fischel W. Wilhelm Wundt und Emil Kraepelin. Gedanken über einen Briefwechsel. In: Karl-Marx-Universität Leipzig 1409–1959. Beiträge zur Universitätsgeschichte. Leipzig: Verlag Enzyklopädie; 1959. p. 382–91.
24. Forel A. Rückblick auf mein Leben. Zürich: Gutenberg; 1935.
25. Steinberg H. Paul Flechsig (1847–1929) – ein Hirnforscher als Psychiater. In: Angermeyer MC, Steinberg H, editors. 200 Jahre Psychiatrie an der Universität Leipzig. Personen und Konzepte. Heidelberg: Springer; 2005. p. 81–120.
26. Kolle K. Emil Kraepelin 1856-1926. In: Kolle K, editor. Grosse Nervenärzte, vol. 1. Stuttgart: Thieme; 1956. p. 175–86.
27. Kolle K. Kraepelin und Freud: Beitrag zur neueren Geschichte der Psychiatrie. Stuttgart: Thieme; 1957.
28. Havens LL. Emil Kraepelin. J Nerv Ment Dis. 1965;141:16–28.
29. Alexander FG, Selesnick ST. Geschichte der Psychiatrie. Konstanz: Diana; 1969.
30. Güse HG, Schmacke N. Psychiatrie zwischen bürgerlicher revolution und Faschismus. Kronberg: Athenäum; 1976.
31. Universitätsarchiv Leipzig. Bestand: Personalakten 1461. E. Kraepelin.
32. Kraepelin E. Ueber die Dauer einfacher psychischer Vorgänge. Biol Centralbl. 1881-1882;1:654–72, 721–33,751–66.
33. Kraepelin E. Ueber die Einwirkung einiger medicamentöser Stoffe auf die Dauer einfacher psychischer Vorgänge. Philos Stud. 1881–1883;1:417–62, 573–605.
34. Kraepelin E. Ueber den Einfluss acuter Krankheiten auf die Entstehung von Geisteskrankheiten. Archiv für Psychiatrie und Nervenkrankheiten. 1881;11:137–83, 295–350, 649–77 and 1882;12:65–121, 287–336.
35. Universitätsarchiv Leipzig. Bestand: Medizinische Fakultät. B IV 3, vol. 1. Akten die Prüfungen pro venia legendi betr. 1834–1943.
36. Kraepelin E. Compendium der Psychiatrie. Zum Gebrauche für Studirende und Aerzte. Leipzig: Abel; 1883.

37. Doucet F. Forschungsobjekt Seele. Eine Geschichte der Psychologie. München: Kindler; 1971.
38. Steinberg H, Angermeyer MC. Der Aufenthalt Emil Kraepelins an der schlesischen Provinzial-Irrenanstalt Leubus. Fortschritte der Neurologie · Psychiatrie. 2002;70:252–8.
39. Alter W. Jahresbericht für 1885 der Provinzial-Irren-Anstalt zu Leubus in Schlesien. Breslauer Aerztliche Zeitschrift. 1886;8:238–41.
40. Allik J. History of experimental psychology from Estonian perspecitve. Psychol Forsch. 2007;71:618–25.
41. Rogovin MS. Emil Kraepelin. Derptskij period. Zh Nevropatol Psikhiatr Im S S Korsakova. 1974;74:1244–53.
42. Jaroševskij MG. Istoria psicholigii. Moskva: Mysl; 1976.
43. Kraepelin E. Cytisin gegen Migräne. Neurol Centralbl. 1888;7:1–5.
44. Kraepelin E. Ueber den Einfluss der Uebung auf die Dauer von Associationen. St Petersburger Medicinische Wochenschrift. 1889;1:9–10.
45. Kraepelin E. Zur Kenntnis der psychophysischen Methoden. Philos Stud. 1890;6:493–513.
46. Kraepelin E. Ueber psychische Funktionsstörungen. Allgemeine Zeitschrift für Psychiatrie. 1890;46:522–4.
47. Kraepelin E. Der psychologische Versuch in der Psychiatrie. Psychologische Arbeiten. 1895/1896;1:1–91.
48. Kraepelin E. Ueber die Beeinflussung einfacher psychischer Vorgänge durch einige Arzneimittel. Jena: Fischer; 1892.
49. Trömner E. Nachruf auf Emil Kraepelin. Dtsch Z Nervenheilkd. 1927;96:1–7.
50. Berrios GE, Hauser R. The early development of Kraepelin's ideas on classification: a conceptual history. Psychol Med. 1988;18:813–21.
51. Hildebrandt H. Der psychologische Versuch in der Psychiatrie. Was wurde aus Kraepelins (1895) Programm? Psychol Gesch. 1993;5:5–30.
52. van Bakel AHAC. "Ueber die Dauer einfacher psychischer Vorgänge". Emil Kraepelins Versuch einer Anwendung der Psychophysik im Bereich der Psychiatrie. In: Hagner M, Rheinberger HJ, Wahrig-Schmidt B, editors. Objekte – Differenzen – Konjunkturen. Experimentalsysteme im historischen Kontext. Berlin: Akademie; 1994. p. 83–105.
53. Kraepelin E. Psychiatrie. Ein kurzes Lehrbuch für Studirende und Aerzte. Leipzig: Abel (Meiner); 1893.
54. Kraepelin E. Psychiatrie. Ein Lehrbuch für Studirende und Aerzte. 6th ed. Leipzig: Barth; 1899.

Open Access This chapter is licensed under the terms of the Creative Commons Attribution 4.0 International License (http://creativecommons.org/licenses/by/4.0/), which permits use, sharing, adaptation, distribution and reproduction in any medium or format, as long as you give appropriate credit to the original author(s) and the source, provide a link to the Creative Commons license and indicate if changes were made.

The images or other third party material in this chapter are included in the chapter's Creative Commons license, unless indicated otherwise in a credit line to the material. If material is not included in the chapter's Creative Commons license and your intended use is not permitted by statutory regulation or exceeds the permitted use, you will need to obtain permission directly from the copyright holder.

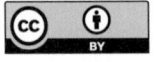

Kraepelin and the Development of Physical Treatments in Psychiatry

2

I. N. Ferrier

2.1 Introduction

The relationship between the work of Emil Kraepelin and the development of physical treatments in psychiatry is complex and multi-faceted. Here an assessment of his contribution and impact has been divided into three phases. First, the period as a student and a trainee when he became very enthused with the burgeoning science of experimental psychology and used its techniques to examine the central effects of psychoactive substances. His contribution to this field was considerable, particularly his discussion of research design and methodology and, in a sense, he can be considered as one of the founding fathers of psychopharmacology. Next, during his seminal years of collecting information on large cohorts of patients which led to his nosological theories, there was relatively limited research or study of drugs and other therapeutic agents, which he perceived only to provide some symptomatic relief. This dearth stemmed from the all-consuming nature of his clinical research but was also related to his predominantly negative view about curability and his views about the role of factors such as alcoholism, venereal disease and degeneration, which led him to believe that prevention was likely to be the more fruitful approach than therapy. He did study the effects of hormonal tissue extracts and, to a lesser extent, lithium but was unimpressed with both, which, given his powerful influence on the field and the potential toxicity of these approaches at the time, was probably just as well. One can argue that the discovery of the benefits of drugs in psychiatry, with all its limitations, requires more understanding of biochemistry and pharmacology than was available in Kraepelin's day. Finally, there is the question of whether Kraepelin's nosological legacy has helped or hindered the fields of biological psychiatry and psychopharmacology. As outlined below, the argument can be made that while the categorical classification diagnostic systems that most

I. N. Ferrier (✉)
Department of Psychiatry, Newcastle University, Newcastle upon Tyne, UK
e-mail: nicol.ferrier@newcastle.ac.uk

© The Author(s) 2026
G. Ikkos, T. Becker (eds.), *Psychiatry after Kraepelin*,
https://doi.org/10.1007/978-3-032-09475-9_2

19

psychopharmacological research is based on have been shown to be theoretically and scientifically flawed, nonetheless useful data have been collected on the well-characterised cohorts that this approach encourages.

2.2   Kraepelin and Pharmaco-Psychology

Emil Kraepelin studied medicine in Leipzig and Würzburg from 1874 until 1878. In 1877, while a student in Leipzig, he did an attachment with Willhelm Wundt (1832–1920), Professor of Philosophy and one of the founders of experimental psychology. After qualifying Kraepelin worked in a District Mental Hospital in Munich until 1882, when he returned to Leipzig. He started a research programme with Wundt leading to a promotion to Lecturer in 1883 and he also established a clinical appointment with Dr Paul Flechsig (1847–1929) [1]. Hoff reports that Wundt influenced Kraepelin in a way 'that can hardly be overestimated' [2] (eds: see Chap. 1). Engstrom and Kendler underline the attraction Kraepelin felt for Wundt by quoting Kraepelin's remark in his autobiography: 'I decided to become a psychiatrist as it seemed that this was the only possibility to combine psychological work with an earning profession' [3]. Wundt had developed experimental techniques to study various cognitive functions in humans and Kraepelin deployed these techniques to investigate the effects of psychoactive drugs on reaction time. Wundt advised that he restrict his studies to only a very few substances and accordingly most of Kraepelin's work in Leipzig focussed on alcohol although his later studies in Dorpat and Heidelberg covered a much wider range of drugs including morphine, chloral hydrate, paraldehyde and caffeine.

Kraepelin published the results of these studies in three long papers written in Leipzig between 1881 and 1883 and in an extensive monograph (*On the Modulation of Simple Psychological Processes by Some Medicines*) written in Dorpat and Heidelberg in 1892 [1, 4]. These studies, while having their intrinsic merit, are also revealing for what they tell us about Kraepelin the scientist. Firstly, they demonstrate his powerful commitment to research. As Muller and Fletcher argue, the papers are part of the evidence that shows he was aware of practical issues such as funding, time constraints and the likelihood (and importance) of publications emerging. Muller and Fletcher also demonstrate that Kraepelin's pharmacological work showed the same creativity that his later work exemplified. They show how the studies were methodologically innovative, for example by demonstrating Kraepelin's clear understanding of the imperative for placebo and control conditions [1]. The papers also evidence Kraepelin's early grasp of the importance of statistical issues in such studies. Mayer-Gross, in a 1957 review of these papers, notes that the 'improvement and elaboration of statistical methods … lay close to Kraepelin's heart' and that 'he discusses … the limited certainty with small sample sizes' [5]. Several of these commentators describe Kraepelin's enthusiasm and aptitude for what he dubbed 'pharmaco-psychology' [1–4]. Muller and Fletcher suggest that he spent 'every free minute' in Wundt's laboratory.

As discussed in more detail below, Kraepelin abandoned pharmaco-psychological research during the pursuit of his famous nosographic research projects in Heidelberg and Munich. But experimental psychology was, in his own words, his 'true obsession' and he returned to lead psychology research after his retirement from his psychiatric clinic post in Munich [1]. Kraepelin's innovations in pharma-psychological methodologies can be seen as important in the development of modern cognitive neuroscience. The modern term psychopharmacology was first used in the early twentieth century and came to prominence with the discovery of chlorpromazine in the 1950s but in many ways Kraepelin can be seen as one of its founding fathers. Kraepelin's contributions to psychopharmacology and clinical neuropsychology were far ahead of his time but his conceptual achievements have been largely neglected by modern psychiatry and cognitive neuroscience [4, 5].

2.3   Kraepelin and Therapeutics

Despite Kraepelin's interest in the psychological effects of drugs, his insistence on the importance of applying the new science of psychology to morbid mental states and his use of this science to study the effects of the drugs described above, Kraepelin did not pursue these kinds of studies with the patients he examined in depth in Heidelberg and Munich where his main focus was on clinical psychopathology and nosology rather than therapeutics. As far as patient management was concerned, he was a firm advocate of non-restraint that was, belatedly compared with England, being introduced into German psychiatric practice in hospitals. He spoke positively about innovations to improve the atmosphere in hospitals such as bed treatment, long soothing baths, farming, good heating and plumbing, 'family nursing' and aftercare by 'benevolent associations' and negatively about features like isolation rooms [6]. Sedatives like chloral hydrate were becoming much more in use in German institutions but Kraepelin considered them 'expedients' whose only benefit was in bringing 'a quiet atmosphere' to the wards. In clinical work, his medication of choice was potassium bromide to promote sleep and calm agitated patients, but it seems clear that he only saw such drugs as alleviating some symptoms and improving the milieu.

Kraepelin spoke of his long-term aim of promoting therapeutic advances but seems to have put more emphasis on the potential value of prevention. The lack of focus on therapeutics may have been linked to his belief in the incurability of most major mental disorders. Bruckner describes how Kraepelin considered only 'fever delirium', 'intoxications, infectious and thyreogenic mental disorders' or 'certain psychogenic diseases' as curable but deemed all 'other forms of insanity incurable' [6]. He was sceptical of therapeutics partly due to his conviction, a 'fatalistic determinism' as Shepard puts it, that much of mental illness was secondary to alcoholism, venereal disease and 'hereditary degeneration' [7]. While he talked forcibly about the benefits of education, particularly temperance, and welfare as preventative strategies, Bruckner argues that he put most faith in eugenic strategies, such as marriage bans and castration, and he urged legal and health policy changes to further these ends [6]. His attitudes to degeneration and the impact of those beliefs are discussed more fully elsewhere in this volume (eds: see Chaps. 4 and 5).

Noll argues that Kraepelin's belief that degeneration was central to the development of dementia praecox was more nuanced than that of classical degeneration theorists [8]. Kraepelin believed in a chronic autointoxication that led to a 'self-poisoning' and that the development of rational therapies was possible only if the underlying mechanisms of this process could be elucidated. According to Noll, Kraepelin was particularly intrigued by the findings of the late nineteenth century of how thyroid extract could cure myxoedema. This finding led him to believe that abnormal secretions of internal glands could cause disease, and he placed dementia praecox firmly within these new medical paradigms as a metabolic autointoxication. Kraepelin believed that in dementia praecox there was a 'tangible morbid process in the brain'. He largely rejected the notion that this process was consequent on hereditary degeneration but posited that, in view of the temporal relationship between the disease onset and sexual development, there may be 'some processes taking place in the sexual organs'. He largely rejected the then popular notion that mental disease was caused by toxins from infections in the gastro-intestinal tract.

Kraepelin was active in examining his patients from a physiological perspective. He reported changes in heart rate and temperature regulation, which he opined were secondary to derangement in central control. He implicated increased central sympathetic output with decreased parasympathetic modulation both of which would speed the heart up, potentially erratically. He ascribed these abnormalities to changes in the thyroid gland as he also did with the skin and pupil size changes he recorded. Organotherapy, particularly thyroid organotherapy, became popular in the 1890s across Europe, and Noll reports that Kraepelin introduced preparations 'of every possible organ' but as Kraepelin himself reported in 1919 'unfortunately without any effect' [8]. Later Kraepelin became agnostic about autointoxication theories and removed dementia praecox from this category placing it in a category of its own (see Heckers, Chap. 14). This change of view, combined with his inherent therapeutic scepticism and caution, stopped him from carrying out surgery on his patients, which however became commonplace in some parts of Europe and North America in the early decades of the twentieth century, preceding the heroic somatic therapies of the 1930s (insulin and malaria therapies, for example). Given Kraepelin's dominant influential position in psychiatry at the turn of the twentieth century, his reservations must have prevented even more widespread use of harmful surgery in that era.

Finally, with respect to therapeutics, Kraepelin took some interest into lithium salts. Schioldann describes the long history of Danish research on and use of lithium. Lithium salts entered the Danish *Materia Medica* in 1863 [9]. Carl Lange (1834–1900) was a Danish academic neuropathologist in private neurology practice and his younger brother, Fritz Lange (1842–1907), was an asylum psychiatrist. Carl propounded his thesis on 'periodic depression' and its response to lithium treatment. Lange distinguished it from manic depressive illness because 'lack of spirits and *joie de vivre* is their constant complaint' and from melancholia due to an absence of delusions and hallucinations. His theory of aetiology included both heritability, of 'decisive significance', and 'a constant tendency of the urine to deposit uric acid sediment'. He posited that the rational treatment to counteract this underlying diathesis required the 'alkaline treatment method'. This included lithium as well as dietary restriction to eliminate sources of uric acid. Fritz Lange focussed more on the theory of 'autointoxication' due to the uric acid diathesis [10]. Kraepelin's verdict was to dismiss outright Lange's beliefs about periodic depression. He did not confirm it by clinical observations. He also considered that the conceptual framework for the use of lithium was not consistent with his own experience that only a few patients had co-occurring gout. He viewed the diagnosis of periodic depression as more likely being manic depressive disorder in which the manic phase had been missed. While he did not support lithium in the treatment of affective disorder, he did employ it for epilepsy and acknowledged that 'at some stage in the future light might be shed on this question by means of metabolic investigations' [11].

2.4   Kraepelin's Psychopharmacological Legacy

Shepard comments that a strong case could be made that the impetus he gave to psychiatric research was Kraepelin's greatest legacy to psychiatry [7]. Kraepelin provides the model of how to combine research into nosology but also in related disciplines like neuropathology, psychophysiology, psychopharmacology and epidemiology with psychiatry's clinical practice and education [3]. Another legacy is his Deutsche Forschungsanstalt für Psychiatrie, the world's first multi-disciplinary psychiatric research institute which opened in 1917, and which later became the Max Planck Institute of Psychiatry, a world leading centre for all aspects of psychiatric research, including therapeutics, which, as Francis says, 'embodies his insistence on rigor and excellence' [6, 12].

The more specific question arises whether the nosological guidelines proposed by Kraepelin have helped or hindered research and productivity in psychopharmacology. Van Praag and Rybakowski for example argue that the adoption of Kraepelinian traditions in nosology has been unsatisfactory for both biological psychiatry and for psychopharmacology [13, 14]. Most scholars in the field now believe that the so-called Kraepelinian dichotomy cannot be supported by a variety of neurobiological and genetic evidence and this would suggest, on first principles, that the outcome of any clinical therapeutic trial based on diagnoses made dichotomously must also be flawed.

However, there are important caveats to this sweeping statement. As elegantly demonstrated by Engstrom and Kendler, Kraepelin himself had major reservations about his disease categories [3]. He did not claim they had validity or scientific value and was clear he was not attempting a 'true classification'. In later editions of his textbook, he reported the 'impossibility of any comprehensive delineation of mental disorders', that the boundary zone between mental health and illness was 'more or less arbitrary' and that 'despite best efforts, we are entirely unable to classify many cases'. In the middle part of the twentieth century, Kraepelin's ideas were challenged and lost influence but were resurrected by clinician scientists, sometimes called neo-Kraepelinians, in the later decades of the century where they formed the basis of diagnostic systems such as the DSM and ICD [2]. These systems made categorical diagnoses. Many argue that these diagnostic schemes have pragmatic usefulness particularly in providing a common language that can be understood by clinicians and researchers from different times and backgrounds and that they have helped reduce the major problem of over-diagnosis, which was an increasing issue, particularly in the USA, when diagnosis had no accepted or acceptable criteria. It is also manifestly true that the adoption of these categorically defined conditions was a major influence on and stimulus to the promotion and burgeoning of research and publication. While the psychiatric conditions being studied might lack validity, at least there was some conformity in the patients chosen for study. However, it can also be argued that the proliferation of diagnoses in subsequent editions of the DSM, and the emergence of so-called multiple comorbidities, has counteracted these benefits. It is worthwhile recalling that Kraepelin himself understood something the Neo-Kraepelinian seemed not to—that there are no pathognomonic symptoms for individual mental disorders (eds: see Foreword). There are no boundaries but rather they, and their complex and interacting causes, lie on various spectrums.

Some argue that because, for example, schizophrenia, unipolar depression and bipolar disorder are not separate disease entities but are on a variety of continua, it is fruitless to look for therapeutic signals in these diagnoses. While it is true that response to medication cannot be used as a diagnostic tool, some important findings have been made using the categorical diagnosis schemes. The fact that all these conditions respond to antipsychotics has been taken to show that these conditions are basically similar but closer inspection shows that while DSM diagnosed schizophrenia responds to both first- and second-generation antipsychotics, the clinical benefits in the affective disorders are solely associated with second-generation antipsychotics and first-generation antipsychotics may if anything worsen their outcome [15]. Similarly, antidepressants have a positive signal in unipolar depression but no signal in bipolar depression [16]. There may be no demarcation between bipolar disorder and schizophrenia, but detailed research has shown an enormous, and clinically relevant, difference in how these 'conditions' respond to lithium so that the latter is the 'gold standard' of prophylactic treatment in bipolar disorder while being virtually ineffective in schizophrenia [17]. All of these examples demonstrate the likelihood of differing neurobiology underlying these 'diagnoses' and, more importantly, flag up neurobiological spectrums which encompass these conditions which require closer inspection and more research. It can be argued that if Kraepelin had not employed course and outcome as a way of delineating the extremes of these spectrums, then such important psychopharmacological advances would not have been made. No model lasts forever, and all must be evaluated regularly, a point, as Van Praag comments, Kraepelin, given his 'intellectual stature', would have readily agreed to [13].

2.5   Discussion

As Shepard comments, since his death, almost a hundred years ago, Kraepelin's reputation has become iconic [7]. It is hard to disagree with the judgement of Mayer-Gross and colleagues in 1969 that 'modern psychiatry begins with Kraepelin' and Hoff's assertion that Kraepelin's work has been one of the most influential over that period [2, 18]. Virtually all commentators agree that Kraepelin's main influence lies in the now accepted perception that detailed clinical assessment, including measuring outcome, is the cornerstone of good clinical research, and that Kraepelin himself and the diagnostic schemes constructed in his name have been stimuli for a great deal of productive research. And, more directly, some of his ideas about experimental psychology have become central to contemporary cognitive neuroscience.

But of course, as with any research and any new conceptual framework, the Kraepelinian perspective has what Hoff calls 'its pitfalls and limitations'. There are major questions about Kraepelin's determination that mental disorders are categorically distinct objects, 'natural kinds' as he put it [2]. A critique of this emphasis is outside the scope of this chapter, focussed as it is on his impact on the development of physical treatments, but is to be found elsewhere in this volume (eds: see Chaps. 6, 8, and 13). Another critique, also discussed elsewhere, is the lack of emphasis Kraepelin puts on the experiences, particularly social and psychological, of the individual patient. In respect of his impact on physical treatment development, his therapeutic nihilism about dementia praecox and his notions about its incurability merit serious questioning as indeed took place contemporaneously, particularly in Germany, and later elsewhere [6]. Similarly, his conviction about the excellent prognosis for bipolar disorder is not supported by current data. Improving the outcome of both Kraepelin's major diagnostic pillars remains an important therapeutic target.

More recently there have been attempts to move away from the rigidity of the categorical approach to psychiatric and psychopharmacological research. For example, Owen and Craddock proposed a move towards a classification that maps the expression of mental illness onto underlying biological systems, and they suggested a series of spectrums from clinical through various cognitive domains to neurobiological and genetic variables along which various disorders, as currently defined, lie [19] (eds: see Chap. 5). Insel and colleagues proposed that neurobiological and therapeutic research should focus on five transdiagnostic general cognitive and motivational domains, the so-called RDoC criteria [20]. In the field of psychopharmacology, it has been proposed that drugs be named on the basis of their neurochemistry rather than their confusing and often limited descriptors such as antipsychotic and antidepressant—the Neuroscience Based Nomenclature [21]. These initiatives, and many other nascent ones, are the beginning of a new 'non-Kraepelinian' classification and one can profoundly hope that these systems or, more probably, their successors will lead to major therapeutic advances in a currently stalled field. However, these newer classification systems are complex and likely to generate a vast amount of data, much of it hard to interpret. As Palm and Moller describe, Kraepelin's views and concepts have been challenged for 100 years but what Berrios and Hauser call their 'binding embrace' persists perhaps because of their pragmatic useful simplicity, something that Kraepelin strived for and which has, on balance, been a pivotal step forward [22, 23].

Key Points

1. Kraepelin was an early pioneer in pharmaco-psychology and made important contributions to its methodology.
2. Kraepelin was sceptical that drugs could help or ameliorate dementia praecox, partly related to his beliefs in the condition's underlying degeneration and incurability.
3. Kraepelin's work led to the use of diagnostic schedules that have acted as a stimulus to research though their rigidity has also led to false premises.
4. A key legacy of Kraepelin is the acceptance that detailed clinical assessment, including that of illness course, is the cornerstone of good research, especially that on outcome.
5. Another major contribution that Kraepelin made was his drive and determination to establish and foster multi-disciplinary research in psychiatry.

References

1. Müller U, Fletcher PC. The origin of pharmacopsychology: Emil Kraepelin's experiments in Leipzig, Dorpat and Heidelberg (1882–1892). Psychopharmacology. 2006;184:131–8.
2. Hoff P. The Kraepelinian tradition. Dialogues Clin Neurosci. 2015;17:311–41.
3. Engstrom EJ, Kendler KS. Emil Kraepelin: icon and reality. Am J Psychiatry. 2015;172:1190–6.
4. Steinberg H, Himmerich H. Emil Kraepelin's habilitation and his thesis: a pioneer work for modern systematic reviews, psychoimmunological research and categories of psychiatric diseases. World J Biol Psychiatry. 2013;14:248–57.
5. Mayer-Gross W. Kraepelins Arzneimittelstudien und die pharmakologische. Psychiatrie der Gegenwart. Nervenarzt. 1957;28:97–100.
6. Brückner B. Emil Kraepelin as a historian of psychiatry – one hundred years on. Hist Psychiatry. 2023;34:111–29.
7. Shepherd M. Kraepelin and modern psychiatry. Eur Arch Psychiatry Clin Neurosci. 1995;245:189–95.
8. Noll R. Kraepelin's 'lost biological psychiatry'? Autointoxication, organotherapy and surgery for dementia praecox. Hist Psychiatry. 2007;18:301–20.
9. Schioldann JA. Did lithium therapy of affective disorders turn one hundred and forty or fifty? Aust N Z J Psychiatry. 2000;34(sup1):A60.
10. Schioldann J. 'On periodical depressions and their pathogenesis' by Carl Lange (1886). Hist Psychiatry. 2011;22:108–15.
11. Kraepelin E. Psychiatrie. Ein Lehrbuch für Studirende und Aerzte. 6th ed. Leipzig: Barth; 1899. p. 408.
12. Francis X, Introduction. This volume.
13. van Praag HM. Kraepelin, biological psychiatry, and beyond. Eur Arch Psychiatry Clin Neurosci. 2008;258:29–32.
14. Rybakowski JK. 120th anniversary of the Kraepelinian dichotomy of psychiatric disorders. Curr Psychiatry Rep. 2019;21:1–8.
15. Licht RW. Typical and atypical antipsychotics in bipolar disorder. Acta Neuropsychiatrica. 2000;12:115–9.

16. Köhler-Forsberg O, Sylvia LG, Fung V, Overhage L, Thase M, Calabrese JR, Deckersbach T, Tohen M, Bowden CL, McInnis M, Kocsis JH. Adjunctive antidepressant treatment among 763 outpatients with bipolar disorder: findings from the Bipolar CHOICE and LiTMUS trials. Depress Anxiety. 2021;38:114–23.
17. Leucht S, Helfer B, Dold M, Kissling W, McGrath JJ. Lithium for schizophrenia. Cochrane Database Syst Rev. 2015;10:CD003834.
18. Mayer-Gross W, Slater E, Roth M. Clinical psychiatry. London: Baillière, Tindall & Cassell; 1969. p. 10.
19. Craddock N, Owen MJ. The Kraepelinian dichotomy–going, going... but still not gone. Br J Psychiatry. 2010;196:92–5.
20. Insel TR. The NIMH research domain criteria (RDoC) project: precision medicine for psychiatry. Am J Psychiatry. 2014;171:395–7.
21. Zohar J, Stahl S, Moller HJ, Blier P, Kupfer D, Yamawaki S, Uchida H, Spedding M, Goodwin GM, Nutt D. A review of the current nomenclature for psychotropic agents and an introduction to the Neuroscience-based Nomenclature. Eur Neuropsychopharmacol. 2015;25:2318–25.
22. Palm U, Möller HJ. Reception of Kraepelin's ideas 1900–1960. Psychiatry Clin Neurosci. 2011;65:318–25.
23. Berrios GE, Hauser R. The early development of Kraepelin's ideas on classification: a conceptual history. Psychol Med. 1988;18:813–21.

Open Access This chapter is licensed under the terms of the Creative Commons Attribution 4.0 International License (http://creativecommons.org/licenses/by/4.0/), which permits use, sharing, adaptation, distribution and reproduction in any medium or format, as long as you give appropriate credit to the original author(s) and the source, provide a link to the Creative Commons license and indicate if changes were made.

The images or other third party material in this chapter are included in the chapter's Creative Commons license, unless indicated otherwise in a credit line to the material. If material is not included in the chapter's Creative Commons license and your intended use is not permitted by statutory regulation or exceeds the permitted use, you will need to obtain permission directly from the copyright holder.

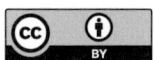

Beyond Conceptual History: Emil Kraepelin's, Karl Jaspers' and Arthur Kronfeld's Views on Psychiatry May Not Only *Inform* But Also *Guide* Our Present-Day Debate

3

Paul Hoff

3.1   Introduction

The title of this chapter could be misunderstood: To say that authors such as Emil Kraepelin, Karl Jaspers and Arthur Kornfeld, who shaped the intellectual history of psychiatry, may not only *inform* but also *enrich* the content of today's debate on the truly fragile identity of the discipline is not an expression of hagiography. The latter merely demonstrates a lack of critical distance and never advances the matter. Careful reception and contextualisation of classical texts, however, bring us closer to their core ideas to offer a historical perspective to build bridges to the current debate.

All scientific approaches are time-bound, including our own today. But to prematurely dismiss historically significant authors as outdated or even ignore them simply because they are part of the history of ideas would grossly underestimate the rich intellectual heritage of psychiatry and, in particular, psychopathology. It should be noted that this is not primarily a matter of theory, but rather action-relevant, that is, practical foundations of psychiatry, whether in diagnosis or therapy, in research or teaching. Within the canon of medical disciplines, psychiatry works with a particularly broad array of heterogeneous theoretical assumptions, whether those involved are always aware of this or not. These assumptions have a considerable influence on the actual work of psychiatrists. For this reason alone, attempts to view the theory and practice of psychiatry separately cannot be successful.

P. Hoff (✉)
University Hospital of Psychiatry Zurich, Zurich, Switzerland

© The Author(s) 2026
G. Ikkos, T. Becker (eds.), *Psychiatry after Kraepelin*,
https://doi.org/10.1007/978-3-032-09475-9_3

The undeniable complexity of psychiatric issues, rooted in the very complexity of the mentally ill person, must not be perceived as an obstacle or scientific disadvantage. On the contrary, it encompasses a fruitful conceptual and methodological diversity that must be respected and constantly re-examined. In this sense, reflecting upon the work of influential earlier authors is not merely of historical interest. Rather, in a form adapted to twenty-first-century discourse, it has the potential to stimulate the contemporary development of psychiatry's self-image and to substantially deepen the necessary debate. This shall be illustrated here.

3.2   Why We Should Have Taken the Biopsychosocial Model More Seriously

The biopsychosocial model of the development and the course of diseases, introduced into the medical debate by George Engel in 1977 [1], soon became a widely recognised point of reference, not only for psychiatry, but, as the title of Engel's work explicitly states, for 'biomedical science' in general. Yet with regard to mental disorders the model is particularly illuminating: it understands their development as the end-point of interacting biological, psychological and social factors, thus touching on the fields of neuroscience, psychology, psychopathology and the social sciences.

However, the prima facie high persuasiveness of this model harbours risks, as cautionary or openly critical voices have insisted, particularly in the last two decades. Ghaemi [2], for example, has written pointedly of the 'rise and fall of the bio-psycho-social model'. In condensed form, two strikingly different, even contradictory interpretations of the model can be identified: The *positive* interpretation, Engels' declared objective, calls for a serious and respectful exchange between the three pillars. The aim here is to broaden the scientific horizon and not to replace one pillar with another or to 'explain away' the contents of one pillar with those of another. In the *negative* interpretation, the model does lead to the recognition of the three pillars, but these stand passively side by side, a merely additive and not a dialogical-constructive approach that lacks a significant exchange of ideas between the perspectives. The logic of power plays no small role here in the sense of the implicit or explicit tendency of one perspective to assert its *fundamental* superiority over the other two.

The development of psychiatry since the publication of Engels' work in 1977 has led some observers to become disillusioned that the intended respectful dialogue between different perspectives has often fallen by the wayside, whether due to ignorance of or disinterest in other points of view, or—as mentioned above—because of the blunt claim to superiority of a single perspective. Examples of the uncritical overreach of the validity of one's own position could be cited for each of the three pillars. However, the decisive factor here is that a reversal of the original intention of the biopsychosocial model from a cooperative, dialogical approach to an exclusionary one has not served the scientific and clinical self-image of psychiatry—even more so, it has clearly damaged it.

3.3 Psychiatry in the Early Twentieth Century: Three Seminal Approaches, Time-Bound (Like Ours), But Still Thought-Provoking and Fruitful (for Us)

3.3.1 Methodology

A key element of each author's thinking is identified and placed in the context of their work. This is based on a careful reading of the relevant historical texts in the sense of 'close reading' [3]. The aim is not to provide a comprehensive overview, but rather to build a convincing bridge between the basic positions of Kraepelin, Jaspers and Kronfeld and the current debate on the self-image of psychiatry. To this end, this chapter formulates three specific questions that relate specifically to the approaches of the earlier authors that should be addressed today.

3.3.2 Emil Kraepelin

Emil Kraepelin (1856–1926) is often perceived primarily as the founder of a psychiatric nosology that exerted a formative influence on the field throughout the twentieth century and up to the current diagnostic manuals International Classification of Diseases 11th revision (ICD-11) and Diagnostic and Statistical Manual of Mental Disorders, Fifth edition, text revision (DSM-5 TR). This is factually correct. However, it fails to recognise the real motivation that drove Kraepelin throughout his nearly five decades of work. At the beginning of his career, psychiatry was still a very young academic discipline, and he wanted to establish it as a *respected*, or better still, an *indispensable element* of medical faculties.

Kraepelin was convinced that this goal could only be achieved if psychiatry was conceptually oriented towards the rules of empirical scientific work.[1] For him, this necessarily included a clear idea of what was meant by mental illness, how it could be reliably diagnosed and how various types of mental illness could be differentiated from each other. He thus entered the fields of clinical nosology and the diagnostics based on it, but he never regarded these as ends in themselves. Instead, rather as concrete, practical applications of his theoretical concept of illness. The latter is now outlined in its main features.

Kraepelin's central point of reference was and remained the concept of 'natural disease entities' ('natürliche Krankheitseinheiten'), which he repeatedly emphasised as the foundation of all psychiatric research. He regarded these entities as predetermined 'by nature', in today's terminology: neurobiologically. Since, according to Kraepelin, they existed completely independently of research, it was the task of research to *discover* them—and *not to construct them conceptually*. He consistently assumed that research would always encounter the same 'natural entities', regardless of the scientific methodology chosen, be it pathological anatomy of

---

[1] A pioneer of scientific psychiatry in the nineteenth century, Wilhelm Griesinger (1817–1868) had taken very similar positions in this regard, but is rarely mentioned by Kraepelin [4].

the central nervous system, aetiological research or long-term clinical observation (which became the focus of Kraepelin's own work for decades).

From the second edition of his textbook (1887) to its ninth edition, published 1927, that is, posthumously, this basic idea remained unchanged, even though significant objections were raised over time. This is the decisive passage from the second edition:

> If we had a thoroughly exhaustive knowledge of all details in one of the three fields, pathological anatomy, aetiology or symptomatology of insanity, it would not only be possible to find a uniform and comprehensive classification of psychoses from each of them, but each of these classifications would also—this requirement is the *foundation of our scientific research in general*—essentially coincide with the other two. ([5], p. 211; translated and italics by P.H.)

In order to demonstrate the remarkable consistency of Kraepelin's basic stance on this issue, given the four decades (!) that have passed and the critical voices that have certainly been heard,[2] I would also like to quote the relevant passage from the ninth edition:

> If we are actually able to achieve the goal, we have in mind, of capturing the real disease processes through our nosological categories, then the various delimitations, whether they are made from the pathological-anatomical, causal, or purely clinical point of view, should ultimately coincide. I regard this requirement as the *cornerstone of our scientific research into mental disorders in general.* ([7], p. 17; translated and italics by P.H.)

In his late programmatic works from the years 1918 to 1920, especially in the essay 'Die Erscheinungsformen des Irreseins' [8],[3] Kraepelin dealt extensively with objections to his nosological approach. As an experienced clinician, he now made the rather far-reaching concession that clinically observable symptoms (including the long-term course of illness) might not be a reliable enough way of identifying the postulated underlying disease entities, but that further scientific methods beyond descriptive psychopathology needed to be developed. However, Kraepelin never abandoned his conceptual foundation, the idea of the existence and scientific recognisability of 'natural disease entities' that do exist in psychiatry as well as in somatic medicine [10].

In a nutshell, Kraepelin's nosology can be described as *well-structured, comparatively easy to comprehend* and *based on pragmatic clinical considerations.* Notwithstanding the existence of critical voices, this self-assured decisiveness, combined with an explicit scientific claim, led to Kraepelin's concept being perceived as 'modern', that is, timely, clinically practicable and research oriented during his lifetime. After his death (1926), this assessment remained unchanged, which explains Kraepelin's significant international influence on psychiatry in the twentieth century and, albeit with increasingly sceptical objections, in the early twenty-first century.

---

[2] One example worth mentioning is Karl Birnbaum (1878–1950), who presented a study—characterised by a differentiated psychopathological approach—entitled 'Structural analysis as a clinical research principle' ('Die Strukturanalyse als klinisches Forschungsprinzip') [6].

[3] This has been translated in English as 'Patterns of Mental Disorder (1920)' [9].

Emil Kraepelin stands in a tradition of nature observation and research the roots of which can be traced back to Plato's 'Phaedrus'. There, Socrates speaks of a good butcher who does not cut up the animal arbitrarily, but deliberately along its *natural* joint structure. Campbell et al. [11] explicitly refer to this vivid image when choosing the title for their rich, pluralistic analysis: 'Carving nature at its joints: Natural kinds in metaphysics and science'. Precisely because of the complexity of their research 'objects',[4] psychiatry and psychology are included in their consideration, but without direct reference to Kraepelin.

3.3.3 Karl Jaspers

Karl Jaspers (1883–1969) published one of the fundamental texts in our field, 'Allgemeine Psychopathologie' ('General Psychopathology'), at the age of 30 in 1913. However, he only worked in clinical psychiatry for a few years before devoting himself to psychology and later philosophy.[5] His personal life path thus points to the close proximity of psychiatry to epistemological, ethical and cultural issues.

I have discussed Jaspers' differentiated examination of Kraepelin's concept of illness elsewhere [14]. Since the focus here is not on nosology, but on the self-image of psychiatry, I will now concentrate on a cautionary note that is especially prominent in the late Jaspers: In his view, particular scientific diligence, even modesty, must be exercised as soon as psychiatric research is confronted with issues of *conditio humana*, that is, with the image of man and the status of the person.

For Jaspers, all psychiatric activities, especially diagnostic and therapeutic processes, were never merely technical procedures that had to follow a set of rules. Rather, they were always interpersonal, dialogical acts. He warned against transferring patterns of thought prevalent in the natural sciences uncritically to psychological, social and cultural phenomena, which can be read as a criticism of Kraepelin's naturalistic nosology. By this he meant above all the idea of an object of research existing completely independently of the investigation and the investigator. In the fourth edition of 'Allgemeine Psychopathologie' ('General Psychopathology') (1946), published immediately after the Second World War, which, unlike the first edition of 1913, was strongly influenced by his now fully developed existential philosophy, Jaspers expressed himself very clearly:

> *In the world* I can move forward recognising all sides. *The world* I cannot recognise. It is no different with humanity. … I never capture a person in their entirety, once this person has become an object for me.
> There is *no system of being human*. In whatever wholeness we think we grasp humanity, it has slipped away from us. ([15], pp. 468, 641; translated and italics by P.H.)

---

[4]The decisive object of research in psychiatry is precisely not an 'object', but the mentally ill person (cf. [12].

[5]Jaspers' early departure from acute clinical psychiatry may have been motivated by physical limitations resulting from his chronic lung disease [13].

On the one hand, Jaspers was concerned with the scientific rigour of psychiatry, which he believed should use clear and consistent terminology. This was of particular importance for psychopathology, for him the indispensable basis for clinical practice and for research. On the other hand, he defended the person, whether mentally healthy or not, against any attempt to appropriate him or her through objectifying, reductive or even one-dimensional scientific models [16].

3.3.4 Arthur Kronfeld

Arthur Kronfeld (1886–1941) was a contemporary of the other two authors, but thirty years younger than Kraepelin and three years younger than Jaspers. Unlike the latter two, Kronfeld is largely unknown today, even among experts. This is all the more regrettable given that Kronfeld made significant contributions to the debate on the identity of psychiatry. During his 25 years as a psychiatrist before being forced into exile by the Nazis in 1935,[6] he developed an independent position based on a comprehensive knowledge of historical and contemporary literature [17]. However, Kronfeld was anything but a pure theorist: After working in various psychiatric clinics, he ran a psychotherapeutic private practice in Berlin in the 1920s and was heavily involved in continuing medical education.

His particular interest in psychopathology and a few years spent together with Jaspers as assistant doctors at the Heidelberg Psychiatric University Clinic, created a lasting rivalry, although Kronfeld was never to achieve the same level of scientific recognition and influence, of course.

In philosophical terms, Arthur Kronfeld was a student (and long-time friend) of the neo-Kantian Leonard Nelson (1882–1927).[7] Nelson was the main representative of the 'New Friesian School', a school of thought active at the beginning of the twentieth century and rooted in a wide variety of academic fields, which sought to bring the teachings of the neo-Kantian Jakob Friedrich Fries (1773–1843) back into the consciousness of the philosophical and political public. Kronfeld was a highly committed member of this group for many years and pursued the declared goal of systematically applying Fries' teachings to the epistemological foundations of psychiatry. As his main epistemological work 'Das Wesen der psychiatrischen Erkenntnis' ('The Nature of Psychiatric Knowledge') [18] impressively demonstrated, it was crucial for Kronfeld that psychiatry, like all other sciences, committed themselves to a consistent and justifiable terminology and methodology.

---

[6] Kronfeld first emigrated to Switzerland and from there to Moscow, where he and his wife completed suicide on 16 October 1941, as Nazi troops approached the city. However, a careful biographical account of his years in exile has yet to be written.

[7] The term 'Neo-Kantianism' suggests a theoretical unity that never existed. On the contrary, the 'Marburg School' of Neo-Kantianism focused strongly on *scientific theory and mathematical-logical topics*. Its main representative was Hermann Cohen (1842–1918). Leonard Nelson was much closer to this current than to the competing 'Southwest German School' around Wilhelm Windelband (1848–1915) and Heinrich Rickert (1863–1936). They emphasised the systematic importance of *values* for the scientific process of generating knowledge.

However, he did not limit this to the empirical-quantitative field of natural sciences and experimental psychology but also applied it to the study of qualitative phenomena at the levels of subjectivity, personhood and responsibility.

One of the reasons why Kronfeld's work is hardly known today is the nature of his writing. His texts are not easily accessible, even for experts. Kronfeld often used complicated language, and there are frequent redundancies.[8] At the same time, he valued concise formulations in both speech and writing. He did not shy away from academic controversy[9] and, when he deemed it appropriate, resorted to exaggeration and sometimes even polemics.

Kronfeld demanded recognition of the psyche (in health and illness) as a genuine field of scientific research. However, he argued that it should be studied in a verifiable manner and with methodological rigour, and that speculative approaches were worthless or even harmful. To put this into concrete terms and in keeping with the neo-Kantianism he espoused, Kronfeld repeatedly spoke of inherent structures and laws of the psyche that needed to be understood. In doing so, he explicitly drew an analogy between the scientific rigour required in psychiatry on the one hand and the empirical natural sciences on the other hand. However—and this is crucial—this analogy was methodological rather than substantive: Even if psychiatric research makes use of empirical methods from neighbouring sciences, such as neurobiology, which in Kronfeld's view it should certainly do under defined conditions, this in no way affects the epistemological independence of the psyche.[10]

Kronfeld described his field of conceptual tension, which he considered to be central to psychiatry, with—at his time and today—quite unfamiliar terms: 'autology' and 'heterology'. In his view, psychiatry works heterologically when it draws on concepts and methods from related sciences, such as neuroanatomy or neurophysiology, for its own research. It proceeds autologically when pursuing its clinical and scientific approaches to the realm of the psyche with *psychological* means as far as possible without resorting prematurely to other methods.

As was typical of Kronfeld when he wanted to give special weight to an argument, he formulated the core statements on the autology of psychiatry very decisively: He claimed that an exclusively 'somatological', that is, neurobiological, approach suffers from

---

[8] One reason for this may be that his main epistemological work from 1920 had not been written in a continuous process. Rather, due to disruptions in Kronfeld's life plans during the First World War, it brought together earlier texts, some of which were thoroughly reworked, with newly written ones.

[9] Kronfeld expressed vehement criticism of psychoanalysis at the very beginning of his career, at the age of 26, which attracted considerable attention in contemporary debate [19].

[10] This is strongly reminiscent of one of the founders of scientific psychiatry in the nineteenth century, Wilhelm Griesinger (1817–1868). Following the contemporary philosopher Friedrich Albert Lange (1828–1875), he declared 'methodological materialism' to be the most suitable conceptual framework for certain areas of psychiatric research. In contrast, he strictly rejected the much more far-reaching 'metaphysical materialism' as speculative and therefore unscientific [4].

a fundamental flaw: the inherent structure of the mental remains out of play. It does not take place according to its *own law*, but as the accidental product of an imagined physiological associative dynamism. ... This *heterological simplification* of the mental, however, is not science, but the distorted image of it. ([18], p. 248; translated and italics by P.H.)

In addition to this scientific objection, Kronfeld pointed out, with a clearly mocking undertone, the inadequate diagnostic and therapeutic results of the 'somatological' perspective:

We would find it all bearable if only we could get on with it! Now, however, we have had to convince ourselves in our earlier survey that even with this abundance of conscience-pressing concessions to somatology, a period of stagnation threatens to set in, that despite the consistent realisation of those guiding ideas, we are forced to linger on the shore of an unknown sea without a ship to sail on. ([18], p. 249; translated by P.H.)

From this theoretical insight, Kronfeld derived a clear requirement for research practice:

There should be no explanation of psychopathological phenomena by heterological (somatic) causation, before they have fully been worked up autologically including their last, autologically irreducible genuine elements. ([18], p. 248; translated by P.H.)

In order to pave the way for the 'autology' he demanded, psychiatry had to free itself

from the dogma according to which mental phenomena are only random and meaningless epiphenomena from which no information about the underlying brain disorders can be expected. In an autological psychiatry ... the exact psychological analysis of symptoms alone will be able to lead to the criterion of the respective type of illness. ([18], p. 99; translated by P.H.)

Nota bene: Kronfeld saw himself as a scientist. He was very interested in biological (in today's terminology: neuroscientific) psychiatry. However, he emphasised that this approach quickly reached its limits when it came to subjective experiences and a person's value judgements or actions. He believed that the only scientifically viable path was that of consistently 'autological' research focused on the irreducible specifics of the psyche. Only this would be able to identify the structures and laws of the psyche that differ from those of the body. For Kronfeld, any attempt to *replace* the autological perspective with a heterological one was doomed to failure by which he meant the substantial loss of conceptual and clinical depth. He nevertheless had no objections whatsoever to a meaningful mutual complementarity of both approaches.

Overall, Arthur Kronfeld advocated a self-confident psychiatry that emphasised its own competencies, but was methodologically critical and epistemologically informed, a status he called 'autological'. With regard to the question of whether and how we can derive benefits for the current debate from the positions of seminal earlier authors, Kronfeld's respectful yet biting comment on Kraepelin is remarkable. He bluntly accuses Kraepelin of neglecting psychiatry's genuine field of research, its 'autology' in his diction, in favour of 'heterological' methods. This criticism was obviously important to Kronfeld, as he gave it a prominent place in the introduction to his main work on epistemology:

> We do not belittle the outstanding achievement of Kraepelin when we realise that the hypertrophy of clinical viewpoints and dogmatism, which grew from edition to edition in his great textbook, has *watered down and superficialised* this very textbook from edition to edition. … He has exposed psychiatric research to the danger of *conventionalist relativities*; he has more and more eliminated psychiatry as an autochthonous science; at present there is an era of *almost slavish dependence* of psychiatric research on its heterological auxiliary sciences, on their special methods, which grow on the soil of foreign disciplines, expecting to mediate its own progress in an idle, sterile bondage *without finding it.* ([18], p. 8; translated and italics by P.H.)

3.4 Psychiatry in the Twenty-First Century: Three Questions We Should Ask

In terms of the number of patients treated, psychiatry is a major medical specialty, one that makes a significant contribution to the health care of the population. Nevertheless, in public discourse psychiatry is often not perceived as on the same level as internal medicine or surgical specialties. In addition, from an insider point of view, the scientific self-understanding of psychiatry also appears to be significantly less robust than that of neighbouring disciplines. This raises questions: How justified is it in the twenty-first century to maintain psychiatry as a medical entity? How does the discipline define its relationship to neuroscience, data science, psychology or the social sciences? Would it be possible or (to take the most radical version of questioning criticism of the specialty) even advisable to *replace* it with deliberately clinically and therapeutically oriented versions of the latter disciplines, for example in the sense of 'clinical neuroscience' or 'computational psychiatry'?

From my perspective, psychiatry as a clinical and scientific field will continue to be necessary in the future. Of course, this does not refer primarily to the term itself, but rather to the core content it addresses, namely a consistently person-centred approach to people in mental crises and disorders. However, this core must be brought into a constructive dialogue with the relevant neighbouring sciences, must be (or become) linkable.[11] In establishing precisely this process, reflection on the thinking of influential authors in the history of psychiatry can be much more than mere reminiscence.

In conclusion, I present three questions that arise from the work of Kraepelin, Jaspers and Kronfeld with regard to contemporary psychiatry. They concern the levels of *epistemology*, the *image of man* underlying psychiatric work and the *self-understanding* of the field. Every scientific approach, including those of the authors presented here, has its limits and runs the risk of becoming dogmatic if it does not recognise and acknowledge these limits. As a caveat and to give direction to the current debate, a potentially critical aspect is therefore identified for each question.

---

[11] There seems to be no more concise translation of the German expression 'anschlussfähig'.

(i) At the *epistemological level*, it is necessary to clarify what kind of object we mean when we speak of 'mental illness'. Kraepelin's concept of 'natural disease entities' as the basis of all psychiatric research is now convincingly countered by the argument that it tends to be rigid, uncritically reifying and, contrary to its original intention, sometimes even inhibiting scientific progress [20, 21].

This raises the following question: Given the enormous heterogeneity of the scientific methods used in psychiatric research today, how can we find a reasonable balance between the three poles of strict reification analogous to Emil Kraepelin's thinking, of a hermeneutic approach to mental illness that emphasises subjectivity and personhood, and of descriptive, quantitative methods based on the analysis of large amounts of data in the sense of 'computational psychiatry'[12]?

(ii) At the level of the *concept of man*, the role of the person in psychiatry is up for debate. However, this central and complex philosophical issue does carry the risk of straying too far from psychiatric practice and of no longer being (and remaining) relevant to the current scientific discourse.

The resulting question is how, today, in an age of heterogeneity and in a 'Society of Singularities' ('Gesellschaft der Singularitäten') [23], it can be possible to convincingly place the concept of the person—specifically, of the mentally ill person—at the centre of psychiatry. In other words, there is a need for a concise discourse on the *conditio humana* in psychiatry that is credible in practice and useful in everyday treatment. Recognising this as an indispensable framework would be in line with a demand made by Karl Jaspers.

(iii) The *self-understanding of psychiatry*, the third level, must be described as fragile today. This has a lot to do with the striking 'centrifugal forces' of rapidly growing neighbouring sciences, especially neurosciences and computer and data sciences. There is a risk that the core area of psychiatry—subjectivity and the dialogical-interpersonal space—will continue to lose scientific attention, if not be fundamentally questioned or, even, dismissed.

The central issue here is how the status of psychiatry as an independent medical discipline can be more than a mere tribute to academic traditions dating back to the nineteenth century. In other words, how can a methodologically critical—in Arthur Kronfeld's diction, an 'autological'—psychiatry define a genuine field of research that is not claimed step by step by neighbouring disciplines, but follows a person-centred and undogmatic psychopathological approach [24]?

Nota bene: This is not about backward-looking traditionalism or preserving established academic structures for their own sake. The goal is to make the rich history of psychiatric ideas fruitful for the further development of the field in the twenty-first century—and thus to prevent its fragmentation and the loss of intellectual depth.

---

[12] Heinz [22] provides thoughtful insights into the notion of 'computational psychiatry' and its potential clinical and scientific benefits.

3.5   Conclusion

Conceptual history is an essential tool for approaching and understanding psychiatry as a therapeutical and scientific field. This is true from the historical perspective. Beyond this, however, and since the identity of psychiatry nowadays is substantially challenged in different ways, it harbours considerable potential to carefully link the approaches of seminal psychiatric thinkers with the present-day debate. This puts the historical roots of our field into context. But it also inspires and encourages us to ask the 'right' questions—creative, dense and forward-looking questions that will prove valuable for psychiatry in the twenty-first century.

Key Points
- The scientific and clinical identity of psychiatry in the twenty-first century is fragile and requires in-depth debate.
- Emil Kraepelin and Karl Jaspers continue to exert a significant influence on psychiatry and psychopathology to this day.
- The work of their contemporary Arthur Kronfeld has largely been forgotten, even though he dealt with the self-understanding of psychiatry in an original and multi-layered way.
- The careful reception of 'classic' psychiatric texts is much more than 'l'art pour l'art': It provides information about the conceptual history of psychiatry, *and* it significantly contributes to generating fruitful questions about the future development of our field.
- Psychiatry is particularly dependent on a wealth of theoretical assumptions. This may (and will) not be apparent at first glance, but it must be taken into account in order to enable sound psychiatric practice in clinics, research and teaching.

References

1. Engel GL. The need for a new medical model: a challenge for biomedicine. Science. 1977;196(4286):129–36.
2. Ghaemi SN. The rise and fall of the biopsychosocial model. Br J Psychiatry. 2009;195(1):3–4.
3. Greenham D. Close reading: the basics. London/New York: Routledge; 2019. (The basics).
4. Hoff P, Hippius H. Wilhelm Griesinger (1817–1868)–sein Psychiatrieverständnis aus historischer und aktueller Perspektive. Nervenarzt. 2001;72(11):885–92.
5. Kraepelin E. Psychiatrie. Ein kurzes Lehrbuch für Studirende und Aerzte. 2., gänzlich umgearbeitete Auflage. Leipzig: Abel; 1887.
6. Birnbaum K. Die Strukturanalyse als klinisches Forschungsprinzip. Zeitschrift für die gesamte Neurologie und Psychiatrie. 1920;53(1):121–9.
7. Kraepelin E. Psychiatrie. 9., vollständig umgearbeitete Auflage. Leipzig: Barth; 1927.
8. Kraepelin E. Die Erscheinungsformen des Irreseins. Zeitschrift für die gesamte Neurologie und Psychiatrie. 1920;62(1):1–29.
9. Kraepelin E. Patterns of mental disorder (1920). In: Hirsch SR, Shepherd M, editors. Themes and variations in European psychiatry: an anthology. Charlottesville: University Press of Virginia; 1974. p. 7–30.

10. Hoff P. Nosologische Grundpostulate bei Kraepelin-Versuch einer kritischen Würdigung des Kraepelinschen Spätwerkes. Z Klin Psychol Psychopathol Psychother. 1988;36:328–36. Available from: https://cir.nii.ac.jp/crid/1572261550069679488.
11. Campbell JK, O'Rourke M, Slater MH. Carving nature at its joints: natural kinds in metaphysics and science (Topics in contemporary philosophy). Cambridge, MA: MIT Press; 2011. Available from: https://academic.oup.com/mit-press-scholarship-online/book/14515.
12. Fuchs T. Der Begriff der Person in der Psychiatrie. Nervenarzt. 2002;73(3):239–46.
13. Abou Shoak M. Jaspers' Krankheit und die Arzt-Patienten-Beziehung. Basel: Schwabe Verlag; 2022.
14. Hoff P. What kind of «thing» is mental illness? Listening to Kraepelin, Jaspers and Kronfeld. Int Rev Psychiatry. 2024;36(6):557–67.
15. Jaspers K. Allgemeine Psychopathologie. 4. Auflage. Berlin: Springer; 1946.
16. Bormuth M. Karl Jaspers: Leben als Grenzsituation: Eine Biographie in Briefen. Göttingen: Wallstein Verlag; 2019. Available from: http://www.informationsmittel-fuer-bibliotheken.de/showfile.php?id=9944.
17. Hoff P. Arthur Kronfeld und die Identität der Psychiatrie: Denkwege vom 18. bis zum 21. Jahrhundert. 1st ed. Stuttgart: Kohlhammer; 2023.
18. Kronfeld A. Das Wesen der psychiatrischen Erkenntnis: Beiträge zur allgemeinen Psychiatrie, 1. Berlin: Springer; 1920.
19. Kronfeld A. Über die psychologischen Theorien Freuds und verwandte Anschauungen. Systematik und kritische Erörterung. Leipzig: Engelmann; 1912.
20. Fusar-Poli P, Solmi M, Brondino N, Davies C, Chae C, Politi P, et al. Transdiagnostic psychiatry: a systematic review. World Psychiatry. 2019;18(2):192–207.
21. Hoff P. On reification of mental illness: historical and conceptual issues from Emil Kraepelin and Eugen Bleuler to DSM-5. In: Kendler KS, Parnas J, editors. Philosophical issues in psychiatry IV: classification of psychiatric illness. Oxford: Oxford University Press; 2017. p. 107–20.
22. Heinz A. A new understanding of mental disorders: computational models for dimensional psychiatry. Cambridge: MIT Press; 2017. Available from: https://livivo.idm.oclc.org/login?url=https://ebookcentral.proquest.com/lib/zbmed-ebooks/detail.action?docID=5109052.
23. Reckwitz A. Die Gesellschaft der Singularitäten: Zum Strukturwandel der Moderne. Berlin: Suhrkamp; 2017.
24. Stanghellini G, Broome MR. Psychopathology as the basic science of psychiatry. Br J Psychiatry. 2014;205(3):169–70.

Open Access This chapter is licensed under the terms of the Creative Commons Attribution 4.0 International License (http://creativecommons.org/licenses/by/4.0/), which permits use, sharing, adaptation, distribution and reproduction in any medium or format, as long as you give appropriate credit to the original author(s) and the source, provide a link to the Creative Commons license and indicate if changes were made.

The images or other third party material in this chapter are included in the chapter's Creative Commons license, unless indicated otherwise in a credit line to the material. If material is not included in the chapter's Creative Commons license and your intended use is not permitted by statutory regulation or exceeds the permitted use, you will need to obtain permission directly from the copyright holder.

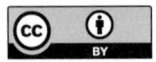

Part II

After Darwin: Biology in the Evolution of Psychiatry

This part examines complex key issues relating to Darwin's legacy in psychiatry, some of them mediated by Kraepelin initially, yet others beyond him. This is not simply about biology but about biology, psychiatry and society more broadly.

Chapter 4 reports how Kraepelin's thinking and practice embraced enthusiastically then widely prevalent but both seriously misguided and socially disastrous theories of degeneration and promoted eugenic ideologies and racial hygiene. Chapter 5 examines Kraepelin's misunderstanding of Darwin's theory of evolution and summarises developments in evolutionary biology since his time and their importance for the current understanding of psychology, medicine and psychiatry. Chapter 6 summarises current evidence emerging from psychiatric genetics. It vindicates Kraepelin's late doubts about his assumption that mental disorders are discrete psychiatric entities and advocates dimensional approaches in psychiatry instead. Chapter 7 offers a comprehensive survey of findings in brain imaging studies of schizophrenia and confirms that they support dimensional and neurodevelopmental rather than categorical models of psychosis.

Degeneration and Eugenics

4

Marius Turda

4.1 Introduction: Eugenics and Racial Hygiene

The social purity and abstinence movements were popular in Europe, Britain and North America from the late 1860s into the 1910s, exerting an important influence on the emergence of eugenics. Eugenicists followed social purists and abstinence campaigners by also advertising themselves as guardians of society's moral behaviour, promoting sexual control, cleanliness, temperance and the ideal of married life, while, at the same time, offering a biological critique of what they perceived to be the degenerative impact of modernity.

When the English scientist Francis Galton coined the term eugenics in 1883, drawing on the Greek expression 'well-born', [1] degeneration was already in use. Its popularisation increased with the publication by the French psychiatrist Bénédict A. Morel of his *Treatise on Degeneration* in 1857 [2], reaching new hights of intensity at the end of the nineteenth century. Cesare Lombroso, Richard von Krafft-Ebing, Max Nordau, August Forel and Edwin R. Lankester are some of the well-known figures associated with the *fin-de-siècle* obsession with degeneration [3, 4]. These authors appealed to different professional and popular audiences, but their writings shared one underlying conviction: that degeneration directly threatened the survival of the race and nation. Therefore, they argued, there was no greater public responsibility than to try to prevent its spread. In search for solutions, many of them turned to eugenics for inspiration and guidance [5].

After 1900, eugenics emerged as a unifying term within debates about the degeneration and regeneration of the race. The institutionalisation which followed certainly helped the spread of eugenic ideas in scientific literature and popular culture. By the time of Galton's death in 1911, eugenic societies had been established in

M. Turda (✉)
Centre for Medical Humanities, School of Education, Humanities and Languages, Oxford Brookes University, Oxford, UK
e-mail: mturda@brookes.ac.uk

© The Author(s) 2026
G. Ikkos, T. Becker (eds.), *Psychiatry after Kraepelin*,
https://doi.org/10.1007/978-3-032-09475-9_4

Germany, Britain, Sweden and the United States. In these and other countries, eugenics found a hospitable environment; it was received, welcomed and embraced by many professions, particularly by physicians, anthropologists, biologists and social educators. During the first decade of the twentieth century, eugenics drew sustenance from many local trations and scientific disciplines. These included not only animal breeding but also modern approaches to medicine, social hygiene and public health. Anthropology and statistics was invoked alongside political efforts to restrict immigration and to prevent racial mixing. And, of course, there was the newly rediscovered Mendelian experiments on plant hybridisation and inheritance [6].

Spurred by important works on Darwinism, evolution and heredity by Ernst Haeckel and August Weismann, eugenic ideas of race improvement travelled fast and wide across Germany during the last decade of the nineteenth century. Wilhelm Schallmayer was among the first German physicians to formulate a theory of race improvement based on the idea of 'Vererbungshygiene' ('hereditary hygiene'). Another complementary concept, 'Rassenhygiene' ('racial hygiene'), was formulated by physician Alfred Ploetz. In his widely acclaimed *Grundlinien einer Rassen-Hygiene* (The Foundations of Racial Hygiene), published in 1895, Ploetz placed the focus of eugenics on the protection of the inherited qualities not just of the individual but, more importantly, of the race. In 1904, together with sociologist Anastasius Nordenholz and zoologist Ludwig Plate, Alfred Ploetz launched the world's first journal devoted solely to the popularisation of racial hygiene, *Archiv für Rassen- und Gesellschafts-Biologie*. A year later, he founded the world's first eugenics society in Berlin [7, 8].

By 1910s, the racial hygiene movement in Germany was already one of the world's most thriving. And psychiatrists contributed significantly to the movement's success, adding medical credibility to the, by then, popular view that society needed to be protected from the growing numbers of those labelled 'unfit', 'feebleminded', 'mentally defective', 'dysgenic' and 'sub-normal' due to their physical and mental disabilities. Many such observations were based on clinical examinations of individuals whose lives the psychiatrists controlled and supervised in asylums, hospitals and private clinics. The implications in the context of a generalised concern with the future of the race were particularly serious, as contemporary observers alarmingly pointed out.

4.2   The Spectre of Alcoholism

Alcoholism is a recurrent theme in both psychiatric and eugenic literature. Racial hygienists considered alcoholism as one of the major factors contributing to individual and collective degeneration [9]. At the IXth International Congress against Alcoholism held in Bremen in 1903, Ploetz and psychiatrist Ernst Rüdin painted alcoholism in dark eugenic terms. Alcoholic intoxication depleted the individual of physical vitality and, in the long term, weakened the race. While prudence, foresight and self-restraint were required from each individual, Ploetz and Rüdin believed that racial hygiene could provide the long-term antidote to degeneration. Among the many features that distinguishes this eugenically infused abstinence narrative from other condemnations of alcoholism was the intensity of its anxiety about the degeneration of the race and the decline of European civilisation [10, 11].

Ploetz reproduced some of these ideas in a pamphlet entitled The Influence of Alcohol upon the Race, published in English in 1907. Alfred Ploetz declared alcohol 'a poison to the race', suggesting that 'from the point of view of racial hygiene' what was needed was 'an absolute cessation of the drinking of alcohol'. Aware that this suggestion to completely eliminate alcohol consumption might be unrealistic, Ploetz recommended other methods for the 'elimination of the unfit', which 'would act more quickly and more thoroughly'. Preventing them from reproduction and denying them marriage might work in practice, he pointed out. The overall responsibility for the prevention of the alcohol-induced degeneration of the race rested on both the expert and the state. It was 'the duty not only of the physician and hygienist, but also of the modern statesman, to keep a sharp lookout for all possible sources of degeneracy and, therefore, for the injuries from alcohol' [12].

Ploetz believed that excessive drinking was a cause for racial degeneration. This view was widely shared by psychiatrists such as Auguste Forel [13], Rudolf Wlassak [14] and Emil Kraepelin. In 1902, Kraepelin's study of the drinking habits of the German students was published in English [15]. It was one of his many public interventions on behalf of the fight against alcoholism [16]. Next to syphilis, he considered 'the abuse of alcohol' as the main contributing factor to the increasing number of 'the insane' admitted to mental institutions. 'The growing degeneration of our race in the future', he noted, was still 'an open question, but certainly it might be very greatly promoted by both these causes' [17]. After the First World War, in a darker mood, Kraepelin would widen the explanation for Germany's ruinous present to include the negative impact of homosexuality on the reproductive capacity of the nation [18] as well as the 'the preponderant influence of the Jewish spirit on German science' [19].

While Kraepelin took up the topic of degeneration caused by alcoholism in his acclaimed lectures on clinical psychiatry and in various editions of his classical textbook, it is the article with the eponym title ('Zur Entartungsfrage'), published in 1908, that is mentioned most frequently in the scholarship [20–22]. But before discussing this article, however, it is worth taking a detour to one of the corners of the Dutch colonial empires.

4.3   A Trip to Java

In 1903, shortly after taking up the chair in psychiatry in Munich, together with his brother, Kraepelin embarks on a trip to western Java, in the Dutch West Indies (Indonesia). During a 3 month-spell in a mental hospital in Buitenzorg (Bogor), he observes and examines 100 European and 100 native Javanese, as well as 25 Chinese patients, hoping to understand whether 'dementia praecox' (schizophrenia)—the psychiatric diagnosis whose understanding and nosology he is most notably associated with—was a 'symptom of civilisation' and of 'race'. What he hoped to demonstrate was, as he recalled in his Memoirs, whether 'the character of a certain race could be demonstrated by the frequency and the individual forms of insanity'. In other words, were the European, the Javanese and the Chinese patients affected by the same mental diseases and in the same way? And if they were not, was that difference due to their race? As he further notes, 'I was able to make a number of observations on the special symptoms of well-known European diseases in the Javanese patients and this seemed to be very important for an understanding of the connection between the type of race and the mental disorder' [23]. The juxtaposition of race and brain diseases reflects his understanding of the dynamics of degeneration.

His objective was not unusual. Many scientists at the time claimed that human mental faculties varied from race to race. On one hand, Kraepelin perpetuates a generally accepted view of racial difference, typical of European colonialism at the time [24]; on the other, as noted already, he shares with the eugenicists the view that modernity has drained the natural abilities of the Europeans and that the increase in 'defective' heredity was a threat to the future of the race.

Upon his return, Kraepelin publishes a short summary of his clinical observations in Centralblatt für Nervenheilkunde und Psychiatrie (*Central Journal for Nervous Diseases and Psychiatry*). The findings were sombre. Severe cases of paralysis and neurosyphilis were found only among the Europeans. While syphilis did exist amongst the indigenous population, it was 'about five times less common'. Furthermore, Kraepelin did not find any cases of alcoholism 'amongst the natives either, whilst among the 50 European men, two, both Germans, were suffering from severe alcoholism.' These clinical observations seem to paint a clear picture. The 'mental morbidity' ('psychische Morbidität') of the Europeans, Kraepelin concludes, was caused by alcohol and syphilis, two hallmarks of the modern, Western civilisation.

Kraepelin is using the prevalence of these two conditions to highlight the contrast 'in character' between indigenous and European patients but also to explain the difference between various stages of civilisation. He clearly recognises that some indigenous people display degenerative proclivities similar but the crucial term here is 'degeneration' ('Entartung'). This was an explicitly European condition, caused by particular historical conditions. Accordingly, the possible solution to this problem needed to be one borne out of modern scientific rationality and the belief that 'unwanted' hereditarian traits could be passed on from one generation to another, progressively weakening the race, until its complete demise. Racial hygiene (eugenics) served this purpose. A 'reasonable racial hygiene' ('verständige Rassenhygiene') was needed, Kraepelin believes, to 'combat degeneration' [25].

4.4   On Degeneration

In 1908, Kraepelin published 'On the Question of Degeneration' ('Zur Entartungsfrage') [26]. From the outset his message is clear: 'One of the most disturbing phenomenon of our cultural life is the rapid and continuous rise of mentally ill people who need institutional care' [27]. This was a phenomenon which characterised countries such as Germany, Holland and Britain and the white European race, more generally. His research trip to Java, as noted, has fortified this conviction.

The focus is 'paralytics, alcoholics, epileptics and alcoholic psychopaths'; as for the causes contributing to this phenomenon, Kraepelin mentions alcohol and syphilis, the two 'epidemic toxins' ('Volksgifte') which, especially in the large urban centres, have contributed significantly to asylum expansion and to a surge in psychiatric institutionalisation. 'Volksgifte', the term used here, suggests that Kraepelin's concern is not solely with the health of the individual but equally with the health of the community. Using a term popularised by the German biologist August Weismann, ('germ-plasm'), but in a nod to Lamarckism, Kraepelin describes an environmentally induced degeneration which could be passed on generationally. Thus, 'The damage to the germ [plasm] ('Keimschädigung')' caused by alcohol and syphilis, 'which in turn can result in the degeneration of entire lineages', was what worried him even more. The prospects for race regeneration were not encouraging, he claims.

'Degenerative psychosis' ('Entartungsirresein'), Kraepelin insists, was widespread amongst the educated urban elites. Rural communities as well as non-European indigenous population were less prone to 'anxieties and phobias' as well as 'obsessive doubt and brooding', features which Kraepelin (and many others at the time) attributed to the decadent urbanites, whose brain had already been softened ('Gehirnerweichung') and whose body was weakened by 'the one-sided cultivation of intellectual faculties'. Not surprisingly, he laments, 'the risk of effeminacy ('Verweichlichung') looms large' [26, 27]. This was at the time a widely shared view. For instance, psychiatrist Richard von Krafft-Ebing had noted in his classic Psychopathia Sexualis, published in 1886, that 'Periods of moral decadence in life of a people are always contemporaneous with times of effeminacy, sensuality, and luxury' [28].

According to Kraepelin, the ruinous impact of modern, Western civilisation was an accomplished fact. As he explains: modern culture led to 'domestication', that is the inability to benefit from the 'natural conditions of life'. Domestication stealthily 'saps our tenacity and our powers of resistance against debilitating influences and reduces our fertility'. It also leads to 'proletarisation', a process defined by urban poverty, malnutrition and dreadful living conditions for the poor working class. Large modern cities, Kraepelin remarks, abound not in physical strength but in 'atrophy and weakened vitality'. These were all threatening signs, for not just the health of the individual was under threat from these degenerative factors, but that of 'our entire race as well'.

What, then, was to be done in order to prevent 'the progressive deterioration of the race in certain directions'? Kraepelin's answer, and indeed his eugenic programme, is to involve the state to apply a nation-wide management of degeneration. With the support of the state, he argued, 'extensive, careful, decades-long studies' of large cities and rural areas can be accomplished. And the scientific guidance for such grand project should come from professionals such as himself, the expert who wished to shape the biological *Weltanschauung* of the race. In short: 'These studies must be undertaken by specially trained commissions comprised of doctors and statisticians whose attention is devoted solely to the task of degeneration. Beyond the number and fertility of marriages, the rates of illness and mortality, the life-expectancy and military fitness, consideration would also need to be given to rates of crime, prostitution, drunkenness, epilepsy, as well as to occurrences of mental illness, idiocy, psychopathy, epilepsy and the transmission of these disorders to progeny'. In other words, all aspects of national life should fall under the purview of racial hygienists working with the state. This was an important assertion of the social role of medicine, in general, and of psychiatry, in particular.

Ultimately, Kraepelin assumes that by reducing the number of 'feeble-minded' people, social problems such as poverty, crime and illegitimacy would be brought under control. But what his psychiatric treatment of degeneration targeted was the 'unfit' and eugenically 'unworthy' individuals seen to be impeding the betterment of the race. And similar to Ploetz, Kraepelin concludes by invoking the duty expected from psychiatrists. 'It is our responsibility to inform the people and the governments, and simultaneously to show them the paths that need to be taken toward the recovery of our race' ('Gesundung unserer Rasse') [26, 27].

Kraepelin's article was well received. In 1909 Ernst Rüdin, at the time Kraepelin's collaborator at the University of Munich, wrote an enthusiastic article for *Archiv für Rassen- und Gesellschafts-Biologie*. The issue of mental degeneration was central to racial hygiene, Rüdin remarked, and to have someone of Kraepelin's academic and international reputation engage with this question sent a very positive message to other psychiatrists willing to become more involved with the movement. Kraepelin is described as the advocate of much-needed eugenic work while at the same time demonstrating a tenaciousness that Rüdin was hoping to be able to emulate [29]. Indeed, in 1917, he became the director of the Department of Genealogy and Demography at the German Institute for Psychiatric Research (Deutsche Forschungsanstalt für Psychiatrie) in Munich, which in 1926 became the Kaiser Wilhelm Institute for Psychiatry. An avid promoter of compulsory sterilisation, Rüdin helped draft the 1933 'Nazi Law for the Prevention of Hereditarily Diseased Offspring'. It seemed that, as Kraepelin had hoped, the German state had finally embraced the regeneration of the race as one of its major goals. The aim was to create a 'new German' purged of degenerative characteristics and decadent tendencies.

4.5   Conclusion

After 1933, the racial hygiene movement in Germany became the world's most infamous. It mixed with racism and anti-Semitism, leading to the murder of thousands of children and adults with disabilities through the 'T4' euthanasia programme, and then to the extermination of millions of people in the Holocaust.

But Kraepelin died in 1926. He might have disliked the racial fanaticism of other eugenically-motivated German psychiatrists, but he shared with them the hope for a racial future, one in which a scientistic model of biological and national engineering was introduced under the guidance of medical and population experts. German historian of medicine Volker Roelke has suggested that Kraepelin was not 'a practitioner of racialist hygiene', [30] an opinion not shared by psychiatrist Sami Timimi. Kraepelin, Timimi notes in *Searching for Normal*, 'was a keen eugenicist and racist' [31]. That Kraepelin's eugenic views continue to receive attention from psychiatrists is important [32]. His exposure to the racial hygiene movement needs to be properly understood. As noted by Eric J. Engstrom: 'There is little doubt that eugenics and racial hygiene inflected especially powerfully in the third stage of Kraepelin's research work' [33]. But we cannot separate his views on degeneration from the historical context in which they were developed. To historicise his contribution to eugenic debates on degeneration requires not only that we enclose it in its specific temporality, but also that we attempt to grasp the meaning of its lingering impact in the writing of other scientists both during and after the demise of Nazism.

Key Points
- It bears repetition: eugenics was constantly sustained by expert knowledge and bolstered by scientific research that poured out of institutes, universities, private and state organisations, and various government agencies. Even a cursory look at any modern state in the twentieth century reveals how popular eugenics was with every ideology and every form of government. Its polymorphous character is truly striking.
- Regrettably, eugenics continues to shape our lives, whether it is forced sterilisation based on ethnicity, gender or criminal record, immigration restrictions and various methods for pursuing prenatal genetic testing for disabilities. It is, therefore, imperative to understand the implications of eugenic thinking and practice for the world today.
- There have been numerous recent and necessary calls for anti-racism by psychiatrists, as well as the wider scientific and medical communities. But while an obsession with degeneration was one of the key drivers of historical eugenics at the beginning of the twentieth century, present-day eugenics functions much more broadly as a set of ideas and practices which continue to stigmatise individuals with developmental and cognitive disabilities.
- Therefore, to combat the legacies of eugenics and scientific racism in psychiatry there must be an even broader, bolder large-scale effort to follow a strict line of respect of the humanity of individuals in psychiatric treatment and care.
- Psychiatrists must put an end to practices that may reflect a de-humanisation of people with developmental and cognitive disabilities by unlearning the eugenic rationalisation of their profession formulated by the 'founding figures' of the discipline at the end of the nineteenth century.

References

1. Turda M. Modernism and Eugenics. Basingstoke: Palgrave; 2010.
2. Morel BA. Traité des dégénérescences physiques, intellectuelles et morales de l'espèce humaine et des causes qui produisent ces variétés maladives. Paris: J. B. Baillière; 1857.
3. Pick D. Faces of degeneration. A European disorder, c. 1848-c.1918. Cambridge: Cambridge University Press; 1989.
4. Chamberlin JE, Gilman SL. Degeneration: the dark side of progress. New York: Columbia University Press; 1985.
5. Turda M. Biology and eugenics. In: Saler M, editor. The fin-de-siècle world. Abingdon: Routledge; 2015. p. 456–70.
6. Bashford A, Levine P. The Oxford handbook of the history of eugenics. New York: Oxford University Press; 2010.
7. Weiss, S. F. Race hygiene and national efficiency: the Eugenics of Wilhelm Schallmayer, University of California Press: Berkeley, 1987.
8. Weindling PJ. Health, race and German politics between National Unification and Nazism, 1870–1945. Cambridge: Cambridge University Press; 1989.
9. Brötz J. Alcohol, abstinence and rationalisation in Germany, c. 1870s–1910s. In: Ernst W, Müller T, editors. Alcohol, psychiatry and society. Comparative and transnational perspectives, ca. 1700–1990s. Manchester: Manchester University Press; 2022. p. 185–219.
10. Ploetz A, Rüdin E. Der Alkohol im Lebensprozeß der Rasse. In: Bericht über den IX. Internationalen Kongress gegen den Alkoholismus, Bremen 14–19. IV. 1903. Jena: Verlag von Gustav Fischer; 1904. p. 70–107.
11. Gruber, M. Die Alkoholfrage in ihrer Bedeutung für Deutschlands Gegenwart und Zukunft, Mässigkeits-Verlag: Berlin, 1909.
12. Ploetz A. The influence of alcohol upon the race. Westerville: American Issue Publishing Company; 1907. p. 20–1.
13. Kuechenhoff B. The psychiatrist Auguste Forel and his attitude to eugenics. Hist Psychiatry. 2008;19:215–23.
14. Wlassak R. The influence of alcohol upon the functions of the brain. Westerville: American Issue Publishing Company; 1907.
15. Kraepelin E. The university man and the alcohol question. Westerville: American Issue Publishing Company; 1902.
16. Kraepelin E. Alkohol und Jugend. Basel: Schriftstelle des Alkoholgegnerbundes; 1910.
17. Kraepelin E. Lecture on clinical psychiatry. In: Johnstone T, editor. , vol. 2. 2nd. Eng. ed. Revised ed. London: Baillière, Tindall and Cox; 1906.
18. Kraepelin E. Geschlechtliche Verwirrungen und Volksvermehrung. Münch Med Woch. 1918;65:117–20.
19. Kraepelin E. Psychiatric observations on contemporary issues. Hist Psychiatry. 1992;3:253–6. [original German 1919].
20. Hoff P. Kraepelin and degeneration theory. Eur Arch Psychiatry Clin Neurosci. 2008;258(Suppl. 2):12–7.
21. Roelke V. Electrified nerves, degenerated bodies: medical discourse on neurasthenia in Germany, circa 1880–1914. In: Gijswijt-Hofstra M, Porter R, editors. Cultures of neurasthenia from beard to the first world war. Amsterdam: Rodopi; 2001. p. 177–97.
22. Engstrom, E. J. Clinical psychiatry in Imperial Germany. A history of psychiatric practice. Ithaca/London. Cornell University Press, 2003.
23. Kraepelin E. Memoirs. Translated by Cheryl Wooding-Deane, Springer Verlag, Berlin, Germany, 1987, 108 and 115.
24. Pols H. The development of psychiatry in Indonesia: from colonial to modern times. Int Rev Psychiatry. 2006;18:363–70.
25. Kraepelin E. Psychiatrisches aus Java. Centralblatt Nerv Psychiatry. 1904;27:468–9.
26. Kraepelin E. Zur Entartungsfrage. Centralblatt Nerv Psychiatry. 1908;31:745–51.

27. Kraepelin E. On the question of degeneration. Hist Psychiatry. 2007;18:399–404.
28. Krafft-Ebing R. Psychopathia Sexualis, authorised trans. of the 7th enlarged and revised German edition by C. G. Chaddock, vol. 6. London: F. J. Rebman; 1894.
29. Rüdin E. [Review of], Kräpelin. Zur Entanrtungsfrage. Archiv Rassen Gesell-Biologie. 1909;6:254–7.
30. Roelke V. Biologizing social facts: an early 20th century debate on Kraepelin's concepts of culture, neurasthenia, and degeneration. Cult Med Psychiatry. 1997;21:383–403. Quote at at p. 399.
31. Timimi, S. Searching for normal. A new approach to understanding mental health, distress and neurodiversity, Fern Press: London, 2025. Quote at p. 53.
32. Yamamura K, Toshiya M. Revisiting Emil Kraepelin's eugenic arguments. Hist Psychiatry. 2024;35:206–14.
33. Engstrom EJ. On the Question of Degeneration' by Emil Kraepelin (1908). Hist Psychiatry. 2007;18:389–98, here at p. 396.

Open Access This chapter is licensed under the terms of the Creative Commons Attribution 4.0 International License (http://creativecommons.org/licenses/by/4.0/), which permits use, sharing, adaptation, distribution and reproduction in any medium or format, as long as you give appropriate credit to the original author(s) and the source, provide a link to the Creative Commons license and indicate if changes were made.

The images or other third party material in this chapter are included in the chapter's Creative Commons license, unless indicated otherwise in a credit line to the material. If material is not included in the chapter's Creative Commons license and your intended use is not permitted by statutory regulation or exceeds the permitted use, you will need to obtain permission directly from the copyright holder.

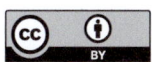

Evolutionary Psychiatry Before, During and After Kraepelin and His Times

5

Paul St John-Smith, Martin Brüne, and Riadh Abed

5.1 Darwin and the History of Evolution with Psychiatry

5.1.1 Introduction

'In the distant future I see open fields for far more important researches. Psychology will be based on a new foundation, that of the necessary acquirement of each mental power and capacity by gradation. Light will be thrown on the origin of man and his history' So ends Darwin's masterpiece 'On The Origin of Species' [1] the first book in his great trilogy. Charles Darwin's landmark book was first published on 24 November 1859. Darwin may have been born 47 years before Kraepelin, but the former's ideas on biology and human behaviour have had a huge impact on biological perspectives and theories right up to and including the present day. Darwin's theories, therefore, indirectly must have had some impact on biological theories such as Kraepelin's, albeit perhaps not explicitly. Be that as it may, the birth of Darwinian psychiatry (also known as evolutionary psychiatry) only really came about in the 1990s with the publication of such books as Randolph Nesse and George Williams book 'Why we get sick' [2] There are accordingly three sections

P. S. John-Smith (✉)
Independent Scholar, Newsletter Editor of the evolutionary group (EPSIG),
The Royal College of Psychiatrists, London, UK

M. Brüne
Department of Psychiatry, Psychotherapy and Preventive Medicine, Division of Social Neuropsychiatry and Evolutionary Medicine, Ruhr University Bochum, Bochum, Germany
e-mail: martin.bruene@ruhr-uni-bochum.de

R. Abed
FRCPsych, Medical Member of the Mental Health Tribunals in England, Ministry of Justice, London, UK

© The Author(s) 2026
G. Ikkos, T. Becker (eds.), *Psychiatry after Kraepelin*,
https://doi.org/10.1007/978-3-032-09475-9_5

in this chapter: first, a brief general chronology of the interaction of psychiatry with evolutionary thinking, secondly the interaction of Kraepelin with evolutionary thinking and thirdly an overview of contemporary (post-Kraepelinian) evolutionary psychiatry.

5.2 Part 1

5.2.1 Chronology

To put both figures in historical context, Charles Darwin was born on 12 February 1809, in Shrewsbury, Shropshire, England and died on 19 April 1882, at the age of 73. Emil Kraepelin was born on 15 February 1856, in Neustrelitz, in the Grand Duchy of Mecklenburg-Strelitz (now part of Germany) and died on 7 October 1926, at the age of 70.

Darwin began formulating the ideas that led to 'On the Origin of Species' [1] in the late 1830s, after his voyage on the HMS Beagle (1831–1836). The main concept was first seen in published form in the joint paper with Wallace in 1858. From his research Darwin formulated the revolutionary idea that there was a demonstrable materialist process (as distinct from supernatural creation myths) by which species and their characteristics evolved. He was not the first to describe Evolution, but along with Alfred Russel Wallace (1823–1913) was the first to publish systematic evidence for evolution and identify a plausible mechanism for it, natural selection. Evolution by natural selection stands as the principal scientific theory that explains how existing species (and their inherited characteristics) came into existence through selective changes over time and how particular adaptations were shaped (because of their survival and reproductive value) due to exposure to certain specific environments (an ongoing process that continues to this day). It is based on the observations that the diversity of life arises through the gradual process driven by variation, inheritance, competition/cooperation resulting in differential reproductive success.

Darwin's theory was first fully spelled out in 1859. It was later refined with the advent of modern genetics, becoming the foundation of modern evolutionary biology or what is now called the Modern Synthesis which transformed evolutionary theory by making genetics central to understanding evolution. It solidified the view that evolution is a change in the genetic composition (frequency) of populations over time, with natural selection acting on any genetic variation within those populations. The theory of evolution by natural selection is currently the cornerstone of all life sciences and this fact has profound implications for psychiatry (and the rest of medicine) regarding any conditions with a heritable component, and we maintain it should be an integral part of psychiatric knowledge and education.

Perhaps of more direct relevance to psychiatry was Darwin's 'Expression of the Emotions in Man and Animals', first published on 26 November 1872. [3]. This work explored the continuity of the biological basis of emotional expressions and their evolutionary significance. It built on the ideas he developed in his earlier works, particularly focusing on the universality of emotions across human cultures and their continuity with expressions observed in animals. This, the third book in the trilogy, has been considered Charles Darwin's forgotten masterpiece and is his only book on psychology. It is also the first ever systematic application of Darwinian theory to the expression of emotions and is considered by some to be the foundational text of evolutionary psychology. Darwin's main objectives were to show how human facial expressions constitute a shared heritage of our species, have parallels with the expressions of other animals and hence provide a behavioural argument for evolutionary continuity. The book was about the expression of emotions and not about the nature or adaptive value of emotions. Darwin's approach in this work is primarily a phylogenetic one, which is to establish the continuity of emotional expression between humans and animals as well as its universality across human populations.

While Darwin had no specific interest or approach to psychiatry, he had significant connections with several prominent figures in the fields of psychiatry and psychology, including James Crichton-Browne, Henry Maudsley and Guillaume Duchenne with whom he engaged in extensive correspondence. These were some of the most important figures in the development of mental health sciences, and their interactions with Darwin helped shape the emerging understanding of human behaviour and emotion. Emil Kraepelin may thus have been influenced by Charles Darwin, particularly by Darwin's ideas about evolution and the biological basis of behaviour.

Kraepelin, a pioneer in psychiatry, also approached mental illness from a biological perspective, possibly reflecting a Darwinian understanding of humans as biological organisms shaped by evolution. By framing mental illness as a biological phenomenon, Kraepelin laid the groundwork for contemporary psychiatric thinking rooted in neuroscience and genetics. This will be discussed further in part 2.

Freud and Jung were also influenced by Darwinian thinking or at least the kudos surrounding the theory. However, they appear to only use selective aspects of evolution as a justification for their own models of mental functioning and therefore have had only a tangential influence on modern post-Kraepelinian evolutionary psychiatry.

John Bowlby is widely considered to be the first clearly systematic evolutionary thinker in clinical psychiatry. He considered the nature of the environment(s) that humans evolved within after separation from the last common ancestor with the other great apes. He named this 'The Environment of Evolutionary Adaptedness' (EEA) a concept fully demarcated by Tooby and Cosmides in the 1980s and which has become a cornerstone of evolutionary thinking in both psychology and psychiatry [4].

Bowlby [5] formulated this idea along with his attachment theory and the result is considered to be the first definitively evolutionary conceptualisation within the field of mental health [5]. Evolutionists emphasise that the EEA does not refer to a single specific time or place but that it is a statistical composite of a range of past human environments in which ancestral humans lived and to which they adapted over time. We may also view each adaptation as having its own unique EEA. For general purposes in humans, the EEA is often thought to be the environment in which our early ancestors (Homo sapiens and earlier hominins) lived during the Pleistocene era, roughly 2.5 million to 12,000 years ago. The EEA is important because, according to evolutionary psychology, the human brain and behaviour evolved to solve the problems faced by our ancestors in that environment. The challenges and conditions of the EEA, such as finding food, avoiding predators, forming social bonds and reproducing, shaped the mental and behavioural traits that we observe in humans today.

Bowlby's attachment theory was deeply influenced by Darwinian evolutionary theory. He believed that attachment behaviours, such as seeking proximity to caregivers, were biologically programmed and evolved because they played a crucial role in survival. Bowlby integrated Darwin's ideas about the adaptive nature of behaviours into his understanding of human development, suggesting that attachment served the evolutionary purpose of ensuring safety and promoting the child's exploration and learning. His work in attachment theory emphasised the innate, evolutionary and adaptive nature of human attachment, borrowing concepts from ethology, comparative psychology and evolutionary biology. Ultimately, Bowlby's ideas helped reshape the understanding of child development and mental health, viewing attachment as a fundamental and evolutionarily derived system critical for human survival.

Other early evolutionary ideas in psychiatry occurred in the twentieth century, including Huxley and Mayr's Schizophrenia paradox [6]. Applying evolutionary thinking they raised the question: 'Why, if it is heritable, does schizophrenia persist and why has it not been eliminated by Natural selection'? The paradox is evident from the observation that schizophrenia, a disorder with severely detrimental effects on reproductive success, persists at quite a high rate around 1% in the overall human population. They suggested that this puzzle might be explained by the genetic trade-offs associated with the disorder, whereby the same genes that predispose to schizophrenia may also confer adaptive advantages in important domains, such as creativity or problem-solving abilities (e.g. in unaffected close relatives). Such hypothetical advantages may be considered as trade-offs and explain why the genes for the disorder persist, despite their negative impact on individuals. This evolutionary question remains valid to this day.

Tim Crow further explored this paradox in the 1980s [7]. Crow's theory also suggested that schizophrenia is a by-product of the evolutionary process that led to the development of the advanced cognitive abilities that characterise humans, especially language and complex thought processes. Schizophrenia might therefore be the result of the selection of genetic changes that although they led to improved human cognitive functions, also increased the risk of mental disorders as a side effect. Thus, the concept of evolutionary trade-offs posits that the same genetic adaptations that enabled humans to develop advanced intelligence and language may have also made the brain more vulnerable to dysfunctions like schizophrenia. Ultimately, Crow's theory emphasises the idea that schizophrenia, rather than being purely maladaptive, might be the price paid by the few for the enormous evolutionary benefits (e.g. language) enjoyed by the vast majority of *Homo sapiens*.

Other notable contributions have been made by Brant Wenegrat in the 1980s regarding sociobiology and mental disorder [8, 9]. Special mention also needs to be made for the pioneering evolutionary work of John Price on depression, dominance hierarchies and the evolution of mental illness [10]. More contemporaneously and spanning the modern era important contributions came from Price's book 'Evolutionary psychiatry: a new beginning' [11]. Further landmark books on the subject include McGuire and Troisi 'Darwinian Psychiatry' in 1998 [12] and Martin Brune's 'Textbook of Evolutionary Psychiatry' 2008 [13]

5.2.2   The Modern Era (Post-2000)

Despite the insights of Darwin and early evolutionists there was no overarching or general evolutionary theory applied to psychiatry until the early 1990s through the introduction of the idea of Darwinian Medicine by Nesse and Williams [2] who laid the foundation for evolutionary psychiatry, emphasising that mental disorders should be studied through an evolutionary lens (see part 3). Their work has had a lasting impact on the way mental disorders are understood, moving away from purely proximate mechanistic models and encouraging a broader, evolutionary (ultimate) perspective on the origins for human vulnerability to mental health conditions. The foundational idea, proposed by pioneering evolutionary psychologists, which now pervades the whole of evolutionary psychology and psychiatry is that natural selection shaped not only our physical bodies but also our psychological systems. Mental health, therefore, must be partly understood as the result of evolutionary pressures. However, because of the limitations of Natural Selection (compared to a designed body/mind) some mental disorders arise as unwanted by-products of the process. This results in various vulnerabilities which are discussed in part 3. Nesse's contributions have helped shape the understanding of mental health in a way that emphasises the interplay between evolutionary pressures, environmental changes and modern psychological well-being.

Ultimately psychiatry is that branch of medicine that deals with mental disorders that manifest themselves through disturbances in cognition, emotions and behaviour. Psychiatrists therefore should have some understanding of the origins of these processes.

Nesse argues that significant benefits of utilising evolutionary thinking include: (1) asking new questions about why evolution has left us all vulnerable to mental disorders, (2) providing a way to think clearly about development and the ways that early experiences influence later characteristics, (3) providing a foundation for understanding emotions and their regulation and (4) providing a foundation for a scientific diagnostic system.

We argue that evolutionary psychology and evolutionary biology can serve as a vital basic science for psychiatry, and we propose in a post-Kraepelinian age that evolution is uniquely well placed to guide psychiatrists in determining what the phenotypic end-products of neurobiological systems are. Importantly, the evolutionary emphasis on function can provide the scientific basis for expanding the concept of the biological to encompass the psychological, social and the cultural domains. Hence, in contrast with mainstream biological psychiatry's rather narrow and 'decontextualized' view of mental disorder as brain disorder (or brain circuit disorder), evolutionists consider the environmental context to be vital in determining the existence of mental disorder.

5.3 Part 2

5.3.1 Emil Kraepelin and Evolutionary Theory

To understand Emil Kraepelin's scientific position and explanatory models of psychiatric illnesses, it is imperative to first consider the socioeconomic environment into which he was born. The middle and late nineteenth century, as well as the early twentieth century, were characterised by tremendous changes, politically, economically and socially. Socially, the industrial revolution brought about a collapse of the system of estates, replaced by a new system of social classes. This was accompanied, on one hand, by politicising the social classes, but also by pauperism of the growing working class. Around the same time, new scientific ideas were published, among which Charles Darwin's theory of evolution by natural selection played a significant role in the social and natural sciences, including medicine. In fact, even though Darwin himself opposed drawing conclusions from his theory regarding societal issues, many, including Darwin's champion, Herbert Spencer, readily mixed biological theory with social developments such as impoverishment and poor physical and mental health among the socially disadvantaged part of society.

Faced with increasing numbers of people with mental illnesses admitted to asylums and psychiatric hospitals, it was quite straightforward for Kraepelin to adopt, like many of his fellow psychiatrists, a Social Darwinist stance. That said, we can conclude from his publications that Kraepelin was aware of Darwin's work. But Kraepelin never seemed to arrive at a full understanding of Darwin's theory, and what the theory could mean for the understanding of mental illnesses. Instead, while readily and uncritically endorsing Spencer's expression of 'survival of the fittest' in its derived and misleading form 'survival of the strongest', Kraepelin's views were also heavily influenced by contemporary views on the impact of modern civilisation on the 'human race', which included the theory of degeneration, and connected to the degeneration paradigm, speculations about human self-domestication. In addition, Kraepelin also held the erroneous view that, as a consequence of degeneration, 'blastophthoria' (i.e. 'germ lesion'; a term coined by Auguste Forel, a Swiss psychiatrist and eugenicist and predecessor of Eugen Bleuler at the famous Burghölzli Hospital) was passed down the generations, an idea resembling Lamarckian inheritance.

Indeed, ideas about human degeneration were already around before the publication of Darwin's work. For example, Jean-Jacques Rousseau [14] argued that civilisation had a negative impact on human nature. A century later, Benedicte Morel [15] proposed that under modern living conditions humankind would suffer 'moral' and physical decline due to progressive deterioration of the 'germ material' (note that the work of Gregor Mendel was lost for several decades, and only re-discovered by Tschermak, Correns and de Vries at the beginning of the twentieth century). Morel introduced the idea that subtle physical abnormalities (asymmetry of facial features, etc.) could serve as biological markers for the alleged deterioration and also provide a biological explanation of delinquent behaviour.

Kraepelin was convinced that degeneration was also responsible for the rapid and steady increase in numbers of the mentally ill [16], whereby he entirely ignored social factors that were clearly causally involved in the rise of mental illnesses. Related to this, Kraepelin adopted the hypothesis of human self-domestication, which he thought would induce 'effeminacy' (German: *Verweichlichung*) and weakening of natural drives in civilised populations, accompanied by a deterioration of physical strength and willpower.

To get an impression of Kraepelin's stance, the following paragraphs illustrate the wording that he used in his publications (translated by MB). These examples also show that Kraepelin's clinical perspectives had shifted from individual well-being of patients to the mental health of the *Volkskörper*.

Kraepelin was concerned, for example, that '*The mass of idiots, epileptics, psycho-paths, criminals, prostitutes, and tramps who descend from alcoholic and syphilitic parents, and who transfer their inferiority to their offspring, is incalculable. Of course, the damage will be balanced in part by their lower viability; however, our highly developed social welfare has the sad side-effect that it operates against the natural self-cleansing of our people. We may barely hope that the degeneration-potential will be strong enough in the long term to eliminate the overflowing sources of germ lesion. … Nevertheless, the well-known example of the Jews, with their strong disposi-tion towards nervous and mental disorders, teaches us that their extraordinarily advanced domestication may eventually imprint clear marks on the race*' (note that Kraepelin's ideas on domestication were included in the 8th edition of his 'Textbook of Psychiatry', published in 1909). [17] (Kraepelin 1908; MB's translation).

Kraepelin held similar views on alcoholism, which he fought vigorously, possi-bly based on his own biography, while again disregarding social factors in the aeti-ology of alcoholism. He tried to buttress his stance by empirical numbers showing that 'the number of acute admissions to the psychiatric hospital in Munich of patients with alcohol-related disorders was thirty-two in 1904, compared with 284 in 1905' [18]. Moreover, nearly 30% of men's acute admissions happened due to alcohol-related disorders compared to only about 6% in women [19].

Kraepelin also believed that he found evidence for degeneration, as 17% of the alcohol-dependent patients had a family history of alcoholism. Moreover, in a study of 29 families of alcoholics there were 33 abortions, and among the surviving 183 infants, 32.7% died within the first year and another 10.9% during early childhood. Among the remaining living children, 35.7% were 'nervous or psychopathic', 8.1% were possibly or probably 'epileptic', 12.2% were mentally retarded (*imbezill*) and 3% were 'idiotic'. In sum, 59% of the children of alcohol-dependent parents were regarded as mentally ill. Of the remaining 40 children, six were diagnosed as 'weak' or otherwise developmentally retarded, seven as 'rickety', three as 'scrofulous' and one child as 'tuberculous'. Only 23 were thought to be free of physical or mental diseases.

Furthermore, Kraepelin, following Morel, described physical signs supposed to indicate degeneration (e.g. anomalies of the skull, ears, teeth, and palate) in 31 of the mentally ill children, in four children who were physically disabled, and in 12 cases among the physically and mentally healthy children [18].

The following passages quoted from Kraepelin's papers on *Der Alkoholismus in München* (Alcoholism in Munich), [19] published in 1906, and *Zur Entartungsfrage* (On the question of degeneration, [16] (1908) illustrate Kraepelin's attitude towards alcoholism and the strong tie to the degeneration paradigm and eventually to Social Darwinism:

'Among all psychiatric questions not a single one is by far as important as the influence of alcohol consumption on the mental health of the people (Volk). ... It seems therefore to be of particular significance, in order to meet an enemy such as alcoholism, which is widely underestimated, to get a reliable impression from the calamity induced by it, in order to take the most suitable action to combat it' (MB's translation). For Kraepelin, it was clear that *'inferior personalities'* such as day labourers (*Tagelöhner*), servants (*Hausknechte*), idlers (*Nichtstuer*), beggars (*Bettler*), tramps (*Landstreicher*), swindlers (*Schwindler*) and annuitant receivers (*Rentenempfänger*) were most likely to become alcohol dependent. Moreover, he readily concluded that *'in at least two thirds of the cases alcohol was the most important reason for "economic sterility"*. Furthermore, he referred to the forensic relevance of the behavioural disturbances associated with alcoholism.

These examples clearly show that Kraepelin utilised a hodgepodge of pseudo-scientific ideas of his time to push forward his biologistic agenda concerning mental illness, which were, at best, loosely connected to Darwin's work. His interest in cross-cultural aspects of psychiatry was no exception to this. In fact, Kraepelin's travel to Indonesia served no other purpose but to seek evidence supporting the degeneration paradigm. His idea was to examine the mental state of individuals belonging to 'primitive' races. To this end, he visited the psychiatric hospital 'Buitenzorg' in Java in 1904 and recognised that the 'paralysis of the insane' and alcoholism were rare despite a high prevalence of syphilitic infections among the Java people. This, he reasoned, would indicate a greater resistance against diseases in these peoples compared to inheritable germ lesions acquired by the forces of civilisation, which ultimately would lead to an increase of degeneration insanity (*'Entartungsirresein'*) [16].

In summary, Kraepelin's thinking and clinical perspective were somehow influenced by Darwin's work, but more indirectly. It is more plausible to conclude that Kraepelin adopted several crude, and even for his time, scientifically poorly supported explanatory models of mental illness, foremost the degeneration paradigm and the idea of human domestication, as well as Lamarckian inheritance as causal factors involved in mental illness. In addition, there is absolutely no doubt that Kraepelin utilised a Social Darwinist perspective to justify eugenic measures, rather than advocating an improvement in social support and healthcare. Kraepelin's pupil and successor as head of the Kaiser Wilhelm Institute for Psychiatric Research in Munich, Ernst Rüdin, who later was involved in the introduction of the 'law of prevention of hereditary-diseased offspring' ('Gesetz zur Verhinderung erbkranken Nachwuchses') in Nazi Germany greatly acknowledged Kraepelin's attitude. In a paper published in 1910 in the *Archiv für Rassen- und Gesellschaftsbiologie* (Archives of Racial and Societal Biology), which back then was one of the leading journals in the field of genetics and eugenics, and of which Rüdin was co-editor-in-chief, he reasoned that 'the medical care for the insane was a distortion of the natural laws of the survival of the fittest and that medicine would be obliged to clean the genetic pool of the *Volk* in order to prevent ongoing degeneration' [20].

Thus, in light of their outstanding position and international recognition it can be argued that the impact of Kraepelin's and Rüdin's views concerning causal mechanisms of mental illness can hardly be overestimated. Rüdin was highly praised as an internationally leading authority in psychiatric genetics and was invited to attend the International Genetic Congress even in summer 1939 (at the brink of WW II). Notably, Rüdin's work on psychiatric genetics was still cited in a textbook of medical genetics in the early 1970 (quoted from Roehlke 2002) [21].

Fortunately for his reputation, one might cynically conclude, Kraepelin died quite conveniently in 1926, at the age of 70. Thus, escaping a potentially harsher historical appraisal on his contributions to psychiatric nosology, treatment, let alone his political aspirations and views [22].

In one thing, he was entirely correct, however, envisioning what we today emphasise as mandatory to improve our understanding of mental disorder:

> The development of human personality has been perfected only after a process characterised by infinitely small, barely perceptible forward steps; retrograde steps have also occurred. Detours have been followed and then left behind. The end result of this unpredictable progress naturally retains traces and vestiges of the various stages of development, even if the vast majority of once-formed then superseded mechanisms have been completely lost. If we therefore try today to fit the expressions of insanity to the individual stages of personality development, then we find the necessary evidence conspicuous only by its absence. Should such attempts ever be successful, it will be necessary to trace back manifestations of our psychological life to their roots in the psyche of the child, of primitive man and of animals. In this way we can discover to what extent certain illnesses reflect a recrudescence of emotions hitherto concealed in our individual or phylogenetic developmental history. Prospects for this seem to me encouraging, despite the poverty of our current knowledge. From this endeavour we may receive help toward our foremost and hardest task: the clinical understanding of disease forms [23].

We will now explore and summarise some of these insights in part 3.

5.4 Part 3

5.4.1 An Outline of Modern Evolutionary Psychiatry

Unlike mainstream psychiatry that focuses on proximate causation, primarily mechanistic explanations of disease and disorder, evolutionary psychiatry extends its scope to include ultimate or evolutionary causation [24]. Evolutionary psychiatry

(EP) has been concisely defined as the subfield of evolutionary medicine that uses the basic science of evolutionary biology to better understand and treat mental disorder [25]. However, this is not to deny the vital contribution to EP of a range of other disciplines including evolutionary anthropology, evolutionary psychology and evolutionary genetics as well as many others. Hence, EP is fundamentally a cross-disciplinary field, drawing on insights from a wide range of seemingly disparate sciences and domains of knowledge.

The evolutionary perspective helps clarify thinking about mental health and mental disorder in a number of unique ways. Three areas stand out as illustrative of the effectiveness of evolutionary theory as a powerful epistemic tool in psychiatry. The first is in helping to clarify the concept of mental disorder. Thus, while the question of what a mental disorder is remains an intractably unresolved issue, utilising the evolutionary concepts of function, dysfunction, adaptation and fitness has led to the formulation of concepts such as Wakefield's 'Harmful Dysfunction' that represent important and promising theoretical advances [26].

The other two unique contributions of evolutionary theory to psychiatry (and medicine generally) include a deeper understanding of biological causation relevant to health and disease and the causal pathways for the human vulnerability to disease and disorder (see below).

5.4.2   Evolution and Causation, Tinbergen's Four Questions

Nikolaas Tinbergen [27], Nobel laureate and co-founder of the science of ethology, building on Ernest Mayr's Proximate-Ultimate causal split [28], proposed that a complete and proper understanding of any biological trait or system should involve understanding its mechanism, developmental history (referred to as proximate causes), phylogenetic history and function (referred to as ultimate or evolutionary causes) (see Table 5.1).

These four causal domains are collectively referred to as Tinbergen's four questions. It should be noted that all four causes apply simultaneously for the proper understanding of any biological phenomenon as they refer to distinct domains.

Table 5.1 Tinbergen's four causal domains'

		Two objects of explanation	
		Sequence (Diachronic)	*Single form* (Synchronic)
Tinbergen's four questions			
Two kinds of explanation	*Proximate* Mechanisms and their ontogeny	*Ontogeny* *How* does the trait develop in individuals?	*Mechanism* What is the trait's structure? *How* does it work?
	Evolutionary Functions and phylogeny	*Phylogeny* What is the evolutionary history of the trait? (*WHY* does the trait exist in this way?)	*Adaptive Significance* How have variations in the trait influenced fitness? (*WHY* does the trait exist?)

Thus, no amount of exploration of brain events, neurobiology or neurochemistry of patients with anxiety or low mood can answer the question as to why the capacity for anxiety and low mood are universal in humans. Such 'why' questions are unique to the evolutionary perspective and are essential if we are to make progress in differentiating distressing normative states from states that are truly dysfunctional.

It is acknowledged that unlike proximate causation which can directly lead to therapeutic interventions, understanding ultimate causation is somewhat removed from direct clinical applications but is no less important. For example, neglecting the question of function (ultimate causation) runs the risk of inadvertently altering psychological functioning through interventions to relieve distressing but adaptive states, leading to potentially negative consequences for some patients. It can also lead us to construct defective models of how and why psychopathology arises.

Focusing exclusively on the proximate is akin to a technician's view of a machine, whereas considering ultimate causation as well is more like an engineer's view [29]. Hence, it may be adequate for a busy clinician to simply recognise the existence of depression or anxiety in a given patient and to dispense standard advice and treatment. However, a clinician who also understands why we have such emotions in the first place and how emotional systems interact with people's current lives is likely to have a deeper understanding of the patient's emotional problems and be able to take greater account of the patient's circumstances that may be contributing to their current state. Ultimate causation also has the potential for influencing the research agenda through testing hypotheses regarding what the normative function is of the system that is giving rise to psychopathology; a question that is seldom asked by mainstream psychiatry [30].

5.4.3 Causal Pathways for the Persistence of Disease and Disorder

It should be noted that selection shapes vulnerability to disease and disorder and not disorders themselves [29]. This applies throughout medicine, including psychiatry, and stems primarily from the fact that bodies and brains are a bundle of traits, systems, organs and adaptations shaped by selection over thousands of generations to increase reproductive success and not necessarily good health, happiness, or longevity.

Evolution helps us recognise that selection (on average) shapes functional systems and not dysfunctional ones. But it is worth remembering that all functional systems, whether biologically evolved or man-made, can malfunction under certain conditions. Also, it should be noted that biological systems frequently have multiple, overlapping functions and this applies particularly to neurobiological systems where the function of many systems remains poorly understood.

The answer to the pivotal conundrum as to why evolution has left humans so vulnerable to disease and disorder has itself been evolving ever since it was first posed by the founders of modern evolutionary medicine [2]. Accordingly, pathways by which evolutionary processes can lead to the existence and persistence of disease or disorder have been proposed (Box 5.1).

Box 5.1: Pathways for the Persistence of Disease and Disorder (Adapted from Abed and St John-Smith [24])
1. Mismatch
2. Life history factors
3. Overactive defence mechanisms
4. Co-evolutionary considerations: consequences of the arms race against pathogens
5. Constraints imposed by evolutionary history
6. Trade-offs
7. Sexual selection and its consequences
8. Balancing selection: maintaining an allele that raises disease risk
9. Mutation load and mutation-selection balance
10. Demographic history and its consequences (path dependency)
11. Selection favours reproductive success at the expense of health
12. Extremes of adaptations

These causal pathways for the persistence of disease and disorder apply to all species including humans and are not mutually exclusive. Several pathways may be implicated concurrently or sequentially in the causation of a given mental disorder. They represent a list of ultimate causes of vulnerability to disease, disorder or dysfunction.

These evolutionary explanations for vulnerability to disorder are based on the recognition that selection is unable to eliminate all harmful mutations and can be too slow to respond to rapidly changing environments, creating states of evolutionary mismatch [31]. The concept of 'mismatch' is arguably one of the most important insights in evolutionary medicine and is crucial for understanding and explaining the existence of 'Diseases of Civilisation' such as obesity, metabolic syndrome, type 2 diabetes, eating disorders (anorexia and bulimia nervosa) and many others. Evolutionary mismatch occurs when the environment changes too rapidly for selection to be able to track it, resulting in residual traits that are no longer suited to the new environmental conditions. Developmental mismatch arises when circumstances alter radically during an individual's lifetime. For example, moving from a state of impoverishment during early development to a state of affluence in adult life can increase the risk of cardiovascular disease, type 2 diabetes and metabolic syndrome [32]. Furthermore, the extreme ends of functional adaptations can become maladaptive, for example, when adaptive personality traits are magnified and intensified [33]. Additionally, over-activation of useful emotional defences (mood states and anxiety) can result in harmful outcomes, leading to what has been termed, defence activation disorders, for example, anxiety and depressive disorders [31].

It is important to recognise that selection inevitably involves trade-offs. Thus, increasing the potency of one trait is often at the expense of worsening performance of another. For example, increasing resistance to infections may increase the risk of autoimmune diseases and improving nutritional conservation can increase the risk of obesity. Also, reducing the threshold for environmental risk avoidance can result in a greater risk of anxiety disorders. Trade-offs are also involved in life history strategies. Life history theory (LHT) deals with species typical solutions for problems associated with survival and reproduction that change over an individual's lifespan [30]. Hence, the choices individuals make as to whether they invest in somatic growth, mating or parental effort entail trade-offs and involve both fitness pay-offs and risks and costs. The trade-offs are the present versus the future, mating versus parenting and quality versus quantity of offspring. This produces a spectrum of LH strategy ranging from the fast (producing a large number of offspring with low levels of parental investment in each) or a slow LH strategy (few offspring with a large investment in each). Thus, LHT provides a framework for understanding how organisms allocate time and energy in achieving core biosocial goals across the lifespan. Differences in life history strategies are partly under genetic control, but it appears that the nature and quality of the individual's early environment may also be important.

5.4.4   The Evobiopsychosocial Model

As noted above, all four of Tinbergen's questions (or causal domains) can simultaneously be asked of all biological systems—including dysfunctional systems. Therefore, applying the same principle to the 3 levels of Engel's biopsychosocial model (BPSM) [32] (Engel, 1980) was a logical next step [34, 35] as the addition of the evolutionary perspective can provide a critical dimension of insights for expanding the medical model beyond Engel's original BPSM. This resulted in the formulation of the evobiopsychosocial model (EBPSM) (Table 5.2).

Hence, the three levels of analysis proposed by Engel's BPSM can each be more deeply and properly understood with Tinbergen's four questions. Combining these parallel frameworks results in a three by four table with 12 cells (Table 5.2).

It should be noted that standard biomedical approaches exclusively ask questions of biological (or 'somatic') mechanism and ontogeny (represented in questions 1 and 2 of Table 5.2). George Engel, being dissatisfied with biomedicine, expanded analysis with the addition of psychological and social dimensions, but did not place them within a comprehensive framework. Hence, the EBPSM firstly clarifies how the BPSM levels relate to each other: despite nominal separation, all three of Engel's levels have a significant biological component—clearly the mechanisms mediating effects at the 'psycho' and 'social' levels are functional biological systems that have been shaped by selection, and psychosocial interventions are effective precisely because of their downstream effects on neurobiological and other somatic systems. Also, the evolutionary perspective draws attention to the fact that biological adaptations can evolve at multiple levels, beyond the strictly somatic. Therefore, the evolutionary questions add critical context elucidating the fact that the biological, psychological and social factors had functions over our deep evolutionary history, which explains their present form. However, we acknowledge that the boundaries

Table 5.2 12 EBPS questions

Engel's 3 BPS levels	Tinbergen's 4 questions			
	Proximate		Evolutionary/Ultimate	
	Mechanism	Ontogeny	Phylogeny	Function
Biological (Somatic)	1. What are the proximate somatic mechanisms?	2. What are the developmental processes that shaped the mechanisms?	3. What are the phylogenetic roots of the mechanism?	4. What function did the somatic mechanism serve in the ancestral environment?
Psychological	5. What are the psychological mechanisms involved?	6. What is the developmental history of the said psychological mechanisms?	7. What are the phylogenetic roots of the psychological mechanism?	8. What function did the psychological mechanism serve in the ancestral environment?
Social	9. What are the immediate social circumstances of importance to the condition?	10. How do the social circumstances affect development over an individual's life-course?	11. What is the phylogenetic history of social arrangements and structures?	12. What functions did such social structures serve in the ancestral environment (if any)?

Adapted from Hunt et al. [36, 41]

between the 12 questions of Table 5.2 can be fuzzy and overlapping. For example, should dysfunctions in pair-bonding (the predominant human mating system) be placed in the psychological or social domains? Clearly, this involves a subjective (psychological) state (romantic love, commitment) as well as an interpersonal (social) state (the formation of a bond between 2 people). Nevertheless, such ambiguities and complexities are ubiquitous in the life and human sciences.

5.4.5   Benefits of EBPSM Over Engel's Original Model

Providing a more coherent, scientifically complete and philosophically sound model of medicine, the EBPSM has specific practical benefits for understanding and improving medical research and practice.

One major insight arising from the evolutionary perspective relates to the propriety of using specific animal models in psychiatry. Current non-evolutionary approaches pay scant attention to the importance of phylogenetics and function. Animal models are often selected based on surface similarities between certain animal behaviours and features of mental disorders in human. For example, animal models of obsessive-compulsive disorder (OCD) focus on features of compulsive behaviour, stereotypy and perseveration in mice and rats, but whether this reflects the same dysfunction involved in OCD in humans is questionable. An evolutionary perspective endorses the utility of animal models to the extent that the system in question is phylogenetically conserved, serves similar functions and is shared between species. For fundamental emotional responses such as fear or anxiety, this suggests laboratory rodents may be useful animal models. For more complex emotional and cognitive states related to recent evolutionary pressures (e.g. related to pair bonds, complex social structures or language), rodent models would be much less useful, and more closely related species such as primates may be more appropriate. The evolutionary perspective distinguishes two different states when making cross-species comparisons regarding phenotypic traits. Traits can be the result of common descent (homologous) or independent/parallel evolutionary processes (convergent traits). Such vital, fine distinctions are entirely invisible to non-evolutionists.

Also, phylogenetic distance between the specific system under investigation is another key factor, almost entirely missing from modern medical research.

A further critical benefit of adopting evolutionary approaches to psychiatric problems is in expanding upon the benefits of holistic perspectives which George Engel endorsed. For example, depression is often clearly biopsychosocial—somatic differences in brain function, debilitating psychological processes and social factors are simultaneously relevant. However, the additional evolutionary perspective asks important questions about those biopsychosocial factors. What is the functional mood system which may be dysregulated? Are there unusual modern environmental factors (e.g. social isolation)—so called 'evolutionary mismatches' which may be causing the dysregulation of that system? This offers novel directions for identifying harmful social environments by contextualising the depressed mood as a psychological state arising within a very different environment to that in which it originally evolved. Unlike Engel's BPSM, the evolutionary approach fully contextualises human psychological functioning within the environment it was designed to function within. Hence, the EBPSM encourages practical holism with crucial additional scientific information relating to human evolutionary history. We suggest this automatically makes clinicians less reductionistic in dealing with patients and can help foster improved clinician–patient empathy and understanding of the problems being faced. Indeed, recent evidence has shown that evolutionary explanations of depression help in reducing self-stigmatisation in patients [37] (Box 5.2).

Box 5.2: Advantages of the Evobiopsychosocial Model
- Embeds the BPS firmly within the Life Sciences, providing a solid scientific grounding
- Combining Tinbergen's 4 causal domains with the BPS's 3 levels provides the opportunity to uncover processes and levels of interaction that otherwise remain hidden
- Has the potential for producing future, novel avenues for theorising, research and interventions on disease and disorder in diverse areas of medicine including mental health
- As is the case with all scientific constructs, the EBPSM is work in progress and it is at early stages of development but holds the promise of important future insights and practical applications

5.4.6   Genomics and Mental Disorder

Box 5.3: Why Do Apparently Harmful Genes Persist in the Gene Pool? (Adapted from Durisko et al. [37])
- De novo mutations
- Mutation-selection balance
- Positive selection in the ancestral environment but mismatched to current conditions
- Selective neutrality (ancestrally neutral)
- Balancing selection
  - Heterozygous advantage
  - Frequency-dependent selection
  - Pleiotropy

Taking an evolutionary perspective, one comes to recognise that viewing the human genome as a static 'blueprint' for the human phenotype is both erroneous and misleading. At the population level and over multiple generations, the frequency of genes is in a state of continuous change with some genes increasing in frequency while others decreasing or are eliminated completely as a result of positive and negative selection pressures (natural, sexual, social) as well as drift (random, chance events) [23, 24]. This raises the question as to why apparently harmful or disease-causing genes exist and persist in the human gene pool [37, 38] (see Box 5.3). We suggest that the question: 'why do disease-causing genes persist in the population?' can only be conceived by taking an evolutionary perspective. Non-evolutionary approaches simply note the existence of such genes and studies their composition and effects. Evolutionists recognise that the human genome is a historical record of past selection pressures. It also recognises that variation is the rule rather than the exception and most importantly, that there is no such thing as a single normative human genome.

With the exception of de novo harmful genes which arise from mutations in the parental germ-line (and not carried by the parent), all other disease-causing genes have been subject to selection pressures of some form. Some harmful genes that are compatible with survival and reproduction will be subject to purifying selection over many generations while others may be eliminated more quickly. However, those that persist within the population over numerous generations may be subject to a process known as balancing selection. Balancing selection takes place where there is a trade-off between the positive and the negative effects of a given genetic variant thus maintaining that variant at a more or less steady level in the population. Examples include where the gene is (1) advantageous in the heterozygous state but harmful in the homozygous state (e.g. sickle cell anaemia); (2) where the gene is subject to frequency dependent selection (potentially advantageous when low in frequency in the population but disadvantageous at higher frequencies, e.g. psychopathy) or; (3) or where the gene has pleiotropic effects (i.e. multiple effects, some advantageous others not at different life stages; e.g. aging).

Other causes for the persistence of harmful genes are ancestral neutrality or positive selection in ancestral times but being mismatched to the current human environment (see sections above).

It should be noted that since the advent of the 'Genomic Revolution' and the advances in the methodologies of the science of genetics, studies have demonstrated that, with very rare exceptions, mental disorders are both highly polygenic and heterogeneous. In other words, there are few, if any, simple Mendelian conditions among the common mental disorders. This finding raises fundamental questions regarding the evolutionary roots of common mental disorders and rules out simplistic one gene-one disorder models.

5.5 Conclusion: Looking Towards the Future

In this chapter, we have outlined some of the theoretical developments underlying evolutionary psychiatry that have been introduced since the time of Kraepelin. Despite Nesse's prescient suggestions of 1984 on Darwinian or Evolutionary psychiatry [39] which predate much evolutionary psychology and medicine, psychiatry has been slow to take up the mantle. However, it is proposed that evolutionary science provides a powerful epistemic tool that can help organise a wide range of facts about human biology and psychology into a coherent narrative that, in time, can lead to insights that give rise to novel models and subsequently, novel treatments and interventions for mental disorders. And given how little is currently known of the aetiology of mental disorder (see Foreword by Allen Frances, this volume) [40] it would be remiss of the psychiatric community to overlook the potential of evolutionary theory in advancing psychiatry especially that evolution forms the cornerstone of all modern life sciences.

On a final note, it is imperative to note that evolutionary psychiatry requires the highest modern ethical standards whereby psychiatrists should work for the benefit of individual patients and their welfare. Medicine, psychiatry, genetics and biomedical research in general should be there to provide treatment and care for individual patients as well as to promote well-being for communities, not to act as guardians of some idealised human genome or act to advance some social construction or opinion as to what humans should be. This lesson should be learned from Kraepelin's legacy.

Key Points
1. Darwin's ideas had some impact on psychiatry and psychology in the late nineteenth century and early twentieth century, although his ideas were often misunderstood and misused.
2. Kraepelin was among those who did not fully appreciate or accurately utilise Darwin's ideas.
3. Neo-Darwinian thinking after World War 2 inspired some important theorising in psychiatry, though no general theory or formal model of evolutionary medicine or psychiatry was envisioned until the 1990s.

4. Evolutionary psychiatry emerged as a framework for understanding mental health and mental disorder in the 1990s.
5. Although evolutionary psychiatry is slowly gaining acceptance among mental health professionals, it has not yet been fully integrated into mainstream medical and psychiatric education and training.

References

1. Darwin, C., 1859. On the origin of species by means of natural selection, or the preservation of favoured races in the struggle for life. Darwin, C., Volume 11 Gale and the British Library.
2. Nesse RM, Williams GC. Why we get sick: the new science of Darwinian medicine. Vintage; 1996.
3. Darwin C. The expression of the emotions in man and animals (1872). In: The portable Darwin; 1993. p. 364–93.
4. Cosmides, L. and Tooby, J., 1997. Evolutionary psychology: a primer (Vol. 13). Center for Evolutionary Psychology, Santa Barbara.
5. Bowlby J, Ainsworth M, Bretherton I. The origins of attachment theory. Dev Psychol. 1992;28(5):759–75.
6. Huxley J, Mayr E, Osmond H, Hoffer A. Schizophrenia as a genetic morphism. Nature. 1964;204(4955):220–1.
7. Crow TJ. Schizophrenia as the price that Homo sapiens pays for language: a resolution of the central paradox in the origin of the species. Brain Res Rev. 2000;31(2–3):118–29.
8. Wenegrat B. Sociobiology and mental disorder. Addison-Wesley; 1984.
9. Wenegrat B. Sociobiological psychiatry. Lexington Books; 1991.
10. Price J. Hypothesis: the dominance hierarchy and the evolution of mental illness. Lancet. 1967;2:243.
11. Stevens A, Price J. Evolutionary psychiatry: a new beginning. Routledge; 2015.
12. McGuire MT, Troisi A. Darwinian psychiatry. Oxford University Press; 1998.
13. Brüne M. Textbook of evolutionary psychiatry. The origins of psychopathology. Oxford University Press; 2008.
14. Rousseau JJ. Discours sur l'origine et les fondemons de l'egalité parmis les hommes. Amsterdam: Marc Michele Rey; 1755.
15. Morel BA. Traite des degenerescences physiques, intellectuelles et morales de l'espece humaine et des causes qui produisent ces varietes maladives par le Docteur BA Morel. chez J.-B. Bailliere. 1857.
16. Kraepelin E. Zur Entartungsfrage. Z Nervenheilk Psychiatr. 1908;31:745–51.
17. Kraepelin E. Psychiatrie. Ein Lehrbuch für Studierende und Ärzte. In: Allgemeine Psychiatrie, vol. I. 8th ed. Leipzig: Johann Ambrosius Barth; 1909.
18. Kraepelin E. Alkoholische Geistesstörungen. In: Jahrbücher der psychiatrischen Klinik München; 1907. p. 22–8.
19. Kraepelin E. Der Alkoholismus in München. Münchener Medizinische Wochenschrift. 1906;53:737–41.
20. Rüdin E. Über den Zusammenhang zwischen Geisteskrankheit und Kultur. Arch Rassen-Gesellschaftsbiologie. 1910;7:722–48.
21. Roehlke V. Zeitgeist und Erbgesundheitsgesetzgebung im Europa der 1930er Jahre. Nervenarzt. 2002;73:1019–30.
22. Engstrom EJ. Emil Kraepelin: psychiatry and public affairs in Wilhelmine Germany. Hist Psychiatry. 1991;2:111–32.
23. Kraepelin E. Die Erscheinungsform des Irreseins. Z Gesamte Neurol Psychiatr. 1920;62:1–29. (translated into English by Dominic Beer, publ. in History of Psychiatry 3 (1992) 509–529.

24. Abed R, St John-Smith P. Evolutionary psychiatry: current perspectives on evolution and mental health. Cambridge: CUP; 2022.
25. Nesse RM, Stein DJ. How evolutionary psychiatry can advance psychopharmacology. Dialogues Clin Neurosci. 2019;21(2):167–75. https://doi.org/10.31887/DCNS.2019.21.2/rnesse.
26. Wakefield JC. The concept of mental disorder: on the boundary between biological facts and social values. Am Psychol. 1992;47(3):373–88. https://doi.org/10.1037/0003-066X.47.3.373.
27. Tinbergen N. On aims and methods of ethology. Z Tierpsychol. 1963;20:410–33.
28. Mayr E. Cause and effect in biology. Science. 1961;134(3489):1501–6. https://doi.org/10.1126/science.134.3489.1501.
29. Nesse RM. Good reasons for bad feelings: insights from the frontier of evolutionary psychiatry. New York: Dutton; 2019.
30. Brüne M. Textbook of evolutionary psychiatry and psychosomatic medicine: the origins of psychopathology. 2nd ed. Oxford: Oxford University Press; 2016.
31. Del Giudice M. Evolutionary psychopathology: a unified approach. New York: Oxford University Press; 2018.
32. Gluckman P, Hanson M. Mismatch: why our world no longer fits our bodies. Oxford/New York: Oxford University Press; 2006.
33. Engel GL. The clinical application of the biopsychosocial model. Am J Psychiatry. 1980;137(5):535–44. https://doi.org/10.1176/ajp.137.5.535.
34. Trull TJ, Widiger TA. Dimensional models of personality: the five-factor model and the DSM-5. Dialogues Clin Neurosci. 2013;15(2):135–46.
35. Abed R, Hunt AS, John-Smith P. Evolutionary theory can advance and revitalise the biopsychosocial model. Br J Psychiatry. 2024;225(4):424–6.
36. Hunt AD, St-John Smith P, Abed R. Evobiopsychosocial medicine. Evol Med Public Health. 2022;11(1):67–77. https://doi.org/10.1093/emph/eoac041.
37. Durisko Z, Mulsant BH, McKenzie K, Andrews PW. Using evolutionary theory to guide mental health research. Can J Psychiatr. 2016;61(3):159–65.
38. Schroder HS, Devendorf A, Zikmund-Fisher BJ. Framing depression as a functional signal, not a disease: rationale and initial randomized controlled trial. Soc Sci Med. 2023;328:115995. https://doi.org/10.1016/j.socscimed.2023.115995.
39. Nesse RM. An evolutionary perspective on psychiatry. Compr Psychiatry. 1984;25(6):575–80.
40. Frances A. Emil Kraepelin and his legacy, foreword. In: Ikkos G, Becker T, editors. Psychiatry after Kraepelin: ambition images practices 1926–2026; 2026.
41. Hunt AD, St John-Smith P, Abed R. The biopsychosocial model advanced by evolutionary theory. In: Abed R, St John-Smith P, editors. Evolutionary psychiatry: current perspectives on evolution and mental health. Cambridge University Press; 2022. p. 19–34.

Open Access This chapter is licensed under the terms of the Creative Commons Attribution 4.0 International License (http://creativecommons.org/licenses/by/4.0/), which permits use, sharing, adaptation, distribution and reproduction in any medium or format, as long as you give appropriate credit to the original author(s) and the source, provide a link to the Creative Commons license and indicate if changes were made.

The images or other third party material in this chapter are included in the chapter's Creative Commons license, unless indicated otherwise in a credit line to the material. If material is not included in the chapter's Creative Commons license and your intended use is not permitted by statutory regulation or exceeds the permitted use, you will need to obtain permission directly from the copyright holder.

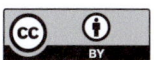

A Genetic Perspective on Kraepelin's Nosology

6

Michael J. Owen

6.1   Introduction

In 1899, Kraepelin divided the psychoses into two distinct diagnostic categories: dementia praecox and manic-depressive insanity [1]. In current practice, following the neo-Kraepelinian perspective adopted in Diagnostic and Statistical Manual of Mental Disorder, Third edition (DSM III), this approach has been retained with the older terms being replaced by schizophrenia (SZ) and bipolar disorder (BD). The so-called Kraepelinian dichotomy thus remains the cornerstone of the modern classification of psychotic disorders and is arguably Kraepelin's most enduring legacy. Kraepelin came to recognise the limitations of this simple categorical approach, and the architects of DSM III never intended their diagnostic system to identify valid disease categories given the lack of understanding of aetiology and pathogenesis [2]. Nevertheless, because of the convenience and reliability of the operationalised diagnostic systems instigated in DSM III and adopted in subsequent iterations of DSM and International Classification of Diseases (ICD), lack of validity was overlooked leading to a process of reification whereby researchers, practitioners and regulators have come to view psychiatric diagnoses as valid categories defining distinct natural disease entities each with their own underlying aetiology and pathogenesis [3, 4]. A glossary of the main terms is available at the end of the chapter. Terms to be found in the glossary are printed in italics when first encountered in the main text.

M. J. Owen (✉)
The Centre for Neuropsychiatric Genetics and Genomics, Division of Psychological Medicine and Clinical Neurosciences, and Neuroscience and Mental Health Innovation Institute, Cardiff University, Cardiff, UK
e-mail: owenmj@cardiff.ac.uk

© The Author(s) 2026
G. Ikkos, T. Becker (eds.), *Psychiatry after Kraepelin*,
https://doi.org/10.1007/978-3-032-09475-9_6

73

6.1.1   The Kraepelinian Dichotomy, A Tradition of Dissent

The limitations of a categorical and dichotomous approach to the classification of the psychoses have been apparent on clinical and epidemiological grounds for some time [5–10]. In brief, there is no symptomatic 'point of rarity' between the two diagnostic categories, which remain syndromic in nature and not distinguishable by diagnostic tests or biomarkers. Individuals with a diagnosis of SZ or BD share many clinical features including psychotic and affective symptoms over the course of their illness and it is not uncommon for patients to receive both diagnoses at different times. It is also not uncommon for clinicians to be unable to place a patient into one category or the other and to label the case as having schizoaffective disorder, an interform of the two prototypical psychoses.

6.2   Genetics and the Kraepelinian Dichotomy

Evidence from genetic epidemiology indicates that SZ and BD are both substantially heritable with *heritability* estimates from twin studies of 0.64–0.81 for SZ and 0.59–0.85 for BD [11]. Genetics has always played a key role in shaping and validating psychiatric nosology [12] and for many years the Kraepelinian dichotomy appeared to be supported by findings suggesting that the two prototypical psychoses appear to 'breed true' [5]. That is to say that the risk of SZ but not BD was increased in the relatives of those with SZ and vice versa in the relatives of bipolar probands. This notion was challenged by a few studies [13, 14], but the case was settled by a large family study of over two million nuclear families from the Swedish population and hospital-discharge registers [15]. The results were clearcut; first-degree relatives of probands with SZ or BD have an increased risk of both disorders. Moreover, evidence from half-siblings and adopted-away relatives indicated that this effect is mainly due to genetic factors. These findings indicate that SZ and BD partly share genetic risk factors and undermine the genetic validity of the Kraepelinian dichotomy. They are in line with a previous proposal that the studies suggesting the two conditions breed true were underpowered to detect shared genetic risk [14].

Since Lichtenstein et al.'s landmark study in 2009 [15], there have been many advances in the *genomics* of SZ and BD. These confirm that they substantially share genetic risk factors and are in line with a continuum of genetic risk. They also point to some distinguishing characteristics that inform our understanding of the nature of the psychosis continuum. Before addressing these, it is necessary to summarise recent advances in genomic studies of SZ and BD. Interested readers can find more detailed treatments elsewhere [11, 16].

6.3   Genomics of SZ and BD

6.3.1   Common Variants

Large collaborative genome-wide associations studies (GWAS) on many thousands of cases and controls have revealed that SZ and BD are among the most *polygenic* of all human disorders with around 10,000 or more common variants estimated to confer risk to each [11]. Moreover, many hundreds of individual common risk loci and genes have been identified at stringent genome-wide levels of significance [11]. Each common variant accounts for a very small amount of risk (odds ratios [ORs] < 1.23) but *en masse* common variants account for around a third of heritability estimates from twin studies and currently constitute the class of genetic variant explaining most of the heritability of SZ and BD.

6.3.2   Rare Variants

Both copy number variants (CNVs) and rare coding variants (RCVs) have been identified that confer risk to psychotic disorders though, as we shall see, this appears to be greater for SZ than BD. The rare risk variants implicated to date confer larger individual risks (ORs: 2–80) than common risk variants. Indeed, there is an approximate inverse relationship between effect size and *allele* frequency [11, 16]. This reflects the fact that SZ and to a lesser extent BD are associated with reduced fecundity [17]. Therefore, alleles that confer high risk will be subject to negative selection and removed from the population before they can increase in frequency, whereas common risk alleles must by evolutionary necessity confer low risk.

6.3.3   Common and Rare Variants Act Together

As discussed below, the *rare risk variants* (*CNVs* and *RCVs*) that confer risk to psychotic disorders are also associated with a variety of other neurodevelopmental disorders (NDDs). There is evidence from several sources [11] that the specific clinical outcomes in individuals who carry such a rare variant reflect the additional influence of common variants that are associated with those outcomes. In other words, the clinical outcomes in rare variant carriers reflect the combined effects of common and rare variants. For example, individuals with SZ who carry a risk CNV also have more common SZ risk alleles than carriers of CNVs who do not have SZ [18, 19]. Importantly, this means that rare and common variants confer risk together rather than there being distinct common and rare variant forms of psychotic disorders.

6.3.4 Evolutionary Considerations

SZ is highly heritable yet persists in the population despite markedly reduced fecundity. Recent genomic findings have helped to explain this 'evolutionary paradox' [16, 20]. Briefly, the population frequency of rare high *penetrance* alleles seems to be determined by the balance between negative selection and the occurrence of new mutations, so-called *mutation-selection balance*. For common risk alleles, the evidence suggests that negative selection predominates, but the effects are weak, allowing risk alleles to achieve high frequencies through genetic drift, so-called *mutation selection-drift*, with this process being facilitated at some loci by a reduction in haplotype diversity due to background selection [20, 21]. These findings do not, however, exclude a role for other mechanisms that might maintain some risk alleles in the population [20]. Whatever the explanation of the evolutionary paradox of SZ, the fact that the disorder persists in the face of markedly reduced fecundity points to the futility of attempts to eradicate it through eugenics and explains why the incidence of SZ was not reduced in subsequent generations following the Nazis' eugenics program [22, 23].

6.4 Implications of Genomic Findings for the Kraepelinian Dichotomy

6.4.1 The Relationship Between SZ and BD: Common Alleles

It is possible to estimate the genetic correlation (rg) between two traits, which is a measure of the average similarity in risk alleles between them. In other words, it is a measure of the genetic overlap between two conditions. The common variant genetic correlation between SZ and BD is 0.7, suggesting a 70% overlap in common risk alleles between them. These findings are unlikely to be accounted for by *assortative mating* or by reciprocal misdiagnosis of distinct categorical disorders [11]. Rather they point to extensive overlap of common risk variants between SZ and BD. This high degree of *pleiotropy* undermines the biological validity of the Kraepelinian dichotomy in line with the results of family studies, the extensive overlap in clinical features and the lack of diagnostic tests and biomarkers distinguishing between the two conditions.

Given that clinical features such as psychosis and affective symptoms are 'transdiagnostic' in that they are seen across the psychotic disorders, one plausible explanation for the extensive pleiotropy observed between SZ and BD is that genetic risk maps better onto transdiagnostic psychopathology rather than onto specific diagnosis. Support for this idea comes from several recent studies that have looked at the relationship between measures of specific genetic risk calculated from GWAS data and diagnostic outcomes or symptom dimensions. SZ common variant liability is highest in people with SZ followed by schizoaffective disorder–bipolar subtype, then BD1 (bipolar disorder type 1) followed by BD2 (bipolar disorder type 2), and then unaffected individuals [24–26]. One of these studies looked at a mixed-diagnosis psychotic disorders group and demonstrated that as SZ genetic risk increased there was a corresponding increase in the proportion of cases with a diagnosis of SZ with a corresponding decrease in the proportion with a diagnosis of BD [24]. Furthermore, in people with BD, SZ liability was highest in those with psychotic symptoms and higher still in those with mood-incongruent psychotic symptoms, the symptoms most akin to SZ [24, 25]. Conversely, in those with SZ, BD liability is associated with the level of manic symptoms [25] and MDD (major depressive disorder) liability is associated with depressive symptoms [27]. Finally, there is evidence that in people with BD, the SZ liability associations seen with mood-incongruent psychosis do not derive from shared SZ and BD alleles but from a component of liability that is relatively specific to SZ [28]. These findings suggest that, at least in part, rather than being genetically and pathogenically distinct disorders, the clinical picture expressed by someone with a psychotic disorder is the result of a confluence of partly orthogonal (non-overlapping) transdiagnostic symptom dimensions and their underlying genetic risk factors.

6.4.2   Rare Variants and the Relationship Between Psychotic Disorders and Childhood Neurodevelopmental Disorders

All the CNVs that confer risk to SZ also confer risk to childhood neurodevelopmental disorders (NDDs) such as intellectual disability (ID), autism and attention-deficit/hyperactivity disorder (ADHD) [16]. Rare coding variants also implicate shared genes and specific mutations between SZ and childhood NDDs [29]. This implies a degree of overlap in the primary molecular pathology and implicates neurodevelopmental process in SZ in line with much other evidence suggesting that SZ is, at least in part, a neurodevelopmental disorder [30]. The overall contribution of CNVs and RCVs to psychiatric and neurodevelopmental conditions is not uniform. Thus, CNVs and RCVs make the strongest contribution to ID, then autism and ADHD, then SZ, followed by BD [16]. Thus, the enrichments of rare mutations are greatest in disorders with the strongest neurodevelopmental contribution as inferred from earlier onset and greater cognitive impairment. Among cases of SZ, the burden of rare mutations is also not uniform being higher in those with more severe cognitive impairment, although it is still elevated in those without it [31].

Evidence that premorbid cognitive and psychomotor impairments are more prominent in SZ than BD suggests that neurodevelopmental insults may contribute to differences between the two conditions [32]. The evidence from rare variants summarised above allowed this conception to be extended to include the relationship between psychotic disorders and childhood NDDs. The neurodevelopmental continuum and gradient model [10, 33] proposes that childhood NDDs and psychotic disorders lie on a neurodevelopmental continuum, whereby there is a gradient of decreasing neurodevelopmental severity running from ID, through childhood NDDs, SZ, schizoaffective disorder and BD [11, 30]. Regarding the Kraepelinian dichotomy, this suggests that while the diagnoses of SZ and BD do not delineate distinct disorders, the two diagnoses differ quantitatively in the extent to which neurodevelopmental processes are involved and that there is a gradient of decreasing neurodevelopmental impairment within the psychotic disorders running from SZ, through schizoaffective disorder to BD.

As well as the accumulating evidence from genomics, the neurodevelopmental gradient model has been supported by several other recent lines of enquiry. First, there is compelling evidence that cognitive impairment in SZ is substantially present before onset and that this premorbid deficit is neurodevelopmental in origin [34]. When cognition is tested across the SZ:BD spectrum, the pattern of impairments seen is similar, but the degree of impairment is most severe in SZ, followed by schizoaffective disorder depressed subtype, followed by schizoaffective disorder bipolar subtype, with BD having the least severe impairments [35]. Second, while large-scale brain imaging studies have not identified circumscribed neuroanatomical differences that allow individuals with SZ and BD to be distinguished from each other or from controls, structural abnormalities have been found including widespread reductions in cortical surface area and thickness, and in the size of subcortical structures [36–39] [Eds: see Ch. 7]. Moreover, across disorders, the effect sizes for different measures are generally in the same direction but are greater in SZ than BD [40]. While some of the measures, particularly cortical thickness, appear to be influenced by environmental factors operating after illness onset including drug treatment, cortical surface area seems to be predominantly neurodevelopmental in origin [37]. Finally, evidence from large-scale epidemiological studies indicates that risk of SZ is better indexed by the extent to which cognitive ability falls short of that expected from familial potential than by cognitive ability per se [34, 41]. This also applies to other conditions and the magnitude of the effect in SZ is substantially higher than in BD but less than in autism [42]. As well as supporting the neurodevelopmental gradient model, these findings point to an important role for non-familial factors such as environmental factors and de novo variants impacting on neurodevelopmental processes.

6.5 The Kraepelinian Dichotomy in 2026

Where does this leave the dichotomous classification of the psychoses 100 years after Kraepelin's death? The evidence that I have reviewed, particularly from genetics and genomics, has built on older evidence from a variety of sources that the current diagnostic categories of SZ and BD do not define disorders that are distinct or homogeneous whether regarding psychopathology, aetiology or mechanisms. Rather, the evidence suggests that psychotic disorders are currently best conceived as lying on a continuum that contains several dimensions (Fig. 6.1).

The first important dimension along which psychotic disorders vary is neurodevelopmental with a gradient of decreasing neurodevelopmental impairment going from SZ, through schizoaffective disorder to BD. Here there are contributions from inherited genetic variants, both rare and common, but also evidence for a substantial involvement of non-*familial* factors such as rare de novo risk variants and environmental factors (Fig. 6.1). The latter are indexed by the degree of cognitive

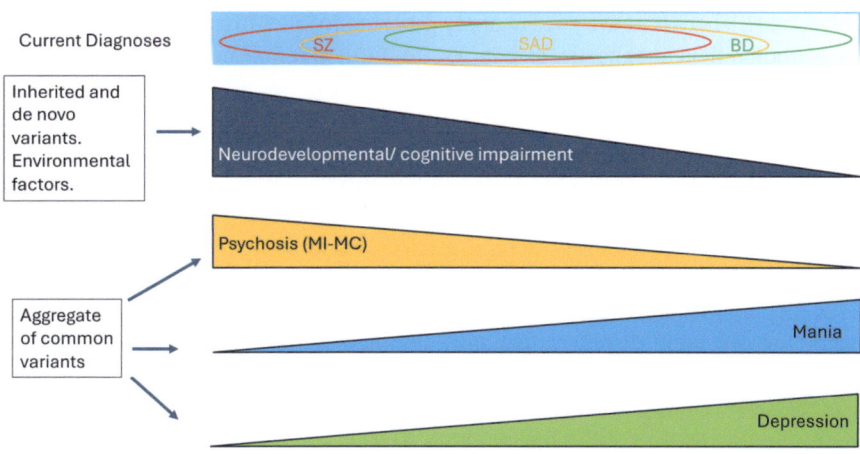

Fig. 6.1 The Psychosis Continuum 2025. Figure shows the overlap between current diagnostic categories (SZ: schizophrenia; SAD: schizoaffective disorder; BD: bipolar disorder). The coloured ovals illustrate the lack of clear diagnostic boundaries between the three diagnoses. Individuals towards the left of the continuum are more likely to experience psychotic, negative and disorganised symptoms and to receive a diagnosis of SZ. As we move to the right the probability of manic and depressive symptoms increases as does the likelihood of an individual receiving a diagnosis of SAD and then BD. Also, moving to the right the prevalence of mood congruent (MC) as opposed to mood incongruent (MI) psychotic symptoms increases. The psychotic continuum contains several dimensions. First, there is a gradient of decreasing neurodevelopmental impairment going from SZ, through SAD to BD. This is the result of contributions from inherited genetic variants, both rare and common, but also reflects a substantial involvement of non-familial factors such as rare de novo risk variants and environmental factors. The degree of neurodevelopmental impairment is indexed by the degree of cognitive impairment but more particularly by the extent to which cognitive function deviates from that expected from familial potential. Second, psychotic disorders vary across several symptomatic dimensions including psychosis, depression and mania that are transdiagnostic in the sense that they cut across the current categorical diagnoses. Each symptom dimension is the result of different combinations of common genetic risk variants that are partly independent. The mix of symptoms experienced by an individual depends upon the mix of risk variants they inherit.

impairment but more particularly by the extent to which cognitive function deviates from that expected from familial potential.

Second, the psychotic disorders vary across several symptomatic dimensions including psychosis, depression and mania that are transdiagnostic in the sense that they cut across the current categorical diagnoses (Fig. 6.1). The clinical picture expressed by an individual seems to be the result of a confluence of partly transdiagnostic symptom dimensions and their underlying common genetic risk factors. In other words, common variant genetic risk maps better onto symptom domains than diagnoses and the resulting clinical picture depends upon the pattern of genetic risk across each of these. There is currently considerable interest in so-called transdiagnostic genomic research including using approaches modelling the latent structure of the pleiotropic relationships between multiple psychiatric disorders and these have identified broad factors that may underlie some cross-disorder correlations [28, 43, 44]. There is now a need to apply these approaches to transdiagnostic symptoms, rather than diagnostic categories, to further refine biologically informed dimensions that cross-existing diagnostic boundaries.

6.6   Biological Insights from Genomics

The genetic findings reviewed so far have focussed on those that inform our understanding of the relationship between different diagnostic categories and the implications for classification and nosology. However, given that genetics is the biggest risk factor for psychotic disorders, genomic findings might therefore be expected to inform our understanding where key pathogenic events might be unfolding. For example, we can ask whether psychotic disorders are fundamentally disorders of brain biology, despite still being referred to as 'functional' psychoses, and if so whether particular brain regions, structures or cell types are implicated. Indeed, one of the strengths of genomics for understanding biological risk is that variation in genomic DNA is 'causally privileged' [45] in that, unlike other biological markers, it is not subject to reverse causation, whereby a supposed risk factor is actually a consequence of the disorder or its treatment rather than a cause, and thus allows causation to be inferred with greater confidence.

This work, called functional genomics, essentially seeks to determine whether the genes implicated by genomic studies are enriched for those specifically expressed in different tissues, brain regions, cell types or neuronal structures. The methodology on which such studies are based is rapidly evolving but so far it appears that a substantial proportion of genetic risk for psychotic disorders involves genes that are specifically expressed in the brain and particularly in neurons rather than glia [11]. There is evidence for important roles for neurodevelopmental processes and perturbation of neuronal and synaptic function, particularly of glutamatergic and GABAergic neurons across many regions of the forebrain [11]. This is consistent with findings from brain imaging studies reviewed above suggesting that psychotic disorders result from subtle but widespread neuronal pathology. It is also consistent with the fact that psychotic disorders are broad multi-domain conditions that impact on many aspects of behaviour, brain function and cognition [16].

Functional genomics studies thus support the view that genetic risk for psychotic disorders is manifest largely in the neurons of the brain. Moreover, they point to fundamental disturbances of neuronal function that are not confined to a small number of brain regions or structures. This would explain the diverse psychopathology of psychotic disorders, their association with a broad range of cognitive impairments and the lack of regional specificity in associated neuroimaging findings. While psychotic disorders may result from widely distributed neuronal pathology, it is likely that individual symptoms, cognitive impairments and other features are associated with dysfunction in specific brain regions and circuits with the variation between individuals reflecting regional and circuit level variability in the downstream impact of these disturbances in neuronal function. If this is the case, there are important implications for research aiming to identify neurobiological mechanisms mediating the effects of genetic risk on behavioural or symptomatic outcomes [46].

6.7   Implications

It seems as if, in the clinic at least, Kraepelin's legacy is here to stay until the next iterations of DSM and ICD, perhaps beyond them too. It is often claimed that we should retain the current categories of SZ and BD until there is convincing evidence for new diagnoses to replace them. But an alternative is for psychiatry to admit that the current diagnostic system is not fit for purpose either for clinical classification or research purposes, and to replace it with a single diagnostic category encompassing SZ, schizoaffective disorder and BD. In the meantime, we must be advocating for a diagnostic system that encourages clinicians and regulators to take a broader view of psychotic disorders than simply assessing the presence or not of the symptoms necessary to make a diagnosis. We need to ensure that clinicians can capture the dimensional variety of symptoms and associated features and how they change over time. Developing and implementing reliable and clinically applicable dimensional measures of the major domains, which clinicians are required to assess, should be a priority and will benefit clinical management allowing more individualised treatment selections to be made [47].

Among researchers there is now a consensus that the current diagnostic systems do not define distinct disorders and there is an increasing focus on research across the current diagnostic categories. As we have seen, this is beginning to reveal partly separate genetic risk for the major symptom categories, but there is a need now for similar approaches to be taken in relation to other risk factors, to integrate neuroscience research and to identify potential biomarkers. These approaches have the potential to identify valid, biologically informed diagnoses that cross existing diagnostic categories. However, they will require sufficiently granular *phenotype* data including measures of symptom domains, as well as measures of clinical and functional outcomes, and for these to be combined with potential biomarkers such as cognition, neuroimaging and blood-based assays. Pioneering work combining clinical and neurobiological data in the psychoses transdiagnostically has identified evidence for different 'biotypes' that transcend current diagnostic categories [48], and further work of this kind incorporating genomic data is likely to be fruitful.

6.8   Conclusion

Kraepelin's dichotomous syndromic classification remains the foundation of current diagnostic practice in psychotic disorders nearly 100 years after his death. That this is the case is clearly evidence of his significance in the history of psychiatry. However, it is not evidence for a century of stasis in understanding the psychotic disorders or in the lack of evidence against the dichotomous classification. Rather, given the strength of the evidence undermining the dichotomy, it represents the innate conservatism of the bodies regulating international diagnostic practice and psychiatry's lack of confidence in admitting to its flawed diagnostic processes.

Key Points
- The diagnostic categories currently applied to psychotic disorders do not define conditions that are distinct or homogeneous whether regarding psychopathology, aetiology or mechanism.
- The evidence suggests a continuum with several dimensions.
- One dimension is a gradient of neurodevelopmental impairment which is greatest in cases diagnosed with SZ, followed by schizoaffective disorder, then by BD. This is indexed by cognitive impairment and particularly the degree to which cognitive function deviates from that expected based on family history.
- Current evidence suggests that the clinical picture expressed by an individual with a psychotic disorder is the result of a confluence of partly orthogonal transdiagnostic symptom dimensions and their underlying genetic risk factors. Genetic risk maps better onto symptom domains than diagnoses and the resulting clinical picture depends upon the pattern of genetic risk for each of these.
- Psychotic disorders as syndromes are fundamentally disorders of neuronal function and development across multiple brain regions with broad impacts on brain function. The pattern of symptoms, cognitive impairments and other features in each case likely reflects the pattern of resulting dysfunction in specific brain regions or circuits depending on the individual mix of genetic and other risk or modifying factors.

Acknowledgements I am very grateful to Nick Craddock, Mick O'Donovan and James Walters who have contributed to the ideas expressed in this chapter.

Glossary

Allele The different versions of a gene variant.

Assortative mating The phenomenon whereby individuals with similar phenotypes or genotypes mate with each other more often than would be expected by chance.

Common variants These are defined as those in which the minor (less frequent) allele is present in the population at frequencies of 1% or more. In particular, they include single-nucleotide polymorphisms (SNPs) that can be assayed in parallel across the genome in what are called genome-wide associations studies (GWAS).

Copy number variants (CNVs) Variants in which the number of copies of a specific segment of DNA varies in the population. These structural differences may have come about because of duplications, deletions or other changes.

De novo variant A change in the DNA sequence of an individual that was not inherited from its parents but rather is the result of a new mutation.

Familial An adjective referring to phenomena that relate to, or occur in, a family or its members. In genetics, it is often used to refer to a characteristic (phenotype) that occurs with greater frequency in a family than in the general population.

Genomics A branch of molecular biology which studies the genome, which is an organism's complete set of DNA including all its genes.

Heritability The proportion of variation in disease risk in a population that is due to inherited genetic variation. It can be estimated through the familial occurrence of disease in family, twin and adoption studies.

Mutation-selection balance The phenomenon whereby deleterious alleles are maintained in the population because the rate at which they are eliminated by selection is balanced by the rate at which they are created by new mutation.

Mutation-selection drift An explanation for genetic variation in traits that are associated with reduced reproductive fitness that particularly applies to highly polygenic traits where the effects of individual alleles are small. It proposes that mildly deleterious alleles can drift to high frequencies through chance events as well as being subject to the opposing effects of new mutation and selection.

Penetrance In the context of human disease genetics, this refers to the proportion of individuals with a particular genetic variant who exhibit the disorder in question.

Phenotype A set of observable characteristics. In human genetics, this can cover traits such as hight or hair colour, the presence or absence of disease, or disease attributes such as symptoms, signs and the results of special investigations.

Pleiotropy The phenomenon when a variant or a gene influences more than one phenotype.

Polygenic A polygenic trait or disorder is one that reflects the combined effects of multiple genetic variants. They are to be distinguished from traits or disorders that result from variants in a single gene that show clearer inheritance patterns.

Single-nucleotide polymorphisms (SNPs) These are the most common type of human genetic variation. Each SNP represents a difference in a single nucleotide base. Nucleotide bases are the building blocks of DNA.

Rare coding variants (RCVs) Variants in the coding sequence of a gene that are present in less than 1% of the population. They can be detected by genome-wide sequencing studies.

Variant A DNA site which varies between individuals in the population.

References

1. Kraepelin E. Psychiatrie: ein Lehrbuch für Studirende und Aerzte. 6th ed. Leipzig: Johann Ambrosius Barth; 1899.
2. Owen MJ. New approaches to psychiatric diagnostic classification. Neuron. 2014;84(3):564–71.
3. Kendell R, Jablensky A. Distinguishing between the validity and utility of psychiatric diagnoses. Am J Psychiatry. 2003;160(1):4–12.
4. Hyman SE. The diagnosis of mental disorders: the problem of reification. Annu Rev Clin Psychol. 2010;6(1):155–79.
5. Kendell RE. Diagnosis and classification of functional psychoses. Br Med Bull. 1987;43(3):499–513.
6. Brockington IF, Meltzer HY. The nosology of schizoaffective psychosis. Psychiatr Dev. 1983;1(4):317–38.
7. Marneros A, Akiskal HS. The overlap of affective and schizophrenic spectra. Cambridge: Cambridge University Press; 2006.
8. Craddock N, Owen MJ. The beginning of the end for the Kraepelinian dichotomy. [Editorial]. Br J Psychiatry. 2005;186(5):364–6.
9. Craddock N, Owen MJ. Rethinking psychosis: the disadvantages of a dichotomous classification now outweigh the advantages. World Psychiatry. 2007;6(2):84–91.
10. Craddock N, Owen MJ. The Kraepelinian dichotomy - going, going... but still not gone. Br J Psychiatry. 2010;196(2):92–5.
11. Owen MJ, Bray NJ, Walters JTR, O'Donovan MC. Genomics of schizophrenia, bipolar disorder and major depressive disorder. Nat Rev Genet. 2025; 26(12):862-877.
12. Robins E, Guze SB. Establishment of diagnostic validity in psychiatric illness: its application to schizophrenia. Am J Psychiatry. 1970;126(7):983–7.
13. Cardno AG, Rijsdijk FV, Sham PC, Murray RM, McGuffin P. A twin study of genetic relationships between psychotic symptoms. Am J Psychiatry. 2002;159(4):539–45.
14. Bramon E, Sham PC. The common genetic liability between schizophrenia and bipolar disorder: a review. Curr Psychiatry Rep. 2001;3(4):332–7.
15. Lichtenstein P, Yip BH, Björk C, Pawitan Y, Cannon TD, Sullivan PF, Hultman CM. Common genetic determinants of schizophrenia and bipolar disorder in Swedish families: a population-based study. Lancet. 2009;373(9659):234–9.
16. Owen MJ, Legge SE, Rees E, Walters JTR, O'Donovan MC. Genomic findings in schizophrenia and their implications. Mol Psychiatry. 2023;28(9):3638–47.
17. Power RA, Kyaga S, Uher R, MacCabe JH, Langstrom N, Landen M, et al. Fecundity of patients with schizophrenia, autism, bipolar disorder, depression, anorexia nervosa, or substance abuse vs their unaffected siblings. JAMA Psychiatr. 2013;70(1):22–30.
18. Tansey KE, Rees E, Linden DE, Ripke S, Chambert KD, Moran JL, et al. Common alleles contribute to schizophrenia in CNV carriers. Mol Psychiatry. 2016;21(8):1085–9.
19. Bergen SE, Ploner A, Howrigan D, CNV Analysis Group and the Schizophrenia Working Group of the Psychiatric Genomics Consortium, O'Donovan MC, Smoller JW, et al. Joint contributions of rare copy number variants and common SNPs to risk for schizophrenia. Am J Psychiatry. 2019;176(1):29–35.
20. Keller MC. Evolutionary perspectives on genetic and environmental risk factors for psychiatric disorders. Annu Rev Clin Psychol. 2018;14(1):471–93.
21. Pardinas AF, Holmans P, Pocklington AJ, Escott-Price V, Ripke S, Carrera N, et al. Common schizophrenia alleles are enriched in mutation-intolerant genes and in regions under strong background selection. Nat Genet. 2018;50(3):381–9.
22. Torrey EF, Yolken RH. Psychiatric genocide: Nazi attempts to eradicate schizophrenia. Schizophr Bull. 2010;36(1):26–32.
23. Haefner H. Comment on E.F. Torrey and R.H. Yolken: "Psychiatric genocide: Nazi attempts to eradicate schizophrenia" (Schizophr Bull. 2010;36/1:26–32) and R.D. Strous: "Psychiatric genocide: reflections and responsibilities". Schizophr Bull. 2010;36:450–4.

24. Allardyce J, Leonenko G, Hamshere M, Pardiñas AF, Forty L, Knott S, et al. Association between schizophrenia-related polygenic liability and the occurrence and level of mood-incongruent psychotic symptoms in bipolar disorder. JAMA Psychiatry. 2018;75(1):28–35.
25. Ruderfer DM, Ripke S, McQuillin A, Boocock J, Stahl EA, Pavlides JM, et al. Genomic dissection of bipolar disorder and schizophrenia, including 28 subphenotypes. Cell. 2018;173(7):1705–15.
26. Charney AW, Ruderfer DM, Stahl EA, Moran JL, Chambert K, Belliveau RA, et al. Evidence for genetic heterogeneity between clinical subtypes of bipolar disorder. Transl Psychiatry. 2017;7(1):e993.
27. Dennison CA, Legge SE, Hubbard L, Lynham AJ, Zammit S, Holmans P, et al. Risk factors, clinical features, and polygenic risk scores in schizophrenia and schizoaffective disorder depressive-type. Schizophr Bull. 2021;47(5):1375–84.
28. Richards AL, Cardno A, Harold G, Craddock NJ, Di Florio A, Jones L, et al. Genetic liabilities differentiating bipolar disorder, schizophrenia, and major depressive disorder, and phenotypic heterogeneity in bipolar disorder. JAMA Psychiatry. 2022;79(10):1032–9.
29. Rees E, Creeth HD, Hwu HG, Chen WJ, Tsuang M, Glatt SJ, et al. Schizophrenia, autism spectrum disorders and developmental disorders share specific disruptive coding mutations. Nat Commun. 2021;12(1):5353.
30. Owen MJ, O'Donovan MC. Schizophrenia and the neurodevelopmental continuum: evidence from genomics. World Psychiatry. 2017;16(3):227–35.
31. Singh T, Walters JTR, Johnstone M, Curtis D, Suvisaari J, Torniainen M, et al. The contribution of rare variants to risk of schizophrenia in individuals with and without intellectual disability. Nat Genet. 2017;49(8):1167–73.
32. Murray RM, Sham P, van Os J, Zanelli J, Cannon M, McDonald C. A developmental model for similarities and dissimilarities between schizophrenia and bipolar disorder. Schizophr Res. 2004;71(2–3):405–16.
33. Owen MJ, O'Donovan MC, Thapar A, Craddock N. Neurodevelopmental hypothesis of schizophrenia. Br J Psychiatry. 2011;198(3):173–5.
34. Owen MJ, O'Donovan MC. The genetics of cognition in schizophrenia. Genom Psychiatry. 2024;1:1–8.
35. Lynham AJ, Hubbard L, Tansey KE, Hamshere ML, Legge SE, Owen MJ, Jones IR, Walters JTR. Examining cognition across the bipolar/schizophrenia diagnostic spectrum. J Psychiatry Neurosci. 2018;43(4):245–53.
36. van Erp TG, Hibar DP, Rasmussen JM, Glahn DC, Pearlson GD, Andreassen OA, et al. Subcortical brain volume abnormalities in 2028 individuals with schizophrenia and 2540 healthy controls via the ENIGMA consortium. Mol Psychiatry. 2016;21(4):547–53.
37. van Erp TG, Walton E, Hibar DP, Schmaal L, Jiang W, Glahn DC, et al. Cortical brain abnormalities in 4474 individuals with schizophrenia and 5098 control subjects via the enhancing neuro imaging genetics through meta analysis (ENIGMA) consortium. Biol Psychiatry. 2018;84(9):644–54.
38. Hibar DP, Westlye LT, van Erp TG, Rasmussen J, Leonardo CD, Faskowitz J, et al. Subcortical volumetric abnormalities in bipolar disorder. Mol Psychiatry. 2016;21(12):1710–6.
39. Hibar DP, Westlye LT, Doan NT, Jahanshad N, Cheung JW, Ching CR. Cortical abnormalities in bipolar disorder: an MRI analysis of 6503 individuals from the ENIGMA Bipolar Disorder Working Group. Mol Psychiatry. 2018;23(4):932–42.
40. Cheon EJ, Bearden CE, Sun D, Ching CR, Andreassen OA, Schmaal L, et al. Cross disorder comparisons of brain structure in schizophrenia, bipolar disorder, major depressive disorder, and 22q11.2 deletion syndrome: a review of ENIGMA findings. Psychiatry Clin Neurosci. 2022;76(5):140–61.
41. Kendler KS, Ohlsson H, Mezuk B, Sundquist JO, Sundquist K. Observed cognitive performance and deviation from familial cognitive aptitude at age 16 years and ages 18 to 20 years and risk for schizophrenia and bipolar illness in a Swedish national sample. JAMA Psychiatry. 2016;73(5):465–71.

42. Kendler KS, Ohlsson H, Keefe RSE, Sundquist K, Sundquist J. The joint impact of cognitive performance in adolescence and familial cognitive aptitude on risk for major psychiatric disorders: a delineation of four potential pathways to illness. Mol Psychiatry. 2018;23(4):1076–83.
43. Cross-Disorder Group of the Psychiatric Genomics Consortium. Genomic relationships, novel loci, and pleiotropic mechanisms across eight psychiatric disorders. Cell. 2019;179(7):1469–82.
44. Grotzinger AD, Mallard TT, Akingbuwa WA, Ip HF, Adams MJ, Lewis CM, et al. Genetic architecture of 11 major psychiatric disorders at biobehavioral, functional genomic and molecular genetic levels of analysis. Nat Genet. 2022;54(5):548–59.
45. Kendler KS. Are psychiatric disorders brain diseases?—a new look at an old question. JAMA Psychiatry. 2024;81(4):325–6.
46. O'Donovan MC, Owen MJ. The implications of the shared genetics of psychiatric disorders. Nat Med. 2016;22(11):1214–9.
47. Barch DM, Bustillo J, Gaebel W, Gur R, Heckers S, Malaspina D, et al. Logic and justification for dimensional assessment of symptoms and related clinical phenomena in psychosis: relevance to DSM-5. Schizophr Res. 2013;150(1):15–20.
48. Clementz BA, Assaf M, Sweeney JA, Gershon ES, Keedy SK, Hill SK, et al. Categorical and dimensional approaches for psychiatric classification and treatment targeting: considerations from psychosis biotypes. In: Javitt DC, McPartland JC, editors. Neurophysiologic biomarkers in neuropsychiatric disorders: etiologic and treatment considerations. Cham: Springer; 2024. p. 685–723.

Open Access This chapter is licensed under the terms of the Creative Commons Attribution 4.0 International License (http://creativecommons.org/licenses/by/4.0/), which permits use, sharing, adaptation, distribution and reproduction in any medium or format, as long as you give appropriate credit to the original author(s) and the source, provide a link to the Creative Commons license and indicate if changes were made.

The images or other third party material in this chapter are included in the chapter's Creative Commons license, unless indicated otherwise in a credit line to the material. If material is not included in the chapter's Creative Commons license and your intended use is not permitted by statutory regulation or exceeds the permitted use, you will need to obtain permission directly from the copyright holder.

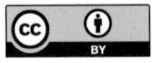

Brain Imaging in Schizophrenia

7

Stephen M. Lawrie

Box 7.1 Here—Lay Summary
Brain imaging studies have advanced our understanding of the structure, chemistry and function of the brain in schizophrenia. Grey matter is reduced, and these reductions are related to the severity of some symptoms. White matter is also reduced and correlates with reductions in cognitive function. The clearest evidence for altered brain chemistry is of increased dopamine synthesis and turnover, which drives hallucinations and delusions. In terms of brain function, the frontal lobes are underactive (so-called 'hypofrontality') and the connections between different parts of the brain are less well organised than in healthy controls. Some of these changes are present before the onset of illness, get worse as schizophrenia develops and get worse still in those who go on to have a poor outcome. This raises the possibility that brain imaging could help in making an early diagnosis or prognosis in clinical practice.

7.1 Introduction

The first direct suggestions that the structure and function of the brain in schizophrenia might be different from controls came from pneumoencephalography in the early years of the twentieth century and from the first functional imaging studies in mid-century [1, 2]. These were, however, qualitative impressions.

The modern era of quantitative neuroimaging in psychiatry arguably began about 50 years ago with the publication of a landmark report by Eve Johnstone, Tim Crow

S. M. Lawrie (✉)
Department of Psychiatry, Edinburgh University, Edinburgh, Scotland
e-mail: S.Lawrie@ed.ac.uk

© The Author(s) 2026
G. Ikkos, T. Becker (eds.), *Psychiatry after Kraepelin*,
https://doi.org/10.1007/978-3-032-09475-9_7

87

and colleagues. Motivated by finding that ~20% of long stay patients had age disorientation, they used computerised tomography and showed greater ventricular size in schizophrenia than healthy controls on computerised tomography [3]. Many replications followed. Some studies found similar changes in first episode patients, but others found correlations with duration of illness, suggesting both pre-morbid alterations and progression. After some 15 years, a meta-analysis of 53 studies of 3810 patients and controls found evidence for both [4]. Around the same time, a narrative literature review showed that the most consistent associate of ventriculomegaly was cognitive impairment [5].

The advent of sensitive, commercially available MRI machines, which did not expose participants to X-rays, led to an explosion of research, complemented by PET and MRS studies, of differences in schizophrenia and in those at high risk, with the prospect of being able to provide quantitative assessments of diagnosis and prognosis.

In this chapter, I shall review the landmark papers using each technology and the most recent systematic reviews, meta-analyses and mega-analyses of the literature comparing participants with schizophrenia versus controls, those at familial or clinical high risk versus patients and/or controls, and studies of those at high risk and with schizophrenia over time using each method. These studies typically report any such differences in terms of an overall effect size in standard deviation (sd) units, either as Cohen's 'd' or Hedge's 'g'. Note, however, that much of the functional imaging literature reports areas of differential activation beyond a statistical threshold, rather than quantitative differences, constraining quantitative reviews to coordinate-based meta-analyses (CBMAs) of common effects rather than calculating overall effect sizes.

In doing so, I will follow explicit criteria [6] for rating the quality of the evidence, which are as follows:

- 'Convincing' if N cases >1000, $P < 10^{-6}$, $I^2 < 50\%$, the 95% confidence interval (CI) excludes the null, with no evidence of publication bias
- 'Highly suggestive' if $N > 1000$, $P < 10^{-6}$, and the largest study has a significant effect
- 'Suggestive' if $N > 1000$ and $P < 10^{-3}$
- Otherwise 'weak'

This review will therefore provide an overview of what we do and don't know about brain structure, chemistry and function in schizophrenia and suggest a course towards solidifying that knowledge and evaluating clinical applications. I will also touch upon the main replicated findings in bipolar disorder and those at elevated risk of that condition.

Figure 7.1 illustrates the regions of the brain consistently implicated in schizophrenia, and Box 7.2 refers to a list of abbreviations used in the review. (From Ref. [7])

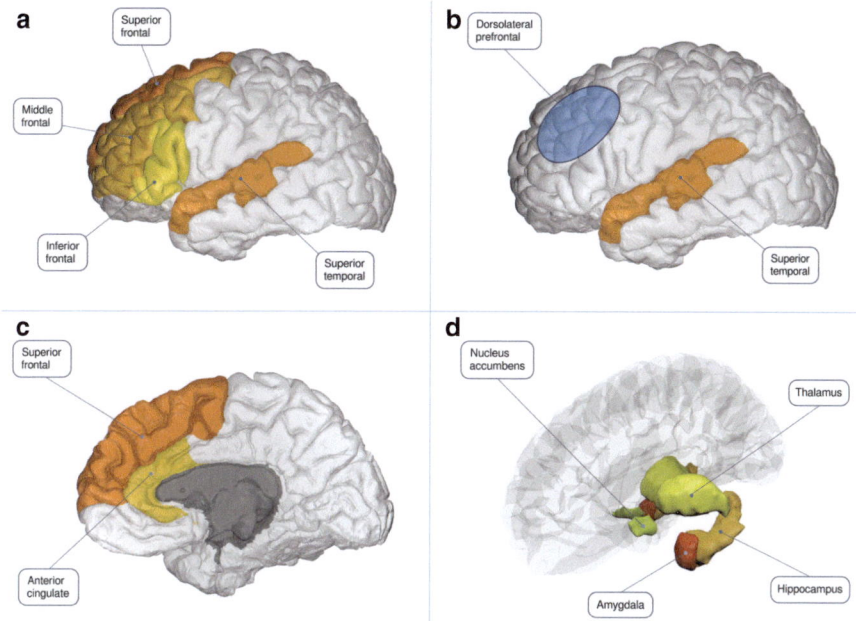

Fig. 7.1 Regions of the brain consistently implicated in schizophrenia. (**a**) Lateral view of key frontal and temporal gyri on cortical surface. (**b**) Lateral view showing cytoarchitecturally defined DLPFC. (**c**) Medial view of cortex. (**d**) Sub-cortical structures. Acknowledgement: This figure was prepared by Aleks Stolicyn, using a tool called BrainPainter. (Reference: Marinescu et al. [7])

Box 7.2 Here—List of Abbreviations in Alphabetical Order
AI   artificial intelligence
AVH   auditory verbal hallucination
BOLD   blood oxygen level-dependent imaging (fMRI)
CA 1–4   cornu ammonis 1–4 (regions of hippocampus)
CBMA   coordinate-based meta-analysis
CHR   clinical high risk (participants)
CNS   central nervous system
CT   cortical thickness
d   measure of effect size (Cohen's d)
D2   dopamine 2 receptor
DLPFC   dorsolateral prefrontal cortex
dMRI   diffusion (weighted) MRI
DOPA   dihydroxyphenylalanine (amino acid dopamine precursor)
DSD   dendritic spine density
DTI   diffusion tensor imaging
ENIGMA   enhancing neuro imaging genetics through meta-analysis
   (consortium)

(continued)

Box 7.2 (continued)

FA   fractional anisotropy (MRI)

FDR   first-degree relative

FEP   first-episode psychosis

FHR   familial high risk (participants)

fMRI   functional MRI

FTD   formal thought disorder

FWER   family-wise error rate

g   gram (unit of mass in metric system)

g   measure of effect size (Hedges'g)

GABA   gamma aminobutyric acid (CNS transmitter)

GABAA/BZR   GABAA/benzodiazepine receptor

Glu   glutamic acid

Glx   combined levels of glutamate and glutamine

GM   grey matter

GMV   grey matter volume

99mTc-HMPAO   radioactive tracer used in SPECT

[123I]IBZM   radiotracer iodobenzamide

ICC   intra-class correlation coefficient

ICV   intracranial volume

ILF   inferior longitudinal fasciculus (brain WM tract)

IQ   intelligent quotient

k   number of groups of categories compared in statistical analysis (ANOVA)

MCC   midcingulate cortex

MOFC   medial orbitofrontal cortex

MPFC   prefrontal cortex

MR   Mendelian Randomisation

MRI   magnetic resonance imaging

MRS   magnetic resonance spectroscopy

N   number

NAA   N-acetyl aspartate

NMDA   N-methyl D-aspartate (amino acid)

P   probability (measure of statistical significance)

PET   positron emission tomography

PFC   prefrontal cortex

PM   post-mortem

15O or 18F   radionuclides oxygen15 or fluorine18 radionuclides

rCBF   regional cerebral blood flow

RDoC   National Institute of Mental Health Research Domain Criteria

ROI   region of interest

rs-fcMRI   resting-state functional connectivity MRI

SA   surface area

s&dMRI   structural and diffusion (weighted) MRI

SD   standard deviation

(continued)

Box 7.2 (continued)

SLF   superior longitudinal fasciculus (brain WM tract)
sMRI   structural MRI
SPECT   single photon emission computed tomography
STG   superior temporal gyrus
SUD   substance use disorder
SV2A   synaptic vesicle glycoprotein (brain marker)
T   Tesla (unit of strength of magnetic field in MRI)
TBSS   tract-based spatial statistics
TPJ   temporo-parietal junction
TSPO   translocator protein (brain ligand)
VBM   voxel-based morphometry
VLPFC   ventrolateral prefrontal cortex
VS   ventral striatum
WBV   whole brain volume
WM   white matter

7.2   Structural MRI (sMRI)

sMRI of the brain for volumetry usually acquires 'T1 data' in 1–2 mm thick 'slices'. Regions of interest (ROIs) used to be delineated manually or semi-automatically, and summed to produce volumes, with some arbitrary neuroanatomical boundaries to facilitate measurement reliability, but this was a very laborious process. Various types of 'computational morphometry' were developed—of which VBM became the industry standard—to automatically survey the whole brain, including complex structures such as the insula. Assaying tens of thousands of volume elements ('voxels') is, however, anatomically imprecise and requires correction for multiple hypothesis testing. More recently, the ENIGMA (Enhancing Neuro Imaging Genetics through Meta-Analysis) consortium has facilitated neuroimaging groups to use the same software 'Freesurfer' to identically analyse sMRI scans and pool results in a 'mega-analysis'. Freesurfer uses high-resolution automatic surface-based techniques to return measures of cortical thickness (CT) and surface area (SA) for 32 bilateral cortical 'parcels' and 8 bilateral subcortical volumes, and is now the 'industry standard' approach to sMRI analysis.

7.2.1   Schizophrenia Compared to Healthy Controls

The landmark sMRI report in schizophrenia didn't exactly use healthy controls, but unaffected identical twins of those with schizophrenia [8]. Controlling for genetic influences on brain structure in this way meant that increases in the volumes of the ventricles and reductions in, for example, hippocampus could actually be seen with the naked eye in the sense that a blinded radiologist could almost always identify the scan that came from a given patient rather than their healthy twin. Given the essentially identical genetic and environmental upbringing these twins would have had, however, the finding raised issues as to whether the differences were attributable to some sort of 'disease process' or might reflect differential exposure to risk factors or post-onset effects of the illness, such as antipsychotic medication, alcohol excess or 'social drift' to unemployment and poverty. These questions remain to be fully resolved (see Sect. 7.6).

Meta-analytical reviews followed around a decade later and delivered some consensus about the brain regions most affected [9, 10], tried to explain differences ('heterogeneity') between studies [10], highlighted the issue of publication bias [9, 11], and found some evidence of antipsychotic medication effects in terms of enlarged components of the basal ganglia [9, 10]. Some commentators even suggested that structural neuroimaging in schizophrenia was inconclusive and potentially artefactual or epiphenomenal [12]. This view is now, however, difficult to sustain given the volume and strength of the evidence available.

There is for example a meta-analysis of 387 ROI studies of 9098 patients [13], which reported a small but highly significant reduction of 2% in intracranial volume (ICV), especially in male patients, suggesting some neurodevelopmental underpinnings, with greater reductions in whole brain volume (WBV) (reduction at 2.6% and in grey matter (GM, 4.3%, effect size Cohen's $d = -0.49$). Other moderate effect sizes included lateral and third ventricular (and pallidum) increases and reduced GM in prefrontal ($d = -0.49$) and temporal lobes ($d = -0.43$), hippocampus ($d = -0.52$), fusiform ($d = -0.52$) and superior temporal gyrus (STG, $d = -0.58$). By the standards of clinical epidemiology, some of these results are 'convincing' (e.g. amygdala, thalamus) or 'highly suggestive' (e.g. WBV, GM, hippocampus), but some are only 'suggestive' (anterior cingulate, STG, insula).

The largest available co-ordinate based meta-analysis (CBMA) of VBM data reports GM reductions in very similar regions, plus the anterior cingula [14].

The largest ENIGMA studies of schizophrenia to date further reinforce these findings. Comparing 4474 patients and 5098 controls, widespread reductions in CT ($d = -0.52$) and SA ($d = -0.25$) were found, with larger effect sizes for prefrontal and temporal regions (all $P < 0.00001$, 'highly suggestive') [15]. Sub-cortical volume reductions, in 2028 patients and 2540 controls, include bilateral hippocampus, amygdala, thalamus, as well as ICV, with volume increases in the pallidum and lateral ventricles (all $P < 0.00001$, 'highly suggestive'), but these results were subject to notable heterogeneity, only partly explained by age, sex, medication and other effects [16].

Overall, ROI, VBM, CBMA and Freesurfer ENIGMA results provide complementary evidence, which is likely to become stronger as more patients are added, and the similarities in the regions affected and their effect sizes are striking. This provides measurement validity and argues against the results being artefactual. Some of the highlighted regions are illustrated in Fig. 7.1.

7.2.2   sMRI Symptom Localisation

Finding correlations between volume reductions and symptoms (or cognitive impairment, see below) supports the view that these changes are relevant to the disorder and not epiphenomenal. Shenton et al. produced the initial landmark report of structural associations with positive symptoms [17]. They studied 15 patients and controls and found reduced volumes of the left STG (15%), among other regions. The volume of left posterior STG correlated with thought disorder severity.

A systematic review of ROI studies found that 18 of 30 studies which reported analyses found negative correlations of ~0.3 between STG volume, especially on the left, with positive symptom severity, particularly of hallucinations—although the strength of this association is probably elevated by publication bias [18]. A CBMA of 13 correlational studies of GM and hallucinations found that hallucination severity correlated with decreased GM in left STG and left posterior insula, and 11 studies of a total of 504 hallucinating patients had reduced GM in the left anterior insula and left inferior frontal gyrus compared to controls [19].

Several ENIGMA mega-analyses have reported on the sMRI associations of symptoms. Positive symptoms are negatively related to STG thickness in 1987 patients (left: β std -0.052, $P = 0.021$; right: β std -0.073, $P = 0.001$, 'weak'), robust to controlling for duration of illness and antipsychotic medication [20]. Negative symptom severity is associated with left orbito-frontal cortex and pars opercularis thickness ($N = 1985$, β std. -0.075, $P = 0.019$, 'weak') [21], while patients with the 'deficit syndrome' have more pronounced CT reductions in the right fronto-parietal cortices [22].

Symptoms are, however, not attributable to reduced GM in lone brain regions (see fMRI below). In a recent analysis of neural networks for positive and negative formal thought disorder (FTD) in 752 patients, both networks encompassed fronto-occipito-amygdala regions, while positive FTD included lateral temporal cortices [23].

Thus, positive symptoms and particularly hallucinations have been related to STG reductions by three methods, but these are all 'weak' associations, and the direction of causality is unknown.

7.2.3   Specificity

There are some suggestions of some disorder specificity with respect to diagnosis [14], but in the main, these reflect less significant changes, for example, in bipolar disorder than schizophrenia, rather than complete separation. For example, Goodkind et al. [24] reported greater reductions in the anterior cingulate in schizophrenia than in other disorders, but this was related to impairments in executive function, which are greater in schizophrenia. On the other hand, McCutcheon et al. [25] recently provided evidence for an identifiable psychosis anatomical component, albeit relevant to all psychotic disorders.

7.2.4 High-Risk Studies and Predicting Psychosis

Studying people at high risk of schizophrenia can reveal pre-morbid differences, and possible predictors of or changes with the transition to a psychotic disorder. The two main approaches are to sample young people with affected relatives at 'familial high risk' (FHR), or those at 'clinical high risk' (CHR) with psychotic symptoms short of a diagnosis. Each approach led to landmark reports of differences in those at FHR before they became ill [26], with further changes in those at CHR leading up to and after diagnosis [27]. Replications were, however, inconsistent, necessitating systematic reviews of the literature.

Boos et al. [28] reviewed 25 ROI studies of 1065 first-degree relatives (FDRs). GM was slightly reduced ($d = -0.21$), and the third ventricle was slightly larger in relatives than in controls ($d = -0.21$). Consistent differences were also found in the hippocampus ($d = -0.31$), but all these results are 'weak'. A slightly larger effect in combined amygdala-hippocampal volumes was subject to significant, unexplained heterogeneity. Importantly, a larger hippocampal volume in 511 relatives than 335 patients ($d = 0.43$, $k = 9$), with heterogeneity attributable to one outlier study ($d = 0.29$, $k = 8$), suggests changes between being at FHR and schizophrenia.

The largest CBMA in FHR [29] found similar GM reductions in the left amygdala extending to left STG, but this was not significant after correction for multiple comparisons. Similarly, those at CHR had reduced GM in the medial frontal gyrus not statistically significant after correction.

An ENIGMA analysis [30] of 1228 FDRs of 1016 patients with schizophrenia, found reductions in the relatives in ICV (and controlling for that) in cortical GM, WM, amygdala and hippocampus, but the effects were all small and non-significant after correction, except for the thalamus ($d = -0.13$, $P < 0.05$, 'weak') and third ventricle. ENIGMA has also performed the largest pooled study of CHR individuals to date [31], in 1792 CHRs and 1377 controls. CHRs had widespread lower CT ($d = -0.18$, $P < 0.00001$ corrected, 'highly suggestive'), with similar effects in right hippocampus, fusiform gyri and insula.

7.2.5 Predicting Psychosis

There is as yet no meta-analysis of ROI studies. A CBMA of 1248 at CHR [32], found that later transition to psychosis over 7–71 months ($N = 153$, mean age 21) was associated with less GM in the right STG and left anterior cingulate, unrelated to medication exposure, but neither result survived correction (FWER >0.05). Similarly, in the ENIGMA study already cited [31], lower CT in fusiform, STG and paracentral regions were non-significantly associated with subsequent psychosis, but 'resembled' patterns of CT differences in schizophrenia ($\rho = 0.35$; 95% CI, 0.12–0.55).

In sum, ROI and CBMA meta-analyses, and Freesurfer mega-analyses, provide consistent but weak evidence of small effects in the medial temporal lobes in FHR, and stronger evidence of wider effects in CHR populations, but are equivocal about prediction.

7.2.6   Longitudinal Changes and Outcome

The first suggestions of progressive sMRI changes in established schizophrenia emerged in the early 1990s and tended to show associations with some form of poor outcome, but none of the studies were large enough to be definitive. Many reviews of cross-sectional studies of people in their first episode and those with chronic schizophrenia report greater differences in chronic patients, suggesting possible changes over time, although these do not, of course, directly measure progression.

Olabi et al. [33] reviewed 27 longitudinal studies of 928 patients (mean age 13–42 years) and 867 controls over 1–10 years. Those with schizophrenia showed significantly greater longitudinal decreases in whole brain volume (annualised percentage volume change −0.07%,) whole brain (−0.59%) and frontal (−0.32%) GM, and frontal (−0.32%), parietal (−0.32%), and temporal (−0.39%) WM volume, as well as larger increases in bilateral lateral ventricular volume (+0.36%)—but the evidence is 'weak' and there was notable heterogeneity between studies that was only partly explained by differences in patient age and illness duration. There was no evidence to suggest progressive medial temporal lobe reductions. Vita et al. [34] focused on GM changes after the first episode and found a moderate effect ($d = -0.50, N = 532$, 'weak') but with heterogeneity related to age at onset, proportion on second generation antipsychotics and MRI slice thickness (one of the few reviews to find an effect of image acquisition/processing). Studies of parts of the STG showed potentially larger effects, but in fewer studies, with heterogeneity and/or publication bias.

Clearly, ~0.3–0.6% annual reductions cannot continue indefinitely when overall reductions are ~3–5% depending on the region. It is possible that some changes occur around the time of onset, and that further changes occur, possibly for longer, in those with a poor outcome.

7.2.7   Neuropathology

Macroscopic post-mortem (PM) studies of the brain offer a directly comparable approach to ROI sMRI, but the PM studies tend to be even smaller. Harrison et al. [35] combined data from 17 studies and found that the brains in 540 people with schizophrenia were, on average, 2% (24 g) lighter than those from the 794 controls. In a meta-analysis of 32 even smaller studies of hippocampal volumes, in 413 patients and 415 controls, volume (and neuron number) was significantly reduced in multiple hippocampal subfields in the left hippocampus, but not on the right (of which there were fewer studies with more heterogeneity). Neuron size (but not density), averaged bilaterally, was significantly reduced in all calculated subfields. The effect sizes (g) were generally around 0.4–0.6, although that for CA4 was −0.74 [36]. These results are 'weak' in themselves but are compatible with ROI meta-analyses, VBM, CBMAs and ENIGMA mega-analyses and provide measurement validity of those findings.

Microscopically, a review of 31 studies of dendritic spine density (DSD), post-synaptic density and protein expression revealed an overall decrease in all such postsynaptic elements in schizophrenia (Hedge's $g = -0.33$) [37]. Subgroup analyses showed a significant reduction of them all in cortical ($g = -0.44$) but not subcortical tissues ($g = -0.11$), and a large decrease for DSD ($g = -0.81$), but substantial heterogeneity was present. These consistent findings of smaller, less connected neurons in schizophrenia likely represent the cellular underpinnings of the reduced GM observed in both PM and sMRI studies, given that axons and dendrites each make up ~30% of human GM [38]. Disrupted neurodevelopmental, apoptotic, synaptic, GABA and glutamatergic, inflammatory and stress responses are, however, also implicated.

7.3   Diffusion MRI (dMRI)

Cerebral white matter (WM) is organised in fibre bundles, and dMRI is the standard approach for examining WM tracts. The most commonly used imaging technique has been diffusion tensor imaging (DTI), analysed with tract-based spatial statistics (TBSS). TBSS averages and compares DTI data from a thin WM skeleton to estimate water diffusion along up to 23 key tracts in the brain, but dMRI has limitations in dealing with crossing fibres and tracts near the cortex. The most common index is fractional anisotropy (FA), which ranges from 0 to 1 (from isotropic water diffusion to anisotropic as constrained by tracts). A systematic review and meta-analysis of six dMRI quantities found that all, including FA, were related to myelin content on direct histological examination [39].

Early notable studies showed reduced FA in PFC, corpus callosum and indeed across the whole brain [40, 41], and in specific tracts such as the uncinate fasciculus [42] and in the cingulate bundle, which correlated with cognition [43]. The largest CBMA of DTI studies [44] examined 1543 people with schizophrenia, and found decreased FA (and WM volume) in the bilateral corpus callosum, extending to the anterior and superior corona radiata, correlated with both illness duration and medication usage. There were also negative symptom correlations in the inferior longitudinal fasciculus (ILF) connecting the inferior temporal and occipital lobes.

That review also found some potentially schizophrenia specific alterations in the left cingulum and in the right anterior limb of the internal capsule compared to bipolar disorder, but these were also related to the frequency of antipsychotic medication.

There is also a review [45] of five DTI studies comparing 106 patients with hallucinations and 150 controls, which showed reduced FA in the left arcuate fasciculus of hallucinators ($g = -0.42$), a tract connecting inferior PFC with STG.

An ENIGMA mega-analysis of DTI compared 1963 people with schizophrenia and 2359 healthy controls with harmonised TBSS processing. It found significant FA reductions in 20 of 25 major WM tracts. Effect sizes varied by region, peaking with average FA ($d = -0.42$, $P < 0.002$, 'suggestive') for the entire WM skeleton. The anterior corona radiata ($d = -0.40$) and corpus callosum ($d = -0.39$) showed the largest effects. No significant effects of age at onset, duration of illness, cigarette smoking or medication dosage were detected, but there were again associations with negative symptom severity [46]. A further ENIGMA analysis of 760 patients and 957 controls with cognition data found that a global FA component accounted for a significant amount of variation in IQ and processing speed in the full sample ($g = 0.27$, $P < 0.001$, 'suggestive'), with similar effects in patients ($g = 0.20$) and controls ($g = 0.32$). Comparable associations were also found between a FA component for six long association tracts and cognition for the full sample ($g = 0.28$), the patients ($g = 0.23$), and controls ($g = 0.31$) [47].

There are also systematic reviews of high-risk DTI studies. These provide 'weak' evidence for decreased FA in the genu and splenium of the corpus callosum in FHR [48], and for reduced FA in the SLF, the ILF and the inferior fronto-occipital fasciculus in CHR [49]. There are only isolated reports of possible further longitudinal changes with the development of psychosis or a poor outcome. Similarly, there is some evidence that DTI could predict treatment resistance in established schizophrenia [50].

Overall, there is 'suggestive' evidence that FA is generally reduced in schizophrenia and correlates with cognition, mediated by processing speed, with lesser evidence for some more regionally specific associations with positive and negative symptoms, and alterations in those at high risk for familial or clinical reasons.

7.4   Neurochemical Imaging with MRS and SPECT/ PET Ligands

Magnetic resonance spectroscopy (MRS) is the third commonly used adaptation of MRI to study schizophrenia and other conditions. It can be used to study the levels of various cellular metabolites in body tissues, producing a spectrum of resonances that correspond to the amount of different molecules, such as phosphorus-containing compounds, N-acetyl aspartate (NAA) and glutamate. The technique, however, has low resolution, requiring a focus on regions of interest such as DLPFC and hippocampus with a 5–10 mm cubed search volume, and has low reproducibility at lower field strengths.

MRS studies of schizophrenia in the 1990s, conducted with 1–1.5 T magnets, suggested reduced phosphomonoesters and increased phosphodiesters in PFC on phosphorus spectroscopy, and reduced NAA in frontal and temporal lobes on proton spectroscopy, with possibly greater reductions in NAA in the basal ganglia in bipolar disorder [51]. In a grand total of 182 studies, NAA levels were significantly lower in chronic schizophrenia than controls in the frontal lobe (Hedge's $g = -0.36$, $P < 0.001$, $N = 1362$, 'suggestive'), with other consistent but evidentially 'weak' reductions in hippocampus ($g = -0.52$, $P < 0.001$), temporal lobe ($g = -0.35$, $P = 0.031$), thalamus ($g = -0.32$, $P = 0.012$) and parietal lobe ($g = -0.25$, $P = 0.028$). They were also lower in first episodes than controls in the frontal lobe ($g = -0.26$, $P = 0.002$), anterior cingulate cortex ($g = -0.24$, $P = 0.016$) and thalamus ($g = -0.28$, $P = 0.028$), and lower in those at high-risk in the hippocampus ($g = -0.20$,

$P = 0.049$), suggesting a possible progression of NAA alterations from hippocampus, to frontal cortex and thalamus, and other regions [52]. It is, however, difficult to interpret NAA reductions in terms of what they mean about the pathophysiology of schizophrenia, other than as non-specific markers of impaired neuronal metabolic function.

The advent of widely available 3 T machines has facilitated the study of absolute levels of glutamate and GABA, which convey more obvious neurobiological meaning as the major excitatory and inhibitory neurotransmitters, even if glutamate is often combined with glutamine as 'Glx'. The largest systematic review and meta-analysis to date included 134 studies, including 7993 participants with schizophrenia-spectrum disorders (including high-risk, first episodes, unmedicated, established and treatment-resistant cases) and 8744 healthy controls, although no more than 88 patients contributed data to any analysis, and the associations are accordingly 'weak'. Glx levels in the basal ganglia ($g = 0.32$) were elevated overall. Subgroup analyses showed elevated Glx levels in the hippocampus ($g = 0.47$) and dorsolateral prefrontal cortex (DLPFC, $g = 0.25$) in unmedicated patients than in controls. GABA levels in the midcingulate cortex (MCC) were decreased in the first-episode psychosis (FEP) group compared with controls ($g = -0.40$). Intriguingly, the treatment-resistant schizophrenia (TRS) group had elevated Glx and Glu levels in the MCC (Glx: $g = 0.7$; Glu: $g = 0.63$), while MCC Glu levels were decreased in the patient group except TRS ($g = -0.17$) [53]. Another review has reported evidence of increased Glx in the thalamus in genetically high-risk people ($g = 0.36$, $P = 0.003$, $N = 113$, $k = 5$, 'weak') [54]. Increased glutamatergic metabolite levels are consistent with animal data suggesting that this is secondary to NMDA hypofunction and may actually drive increased dopaminergic activity.

Positron emission tomography (PET) and single photon emission computerised tomography (SPECT) are typically employed to study blood flow, and glucose uptake with PET (see below), but can also study neurotransmission with the addition of radioactive ligands for brain receptors. In the 1970s and 1980s, competing research groups in the USA and Sweden used different PET D2 receptor ligands to assay D2 receptor density in the striatum and could not agree as to whether D2 receptors were increased or not. The data overall suggests not, but there may be other regional differences.

Examinations of dopamine turnover have been much more revealing. In one particularly elegant study, Laruelle et al. [55] measured amphetamine-induced dopamine release, estimated by the amphetamine-induced reduction in dopamine D2 receptor availability, measured as the binding potential of the specific D2 receptor radiotracer iodobenzamide ([123I]IBZM). The amphetamine-induced decrease in [123I]IBZM binding potential was significantly greater in a group of people with schizophrenia who were not taking antipsychotic medication (-19.5 +/$-$ 4.1%) compared with a healthy control group (-7.6 +/$-$ 2.1%). Moreover, in the schizophrenia group, the elevated amphetamine effect on [123I]IBZM binding potential was associated with the emergence or worsening of positive psychotic symptoms, providing a direct neurochemical-symptom link and support for the dopamine hypothesis of schizophrenia.

By far the most compelling evidence comes from the use of the PET ligand fluoro-DOPA, which is incorporated into neurones to synthesise dopamine, particularly in the striatum and as such measures dopamine activity in pre-synaptic neurones. In a systematic review and meta-analysis of 21 such studies [56], presynaptic dopamine function was significantly elevated in individuals with schizophrenia relative to controls with a summary effect size of 0.68 ($N = 269$, $P < 0.001$, 'weak'), with, if anything, a slightly larger effect in drug-naive patients ($g = 0.78$). Intriguingly, the effect is primarily seen in the associative (dorsal) striatum (caudate and putamen) rather than the limbic (ventral) striatum (nucleus accumbens etc), which has implications for how this may drive psychotic symptoms and is in keeping with fMRI studies (see below). A few small studies also suggest that such changes are seen to a lesser extent in people at high risk of psychosis, and that the risk of transition is higher in those with higher levels, with some possible further increases as they develop schizophrenia, although these results are not significant on meta-analysis [54]. Note, however, that increased fluoro-DOPA synthesis and release is also seen in bipolar disorder with psychotic symptoms [57]. Elevated dopamine turnover is therefore a non-specific marker of psychosis.

A few other PET ligands have been studied in a few small studies of schizophrenia. There is preliminary evidence from 5 studies of 61 people with psychotic disorders, using the synaptic vesicle glycoprotein 2A (SV2A) marker, that there may be widespread and large reductions in synaptic density, which could underlie GM reductions [58]. There is equivocal evidence for neuroinflammation using the 18-kDa translocator protein (TSPO) ligand, from 12 studies comprising 190 patients with schizophrenia and 200 healthy controls, in that there was a significant elevation in tracer binding potential ($g = 0.31$; $p = 0.03$) but no significant differences when volume of distribution was used (as the outcome ($g = -0.22$; $p = 0.29$) [59]. Finally, a review of seven PET/SPECT studies of GABAA/benzodiazepine receptor (GABAA/BZR) availability (118 controls, 113 patients) did not suggest replicable group differences in regional GABAA/BZR availability [60].

Overall, therefore, the best available neurochemical imaging evidence in schizophrenia is for increased glutamatergic neurotransmission in the cingulate cortex and increased dopamine turnover in the striatum. On its own, this is rather 'weak' evidence, but it finds a lot of support from other studies and can be blended into a coherent account of the condition (see below).

7.5 Functional Imaging with SPECT, PET and fMRI

Functional imaging is attractive because it can capture objective evidence of cognitive processes and subjective thoughts, feelings and emotions. Functional brain images are, however, indirect measures of neuronal activity, indexed by blood flow and metabolism. Synaptic excitation and inhibition, somal action potentials and local field potentials are indexed by just one dimension of haemodynamic and metabolic response according to energy need.

SPECT imaging uses intravenous radioactive tracers, typically 99mTc-HMPAO, which omit gamma rays that are detected by rotating gamma cameras. These include a sodium iodide crystal, which 'scintillates' on contact. Thus, the origin of the signal is calculated. A PET scan, in contrast, typically uses injectable 15O or 18F radionuclides (incorporated into, e.g. water or glucose), which are unstable, have an excess of positrons and travel 1–3 mm before colliding with electrons. An annihilation reaction follows, releasing two gamma ray photons at 180 degrees to each other, picked up by a ring of radiation detectors and thus providing greater spatial resolution (2–3 mm) than SPECT. Functional MRI (fMRI) uses the blood oxygen level dependent (BOLD) contrast between oxygenated and deoxygenated haemoglobin in blood flow to active brain regions, with a similar resolution. Analysis of fMRI typically follows five key stages: alignment of 3–4 s each scan with each other, co-registration with a structural imaging, spatial normalisation so that each brain fits a standardised template, spatial smoothing over 8–10 mm for valid signal detection, and then the statistical analysis.

7.5.1 'Hypofrontality'

The first demonstrations of quantitative reductions in regional CBF (rCBF) blood flow to the frontal lobes [61] and glucose use [62] in schizophrenia came from cognitive/pain activation studies, the latter including those with 'affective disorders'. Weinberger et al. [63] localised this to the DLPFC during the Wisconsin Card Sort Test. Generally, hypofrontality was most clearly evident in chronic patients with negative symptoms. It was, however, difficult to distinguish a 'hypofrontality' due to a primary reduction in blood flow/glucose uptake from patients simply not doing the task, and when researchers purposefully paced tasks or otherwise ensured patients did them hypofrontality was less evident and a tendency to 'hyperfrontality' emerged if the patients were able to do that task [64], with a progressive loss of frontal activity as the task becomes more difficult and performance failed [65].

Hypofrontality fell out of favour as a consequence but remains one of the best replicated findings in the functional imaging literature on schizophrenia, although antipsychotic medication is a confound. An early quantitative review found that resting and activation frontal flow/metabolism were both reduced with a medium effect size, with a small effect of neuroleptic treatment. The most robust result is a relative resting reduction in blood flow/glucose uptake ($d = -0.32$, $N = 1474$, $P = 0.01$, 'suggestive') [66]. A recent systematic review and meta-analysis [67], reporting on 36 studies in 1335 subjects overall, found reduced frontal absolute glucose uptake ($g = -0.74$; $P = 0.01$; $N = 209$, but with heterogeneity, 'weak'), and relative to whole brain ($g = -0.44$: $P = 0.01$; $N = 195$, 'weak'), in schizophrenia than controls. Absolute frontal glucose uptake was lower in chronic ($g = -1.18 \pm 0.73$) than in first-episode patients ($g = -0.09 \pm 0.88$) and controls. Medicated patients showed frontal 'hypometabolism' relative to controls (-1.04 ± 0.26), but drug-free patients did not differ significantly from controls.

7.5.2   Episodic Memory

Long-term declarative ('episodic') memory is arguably the main specific cognitive function that may show a greater deficit than general cognition in schizophrenia. It depends on interactions between the hippocampus and parts of the PFC. There is a consistent thread in the functional imaging literature on schizophrenia of an increased activation of the (para)hippocampus, with reductions of PFC activity, during encoding and retrieval [68].

7.5.3   Emotion and Social Cognition

The amygdala, another region that is reduced in volume in schizophrenia, is central to the perception and expression of emotion, especially fear. Amygdala activation to emotional images (especially faces) is consistently reduced in schizophrenia, but may be partly attributable to an over-activation to neutral faces [69, 70]. A CBMA found that patients with chronic schizophrenia demonstrated attenuated activations in the limbic emotional system, along with compensatory over-activation in the medial pre-frontal cortex (MPFC) during threatening faces processing. It is, however, unclear whether task instructions in the scanner, such as whether patients are expressly asked to judge fear or simply look at the faces, influence the results [70, 71].

Social cognition, more broadly, during such tasks as theory of mind (appreciating others' mental states), recruits the temporo-parietal junction (TPJ) region as well as MPFC and amygdala. A recent CBMA of emotional attribution and intention/belief inference found that brain activation in patients was significantly decreased in the right ventrolateral prefrontal cortex (VLPFC) during emotional attribution, while there was a significant decrease in the left posterior TPJ during intention/belief attribution [72]. It seems likely that some combination of over-sensitivity to social threat (e.g. facial fear processing) and impaired evaluation of others' intentions could underlie persecutory delusions. The studies that have directly addressed this have not been able to robustly replicate a clear link, but see 'Symptoms' below.

7.5.4   Reward and Salience

A more recent approach shows real promise for bridging the gaps between neuro-physiology, pharmacology and phenomenology—by building on cutting-edge neuroscience approaches to the same using motivational learning paradigms. All human learning arises from prediction errors, that is, the discrepancies between expectations and outcomes, and disruptions of such processes are thought to underlie motivational impairments in schizophrenia. On perceptual salience tasks, judging whether stimuli are relevant versus irrelevant, early landmark studies showed a decrease in midbrain and ventral striatal (VS) signals in first episode psychosis [73]. Overall, the literature shows a clear (albeit 'weak') VS hypoactivation during reward anticipation (23 studies, 917 patients, left/right $d = -0.5/-0.7$, $P < 0.001$), which correlates on the left side with the severity of negative symptoms ($r - 0.41$). VS hypoactivation is also evident on reward feedback [74]. Moreover, a meta-analysis of whole-brain neuroimaging studies that investigated prediction error signal processing in schizophrenia using reinforcement learning paradigms (14 studies of 324 schizophrenia patients) found reduced activity in the mesolimbic circuit, including the striatum, thalamus, amygdala, hippocampus, anterior cingulate cortex, insula, superior temporal gyrus, and cerebellum, when processing prediction errors— which reads like a list of brain regions recurrently implicated in the disorder [75]. That review also found hyperactivity in frontal areas and hypoactivity in mesolimbic areas when encoding prediction error signals in schizophrenia patients, in keeping with abnormal dopamine signalling of reward prediction error and failures representing the value of alternative responses during prediction error learning and decision making.

7.5.5   Connectivity and Resting State fMRI

fMRI is well-suited to measuring the inter-relations between brain regions during neuronal activity and provides complementary information to dMRI-measured structural connectivity. The simplest approach is to estimate 'functional connectivity', which is the temporal correlation fMRI time series between two regions, while 'effective connectivity' adds a causal consideration through a more complex multivariate modelling procedure. One would expect, for example, that fronto-hippocampal interactions during memory tasks and/or fronto-amygdala interactions during socio-emotional processing would be disrupted in schizophrenia. Indeed, there are studies which demonstrate such dysconnectivity, but the literature is inconsistent [76].

Much more consistency has been forthcoming from analyses of resting-state functional connectivity MRI (rs-fcMRI), when participants are asked to lie still, with eyes closed. Most (about three-quarters) of brain metabolism occurs at rest, and this approach has the advantage that task performance is not a consideration, even if resting brain activity is less constrained than active brain and may amount to 'random episodic spontaneous thoughts'. If one takes a data-driven approach, using independent component analysis, noise and movement-related nuisance components can be separated out, leaving components of interest. Hypoconnectivity within the default mode network that is most active during rest is a common rs-fcMRI finding in schizophrenia—as is reduced connectivity across others, including frontoparietal (attentional), salience and limbic (emotional) networks [77].

7.5.6   Symptoms

Another area of research endeavour where functional imaging has delivered consistent results is in localising psychotic symptoms, especially auditory verbal hallucinations (AVHs). Early studies with SPECT and PET in those with AVHs showed activations of language production areas and a lack of activation of language reception regions, respectively, suggesting a failure of monitoring of inner speech, that is, self-productions are experienced as coming from external space [78, 79]. Silbersweig et al. [80] took this work forward by asking participants to press a button in the PET scanner when experiencing AVHs and reported activations in subcortical nuclei (thalamic, striatal), limbic structures (especially hippocampus), and paralimbic regions (parahippocampal and cingulate gyri, as well as orbitofrontal cortex). In an elegant study, Shergill et al. [81] took advantage of fMRI by measuring spontaneous neural activity without requiring subjects to signal when hallucinations occurred. Approximately 50 individual 3–4 s scans were acquired at unpredictable intervals while participants were intermittently hallucinating. Immediately after each scan, they reported whether they had been hallucinating, and neural activity was compared when patients were and were not experiencing hallucinations in each person and the group. AVHs were associated with activation in the inferior frontal/insular, anterior cingulate, and temporal cortex bilaterally (with greater responses on the right), the right thalamus and inferior colliculus, and the left hippocampus and parahippocampal cortex.

These results have held up in meta-analyses [82]. Activations in the medial temporal lobe highlight a role for memory intrusions in the provision of content for AVHs, insula activation may relate to the involvement of awareness and self-representation, and activation in the paracingulate region of medial PFC during AVHs is consistent with models implicating reality monitoring impairment in the misattribution of self-generated information as externally perceived. It should be noted, however, that very similar activations are seen in non-clinical 'voice hearers'.

Goghari et al. [83] quantitatively reviewed 25 task-related fMRI studies and found small to moderate associations between specific symptom dimensions and regional brain activity. Negative symptoms were related to the functioning of the ventrolateral PFC and ventral striatum. Positive symptoms, particularly persecutory ideation, were related to the functioning of the medial prefrontal cortex, amygdala, and hippocampus/parahippocampal region. Disorganisation symptoms, although less frequently evaluated, were related to the functioning of the DLPFC. Surprisingly, no symptom domain had a consistent relationship with the middle or superior temporal regions, presumably because the early focus on tasks activating PFC precluded such findings.

Delusions are arguably more variable than AVHs in form and content and correspondingly less amenable to group studies, but a recent narrative review suggests that the predictive processing framework discussed above (in reward and salience) can accommodate the 95 studies they synthesised. Aberrant prediction errors signalling during processing of social, self-generated and sensory information could lead to inaccuracies in assessing the intentions of others, judging the self-relevancy of ambiguous stimuli, and misattribution of self-generated actions and unusual sensations, which could provoke delusional ideation with persecutory, referential, control and somatic content respectively [84].

7.5.7 High-Risk Studies

FHR and CHR studies have consistently found altered PFC activation in those at high risk, as well as altered connectivities between PFC and thalamus, which are associated with positive symptoms and indeed transition to a psychotic disorder [85, 86]. These alterations are usually increases on tasks and reductions on rs-fcMRI. There are also intriguing reports of different patterns, such as increased amygdala activation in those at FHR of bipolar disorder [87].. Quantitative reviews have, however, not yet been able to find any clear results overall, probably as a result of the long-standing issues with small numbers, various tasks and variable implementations.

7.5.8 Specificity

Several massive reviews of hundreds of studies in thousands of patients have searched for common and distinct activation and connectivity patterns in schizophrenia, bipolar disorder, depression, anxiety and substance use disorders (SUDs). Generally, the similarities are greater than the differences. A greater degree of (left) PFC hypoactivation ('hypofrontality') was evident in schizophrenia in one such CBMA [88], but potentially attributable to more pronounced cognitive difficulties in psychosis. Another CBMA found an effect of diagnosis for the amygdala and caudate nucleus and an effect of RDoC (National Institute of Mental Health Research Domain Criteria) fundamental neuroscience domains and constructs for the amygdala, hippocampus, putamen and nucleus accumbens [89]. In terms of connectivity, rs-fcMRI hypoconnectivity across the default mode network as well frontoparietal, salience and limbic networks, is substantially more evident in schizophrenia than other disorders [77].

7.5.9 Treatment Response and Illness Course

Just as striatal hyperactivity and hyperdopaminergia on PET are associated with positive symptom severity, predict treatment response to antipsychotic drugs and are normalised by them, so does rs-fcMRI of cortico-striatal connectivity [86, 90]. Indeed, the two are related. Several studies have found that a 'striatal connectivity index' (and indeed rs-fcMRI connectivity) predicts antipsychotic drug response. Many of these studies show ~80% sensitivity and specificity in doing so, a figure that is sometimes sufficient for routine clinical use in medicine. What is needed, however, for clinical practice is to be able to predict treatment-resistance—or, better still, clozapine response.

7.6   Discussion

This review has taken an 'umbrella review' approach in focusing on systematic reviews and meta-analyses, complemented by large-scale ENIGMA mega-analyses, and grading the overall strength of the evidence. By the standards of clinical epidemiology [6], a few of the sMRI differences between people with schizophrenia and controls (i.e. healthy people volunteering to take part in brain imaging studies) are 'convincing'; some of them and a few sMRI high risk findings are 'highly suggestive'; and some dMRI, MRS NAA and 'hypofrontality' findings are 'suggestive'. All of the fMRI results are 'weak', although this is partly due to difficulties combining the results from published data, and there are consistent bodies of evidence for altered memory, emotional and reward processing in patients. Some of these findings would be strengthened by updated reviews and mega-analyses, by developing techniques to combine the three main sMRI data types, and by being able to pool more of the available functional imaging data.

The main limitations of neuroimaging science generally are that there have been too many studies lacking clear hypotheses and/or the power to test them, due to particular problems with small numbers and variable methods. Very few bodies of work come close to achieving $N > 1000$ and/or $P < 10^{-6}$ required for 'highly suggestive' findings overall. As a result, the field has acquired a reputation for failures of replication–functional neuroimaging and fMRI in particular. Such criticism has at times been rather excessive, such as people citing the famous 'dead salmon experiment' as showing fMRI is artefactual. In actual fact, the brain of the dead salmon only lit up when the authors deliberately failed to adjust the statistical thresholds in their activation study [91]. Most researchers do this and do not try to publish uncorrected results. A much greater problem is that fMRI requires additional processing and greater methodological harmonisation than sMRI or dMRI, and there is still no standardised analysis of functional or effective connectivity [92]—although in recent years notable progress has been made with harmonisation of approaches to rs-fcMRI. The variability in analysis pipelines, which is in the tens of thousands for fMRI, and the researcher 'degrees of freedom' in being able to do multiple analyses with the same data set, are the main problems. The solution is to promote the use of Open Science principles of the preregistration of study aims, hypotheses, endpoints and analyses.

Nevertheless, clear progress has been made over the past 30 years or so. Overall, three different approaches to analysing sMRI (ROI, VBM and Freesurfer) in schizophrenia consistently point towards small reductions in ICV and SA, implicating neurodevelopmental processes, and greater reductions in WBV, GMV, and CT, particularly in prefrontal and temporal lobes. All three techniques have been validated against each other and in other conditions such as ageing and dementia [93]. These compatible findings with different methods provide measurement validity and make it clear that the results are not an artefact of image processing or statistical approach, as some have argued. Diffusion MRI also finds consistent differences of a modest size for reduced FA in WM, related in particular to cognition. sMRI and dMRI have also been validated by macro- and micro-scopic neuropathological studies,

providing further measurement validity and arguing against some artefactual alteration of the T1 signal. Further, some differences evident across sMRI, dMRI, PET
and fMRI are associated with key features of schizophrenia, especially positive
symptoms in the STG. Functional mapping of auditory hallucinations with fMRI
and PET reinforces the s/dMRI findings implicating STG and can assay interconnected neuronal populations [94].

7.6.1 Potential Causes and Confounders

A key question arises for the field is the extent to which causal factors and potential
confounders account for these results. Schizophrenia is highly heritable, as is brain
structure and to a lesser extent, chemistry and function, although showing clear
associations between neuroimaging measures and known genetic risk factors has
proven somewhat elusive—again, probably because the studies to date have been
too small to have sufficient power to detect effects. Thousands of scans are required
to find what are probably small effects. Some cutting-edge studies have taken
advantage of the progress in identifying genetic risk factors for schizophrenia and
used a technique called Mendelian Randomisation (MR) in large combined neuroimaging and genetic data-sets, such as the UK Biobank, to show possible genetic
impacts on sMRI and dMRI. Equally, however, there is MR evidence that alcohol,
coffee and tea, smoking, and education alter brain structure [95].

Environmental risk factors for schizophrenia with effects on brain development
and/or function could also account for some alterations. A few studies suggest that
obstetric complications impact on, for example, hippocampal volumes, but they are
too small and underpowered to detect interactions [96]. A narrative review of 15
studies on the impact of childhood adversity reported that the most replicated result
was an association with decreased total GM, particularly in the PFC [97] [Eds: see
also Chap. 13] Any such effects on PET or fMRI have been much less frequently
studied.

Risk factors with ongoing effects or later exposure could also account for some
of the differences between being at high risk and developing schizophrenia, and any
progression. An ENIGMA cross-disorder comparison of sMRI in substance use disorders (SUDs) showed alcohol-related brain changes (7 studies) equivalent to those
in schizophrenia in several subcortical and cortical regions [98]. More modest cannabis use disorder effects (7 studies) overlapped with those findings, with a strong
association with reduced CT of the MOFC.

It is concerning that the impact of SUDs on brain structure (and function) can be
as substantial as in schizophrenia, even though neuroimaging studies typically
exclude people with SUDs, and brain changes associated with alcohol are concentrated on PFC and WM [99]. Alcohol, cannabis and cigarette consumption is, however, generally greater in people with schizophrenia than healthy controls and
should be controlled for in future studies.

There is a long list of potential confounders of these associations [9, 12]. There
are known effects from animal and human studies of pre- and peri-natal stress on

GM and WM [100], low socio-economic position on s&dMRI across the lifespan [101], and of childhood adversity on sMRI and dMRI, some with likely time- and region-specific effects [102–104]. Although most schizophrenia scanning studies control for age, educational attainment and socio-economic factors in some way, residual confounding is likely. As a one-off scan, rs-fcMRI is also vulnerable to such confounding (in a way that task-activated fMRI is not, as it has an internal control scan). It also indexes brain development. Cortical networks develop through processes of increasing integration and decreasing segregation, and the extent of these can be used to measure brain maturity. The promising and potentially specific disruptions on rs-fcMRI of schizophrenia could therefore reflect, at least in part, the neurodevelopmental disruptions seen much more frequently in schizophrenia than most others. It is therefore complementary to task-based imaging, not a replacement.

7.6.1.1 Antipsychotic Medication Effects

Early reviews suggested that antipsychotic medication may underlie increases in caudate and putamen volumes [10]. On the other hand, clozapine may reduce these and increase PFC volumes. In the ENIGMA analysis, CT reductions were two to three times larger in medicated than unmedicated patients, and associated with medication type and dose, but the overall effect was actually small, and associations were also evident with symptom severity and duration of illness [15]. Fusar-Poli et al. [105] reviewed the sMRI ROI studies and found a small relationship between reducing GMV and cumulative exposure to antipsychotics ($\beta - 0.013$, $P = 0.048$, 'weak'). There was no significant association with duration of illness in that review, but even if one assumes the relationship with medication is causal, antipsychotic medication accounts for at most a few per cent of the variance in progressive GMV loss. It will be very difficult, if not impossible, to tease apart the relative contributions of illness severity and antipsychotics without randomised data. The acid test would be to randomise people with schizophrenia (or at high risk) to treatment or placebo, with longitudinal neuroimaging, but the data available are from small studies prone to drop-outs. Antipsychotic medication generally normalises functional neuroimaging measures, with the notable exception of 'hypofrontality'.

7.6.2   Towards Neuroimaging Biomarkers

Given the modest effect sizes of ~0.5 between cases and controls, smaller differences between those at high risk who do and do not make the transition to psychotic disorder, uncertain rates of progression to poor outcome, and the non-specificity of such changes to schizophrenia, it is unlikely that current neuroimaging approaches will provide a diagnostic or prognostic test. Machine learning approaches have improved accuracy [106], Deep learning or AI techniques may do more so [107], and multimodal neuroimaging may bring greater predictive power [108], but better results still are likely by including other clinical, behavioural and cognitive predictors of schizophrenia [109]. Neuroimaging biomarker studies have typically been conducted without clinical predictors, and vice-versa, and both literatures tend to neglect truly independent external validation in building predictive models. Future studies also need to be much larger to build robust predictive models.

These studies also need to be planned and powered, considering measurement reliability. Critical issues include the sensitivity of neuroimaging to biological variation (subject variance, which is always higher in disease) and the precision (or measurement error) with which that can be measured [93]. The intra-class correlation coefficient (ICC) quantifies biological variation relative to measurement error and approaches 1 if the latter is relatively small. The ICC for Freesurfer global CT is very good at ~0.99, but it is only moderate for smaller structures and TBSS global FA and FluoroDOPA-PET, and very low for fMRI [86].

One such obvious potential clinical application is for predicting treatment response to antipsychotics, but this would be more useful for drug development than clinical practice, where one is likely to treat anyway. It would be more clinically useful to predict treatment resistance, but there are as yet no clear neuroimaging associations for that or clozapine response [110]. Novel PET ligands are likely required of,for example, glutamatergic or muscarinic receptors.

7.6.3   Connectomics

One exciting, innovative approach is 'connectomics'. This has the appeal that 'small world networks' are a general organising property across all of nature, and connectomic approaches can quantitatively map relationships across 'levels of explanation' from genes and synapses to structure and function, to behaviour and experience. These may relate more closely to underlying neurobiology and could have stronger relationships with clinical measures and outcomes than current measures, but the best methods are still under development. In a meta-analysis of 48 sMRI studies, there was a significant decrease in network segregation with a large reduction in local efficiency ($g = -0.86$) in schizophrenia, but all results had very high heterogeneity, and methodological factors altered the graph theoretical characteristics [111]. Further, in an ENIGMA direct comparison of two network susceptibility models—highly interconnected hub vulnerability to cortical thinning, and epicentre mapping of connectivity profiles implicating fronto-temporal regions—there was evidence for both [112].

Graph theoretical approaches have also been applied to fMRI connectivity data. These generally point to aberrant network properties, including reduced efficiency, disrupted hub connectivity and altered modularity in schizophrenia compared to controls. These suggest an overall disruption in the balance of regional integration and separation, that is, reduced small-worldness [86]. Two fMRI connectomics meta-analyses are available. In 121 studies that reported both under- and over-activations in the same patients, in network terms, these abnormalities were located in close topological proximity to each other. Under-activation in a peripheral node was more frequently associated specifically with over-activation of core nodes than with over-activation of another peripheral node. In other words, abnormal responses are concentrated in hubs of the normative connectome [113]. Finally, in a total of 13 small functional neuroimaging studies (8 fMRI, 5 EEG), brain networks in patients with schizophrenia exhibited significant decreases in measures of local organisation ($g = -0.56$) and significant decreases in small-worldness ($g = -0.65$), but with notable levels of heterogeneity between studies [114].

7.7   Conclusions

Neuroimaging in schizophrenia has established several robust and validated findings, including brain-behaviour relations, but many associations are weak or nonspecific. Further progress will require targeted scientific research and clinical studies that should observe the principles of open science in terms of clear hypotheses, adequate power, reproducible methods and analysis [115], while following guidelines for the conduct and reporting of diagnostic and prognostic studies if relevant.

Key Points
- Meta-analyses and mega-analyses of structural magnetic resonance imaging (sMRI) in thousands of people with schizophrenia have shown reduced brain volumes (general or specific), relative to healthy controls, some of which are present before onset and consistently correlate with the severity of symptoms.
- ENIGMA mega-analyses of diffusion MRI (dMRI) studies in hundreds of patients demonstrate a general reduced structural connectivity of white matter, which correlates with the severity of cognitive impairment.
- MRS reductions in N-acetyl-aspartate in some regions and reduced glucose uptake in the pre-frontal cortex (PFC) on PET both suggest impaired cerebral mitochondrial metabolism.
- MRS studies also suggest glutamatergic abnormalities, while fluorodopa PET shows increased dopamine turnover in the striatum as the likely cause of psychotic symptoms.
- The functional imaging literature in schizophrenia suggests 'hypofrontality', disrupted processing during memory, emotional and reward tasks, and at rest, with consistent network associations of psychotic symptoms, especially auditory hallucinations.

Acknowledgements I would like to thank Mark Bastin, Simon Cox, Dominic Job, Andrew McIntosh, Bill Moorhead, Liana Romaniuk, Danny Smith and Heather Whalley for helpful discussions about neuroimaging data and their interpretation.

Conflicts of Interest SML has been paid by Kynexis and Wellcome for giving educational talks to their staff.

Funding SML acknowledges financial support from Wellcome (218493/Z/19/Z; 223615/Z/21/Z; 324532/Z/25/Z) and UKRI (APP4419).

References

1. Weinberger DR, Wagner RL, Wyatt RJ. Neuropathological studies of schizophrenia: a selective review. Schizophr Bull. 1983;9:193–212.
2. Kety SS, Woodford RB. Cerebral blood flow and metabolism in schizophrenia; the effects of barbiturate semi-narcosis, insulin coma and electroshock. Am J Psychiatry. 1948;104:765–70.
3. Johnstone EC, Crow TJ, Frith CD, Husband J, Kreel L. Cerebral ventricular size and cognitive impairment in chronic schizophrenia. Lancet. 1976;ii:924–6.
4. Raz S, Raz N. Structural brain abnormalities in the major psychoses: a quantitative review of the evidence from computerized imaging. Psychol Bull. 1990;108:93–108.
5. Lewis SW. Computerised tomography in schizophrenia 15 years on. Br J Psychiatry Suppl. 1990;9:16–24.
6. Radua J, Ramella-Cravaro V, Ioannidis JPA, et al. What causes psychosis? An umbrella review of risk and protective factors. World Psychiatry. 2018;17:49–66.
7. Marinescu RV, Eshaghi A, Alexander DC, Golland P. BrainPainter: a software for the visualisation of brain structures, biomarkers and associated pathological processes. arXiv. 2019; Available from: https://arxiv.org/abs/1905.08627
8. Suddath RL, Christison GW, Torrey EF, Casanova MF, Weinberger DR. Anatomical abnormalities in the brains of monozygotic twins discordant for schizophrenia. N Engl J Med. 1990;322:789–94.
9. Lawrie SM, Abukmeil SS. Brain abnormality in schizophrenia. A systematic and quantitative review of volumetric magnetic resonance imaging studies. Br J Psychiatry. 1998;172:110–20.
10. Wright IC, Rabe-Hesketh S, Woodruff PW, David AS, Murray RM, Bullmore ET. Meta-analysis of regional brain volumes in schizophrenia. Am J Psychiatry. 2000;157:16–25.
11. Ioanniddis JP. Excess significance bias in the literature on brain volume abnormalities. Arch Gen Psychiatry. 2011;68:773–80.
12. Weinberger DR, Radulescu E. Finding the elusive psychiatric "lesion" with 21st-century neuroanatomy: a note of caution. Am J Psychiatry. 2016;173:27–33.
13. Haijma SV, Van Haren N, Cahn W, Koolschijn PCMP, Hulshoff Pol HE, Kahn RS. Brain volumes in schizophrenia: a meta-analysis in over 18000 subjects. Schizophr Bull. 2013;39:1129–38.
14. Ellison-Wright I, Bullmore E. Anatomy of bipolar disorder and schizophrenia: a meta-analysis. Schizophr Res. 2010;117:1–12.
15. van Erp TGM, Walton E, Hibar DP, et al. Cortical brain abnormalities in 4474 individuals with schizophrenia and 5098 control subjects via the Enhancing Neuro Imaging Genetics Through Meta Analysis (ENIGMA) consortium. Biol Psychiatry. 2018;84:644–54.
16. Van Erp TGM, Hibar DP, Rasmussen JM, et al. Subcortical brain volume abnormalities in 2028 individuals with schizophrenia and 2540 healthy controls via the ENIGMA consortium. Mol Psychiatry. 2016;21:547–53.
17. Shenton ME, Kikinis R, Jolesz FA, et al. Abnormalities of the left temporal lobe and thought disorder in schizophrenia. A quantitative magnetic resonance imaging study. N Engl J Med. 1992;327:604–12.
18. Sun J, Maller JJ, Guo L, Fitzgerald PB. Superior temporal gyrus volume change in schizophrenia: a review of region of interest volumetric studies. Brain Res Rev. 2009;61:14–32.
19. Romeo Z, Spironelli C. Hearing voices in the head: two meta-analyses on structural correlates of auditory hallucinations in schizophrenia. Neuroimage Clin. 2022;36:103241.
20. Walton E, Hibar DP, van Erp TG, et al. Positive symptoms associate with cortical thinning in the superior temporal gyrus via the ENIGMA Schizophrenia consortium. Acta Psychiatr Scand. 2017;135:439–47.
21. Walton E, Hibar DP, van Erp TGM, et al. Prefrontal cortical thinning links to negative symptoms in schizophrenia via the ENIGMA consortium. Psychol Med. 2018;48:82–94.

22. Banaj N, Vecchio D, Piras F, et al. Cortical morphology in patients with the deficit and non-deficit syndrome of schizophrenia: a worldwide meta- and mega-analyses. Mol Psychiatry. 2023;28:4363–73.
23. Sharkey RJ, Bacon C, Peterson Z, et al. Differences in the neural correlates of schizophrenia with positive and negative formal thought disorder in patients with schizophrenia in the ENIGMA dataset. Mol Psychiatry. 2024;29:3086–96.
24. Goodkind M, Eickhoff SB, Oathes DJ, et al. Identification of a common neurobiological substrate for mental illness. JAMA Psychiatry. 2015;72:305–15.
25. McCutcheon RA, Pillinger T, Guo X, et al. Shared and separate patterns in brain morphometry across transdiagnostic dimensions. Nat Ment Health. 2023;1:55–65.
26. Lawrie SM, Whalley H, Kestelman JN, et al. Magnetic resonance imaging of brain in people at high risk of developing schizophrenia. Lancet. 1999;353:30–3.
27. Pantelis C, Velakoulis D, McGorry PD, et al. Neuroanatomical abnormalities before and after onset of psychosis: a cross-sectional and longitudinal MRI comparison. Lancet. 2003;361:281–8.
28. Boos HB, Aleman A, Cahn W, Hulshoff Pol H, Kahn RS. Brain volumes in relatives of patients with schizophrenia: a meta-analysis. Arch Gen Psychiatry. 2007;64:297–304.
29. Luna LP, Radua J, Fortea L, et al. A systematic review and meta-analysis of structural and functional brain alterations in individuals with genetic and clinical high-risk for psychosis and bipolar disorder. Prog Neuro-Psychopharmacol Biol Psychiatry. 2022;117:110540.
30. de Zwarte SMC, Brouwer RM, Agartz I, et al. The association between familial risk and brain abnormalities is disease specific: an ENIGMA-relatives study of schizophrenia and bipolar disorder. Biol Psychiatry. 2019;86:545–56.
31. Fortea A, Batalla A, Radua J, et al. Cortical gray matter reduction precedes transition to psychosis in individuals at clinical high-risk for psychosis: a voxel-based meta-analysis. Schizophr Res. 2021;232:98–106.
32. ENIGMA Clinical High Risk for Psychosis Working Group. Association of structural magnetic resonance imaging measures with psychosis onset in individuals at clinical high risk for developing psychosis: an ENIGMA working group mega-analysis. JAMA Psychiatr. 2021;78:753–66.
33. Olabi B, Ellison-Wright I, McIntosh AM, Wood SJ, Bullmore E, Lawrie SM. Are there progressive brain changes in schizophrenia? A meta-analysis of structural magnetic resonance imaging studies. Biol Psychiatry. 2011;70:88–96.
34. Vita A, De Peri L, Deste G, Sacchetti E. Progressive loss of cortical gray matter in schizophrenia: a meta-analysis and meta-regression of longitudinal MRI studies. Transl Psychiatry. 2012;2:e190.
35. Harrison PJ, Freemantle N, Geddes JR. Meta-analysis of brain weight in schizophrenia. Schizophr Res. 2003;64:25–34.
36. Roeske MJ, Konradi C, Heckers S, Lewis AS. Hippocampal volume and hippocampal neuron density, number and size in schizophrenia: a systematic review and meta-analysis of postmortem studies. Mol Psychiatry. 2021;26:3524–35.
37. Berdenis van Berlekom A, Muflihah CH, et al. Synapse pathology in schizophrenia: a meta-analysis of postsynaptic elements in postmortem brain studies. Schizophr Bull. 2020;46:374–86.
38. Bennett MR. Schizophrenia: susceptibility genes, dendritic-spine pathology and gray matter loss. Prog Neurobiol. 2011;95:275–300.
39. Lazari A, Lipp I. Can MRI measure myelin? Systematic review, qualitative assessment, and meta-analysis of studies validating microstructural imaging with myelin histology. NeuroImage. 2021;230:117744.
40. Lim KO, Hedehus M, Moseley M, de Crespigny A, Sullivan EV, Pfefferbaum A. Compromised white matter tract integrity in schizophrenia inferred from diffusion tensor imaging. Arch Gen Psychiatry. 1999;56:367–74.
41. Agartz I, Andersson JL, Skare S. Abnormal brain white matter in schizophrenia: a diffusion tensor imaging study. Neuroreport. 2001;12:2251–4.

42. Burns J, Job D, Bastin ME, Whalley H, Macgillivray T, Johnstone EC, Lawrie SM. Structural disconnectivity in schizophrenia: a diffusion tensor magnetic resonance imaging study. Br J Psychiatry. 2003;182:439–43.
43. Kubicki M, Westin CF, Nestor PG, et al. Cingulate fasciculus integrity disruption in schizophrenia: a magnetic resonance diffusion tensor imaging study. Biol Psychiatry. 2003;54:1171–80.
44. Zhao G, Lau WKW, Wang C, et al. A comparative multimodal meta-analysis of anisotropy and volume abnormalities in white matter in people suffering from bipolar disorder or schizophrenia. Schizophr Bull. 2022;48:69–79.
45. Geoffroy PA, Houenou J, Duhamel A, et al. The Arcuate Fasciculus in auditory-verbal hallucinations: a meta-analysis of diffusion-tensor-imaging studies. Schizophr Res. 2014;159:234–7.
46. Kelly S, Jahanshad N, Zalesky A, et al. Widespread white matter microstructural differences in schizophrenia across 4322 individuals: results from the ENIGMA Schizophrenia DTI Working Group. Mol Psychiatry. 2018;23:1261–9.
47. Holleran L, Kelly S, Alloza C, et al. The relationship between White matter microstructure and general cognitive ability in patients with schizophrenia and healthy participants in the ENIGMA consortium. Am J Psychiatry. 2020;177:537–47.
48. Xu M, Zhang W, Hochwalt P, et al. Structural connectivity associated with familial risk for mental illness: a meta-analysis of diffusion tensor imaging studies in relatives of patients with severe mental disorders. Hum Brain Mapp. 2022;43:2936–50.
49. Waszczuk K, Rek-Owodziń K, Tyburski E, Mak M, Misiak B, Samochowiec J. Disturbances in White matter integrity in the ultra-high-risk psychosis state-a systematic review. J Clin Med. 2021;10:2515.
50. Parsaei M, Sheipouri A, Partovifar P, et al. Diffusion magnetic resonance imaging for treatment response prediction in schizophrenia spectrum disorders: a systematic review. Psychiatry Res Neuroimaging. 2024;342:111841.
51. Kraguljac NV, Reid M, White D, et al. Neurometabolites in schizophrenia and bipolar disorder - a systematic review and meta-analysis. Psychiatry Res. 2012;203:111–25.
52. Whitehurst TS, Osugo M, Townsend L, et al. Proton magnetic resonance spectroscopy of N-acetyl aspartate in chronic schizophrenia, first episode of psychosis and high-risk of psychosis: a systematic review and meta-analysis. Neurosci Biobehav Rev. 2020;119:255–67.
53. Nakahara T, Tsugawa S, Noda Y, et al. Glutamatergic and GABAergic metabolite levels in schizophrenia-spectrum disorders: a meta-analysis of (1)H-magnetic resonance spectroscopy studies. Mol Psychiatry. 2022;27:744–57.
54. McCutcheon RA, Merritt K, Howes OD. Dopamine and glutamate in individuals at high risk for psychosis: a meta-analysis of in vivo imaging findings and their variability compared to controls. World Psychiatry. 2021;20:405–16.
55. Laruelle M, Abi-Dargham A, van Dyck CH, et al. Single photon emission computerized tomography imaging of amphetamine-induced dopamine release in drug-free schizophrenic subjects. Proc Natl Acad Sci USA. 1996;93:9235–40.
56. McCutcheon R, Beck K, Jauhar S, Howes OD. Defining the locus of dopaminergic dysfunction in schizophrenia: a meta-analysis and test of the mesolimbic hypothesis. Schizophr Bull. 2018;44:1301–11.
57. Jauhar S, Nour MM, Veronese M, et al. A test of the transdiagnostic dopamine hypothesis of psychosis using positron emission tomographic imaging in bipolar affective disorder and schizophrenia. JAMA Psychiatry. 2017;74:1206–13.
58. Husain MO, Jones B, Arshad U, et al. A systematic review and meta-analysis of neuroimaging studies examining synaptic density in individuals with psychotic spectrum disorders. BMC Psychiatry. 2024;24:460.
59. Marques TR, Ashok AH, Pillinger T, et al. Neuroinflammation in schizophrenia: meta-analysis of in vivo microglial imaging studies. Psychol Med. 2019;49:2186–96.
60. Egerton A, Modinos G, Ferrera D, McGuire P. Neuroimaging studies of GABA in schizophrenia: a systematic review with meta-analysis. Transl Psychiatry. 2017;7:e1147.

61. Ingvar DH, Franzén G. Distribution of cerebral activity in chronic schizophrenia. Lancet. 1974;2(7895):1484–6.
62. Buchsbaum MS, DeLisi LE, Holcomb HH, et al. Anteroposterior gradients in cerebral glucose use in schizophrenia and affective disorders. Arch Gen Psychiatry. 1984;41:1159–66.
63. Weinberger DR, Berman KF, Zec RF. Physiologic dysfunction of dorsolateral prefrontal cortex in schizophrenia. I. Regional cerebral blood flow evidence. Arch Gen Psychiatry. 1986;43:114–24.
64. Frith CD, Friston KJ, Herold S, et al. Regional brain activity in chronic schizophrenic patients during the performance of a verbal fluency task. Br J Psychiatry. 1995;167:343–9.
65. Fletcher PC, McKenna PJ, Frith CD, Grasby PM, Friston KJ, Dolan RJ. Brain activations in schizophrenia during a graded memory task studied with functional neuroimaging. Arch Gen Psychiatry. 1998;55:1001–8.
66. Hill K, Mann L, Laws KR, Stephenson CM, Nimmo-Smith I, McKenna PJ. Hypofrontality in schizophrenia: a meta-analysis of functional imaging studies. Acta Psychiatr Scand. 2004;110:243–56.
67. Townsend L, Pillinger T, Selvaggi P, Veronese M, Turkheimer F, Howes O. Brain glucose metabolism in schizophrenia: a systematic review and meta-analysis of (18)FDG-PET studies in schizophrenia. Psychol Med. 2023;53:4880–97.
68. Ragland JD, Laird AR, Ranganath C, Blumenfeld RS, Gonzales SM, Glahn DC. Prefrontal activation deficits during episodic memory in schizophrenia. Am J Psychiatry. 2009;166:863–74.
69. Hall J, Whalley HC, McKirdy JW, et al. Overactivation of fear systems to neutral faces in schizophrenia. Biol Psychiatry. 2008;64:70–3.
70. Dugré JR, Bitar N, Dumais A, Potvin S. Limbic hyperactivity in response to emotionally neutral stimuli in schizophrenia: a neuroimaging meta-analysis of the hypervigilant mind. Am J Psychiatry. 2019;176:1021–9.
71. Dong D, Wang Y, Jia X, et al. Abnormal brain activation during threatening face processing in schizophrenia: a meta-analysis of functional neuroimaging studies. Schizophr Res. 2018;197:200–8.
72. Vucurovic K, Caillies S, Kaladjian A. Neural correlates of theory of mind and empathy in schizophrenia: an activation likelihood estimation meta-analysis. J Psychiatr Res. 2020;120:163–74.
73. Murray GK, Corlett PR, Clark L, et al. Substantia nigra/ventral tegmental reward prediction error disruption in psychosis. Mol Psychiatry. 2008;13:239, 267–76.
74. Radua J, Schmidt A, Borgwardt S, et al. Ventral striatal activation during reward processing in psychosis: a neurofunctional meta-analysis. JAMA Psychiatr. 2015;72:1243–51.
75. Yang X, Song Y, Zou Y, Li Y, Zeng J. Neural correlates of prediction error in patients with schizophrenia: evidence from an fMRI meta-analysis. Cereb Cortex. 2025;34:bhad471.
76. Whalley HC, Steele JD, Mukherjee P, et al. Connecting the brain and new drug targets for schizophrenia. Curr Pharm Des. 2009;15:2615–31.
77. Brandl F, Avram M, Weise B, et al. Specific substantial dysconnectivity in schizophrenia: a transdiagnostic multimodal meta-analysis of resting-state functional and structural magnetic resonance imaging studies. Biol Psychiatry. 2019;85:573–83.
78. McGuire PK, Shah GM, Murray RM. Increased blood flow in Broca's area during auditory hallucinations in schizophrenia. Lancet. 1993;342:703–6.
79. McGuire PK, Silbersweig DA, Wright I, et al. Abnormal monitoring of inner speech: a physiological basis for auditory hallucinations. Lancet. 1995;346:596–600.
80. Silbersweig DA, Stern E, Frith C, et al. A functional neuroanatomy of hallucinations in schizophrenia. Nature. 1995;378:176–9.
81. Shergill SS, Brammer MJ, Williams SC, Murray RM, McGuire PK. Mapping auditory hallucinations in schizophrenia using functional magnetic resonance imaging. Arch Gen Psychiatry. 2000;57:1033–8.
82. Zmigrod L, Garrison JR, Carr J, Simons JS. The neural mechanisms of hallucinations: a quantitative meta-analysis of neuroimaging studies. Neurosci Biobehav Rev. 2016;69:113–23.

83. Goghari VM, Sponheim SR, MacDonald AW 3rd. The functional neuroanatomy of symptom dimensions in schizophrenia: a qualitative and quantitative review of a persistent question. Neurosci Biobehav Rev. 2010;34(3):468–86.
84. Dudina AN, Tomyshev AS, Ilina EV, Romanov DV, Lebedeva IS. Structural and functional alterations in different types of delusions across schizophrenia spectrum: a systematic review. Prog Neuro-Psychopharmacol Biol Psychiatry. 2025;136:111185.
85. Whalley HC, Simonotto E, Marshall I, et al. Functional disconnectivity in subjects at high genetic risk of schizophrenia. Brain. 2005;128:2097–108.
86. Voineskos AN, Hawco C, Neufeld NH, et al. Functional magnetic resonance imaging in schizophrenia: current evidence, methodological advances, limitations and future directions. World Psychiatry. 2024;23:26–51.
87. Whalley HC, Sussmann JE, Chakirova G, et al. The neural basis of familial risk and temperamental variation in individuals at high risk of bipolar disorder. Biol Psychiatry. 2011;70:343–9.
88. McTeague LM, Huemer J, Carreon DM, Jiang Y, Eickhoff SB, Etkin A. Identification of common neural circuit disruptions in cognitive control across psychiatric disorders. Am J Psychiatry. 2017;174:676–85.
89. Sprooten E, Rasgon A, Goodman M, et al. Addressing reverse inference in psychiatric neuroimaging: meta-analyses of task-related brain activation in common mental disorders. Hum Brain Mapp. 2017;38:1846–64.
90. Li A, Zalesky A, Yue W, et al. A neuroimaging biomarker for striatal dysfunction in schizophrenia. Nat Med. 2020;26:558–65.
91. Bennett CM, Baird AA, Miller MB, Wolford GL. Neural correlates of interspecies perspective taking in the post-mortem Atlantic salmon: an argument for proper multiple comparisons correction. J Serendipitous Unexpected Results. 2009;1:1–5.
92. Botvinik-Nezer R, Holzmeister F, Camerer CF, et al. Variability in the analysis of a single neuroimaging dataset by many teams. Nature. 2020;582:84–8.
93. Tofts P. Quantitative MRI of the brain: measuring changes caused by disease. Wiley; 2003.
94. Jardri R, Pouchet A, Pins D, Thomas P. Cortical activations during auditory verbal hallucinations in schizophrenia: a coordinate-based meta-analysis. Am J Psychiatry. 2011;168:73–81.
95. Andreassen OA, Hindley GFL, Frei O, Smeland OB. New insights from the last decade of research in psychiatric genetics: discoveries, challenges and clinical implications. World Psychiatry. 2023;22:4–24.
96. Costas-Carrera A, Garcia-Rizo C, Bitanihirwe B, Penadés R. Obstetric complications and brain imaging in schizophrenia: a systematic review. Biol Psychiatry Cogn Neurosci Neuroimaging. 2020;5:1077–84.
97. Cancel A, Dallel S, Zine A, El-Hage W, Fakra E. Understanding the link between childhood trauma and schizophrenia: a systematic review of neuroimaging studies. Neurosci Biobehav Rev. 2019;107:492–504.
98. Navarri X, Afzali MH, Lavoie J, et al. How do substance use disorders compare to other psychiatric conditions on structural brain abnormalities? A cross-disorder meta-analytic comparison using the ENIGMA consortium findings. Hum Brain Mapp. 2022;43:399–413.
99. Boer OD, El Marroun H, Muetzel RL. Adolescent substance use initiation and long-term neurobiological outcomes: insights, challenges and opportunities. Mol Psychiatry. 2024;29:2211–22.
100. Avishai-Eliner S, Brunson KL, Sandman CA, Baram TZ. Stressed-out, or in (utero)? Trends Neurosci. 2002;25:518–24.
101. Thanaraju A, Marzuki AA, Chan JK, et al. Structural and functional brain correlates of socioeconomic status across the life span: a systematic review. Neurosci Biobehav Rev. 2024;162:105716.
102. Winter A, Gruber M, Thiel K, et al. Shared and distinct structural brain networks related to childhood maltreatment and social support: connectome-based predictive modeling. Mol Psychiatry. 2023;28:4613–21.

103. Tozzi L, Garczarek L, Janowitz D, et al. Interactive impact of childhood maltreatment, depression, and age on cortical brain structure: mega-analytic findings from a large multi-site cohort. Psychol Med. 2020;50:1020–31.
104. Alex AM, Aguate F, Botteron K, et al. A global multicohort study to map subcortical brain development and cognition in infancy and early childhood. Nat Neurosci. 2024;27:176–86.
105. Fusar-Poli P, Smieskova R, Kempton MJ, Ho BC, Andreasen NC, Borgwardt S. Progressive brain changes in schizophrenia related to antipsychotic treatment? A meta-analysis of longitudinal MRI studies. Neurosci Biobehav Rev. 2013;37:1680–91.
106. Zhu Y, Maikusa N, Radua J, Sämann PG, et al. Using brain structural neuroimaging measures to predict psychosis onset for individuals at clinical high-risk. Mol Psychiatry. 2024;29:1465–77.
107. Di Camillo F, Grimaldi DA, Cattarinussi G, et al. Magnetic resonance imaging-based machine learning classification of schizophrenia spectrum disorders: a meta-analysis. Psychiatry Clin Neurosci. 2024;78:732–43.
108. Porter A, Fei S, Damme KSF, Nusslock R, Gratton C, Mittal VA. A meta-analysis and systematic review of single vs. multimodal neuroimaging techniques in the classification of psychosis. Mol Psychiatry. 2023;28:3278–92.
109. Schmidt A, Cappucciati M, Radua J, et al. Improving prognostic accuracy in subjects at clinical high risk for psychosis: systematic review of predictive models and meta-analytical sequential testing simulation. Schizophr Bull. 2017;43:375–88.
110. Mouchlianitis E, McCutcheon R, Howes OD. Brain-imaging studies of treatment-resistant schizophrenia: a systematic review. Lancet Psychiatry. 2016;3:451–63.
111. Gao Z, Xiao Y, Zhu F, Tao B, Yu W, Lui S. The whole-brain connectome landscape in patients with schizophrenia: a systematic review and meta-analysis of graph theoretical characteristics. Neurosci Biobehav Rev. 2023;148:105144.
112. Georgiadis F, Larivière S, Glahn D, et al. Connectome architecture shapes large-scale cortical alterations in schizophrenia: a worldwide ENIGMA study. Mol Psychiatry. 2024;29:1869–81.
113. Crossley NA, Mechelli A, Ginestet C, Rubinov M, Bullmore ET, McGuire P. Altered hub functioning and compensatory activations in the connectome: a meta-analysis of functional neuroimaging studies in schizophrenia. Schizophr Bull. 2016;42:434–42.
114. Kambeitz J, Kambeitz-Ilankovic L, et al. Aberrant functional whole-brain network architecture in patients with schizophrenia: a meta-analysis. Schizophr Bull. 2016;42(Suppl 1):S13–21.
115. Munafò MR, Nosek BA, Bishop DVM, et al. A manifesto for reproducible science. Nat Hum Behav. 2017;1:0021.

Open Access This chapter is licensed under the terms of the Creative Commons Attribution 4.0 International License (http://creativecommons.org/licenses/by/4.0/), which permits use, sharing, adaptation, distribution and reproduction in any medium or format, as long as you give appropriate credit to the original author(s) and the source, provide a link to the Creative Commons license and indicate if changes were made.

The images or other third party material in this chapter are included in the chapter's Creative Commons license, unless indicated otherwise in a credit line to the material. If material is not included in the chapter's Creative Commons license and your intended use is not permitted by statutory regulation or exceeds the permitted use, you will need to obtain permission directly from the copyright holder.

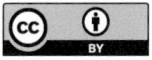

Part III

Psychiatric Diagnosis: Concepts and Challenges

This part examines relevant developments in relation to psychiatric diagnosis both from more narrowly empirical positive scientific and more socially critical points of view. His own late doubts notwithstanding, Kraepelin's early and determined insistence on discrete diagnostic entities and his distinction between schizophrenia and manic depression are perhaps his most enduring legacies in psychiatry and its lasting controversies.

Chapter 8 offers a deep and broad review of conceptual and empirical issues in relation to the diagnosis of schizophrenia. Chapter 9 returns to evolutionary biology and explores both the cognitive advantages and social disadvantages related to the clinical features required to diagnose autism spectrum disorders. It also refers to controversies regarding neurodiversity and its relationship to these diagnoses. Chapter 10 attends to the discriminatory risks arising for citizens from psychiatric diagnoses. It highlights the dialectical relation between psychiatric theories and social and group phenomena and illustrates the catastrophic risks that materialised in the work of Austrian psychiatrist Hans Asperger in relation to autism, especially what came to be called Asperger's Syndrome at one point. Chapter 11 examines an alternative, philosophically well informed and socially inclusive psychiatric tradition which developed in France, namely 'Institutional Psychotherapy'. Chapter 12 details the nature and evolution of the new social movement of Mad Studies and the challenges it brings to psychiatry, including but not limited to diagnosis.

From Dementia Praecox to Autoimmune Psychosis: Diagnostic Challenges of the Schizophrenias

8

Jesus Ramirez-Bermudez and Awais Aftab

8.1 The History of Schizophrenia: A Panoramic View of the Conceptual Problems

A theoretical understanding of schizophrenia must address issues around the historical evolution and the ontological status of this medical construct. If schizophrenia is a brain disease, or even a collection of diseases with clinical similarities, and thus can be regarded as a natural kind, a historical approach should be able to uncover descriptions of cases where the clinical pattern presented itself to human societies throughout history. In his conceptual history of schizophrenia, German E. Berrios refers to this perspective as the 'continuity hypothesis'. This hypothesis suggests that schizophrenia has always existed and that psychiatrists gradually recognised its pattern during the nineteenth and twentieth centuries, with incremental refinements leading to the current clinical definition, as outlined by organisations such as the World Health Organisation and the American Psychiatric Association [1]. This view could be regarded as a strong form of naturalism [2]. However, Berrios also proposes a 'discontinuity thesis', according to which there is insufficient conceptual continuity between the foundational work of figures like Morel, Kraepelin, Bleuler, and Schneider. According to the discontinuity thesis, 'schizophrenia is *not* the result of one definition and one object of inquiry successively studied by various psychiatric teams but a patchwork made out of clinical features plucked from different definitions' [1]. The construction of the schizophrenia concept can be described as the history of a set of research programmes running in

J. Ramirez-Bermudez (✉)
Neuropsychiatry Unit, National Institute of Neurology and Neurosurgery, Mexico City, Mexico

A. Aftab
Department of Psychiatry, Case Western Reserve University School of Medicine, Cleveland, OH, USA

© The Author(s) 2026
G. Ikkos, T. Becker (eds.), *Psychiatry after Kraepelin*,
https://doi.org/10.1007/978-3-032-09475-9_8

parallel, rather than having a linear progression, as each of these programs was based on a different concept of disease, mental symptoms, and mental functioning.

The discontinuity thesis is inconsistent with the idea of schizophrenia as a *natural kind*. If this is true, what are the ontological implications? Although a range of theoretical positions are available, we can simplify them as two varieties of constructivism. A strong constructionist thesis posits that a social process creates the notion of 'schizophrenia' entirely, without reflecting any objective clinical pattern that pre-exists the construct [3]. This form of constructionism is endorsed by critics of psychiatry such as Thomas Szasz, who regards schizophrenia as the 'sacred symbol of psychiatry'—a means of social control artificially constructed by psychiatrists, rather than a legitimate medical diagnosis corresponding to an actual health condition [1]. This view can also be regarded as a strong normativism [2]. Here, schizophrenia is taken as a theoretical fiction. But other theorists, such as Kenneth Kendler and Peter Zachar, also consider a moderate form of constructionism [3]. In this view, schizophrenia is a cluster of clinical and neurobiological features, whose manner of recognition is determined in part by historical and sociocultural factors, and which can be regarded as a practical kind allowing for clinical decision making and scientific research. The concept has a significant amount of coherence, scientific meaning, and a significant part of its referents are real, recognisable, and relatively stable objects of inquiry, but the construct lacks an essence. The clinical phenotype of schizophrenia shows associations with various validators (such as family history, genetics, premorbid development, course of illness, and treatment response) [4] but these associations lack specificity (they overlap with other clinical phenotypes such as bipolar disorder), don't point towards a distinct disease entity, and the phenotype lacks precision, resulting in an excessive number of borderline cases and a heterogeneous population of patients who exhibit varying degrees of resemblance to the clinical prototype.

In this text, we aim to keep in mind the tension between the continuity and the discontinuity hypotheses, and their significance to the epistemology and ontology of schizophrenia. We will provide a historical narrative of the concept, from the earlier conceptions of psychosis, and into the birth of the word 'schizophrenia'. We will deal with the changes in the understanding of the clinical phenomenology and the current challenges to the scientific model. Finally, we will deal with the differential diagnosis, which will lead us to consider the concepts of 'secondary schizophrenia' and 'schizophrenia-like psychosis'. At this point, the problem of autoimmune psychosis and its scientific implications will be considered.

8.2   The Genealogy of the Concept of Psychosis

The Hippocratic tradition outlined five categories foundational to the later emergence of modern psychopathology: phrenitis, lethargy, mania, melancholia, and paranoia. Of these, phrenitis is most relevant to the conceptual ancestry of psychosis. Though the etymology of 'schizophrenia' traces back to *phren*, originally thought to denote the seat of reason, its anatomical referent shifted over time from mind to diaphragm [5]. The term *phrenitis*, combining *phren* with the disease-indicating suffix -*itis*, remained in use to describe acute mental disturbances accompanied by fever—characterised by hallucinations, delirious states, loss of sleep, 'wandering talk', 'irrational talk'; patients are described as 'out of their minds', rambling, laughing, singing, with no power to restrain themselves, sometimes transitioning into a coma state and death [5].

In Roman medicine, *delirium* emerged as a synonym, retaining an emphasis on fever-induced mental disarray. The classical reference for this term was written by Celsus [6]. The term *phrenitis* was still used in the nineteenth century by some European authors. *Delirium* was the more successful term, and it persists in the modern medical taxonomies. While melancholia and mania have garnered extensive historical-philosophical analysis, phrenitis and delirium have remained on the periphery. Yet, as Berrios notes, they are crucial to the conceptual lineage of psychosis. Asclepiades distinguished *furor mentis*—madness as chronic delirium without fever—from acute febrile states, reserving *phrenitis* for the latter [7]. This distinction would prove durable. In the early nineteenth century, European terms for madness—*folie, pazzia, locura, Wahnsinn*—began to give way to the more technical *psychosis* [8]. But prior to its medical formalisation, alienists relied on terms like insanity, alienation, and dementia. Locke's seventeenth-century redefinition of insanity as a disruption of rational coherence laid the groundwork for later conceptions. Pinel's 1801 taxonomy of *aliénation mentale* included mania (generalised delusion), melancholy (partial delusion), idiocy (obliteration of faculties), and dementia (loss of intellect) [9].

By the mid-nineteenth century, the term *psychosis* was used by Ernst von Feuchtersleben to encapsulate disorders such as insanity, fixed delusions, and idiocy [10]. Psychosis was conceptualised as a chronic analogue to delirium—delusions and hallucinations without fever. Feuchtersleben reiterated this point directly: 'acute delirium with fever must be distinguished from the chronic variety which is called insanity' [11]. This was less an innovation than a revival of Stoic and Asclepiadean insights. The eventual split between 'organic' and 'functional' psychoses would anchor psychiatric taxonomies for the next century [8].

In 1810, John Haslam published *Illustrations of Madness*, detailing the case of James Tilly Mathews. Often cited as the first clinical account resembling schizophrenia, Mathews' story predated the term by nearly a century. A tea merchant detained during the French Revolution, Mathews claimed he was targeted by a gang employing a mind-controlling device powered by 'pneumatic chemistry'. The machine, he said, enabled silent cerebral speech and forced facial expressions through the manipulation of magnetic fluids [12]. Mathews' delusions—chronic, bizarre and systematised—bear striking resemblance to the modern schizophrenia prototype: persecutory ideation, thought insertion, and auditory hallucinations. Any retrospective diagnosis must be approached cautiously. It cannot be stated with certainty that schizophrenia would be the correct diagnosis for Mathews. Still, the case appears emblematic of a clinical pattern that psychiatry would eventually name and formalise.

8.3   On the Construction of Dementia Praecox

The nineteenth century was rich in descriptions of patients who were hospitalised in the European asylums and suffered from severe mental illness. The old terms, like mental alienation, the insanities and the vesanic dementias, were gradually substituted by the emerging concepts: *'maladies mentales'* (Esquirol), monomania, *délire de persecutions* (Lasegue), *délire de negations* (Cotard), *délire hallucinatoire*, *délire d'interpretation* [13]. At the end of the century, before Kraepelin's shaping of dementia praecox, Valentin Magnan and Paul Sérioux developed the notion of a 'chronic delusion with systematic evolution (*Le délire chronique a ´volution Systématique*). This concept, reported in 1892, included four stages: (1) incubation (characterised by a delusional mood), (2) crystallisation of the delusion of persecution, (3) emergence of delusions of grandeur, and (4) dementia. The analysis of the cases has resemblances to what later on were called schizophrenia, psychotic depression and delusional disorder [13]. Philippe Chaslin developed the concept of systematised vs incoherent delusions. The best example of systematised delusions could be seen in cases of paranoia. Incoherent delusions could be related to intellectual disability of dementia [13]. This panoramic view of the pre-Kraepelinian era reveals a vibrant landscape of emerging concepts.

The construction of dementia praecox was built on Kraepelin's own observations, but also with the previous studies of Kahlbaum and his student, Hecker. Between 1868 and 1874, the German psychiatrist Karl Kahlbaum described a syndrome relevant to the history of the schizophrenia construct: catatonia. According to Kahlbaum, it is 'a state in which the patient sits quietly or completely mute, motionless, without anything causing them to change position, appearing to be absorbed in the contemplation of an object, with their eyes fixed on a distant point, and without any apparent volition, without any reaction to sensory impressions' [14]. Some patients progressed to intellectual deterioration, while others experienced remarkable recoveries. Kahlbaum suggested to classify these cases as having a catatonic vesania or madness of tension [15]. Wernicke supported Kahlbaum's concept of catatonia, but suggested the term 'akinetic motility psychosis' to characterise the syndrome, which, in his view, was caused by a disruption of a psychomotor path [16].

Kahlbaum emphasised the presence of 'epileptiform and choreiform tonic or clonic convulsions' [16]. This suggests neurological causes in some of his patients. Today, we know that autoimmune encephalitis (e.g. NMDA receptor encephalitis) can cause catatonia, seizures, dyskinesia, and psychosis [14, 17–19]. It is reasonable to hypothesise that at least some of the patients described by Kahlbaum as having catatonia would not meet current diagnostic criteria for schizophrenia.

Kahlbaum's taxonomy included mental disorders affecting only special psychological functions: he used the term 'partial or special psychoses' to describe these cases, exemplified by dysthymia and paranoia. On the other hand, he included mental disorders affecting all psychological functions: total or complex psychoses, represented by typical madness (typical vesania), general paresis of the insane, and tensional or tonic madness (catatonia). When classifying mental illnesses, Kahlbaum stressed that some mental disorders can also be related to specific developmental periods. One of his students, Ewald Hecker, described in 1871 seven cases of a new entity, 'hebephrenia', which started during adolescence. In his monograph, Hecker clarifies that he cared for 500 patients in a 4-year period, collecting 14 patients with the hebephrenia pattern. The report only includes 7 cases (2 women) whose symptoms started between 17 and 23 years. Hecker analyses the precipitating factors, their psychopathology, and the temporal course of the illness [20]. He included letters written by the patients, which allowed for an analysis of thought disturbances. These were chronic cases of adolescents with intellectual deterioration and eccentricities in speech and behaviour [20].

In 1899, Emil Kraepelin proposed the existence of a clinical entity that included Hecker's hebephrenia, Kahlbaum's catatonia, and a third syndrome, 'paranoid dementia', described by him, and characterised by a chronic pattern of hallucinations and delusions. According to Kraepelin, young people with these syndromes shared a common fate: the significant deterioration of cognitive functions. He called this *dementia praecox* [1]. The term *démence précoce* had been used in French by Benedict Morel in 1860 as a way to describe the behaviours of some patients; it was not a formal clinical entity like Kraepelin's *dementia praecox*. Kraepelin admired botany, and his brother Karl was a specialist in the taxonomy of arachnids. Influenced by this, Kraepelin used Latin to name the new clinical entity, as if he were a botanist [21]. Here, we summarise his final perspective, according to the fourth edition of his 1921 *Introduction to Clinical Psychiatry* (*Einführung indie Psychiatrische Klinik*). According to the excellent article by Kenneth Kendler entitled *Kraepelin's Final Views on Dementia Praecox* [22], Kraepelin states that:

1. Dementia praecox was a common disorder in psychiatric asylums: 'The greatest number of uncured patients who accumulate in insane asylums are dementia praecox sufferers' [22].
2. The global psychopathological pattern is 'characterised by more or less advanced disintegration of the mental personality with predominating emotional and volitional disturbances' [22].
3. The pattern has an early onset: 'Dementia praecox as a rule starts in youth, most frequently in the third decade, exceptionally already in childhood…In later years, the illness occurs more rarely' [22].
4. A family pattern is common: 'Often a number of members in a family are afflicted in a similar way' [22].
5. The prodromal phase is important: 'there gradually develops, more rarely rapidly, a transformation of nature, with erratic, idiosyncratic, withdrawn, agitated behaviour' [22].
6. Hallucinatory and delusional symptoms are common in the early phases: 'In many cases hallucinations begin, especially auditory hallucinations, but also of the other senses, with delusional ideas linked to these, above all with a hostile or hypochondriacal content, but later also with a pleasurable content' [22].

7. Thought disorder is frequent: 'The train of thought can initially remain ordered, but later in many cases displays leaps, becomes disjointed, sometimes reaches complete incoherence' [22].

8. The reduction in affective reactions is pervasive, as well as the decline in spontaneous cognitive and goal directed behaviour (the so called negative symptoms): 'Soon the weakening of emotional reactions is very conspicuous, with dull apathy, indifference toward relatives, the environment, their own fate, loss of mental activity, inattentiveness, silence about wishes, hopes, fears' [22].

9. The reduction in psychomotor and interpersonal reactivity can be severe: 'Self-evident and everyday reactions (looking up when spoken to, taking an outstretched hand, answering a greeting, avoiding or defending against a threat) are absent'. In some cases, catatonic signs appear: 'automatism, the limp submission to external influences, the long maintenance of an applied posture (*flexibilitas cerea*), the repetition of words (*echolalia*), the imitation of movements (*echopraxia*)… especially important is the negativism, the impulsive, senseless resistance toward any influence'. 'Sometimes less pronounced disturbances of action are stereotypy …and the mannered behaviour, incorrect convolution and alteration of simple actions...' [22].

10. According to Kraepelin, the loosening of associations explains terms such as 'schizophrenia' and 'intra-psychic ataxia', and the experiences of control of their own will are common, often with a delusional interpretation. 'Often the patients themselves are aware of the feeling of inner lack of freedom, the dependence of thinking and actions on foreign influences, however, which then are interpreted as being due to persecution by means of telepathic and hypnotic effects' [22].

11. The most reliable subtypes of dementia praecox are dementia simplex, hebephrenic dementia, depressive dementia, an agitated and circular form, catatonia or 'tension insanity', and dementia paranoides.

12. The functional and psychopathological outcome is variable, often with a chronic, severe disability, but with some cases with complete recovery and frequent cases with moderate disability: 'The overwhelming majority of pronounced cases of illness end in chronic mental infirmity, often of a high degree (permanent need for institutionalisation). Whether full, enduring recovery occurs in some cases is uncertain, but it cannot be denied with regard to a reliably observed improvement which resembles recovery and has lasted for more than a decade. Often the degree of change brought about by the illness remains moderate' [22].

It has been postulated that Kraepelin's evidence for unifying hebephrenia, catatonia, and paranoid dementia was insufficient. However, the concept of *dementia praecox* was decisive, giving rise to the idea that there were paranoid, catatonic, and hebephrenic forms of the same illness [1].

8.4   Schizophrenia: The Neologism

While Emil Kraepelin was establishing a psychopathological synthesis, something interesting was happening in Vienna: Dr. Sigmund Freud abandoned his neurophysiological research. After attending Charcot's lectures in Paris, he laid the foundations of psychoanalysis through *The Interpretation of Dreams*, *The Psychopathology of Everyday Life*, and *Three Essays on the Theory of Sexuality*. Freud developed the method of free association, believing, unlike Jean-Martin Charcot, that a reliance on hypnosis was unnecessary. Influenced by Freud, Carl Gustav Jung developed a similar but more structured test, the 'word association test', while he worked with Eugen Bleuler. The doctor would present lists of words and ask the patient to say the first response that came to mind. Jung assessed the semantic content of the response, as well as physiological variables and reaction times [23]. Freud and Jung's work on the association of ideas and words was instrumental in the development of the concept of schizophrenia, which explicitly built upon Kraepelin's *dementia praecox* [23]. In 1908, Bleuler publicly coined the neologism 'schizophrenia', which means 'division (or split) of the mind' [24]. To justify this etymological choice, he wrote: 'I call it schizophrenia rather than *dementia praecox* because the splitting of psychic functions is one of its most important characteristics' [1]. To explain the meaning of this statement, Bleuler referred to the severe disturbance in associative processes: 'In all schizophrenic forms, even the mildest, we find a specific disturbance of thought, characterised by a looseness of normal associations' [25]. In this way, it can be said that Bleuler relied on the psychological framework of associationism coming from John Locke, interpreted with the resources of the new psychoanalytical theory, but also with the concepts of dissociation coming from the French psychologist, Pierre Janet, and Jung's word association test [26]. The first academic thesis dedicated to schizophrenia, directed by Bleuler, was entitled *On the Psychological Content of a Case of Schizophrenia (Dementia Praecox)*. It was presented in 1911 by Sabina Spielrein, and it highlights the psychoanalytical influence on the early framing of the schizophrenia concept.

Along with the loose association of ideas, Dr. Bleuler affirmed the existence of other cardinal symptoms: 'In the affective sphere, we observe in severe cases a problem that can be very pronounced: for years, not a single sign of emotion is observed' [25]. Clinicians refer to this as 'affective flattening'. Sometimes, even the instinct of self-preservation is impaired: 'In the case of a fire, patients remain motionless amid the flames and will let the fire burn them if no one comes to their aid' [25]. He described a third cardinal sign: autism. In the early twentieth century, this word did not refer to the verbal communication problems and social reciprocity issues later observed in children by Leo Kanner and Hans Asperger (Eds: see Chaps. 9 and 10). 'Autism' was simply a verbal formula used to indicate that the patient's attention, intentionality, and affectivity were directed inward, toward their private world of experiences; contact with the external world was inadequate and deficient [25].

Apparently, Bleuler was providing refined descriptions of the construct brought to light by Emil Kraepelin, *dementia praecox*, but he likely did something else: he synthesised ideas from different paradigms into a psychopathological metaphor. It has been said that the Swiss master seemed destined to act as a mediator between opposing schools: on one hand, Kraepelin's biological psychiatry, and on the other hand, Pierre Janet's concepts on dissociation and the psychoanalytic approach to the unconscious. Schizophrenia combined mental disturbance arising from a neuropathological disorder, and clinical phenomena that would have a psychodynamic explanation. According to Bleuler, the cardinal symptoms (loose associations, affective flattening, autism) were the result of well-defined anatomical-pathological abnormalities at the brain level, which are not observed in other psychoses [25].

Bleuler proposed the existence of 'secondary symptoms' that emerged as psychological reactions to the disturbing experience of the cardinal symptoms, similar to the defence mechanisms described by psychoanalysis. He stated that delusions and hallucinations were secondary reactions to the cardinal symptoms. Their content was shaped by the patient's desires and fears, which could be repressed and unconscious [25]. Bleuler's conceptualisation was not without the sexism characteristic of his time: 'In the schizophrenic woman, there is not a single delusional idea that is not essentially motivated by sexuality' [25].

The metaphor of a division, separation, split, rupture, or fragmentation of the mind was part of nineteenth-century romantic psychology and became a part of literary culture, as seen in Stevenson's story (*Dr. Jekyll and Mr. Hyde*). This metaphor, which its supporters took as a reality, also penetrated the realms of philosophy, psychoanalysis, and popular culture [1]. This largely explains the almost immediate acceptance of the clinical neologism; it was not just a point of convergence between biological psychiatry and psychoanalysis: it was also an articulation between academic culture and popular culture.

8.5 The Psychopathology of Schizophrenia: Phenomenological, Clinimetric and Neurocognitive Views

At the beginning of the twentieth century, Karl Jaspers, a doctor and philosopher—at the crossroads of phenomenology and existentialism—formulated an ambitious *General Psychopathology* and achieved a phenomenological description of delusions [13]. One of his students at the University of Heidelberg, Kurt Schneider, dedicated himself to the study of schizophrenia: following Bleuler, he conceptualised this disorder as the result of a triple psychological split: in the process of thought, in the development of voluntary activity, and in affective processes [27]. In a person without mental pathology, these psychological dimensions would be the pillars of an integrated sense of selfhood. In contrast, individuals diagnosed with schizophrenia suffered from the 'xenopathy' described by nineteenth-century French psychiatrists: experiencing their own mental activity as if it were foreign [28].

Schneider believed that certain symptoms could have special diagnostic value. These are known as nuclear symptoms, or first-rank symptoms, and they have been summarised as follows: [27, 29] (1) Delusional perception. (2) Thought echo or commentary. (3) Experiences of control and replacement of will, leading to delusions of control. (4) Thought insertion. (5) Thought withdrawal. (6) Thought broadcast. (7) Audioverbal hallucinations of voices that speak to each other and comment on the patient's actions. The hostile, devaluing quality of the hallucinatory messages prompted psychodynamic interpretations, which attribute the genesis of the phenomenon to problematic relationships with the parents and violent communication styles in early development. This conceptual line culminated in the double bind theory postulated by Gregory Bateson and colleagues in 1956. The 'double bind' refers to a style of communication in which a subject receives two or more conflicting messages as a form of control with covert coercion. Bateson postulated that the symptoms of schizophrenia were reactions to conflicting demands in which no matter what a person does, he 'can't win'. This can be particularly distressing in the context of early family relationships [30]. More recently, a large meta-analysis has shown significant associations between childhood adversity and the development of psychosis, with an odds ratio of 2.80 (95% CI = 2.18, 3.60); the highest odds ratio was estimated for emotional abuse (3.54, 95% CI = 3.04, 4.13) [31].

Nuclear symptoms gave rise to influential research programs based on clinical neuropsychology and cognitive neuroscience. According to Chris Frith, the core feature of schizophrenic delusions may be related to a dysfunction in the systems that support self-monitoring. Normally, the brain predicts the sensory consequences of intended movements, allowing the effects of actions to be labelled as self-generated and distinguished from external events. In patients experiencing delusions of control, the intention to perform an action remains unconscious, and they fail to anticipate the action at a conscious level. This unexpected action results in a feeling of not being in control. Such experiences can be conceptualised as a disturbance in the sense of agency [32].

According to Frédérique de Vignemont, the sense of agency, ownership, and presence are fundamental aspects of bodily self-awareness [33, 34]. In recent decades, phenomenological psychopathology has offered a detailed account of the disturbances in self-awareness that constitute the lived experience of schizophrenia [35–37]. These studies suggest that the core disturbance is a qualitative disruption of consciousness often described as a 'loss of natural self-evidence'. This refers to a breakdown in the basic, intuitive sense of reality that typically enables smooth engagement with the world. As a result, everyday experiences may appear strange or confusing. A key aspect of this disruption is diminished self-affection—the fading of the immediate, pre-reflective sense of being a conscious, embodied subject. This is often accompanied by hyperreflexivity, an exaggerated self-focus in which normally implicit processes become objects of intense scrutiny [38, 39].

The formulation of the so-called nuclear symptoms or first rank symptoms of schizophrenia developed by Kurt Schneider has been very influential as a diagnostic anchor and as a window into the neurobiology of schizophrenia. Timothy J. Crow postulated that these symptoms provide a window into the relationship between speech and thought. He suggested that the symptoms are universal and linked to a genetic variation as ancient as modern *Homo sapiens*, associated with the hemispheric lateralisation of language. This formed the basis of his hypothesis that schizophrenia is the price humanity pays for possessing language [40]. Crow also developed the influential division of schizophrenia into two categories: type I, characterised by the so-called positive symptoms (delusions, hallucinations etc.), and type II, characterised by negative symptoms (affective flattening, avolition etc.). However, it was soon observed that many patients had features of both types, so the categorical approach was substituted by a clinimetric approach allowing for dimensionality. Nancy Andreasen developed the *Scale for the Assessment for the Negative Symptoms* (SANS) and later the *Scale for the Assessment of Positive Symptoms* (SAPS). Soon, these instruments were replaced by the *Positive and Negative Syndrome Scale* (PANSS), constructed by Kay, Opler and Fiszbein [41]. This clinimetric instrument has remained as the standard for psychopathological and pharmacological assessment. It includes seven items dedicated to positive symptoms, seven items for negative symptoms, and 16 items of general psychopathology. The factorial analysis of these tools gave rise to different solutions to describe the symptom domains of schizophrenia. Peter F. Liddle proposed three dimensions: (a) reality distortion (delusions and hallucinations), (b) disorganisation (formal thought disorder and disorganised behaviour), and (c) negative symptoms (lack of volition, poverty of speech, and flattening of affect) [42]. A five-factor solution has also been used as a heuristic tool, including negative, positive, excitement, cognitive and depression/anxiety domains of psychopathology [43].

In the Hierarchical Taxonomy of Psychopathology (HiTOP), the leading dimensional classification of mental disorders, the symptom domains are conceptualised as extremes on two spectra: psychoticism and detachment [44–46]. Psychoticism spectrum encompasses phenomena such as reality distortion, disorganisation, and related traits like unusual beliefs and experiences, which appear by adolescence, showing moderate stability over time. Clinical high-risk states often involve subthreshold reality distortion, with 15–25% progressing to full psychotic disorders. Detachment spectrum includes negative symptoms and traits such as emotional detachment and social withdrawal. Detachment remains highly stable across the lifespan, correlating with long-term functional impairments. It is a stronger predictor of functional decline than psychoticism.

Within these spectra, the HiTOP model identifies 14 narrow components that capture more specific aspects of psychopathology. Cognitive impairment and functional decline are recognised as auxiliary domains. From a dimensional lens, what we have traditionally called schizophrenia is a prototypical clinical profile of high psychoticism, high detachment, cognitive impairment and functional decline. Since different mechanisms are responsible for variation along different spectra, and people can show a variety of profiles (e.g. high psychoticism and low detachment, or low psychoticism and high detachment with or without cognitive decline), the resulting syndrome is unsurprisingly heterogeneous and fuzzy. This dimensional, hierarchical structure helps explain both the co-occurrence and heterogeneity of schizophrenia symptoms, their overlap with adjacent disorders such as bipolar disorder, and the existence of subthreshold symptoms and their progression to clinical disorders.

Finally, the neurocognitive approach relies on three aspects of neuropsychological functioning: (A) Basic cognition: The deficits are particularly pronounced in executive function, working memory, and sustained attention, though their severity varies considerably among individuals. These disturbances are present in antipsychotic naïve patients [4, 47, 48]. (B) Social cognition: Individuals with schizophrenia often experience impairments in emotion processing, social perception, attributional style, and theory of mind (mentalising). This affects the capacity to interpret emotions and social cues and norms during interpersonal interactions [49]. (C) Metacognition. New clinical resources are being developed to assess explicit metacognition in clinical practice. Also, a model of implicit and explicit metacognition with heuristic value to understand psychosis has been proposed [50, 51].

8.6   Current Neuroscience Perspectives on Schizophrenia

Scientific developments over the last few decades have increased our understanding of the causes and mechanisms of schizophrenia, but they have also destabilised the very notion of schizophrenia as a distinct and discrete biogenetic disease entity. Increasingly, it is recognised as a multidimensional phenotype existing on a spectrum with other psychotic disorders, with risk factors and mechanisms that are shared with many other psychopathological conditions. Relevant information is reviewed in detail in other book chapters, for example, Chap. 5 (evolutionary psychiatry), Chap. 6 (genetics), Chaps. 7, 13, 14 (brain imaging) and Chaps. 23, 25 (neurophysiology and therapeutics). Here we will briefly summarise our understanding.

The current neuroscientific picture of schizophrenia, which is still very much tentative and in the process of evolution, looks something like follows: schizophrenia is a multidimensional and aetiologically heterogeneous phenomenon. Aberrant information processing and structural and functional brain network alterations appear to be proximally related to the symptom profile of schizophrenia, and these disturbances occur as downstream outcomes of multiple pathways that involve synaptic pruning, immune dysregulation, brain dysconnectivity, and altered neurochemical transmission. Sometimes, a relatively circumscribed genetic or neurological process is sufficient to produce a schizophrenia-like syndrome (e.g. 22q11.2 deletion, interictal psychosis in epilepsy, or anti-NMDA receptor encephalitis), much like congestive heart failure, which can be caused by a single autosomal dominant genetic mutation [4]. In other cases, the causes are more distributed, with the exact combination and accumulation of causes varying from person to person. The hypothesised cascade of causes in schizophrenia goes from complement activation, synapse elimination, and cortical thinning to cognitive impairments and aberrant information processing, and these pathways are disrupted in different individuals through a combination of different factors, including prenatal infections, cannabis use, childhood trauma, and adversity in later life.

8.7 Schizophrenia-like Psychosis and the Problem of Differential Diagnosis

When examining the psychopathological and neurobiological heterogeneity of schizophrenia, some authors propose that the translational research program will eventually identify various diseases that are currently subsumed under the broad category of schizophrenia. This hypothesis is supported partly by the fact that, over the past century, many neurological diseases have been described that can produce clinical manifestations that resemble the schizophrenia phenotype. This pattern, referred to as 'schizophrenia-like psychosis', was categorised by Perminder Sachdev as 'secondary schizophrenia' in his well-known textbook [52]. The estimated lifetime risk of developing any psychotic disorder is approximately 3% in the general population [53]. Among those who suffer from a psychotic disorder, the proportion of psychosis due to any underlying medical cause is approximately 5% (95% CI: 3–9%) [53]. The best-known disease in which a pattern of schizophrenia-like psychosis appears is epilepsy. Psychosis develops in 5–7% of individuals with epilepsy, twice as likely as compared to the general population [54, 55]. In the case of temporal lobe epilepsy, the relationship is stronger, with a prevalence ranging from 10% to 15%. Other risk factors include poorly controlled seizures, hippocampal sclerosis, and a history of status epilepticus [54]. The most used taxonomy includes four primary types: (1) ictal psychosis, in which the psychotic symptoms are a direct expression of the epileptic discharge; (2) postictal psychosis, where psychotic symptoms occur following seizures after a free interval during which the patient returns to normal functioning; (3) psychosis associated with complete seizure control (a phenomenon known as forced normalisation), and (4) interictal psychosis, where psychotic symptoms are related to the presence of epilepsy but are not chronologically linked to the seizures. This form of psychosis is often regarded as schizophrenia-like psychosis, with chronic hallucinations and delusions, as well as cognitive dysfunction [54, 55].

Psychosis is also well established as a frequent phenomenon in some neurodegenerative diseases, although in these cases, a schizophrenia-like pattern is less frequent. In Alzheimer's Disease, psychosis typically represents a symptom of disease progression, being more frequent as dementia severity increases [56]. The current research diagnostic criteria for behavioural variant Alzheimer's Disease (bvAD) include delusions and hallucinations as a supportive clinical feature of the behavioural variant Alzheimer's Disease [57] Schizophrenia-like psychosis with paranoid features has been described as a 'prodromal' manifestation in behavioural variant frontotemporal dementia (bvFTD) [58, 59]. Visual hallucinations are very frequent in Lewy body dementia (LBD), sometimes with a lack of awareness, accompanied by delusional interpretation [60]. Psychotic symptoms are also common in prion disease during the initial stages of the rapidly progressive dementia syndrome [61]. In Parkinson's Disease, the prevalence of psychosis is estimated to range from 16% to 23% [62]. Psychotic symptoms appear gradually, involving visual illusions at earlier stages, and eventually visual hallucinations and delusions as the disease progresses. This may be observed in cases progressing to major neurocognitive disorder [63].

Psychosis can be present in several neurogenetic diseases leading to intellectual disability, such as Down syndrome, X-fragile syndrome, and Prader-Willi syndrome [64]. 22q11.2 deletion syndrome, a common microdeletion syndrome, leads frequently to a schizophrenia phenotype [64]. Huntington's disease, a genetic disorder with an autosomal dominant inheritance pattern, leads to neuropsychiatric symptoms, progressive motor disturbances, and severe cognitive decline [65]. Delusions occur in 10% of patients and may have a chronic course [66]. Metachromatic leukodystrophy is a rare demyelinating genetic disease, caused by an autosomal recessive mutation on chromosome 22q, leading to a near-complete absence of the lysosomal enzyme arylsulfatase A, and prominent psychotic features, sometimes resembling the schizophrenia phenotype [67].

Psychosis can also be observed in patients with acquired brain damage due to cerebrovascular disease and traumatic brain injury. In a 10-year population-based study, psychosis was more frequent in participants with stroke (2.3%) compared to participants without stroke (0.9%), with a fully-adjusted HR of 4.98 (95% CI 2.55–9.72) [68]. In traumatic brain injury, the prevalence of psychosis is two to three times higher in individuals with a history of TBI compared to the general population [69, 70].

Finally, it is well known that some patients with neuroimmunological and inflammatory conditions, such as systemic lupus erythematosus and multiple sclerosis, develop states of psychosis and other neuropsychiatric symptoms [71]. In recent decades, interest in psychosis of autoimmune origin has grown significantly, following the discovery of antineuronal antibodies with pathogenic effects over synaptic receptors, and against ion channels and other cell-surface proteins [72–75]. In 2019, an international consensus recommended specific approaches to facilitate early recognition and treatment of psychosis of autoimmune origin. Clinical features that suggest autoimmune psychosis include severe cognitive disturbances, catatonia, and atypical patterns of psychosis [76, 77]. The most common form is anti-NMDA receptor encephalitis, which can cause psychotic symptoms in 80% of the cases, along with catatonia, severe cognitive impairment, seizures and dyskinesia [78]. Some patients may present with psychosis without overt neurological signs, which may cause misdiagnosis, diagnostic delays and therapeutic errors in general hospitals or mental health services [79, 80].

It is difficult to estimate the frequency of autoimmune psychosis. According to some authors, autoimmune encephalitis could account for 6.5% of first episodes of psychosis and 1% of all psychotic disorders [53, 81]. A taxonomy of autoimmune psychosis has been proposed, including: (a) Psychosis associated with neuronal or synaptic autoantibodies, such as the anti-NMDA receptor antibody; (b) Psychosis associated with classic autoimmune or inflammatory diseases (e.g. systemic lupus erythematosus and Hashimoto's encephalopathy); (c) Psychosis in patients with probable encephalitis in which no antibodies are detected. Despite the lack of detectable antibodies, the presentation is highly suggestive of an autoimmune aetiology due to the following arguments: clinical features as atypical psychosis, the presence of seizures and neurological signs, laboratory and imaging abnormal results (e.g. oligoclonal bands in cerebrospinal fluid, CSF pleocytosis, EEG and MRI abnormalities), a reasonable exclusion of alternative causes, and the response to immunological treatment [77, 80].

Patients with autoimmune psychosis exhibit a polymorphic phenomenology, with disorganised speech, catatonic signs, and severe, disproportionate cognitive impairment. Visual hallucinations slightly outnumber auditory ones. Delusions are fluctuating in severity, usually with changing contents, including paranoid, grandeur, somatic, nihilistic, jealousy, and misidentification themes, and also with affective features such as delirious mania and psychotic depression [80, 82–85]. Current evidence suggests that a significant clinical improvement in psychosis, cognition, and overall functionality is achieved after immunotherapy (including steroids, IVIG, plasma exchange, rituximab, and cyclophosphamide) [80]. Observational studies in anti-NMDA receptor encephalitis show that targeted treatment significantly impacts the longitudinal course of the illness, improving functional outcomes and reducing mortality [86].

8.8   Conclusion

This chapter has traced the evolution of schizophrenia as a diagnostic category, reflecting its enduring and puzzling complexity and heterogeneity. Iterative and overlapping clinical observations, theoretical frameworks, and research programs have shaped, fragmented, and challenged the concept. We examined two competing perspectives on the relationship between the concept of schizophrenia and its underlying reality: the continuity thesis, which views schizophrenia as a stable brain disorder, and the discontinuity thesis, which sees it as a historically shifting, culturally shaped concept.

While the term 'schizophrenia' has persisted for over a century, its referents have remained contested. The heterogeneity of its clinical presentations, the variability of its outcomes, and the multiplicity of underlying mechanisms all complicate efforts to define it as a natural kind or as a unitary disease entity. Clinically, schizophrenia remains a disorder of selfhood and persisting disruptions in cognition, perception, emotion, and social engagement. The heterogeneity that has long troubled clinicians and researchers may in fact be intrinsic to the condition, an outcome of a convergence of aetiological pathways (genetic, neurodevelopmental, inflammatory, environmental) that interact in complex and chaotic ways.

Advances in neuroscience, genomics, and immunology have deepened our understanding of these pathways, offering new scientific models for how schizophrenia-like symptoms can emerge from disruptions in synaptic function, predictive coding, or immune signalling. At the same time, these developments challenge the traditional nosological boundaries of schizophrenia. The growing recognition of autoimmune psychosis (and other neuropsychiatric diseases) as being responsible for a subset of cases of schizophrenia-like presentations reminds us that distinct and treatable neurological diseases continue to hide amidst the heterogeneous and multifactorial syndrome.

The future of schizophrenia research and clinical care depends on our ability to tackle aetiological complexity without collapsing the syndrome into a unitary disease entity nor abandoning the search for mechanistic coherence. This requires a commitment to conceptual clarity, empirical humility, and diagnostic pluralism. Dementia praecox, schizophrenia, psychosis spectrum disorder, or whatever term we may use for it in the future, is best approached as a historically contingent and evolving family of clinical concepts.

Key Points
- Schizophrenia is a historically unstable and conceptually heterogeneous construct, lacking a fixed definition across time.
- Continuity vs. discontinuity historical perspectives reflect deeper philosophical disagreements about the nature of psychotic disorders as natural vs constructed kinds.
- Core symptom clusters discourses have been shaped by diverse traditions, including biological psychiatry, psychoanalysis, and phenomenological psychopathology.
- Advances in genetics, immunology, and computational neuroscience complicate the notion of schizophrenia as a single disease entity.
- A pluralistic and multidimensional diagnostic approach is needed to account for overlapping syndromes and mechanistic heterogeneity.

References

1. Berrios GE, Luque R, Villagran JM. Schizophrenia: a conceptual history. J Int Ther Psychol. 2003;3(2):111–40.
2. Stein DJ, Nielsen K, Hartford A, Gagné-Julien AM, Glackin S, Friston K, et al. Philosophy of psychiatry: theoretical advances and clinical implications. World Psychiatry. 2024;23(2):215–32.
3. Kendler KS. The nature of psychiatric disorders. World Psychiatry. 2016;15(1):5–12.
4. Tandon R, Nasrallah H, Akbarian S, Carpenter WT, DeLisi LE, Gaebel W, et al. The schizophrenia syndrome, circa 2024: what we know and how that informs its nature. Schizophr Res. 2024;264:1–28.
5. McDonald GC. Concepts and treatments of phrenitis in ancient medicine. Newcastle upon Tyne: University of Newcastle upon Tyne; 2009.
6. Thumiger C, Singer PN. Introduction. Disease classification and mental illness: ancient and modern perspectives. In: Thumiger C, Singer PN, editors. Introduction disease classification and mental illness: ancient and modern perspectives; 2018. p. 1–32.
7. Coughlin S. Athenaeus of Attalia on the psychological causes of bodily health. In: Thumiger C, Singer PN, editors. Introduction disease classification and mental illness: ancient and modern perspectives; 2018.
8. Berrios GE. Historical aspects of psychoses: 19th century issues. Br Med Bull. 1987;43(3):484–98.
9. Pinel P. Treatise on mental alienation (1809). Oxford: Wiley-Blackwell; 2008.. 198 p.
10. Beer MD. Psychosis: from mental disorder to disease concept. Hist Psychiatry. 1995;6(22):177–200.

11. Berrios GE. Delirium and confusion in the 19th century: a conceptual history. Br J Psychiatry. 1981;139:439–49.
12. Carpenter PK. Descriptions of schizophrenia in the psychiatry of Georgian Britain: John Haslam and James Tilly Matthews. Compr Psychiatry. 1989;30(4):332–8.
13. Berrios GE, Fuentenebro de Diego F. Delirio. Historia, Clínica, Metateoría. Valladolid: Editorial Trotta; 1996.
14. Armando BP. Cronología histórica de los conceptos clínicos sobre esquizofrenia. Parte 1. Alcmeon. 1990;1:59–77.
15. Berrios GE. "The clinico-diagnostic perspective in psychopathology" by K. Kahlbaum. Hist Psychiatry. 2007;18(2):231–3.
16. Goldar JC, Starkstein SE, Hodgkiss A. Karl ludwig kahlbaum's concept of catatonia. Hist Psychiatry. 1995;6(22):201–7.
17. Zúñiga JFM, Ramirez-Bermudez J, De Rivera JJF, Corona T. Catatonia and klüver-bucy syndrome in a patient with acute disseminated encephalomyelitis. J Neuropsychiatry Clin Neurosci. 2015;27(2)
18. Pérez-González AF, Espinola-Nadurille M, Ramírez-Bermúdez J. Catatonia and delirium: syndromes that may converge in the neuropsychiatric patient. Rev Colomb Psiquiatr. 2017;46:2–8.
19. Espinola-Nadurille M, Ramirez-Bermudez J, Fricchione GL, Ojeda-Lopez MC, Perez-González AF, Aguilar-Venegas LC. Catatonia in neurologic and psychiatric patients at a tertiary neurological center. J Neuropsychiatry Clin Neurosci [Internet]. 2016;28(2):124–30. Available from: http://psychiatryonline.org/doi/10.1176/appi.neuropsych.15090218.
20. Kraam A. 'Hebephrenia. A contribution to clinical psychiatry' by Dr. Ewald Heckerin Gorlitz. 1871. Hist Psychiatry. 2009;20(77 Pt 1):87–106.
21. Garnica R. El botanico del manicomio. Ciudad de Mexico: Salvat; 1997.
22. Kendler KS. Kraepelin's final views on dementia praecox. Schizophr Bull. 2021;47(3):635–43.
23. Jung CG. Recuerdos, sueños, pensamientos. Ciudad de México: Seix Barral; 2001.
24. Fusar-Poli P, Politi P. Paul Eugen Bleuler and the birth of schizophrenia (1908). Am J Psychiatry. 2008;165(11):1407.
25. Bleuler E. Esquizofrenia. In: Francoise-Regin C, Jean G, Denis M, editors. Anthology of French language psychiatric texts. Institut d'edition; 1999.
26. Moskowitz A, Heim G. Eugen Bleuler's dementia praecox or the Group of Schizophrenias (1911): a centenary appreciation and reconsideration. Schizophr Bull. 2011;37(3):471–9.
27. Kurt S. Patopsicología clínica. Traducción de la octava edición alemana, por A. Guera Miralles. Madrid: Editorial Paz Montalvo; 1970.
28. Enric JN, Rafael H. El síndrome de Kraepelin-Bleuler-Schneider y la conciencia moderna: Una aproximación a la historia de la esquizofrenia. Clin Salud [Internet]. 2010;21(3):205–19. Available from: http://www.copmadrid.org/webcopm/resource.do?recurso=4000&numero=20101102130418609000.
29. Crow TJ. Nuclear schizophrenic symptoms as a window on the relationship between thought and speech. Br J Psychiatry. 1998;173(OCT.):303–9.
30. Bateson G, Jackson DD, Haley J, Weakland J. Toward a theory of schizophrenia. Behav Sci. 2007;1(4):251–64.
31. Zhou L, Sommer IEC, Yang P, Sikirin L, van Os J, Bentall RP, et al. What do four decades of research tell us about the association between childhood adversity and psychosis: an updated and extended multi-level meta-analysis. Am J Psychiatry. 2025;182(4):360–72.
32. Frith C. The self in action: lessons from delusions of control. Conscious Cogn. 2005;14(4):752–70.
33. De Vignemont F. Affective bodily awareness. Cambridge University Press; 2023.
34. de Vignemont F. The phenomenology of bodily ownership. In: Self-experience essays on inner awareness; 2023. p. 269–90.
35. Fuchs T. One century of Karl Jaspers psychopathology. Oxford: Oxford University Press; 2013.
36. Stanghellini G, Broome MR. Psychopathology as the basic science of psychiatry. Br J Psychiatry. 2014;205:169.

37. Broome MR. On Jaspers' general psychopathology – reflection. Br J Psychiatry. 2013;203(2):102.
38. Parnas J, Zandersen M. Self and schizophrenia: current status and diagnostic implications. World Psychiatry. 2018;17:220.
39. Nelson B, Parnas J, Sass LA. Disturbance of minimal self (ipseity) in schizophrenia: clarification and current status. Schizophr Bull. 2014;40:479–82.
40. Crow TJ. Is schizophrenia the price that Homo sapiens pays for language? Schizophr Res. 1997;28:127.
41. Kay SR, Fiszbein A, Opler LA. The positive and negative syndrome scale (PANSS) for schizophrenia. Schizophr Bull. 1987;13(2):261–76.
42. Liddle PF. The symptoms of chronic schizophrenia. A re-examination of the positive-negative dichotomy. Br J Psychiatry. 1987;151(AUG.):145–51.
43. Lindenmayer JP, Bernstein-Hyman R, Grochowski S. A new five factor model of schizophrenia. Psychiatry Q. 1994;65(4):299–322.
44. Kotov R, Jonas KG, Carpenter WT, Dretsch MN, Eaton NR, Forbes MK, et al. Validity and utility of hierarchical taxonomy of psychopathology (HiTOP): I. Psychosis superspectrum. World Psychiatry. 2020;19(2):151–72.
45. Jonas KG, Cannon TD, Docherty AR, Dwyer D, Gur RC, Gur RE, et al. Psychosis superspectrum I: nosology, etiology, and lifespan development. Mol Psychiatry. 2024;29(4):1005–19.
46. Aftab A, Banicki K, Ruffalo ML, Frances A. Psychiatric diagnosis: a clinical guide to navigating diagnostic pluralism. J Nerv Ment Dis. 2024;212(8):445–54.
47. Saykin AJ, Shtasel DL, Gur RE, Kester DB, Mozley LH, Stafiniak P, et al. Neuropsychological deficits in neuroleptic naive patients with first-episode schizophrenia. Arch Gen Psychiatry. 1994;51(2)
48. Solís-Vivanco R, Rangel-Hassey F, León-Ortiz P, Mondragón-Maya A, Reyes-Madrigal F, De La Fuente-Sandoval C. Cognitive impairment in never-medicated individuals on the schizophrenia Spectrum. JAMA Psychiatry. 2020;77(5):543–5.
49. Green MF, Horan WP, Lee J. Nonsocial and social cognition in schizophrenia: current evidence and future directions. World Psychiatry. 2019;18(2):146–61.
50. Flores-Medina Y, Ávila Bretherton R, Ramírez-Bermudez J, Saracco-Alvarez R, Flores-Ramos M. On metacognition: overconfidence in word recall prediction and its association with psychotic symptoms in patients with schizophrenia. Brain Sci. 2024;14(9):872.
51. Frith U, Frith C. What makes us social and what does it tell us about mental disorders? In: Cogn neuropsychiatry; 2024.
52. Sachdev PS. Secondary schizophrenia. Cambridge: Cambridge University Press; 2010.
53. Blackman G, Byrne R, Gill N, Fanshawe JB, Bell V, Watson C, et al. How common is secondary psychosis? Estimates from a systematic review and meta-analysis. World Psychiatry. 2024;24:145.
54. Maguire M, Singh J, Marson A. Epilepsy and psychosis: a practical approach. Pract Neurol. 2018;18(2):106–14.
55. de Toffol B. Epilepsy and psychosis. Rev Neurol (Paris). 2024;180(4):298–307.
56. Ballard C, Kales HC, Lyketsos C, Aarsland D, Creese B, Mills R, et al. Psychosis in Alzheimer's disease. Curr Neurol Neurosci Rep. 2020;20(12):57.
57. Ossenkoppele R, Singleton EH, Groot C, Dijkstra AA, Eikelboom WS, Seeley WW, et al. Research criteria for the behavioral variant of Alzheimer disease: a systematic review and meta-analysis. JAMA Neurol. 2022;79(1):48–60.
58. Ducharme S, Pijnenburg Y, Rohrer JD, Huey E, Finger E, Tatton N. Identifying and diagnosing TDP-43 neurodegenerative diseases in psychiatry. Am J Geriatr Psychiatry. 2024;32(1):98–113.
59. Kertesz A, Ang LC, Jesso S, MacKinley J, Baker M, Brown P, et al. Psychosis and hallucinations in frontotemporal dementia with the C9ORF72 mutation: a detailed clinical cohort. Cogn Behav Neurol. 2013;26(3):146–54.
60. McKeith IG, Ferman TJ, Thomas AJ, Blanc F, Boeve BF, Fujishiro H, et al. Research criteria for the diagnosis of prodromal dementia with Lewy bodies. Neurology. 2020;94(17):743–55.

61. Huang B, Shafiian N, Masi PJ, Gordon ML, Franceschi AM, Giliberto L. Creutzfeldt-Jakob disease presenting as psychiatric disorder: case presentation and systematic review. Front Neurol. 2024;15:15.
62. Abdul-Rahman T, Herrera-Calderón RE, Aderinto N, Kundu M, Wireko AA, Adebusoye FT, et al. Clearing the fog: a review of antipsychotics for Parkinson's-related hallucinations: a focus on Pimavanserin, quetiapine and clozapine. J Integr Neurosci. 2024;23(4)
63. Pagonabarraga J, Bejr-Kasem H, Martinez-Horta S, Kulisevsky J. Parkinson disease psychosis: from phenomenology to neurobiological mechanisms. Nat Rev Neurol. 2024;20(3):135–50.
64. Feinstein C, Chahal L. Psychiatric phenotypes associated with Neurogenetic disorders. Psychiatr Clin North Am. 2009;32(1):15–37.
65. Stoker TB, Mason SL, Greenland JC, Holden ST, Santini H, Barker RA. Huntington's disease: diagnosis and management. Pract Neurol. 2022;22(1):32–41.
66. Rickards H, De Souza J, Van Walsem M, Van Duijn E, Simpson SA, Squitieri F, et al. Factor analysis of behavioural symptoms in Huntington's disease. J Neurol Neurosurg Psychiatry. 2011;82(4):411–2.
67. Hyde TM, Ziegler JC, Weinberger DR. Psychiatric disturbances in metachromatic Leukodystrophy: insights into the neurobiology of psychosis. Arch Neurol. 1992;49(4):401–6.
68. Richards-Belle A, Poole N, Osborn DPJ, Bell V. Longitudinal associations between stroke and psychosis: a population-based study. Psychol Med. 2023;53(16):7698–706.
69. Li LM, Carson A, Dams-O'Connor K. Psychiatric sequelae of traumatic brain injury—future directions in research. Nat Rev Neurol. 2023;19(9):556–71.
70. Fujii DE, Ahmed I. Psychotic disorder caused by traumatic brain injury. Psychiatr Clin North Am. 2014;37(1):113–24.
71. Gilberthorpe TG, O'Connell KE, Carolan A, Silber E, Brex PA, Sibtain NA, et al. The spectrum of psychosis in multiple sclerosis: a clinical case series. Neuropsychiatr Dis Treat. 2017;13:303–18.
72. Dalmau J, Graus F. Antibody-mediated encephalitis. N Engl J Med. 2018;378(9):840–51.
73. Pape K, Tamouza R, Leboyer M, Zipp F. Immunoneuropsychiatry—novel perspectives on brain disorders. Nat Rev Neurol. 2019;15:317–28. Springer US.
74. Al-Diwani AAJ, Pollak TA, Irani SR, Lennox BR. Psychosis: an autoimmune disease? Immunology. 2017;152:388–401.
75. Graus F, Titulaer MJ, Balu R, Benseler S, Bien CG, Cellucci T, et al. A clinical approach to diagnosis of autoimmune encephalitis. Lancet Neurol. 2016;15:391–404.
76. Pollak TA, Lennox BR, Müller S, Benros ME, Prüss H, Tebartz van Elst L, et al. Autoimmune psychosis: an international consensus on an approach to the diagnosis and management of psychosis of suspected autoimmune origin. Lancet Psychiatry. 2020;7(1):93–108.
77. Najjar S, Steiner J, Najjar A, Bechter K. A clinical approach to new-onset psychosis associated with immune dysregulation: the concept of autoimmune psychosis. J Neuroinflammation. 2018;15(1):1–8.
78. Espinola-Nadurille M, Restrepo Martinez M, Bayliss L, Flores-Montes E, Rivas-Alonso V, Vargas Cañas S, et al. Neuropsychiatric phenotypes of anti-NMDAR encephalitis: a prospective study. Psychol Med. 2022;53:1–9.
79. Ramirez-Bermudez J, Restrepo-Martinez M, Espinola-Nadurille M, Martinez-Angeles V, Lopez-Hernandez JC, Hernandez-Vanegas LE, et al. Examining the features of neuroleptic malignant syndrome in anti-NMDA receptor encephalitis: a case-control study. J Acad Consult Psychiatry. 2024;65(3):222–30.
80. Ramirez-Bermudez J, Espinola-Nadurille M, Restrepo-Martinez M, Martínez-Ángeles V, Martínez-Carrillo F, Cascante L, et al. Autoimmune psychosis: psychopathological patterns and outcome after immunotherapy. Schizophr Res. 2025;281:10–9.
81. Zandi MS, Irani SR, Lang B, Waters P, Jones PB, Mckenna P, et al. Disease-relevant autoantibodies in first episode schizophrenia. J Neurol. 2011;258:686–8.
82. Ramirez Bermúdez J, Bustamante-Gomez P, Espínola-Nadurille M, Kerik NE, Dias Meneses IE, Restrepo-Martinez M, et al. Cotard syndrome in anti-NMDAR encephalitis: two patients and insights from molecular imaging. Neurocase. 2021;27(1):64–71.

83. Warren N, Siskind D, O'Gorman C. Refining the psychiatric syndrome of anti-N-methyl-d-aspartate receptor encephalitis. Acta Psychiatr Scand. 2018;138:401–8.
84. Al-Diwani A, Handel A, Townsend L, Pollak T, Leite MI, Harrison PJ, et al. The psychopathology of NMDAR-antibody encephalitis in adults: a systematic review and phenotypic analysis of individual patient data. Lancet Psychiatry. 2019;6(3):235–46.
85. Restrepo-Martinez M, Ramirez-Bermudez J, Bayliss L, Espinola-Nadurille M. Delirious mania as a frequent and recognizable neuropsychiatric syndrome in patients with anti-NMDAR encephalitis. Gen Hosp Psychiatry. 2020;64(October 2019):50–5.
86. Titulaer MJ, McCracken L, Gabilondo I, Armangué T, Glaser C, Iizuka T, et al. Treatment and prognostic factors for long-term outcome in patients with anti-NMDA receptor encephalitis: an observational cohort study. Lancet Neurol. 2013;12:157.

Open Access   This chapter is licensed under the terms of the Creative Commons Attribution 4.0 International License (http://creativecommons.org/licenses/by/4.0/), which permits use, sharing, adaptation, distribution and reproduction in any medium or format, as long as you give appropriate credit to the original author(s) and the source, provide a link to the Creative Commons license and indicate if changes were made.

The images or other third party material in this chapter are included in the chapter's Creative Commons license, unless indicated otherwise in a credit line to the material. If material is not included in the chapter's Creative Commons license and your intended use is not permitted by statutory regulation or exceeds the permitted use, you will need to obtain permission directly from the copyright holder.

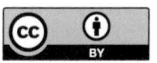

The Origins of Invention and Its Link with Autism

9

Simon Baron-Cohen

9.1 Introduction

What are the origins of invention? And is there a link between our uniquely human capacity for invention, and autism? And what are the implications for understanding the nature and significance of autism and its relation to human evolution and society? In this chapter, I present a personal review summarising my decades long research and some by others and present an overarching perspective.

9.2 Evolution and Autism

If we take the long view of human evolution, we can see evidence of simple tool use going back as far as *Homo habilis*, who lived 2.5 to 1.5 million years ago, and *Homo erectus*, who lived 2.1 million years ago until as recently as 250,000 years ago (Fig. 9.1). Both of these ancestors used simple tools with few functions: to smash, cut and scrape. And even *Homo neanderthalis*, who lived 300,000 years ago until as recently as 40,000 years ago, still only used simple stone axes, with the same limited functions. Although these three early humans showed some differences in their technology, I argue these *simple* tools showed no signs of *generative invention*—that there was little change over this long period of over two million years.

Homo sapiens appears 300,000 years ago and I and others argue a 'cognitive revolution' took place, a change in the modern human brain, between 100,000 and 70,000 years ago. Modern humans appear to have developed the capacity to invent generatively. What is the evidence for this? If we look in the archaeological record, we see the earliest examples of engraving from 77,000 years ago, the first jewellery (in the form of a necklace of beads) from 75,000 years ago (Fig. 9.2), and the first

S. Baron-Cohen (✉)
Autism Research Centre, Cambridge University, Cambridge, UK
e-mail: sb205@cam.ac.uk

© The Author(s) 2026
G. Ikkos, T. Becker (eds.), *Psychiatry after Kraepelin*,
https://doi.org/10.1007/978-3-032-09475-9_9

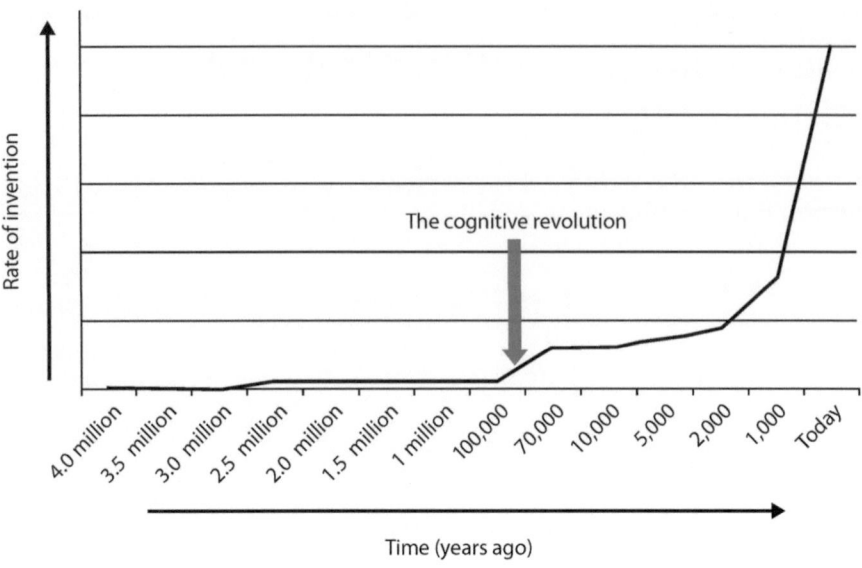

Fig. 9.1 70–100,000 years ago the rate of invention took off. (From Baron-Cohen (2020) The Pattern Seekers)

signs that modern humans were using a bow-and-arrow 71,000 years ago, so-called 'stealth' weapons.

And that is not all. By 43,000 years ago we see the first evidence of counting, in the form of systematic engravings on a bone of what looks like keeping a tally, and the first cave paintings from 40,000 years ago (Fig. 9.3). To me, most striking of all, 40,000 years ago we see the earliest musical instrument—the bone flute (Fig. 9.4). I had the privilege of going to the cave (Hohle Fels) in Schelklingen, Swabia in Germany where this was found, with archaeologist Professor Nicholas Conard, and to his delightful museum in Tübingen (Museum der Universität Tübingen, MUT, www.unimuseum.de), to listen to a recording of the flute being played. Modern humans were not just inventing *complex* tools but were inventing music.

To me, this explosion of artefacts in the archaeological record is a sign that modern humans alone had the capacity for generative invention—not just making one change and sticking with that for millions of years but inventing unstoppably and in a myriad of different ways. By 32,000 years ago we see the first sculpture, by 23,000 years ago the first sewing needles, by 13,000 years ago the first signs of agriculture, by 10,000 years ago the first signs of star gazing as we analysed the movement and changing shape and colour of the moon in relation to the sun, 5000 years ago the first signs of writing, mathematics and the wheel.

As historian Yuval Harari points out in his excellent book *Sapiens*, [1] humans over the last 13,000 years went through the agricultural, industrial and now the digital revolutions. And we are still inventing unstoppably. Fast forward to the twenty-first century, we have invented the first vaccine targeting coronavirus disease 2019

Fig. 9.2 The earliest jewellery, dated 75,000 years ago, made from shells, thought to be a necklace, each drilled with a small hole. (From Baron-Cohen (2020) The Pattern Seekers)

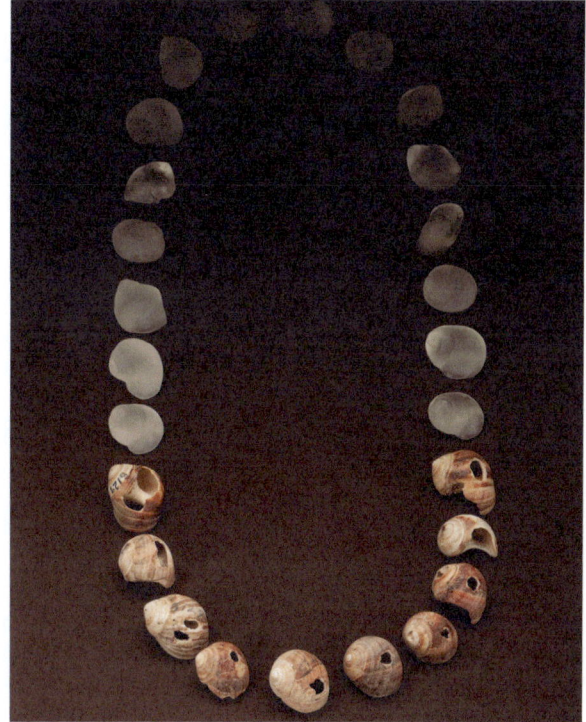

75,000 years ago

Fig. 9.3 A cave painting, dated 40,000 years old. (From Baron-Cohen (2020) The Pattern Seekers)

40,000 years ago

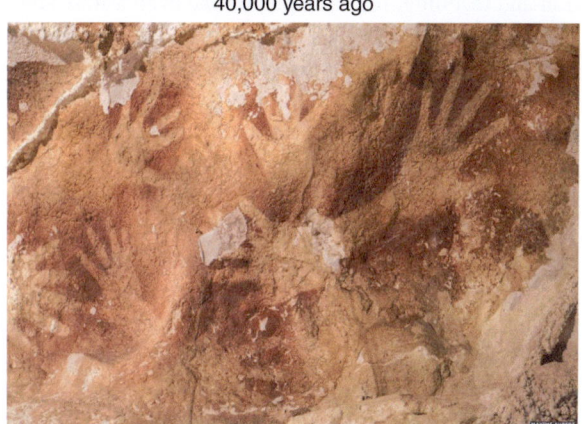

(COVID-19), and NASA are collaborating with Nokia to install 4G on the moon's surface so we can do live streaming when we take our holidays there.

So what was this cognitive revolution in the modern human brain that occurred 100,000 to 70,000 years ago? In my new book *The Pattern Seekers* [2], I argue for

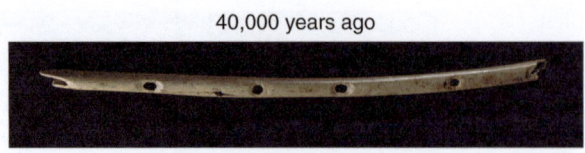

Fig. 9.4 The earliest musical instrument ever found, a flute made from the hollow bone of a bird, dated 40,000 years old. (From Baron-Cohen (2020) The Pattern Seekers)

the evolution of two new circuits in the brain, and surprisingly both seem to have evolved around the same time. One was the *Empathy Circuit*, that enabled a raft of new behaviours, including deception, teaching, self-reflection, advanced social cooperation, social 'chess' and flexible referential communication, including story telling. These explain *why* modern humans could make stealth weapons and jewellery, as we were keeping track of what others might think—using a so-called 'theory of mind', and of what others might know, need to know and believe (including their false beliefs).

The Empathy Circuit recruits a complex network of at least ten brain regions, including the amygdala and the ventromedial prefrontal cortex. It was the subject of my earlier book *Zero Degrees of* Empathy [3] Empathy is also not a single module but has at least two 'fractions': cognitive empathy (also, called Mindreading or theory of mind, and which is defined as the ability to imagine another person's thoughts and feelings) and affective empathy (the drive to respond to another person's mental state with an appropriate emotion). Although we see some evidence of empathy in other non-human animals, there is no convincing evidence that other animals can attribute false beliefs to another animal and engage in flexible deception and teaching, for example, unlike even a four-year old modern human child.

And our recent studies using molecular genetics show that empathy and theory of mind show associations with common genetic variants in our genome, combinations of 'single nucleotide polymorphisms' or SNPs that are associated with where each of us falls on what I call the Empathy Bell Curve of individual differences in this ability. Finding that empathy is partly genetic is a clue that it was the result of natural selection and it is easy to see why it might have been highly adaptive—for example, to build traps into which your prey would fall, or to read the mind of your pre-verbal infant to attend to its emotional and physical needs so that it survived to the age of reproduction to pass on your genes.

This was impressive enough, and the Empathy Circuit could explain *why* we see jewellery, musical instruments, sculpture and cave paintings in the archaeological record—we were thinking about an audience and what they might be interested in—but by itself the Empathy Circuit cannot explain *how* modern humans were capable of invention. I argue that to fully explain the cognitive revolution in our capacity for generative invention, we also needed a second new brain circuit, the *Systemizing Mechanism*.

The Systemizing Mechanism allowed us to seek new patterns in the world—we became pattern seekers of a new kind. Whereas *Homo habilis, erectus* and *neanderthalis* could see patterns using a learning mechanism that is widespread in the

Fig. 9.5 The key steps in systemizing, using the terminology of engineers (input-operation-output) and logicians (if-and-then). (From Baron-Cohen (2020) The Pattern Seekers)

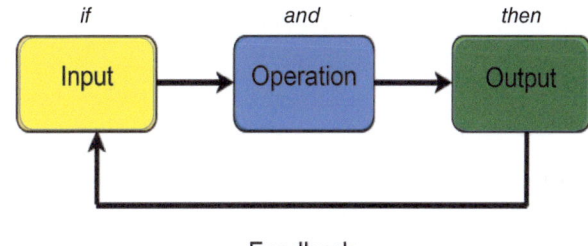

animal kingdom—associative learning—where we can engage in statistical learning of regularities such as A is associated with B (using a hammer to crush a nut is associated with getting the juicy reward, for example), modern humans for the first time from 100,000 to 70,000 years ago were looking for special *if-and-then* patterns (Fig. 9.5). This was a powerful new algorithm in the modern human brain that enabled a new raft of behaviours, all emanating from the capacity for generative invention. So, we could invent music, cooking, medicine, weapons, agriculture, astronomy, sports, business, science, technology, engineering and mathematics (STEM), arts and crafts and even syntax, to name just a few of the benefits of the Systemizing Mechanism.

Humans were looking for *if-and-then* patterns which in engineering terms are equivalent of *input-operation-output* patterns. *If* I take an input, *and* I perform (or observe) an operation on the input, *then* I see a change in the output. An operation could be a wide range of actions, and the most interesting of these would be a *causal* operation. And the job of the Systemizing Mechanism was not only to find such *if-and-then* patterns, but to confirm them through repetition, to confirm their truth, where truth is a regularity that is seen over and over again. Critically, generative invention arises from playing with these *if-and-then* patterns, by changing the input (the *if*) or the operation (the *and*) to observe a change in the output (the *then*). Humans had become *experimentalists*, a skill that is still absent in any other living species today and was absent in our Homo ancestors.

I call this the Systemizing Mechanism because the basis of any system is the *if-and-then* pattern, a powerful regularity or law, whether we are talking about a natural system like the weather, a mechanical system like a bow-and-arrow, an abstract system like music or mathematics, a social system like a business or an army unit, a motoric system like throwing a frisbee or skate-boarding or a collectible system like classifying plants and animals into a taxonomy. None of these behaviours are seen in non-human animals today.

I borrow the *if-and-then* algorithm from the nineteenth century logician George Boole whose analysis of how we think logically is credited with the invention of the modern computer, and his analysis overlaps with other logicians such as Venn (of Venn diagram fame). But when you read Boole's important textbook of logic [4], it seems dry, abstract and hard to relate to the uniquely human capacity for invention. For me, seeing the first musical instrument is a much more concrete example of systemising:

If I blow down this hollow bone,
and I cover one hole,
then I make sound A.

If I blow down this hollow bone,
and I uncover one hole,
then I make sound B.

Beautiful musical sequences of notes, riffs and rhythmic patterns emanating from an *engine* in the brain that enables invention, explaining why humans alone are attracted to listen to and produce music. And you can see the same exquisite logic underlies the invention of any complex tool, defined as a system that does work for us. For brevity, I'll give you just eight more examples:

1. The invention of **stealth weapons** like the bow-and-arrow that could kill from a distance was based on *if* I attach an arrow to a stretchy fibre, *and* release the tension in the fibre, *then* the arrow will fly.
2. The invention of **mechanical systems** such as how to move a heavy rock (explaining how Stone Henge was built for example) involved *if* I have a heavy stone, *and* I harness it to my ox, *then* the heavy stone will move.
3. The invention of **agriculture** involved logic such as *if* I take a tomato seed, *and* plant it in moist soil, *then* I get a tomato plant.
4. The invention of **mathematics** involved logic such as *if* I take the number 3, *and* I cube it, *then* I get the number 27.
5. The invention of **cooking** involved for example that *if* I take an egg, *and* put it in boiling water for 4 min, *then* the yolk will turn from soft yellow to hard yellow.
6. The invention of **medicine** involved observing that *if* I have a headache, *and* I eat the willow tree bark, *then* my headache goes away.
7. The discovery of **astronomy** involved logic such as *if* the moon looks white, *and* the sun, moon and Earth lie in a straight line, *then* the moon looks red.
8. Even the invention of **public health** involved the same beautiful logic: *if* the infection rate is doubling every week, *and* we don't do lockdown, *then* 50,000 people will die this winter.

Like the Empathy Circuit, there are individual differences in the drive to systemise, giving rise to the Systemizing Bell Curve in the population, and there are common genetic variants that are associated with where each of us falls on this bell curve, whether we are barely interested in if-and-then patterns (though all humans are to some extent), or if we are average in systemising or if we systemise non-stop—so called hyper-systemisers. We know less about the brain basis of systemising but at least one brain region that is involved is the intraparietal sulcus. Whilst the Empathy Circuit has been mapped in exquisite detail using functional magnetic resonance imaging over the last 25 years in the field of social neuroscience, the neuroscience underpinning the Systemizing Mechanism awaits more research.

But the fact that where we fall on the Systemizing Bell Curve is even partly genetic again means that this uniquely human ability was the product of natural selection. It is not difficult to see how hyper-systemisers might have had some adaptive advantages, being the persons you would go to in your tribe when your child was sick, or to fix your gadget, and who could invent new and better ways of doing things, amassing significant resources. And we know from anthropology that fertility is associated with reproductive success—surviving long enough to pass on one's genes.

It is time to turn to autism, but there's one more piece of the argument to lay out, which is the relationship between these two new circuits that I argue explain the cognitive revolution 100,000–70,000 years ago. If we plot the Empathy Bell Curve along the Y axis and the Systemizing Bell Curve along on the X axis, so that we can map every individual according to their difference (D) score, we see some interesting patterns (Fig. 9.6).

In our big data study of 600,000 typical people and 36,000 autistic people, we find all humans fall into just five types of brain (a beautiful demonstration of 'neurodiversity'). There are those whose empathy is at a higher level than the systemising, those I call Type E. They are about 30% of the population, and more females (40%) than males (20%) fall into this group. There are those whose systemising is at a higher level than their empathy, those I call Type S. Again, these comprise about 30% of the population, but this time the on average sex difference is flipped over, more males (40%) than females (20%) falling into this group. There are those who

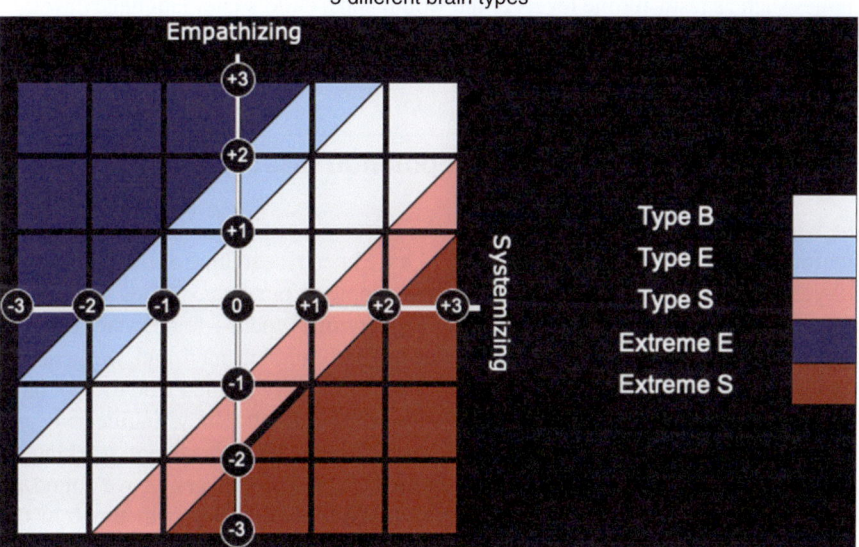

Fig. 9.6 The Empathizing-Systemizing Theory, showing 5 brain types in the population. (From Baron-Cohen (2020) The Pattern Seekers)

show no difference in their drive to empathise or to systemise, being equally good in both, who I call Type B. Again, these comprise about 30% of the population.

And then there are those of us who fall at the extremes [5]: Extreme Type E, whose Empathy Circuit is tuned super high and who empathise non-stop, but their Systemizing Mechanism is tuned to just average levels or below. These comprise about 3% of the population, with more females (4%) than males (1%) falling into this group. And then there are the mirror image, those who are Extreme Type S, whose Systemizing Mechanism is tuned super high and who systemise non-stop, but their Empathy Circuit is tuned to just average levels or below. They also comprise about 3% of the population and the sex ratio is flipped over: more males (4%) than females (2%) fall into this group. I call these the hyper-systemisers, and among these are inventors in history like Thomas Edison, Isaac Newton and Nicholas Tesla, or modern-day inventors like Bill Gates and the musician Glenn Gould. Each of these inventors showed behaviours that suggest they had a higher than average number of autistic traits, even though they did not have or need an autism diagnosis. We will come back to that intriguing connection to autistic traits.

Why are these sex differences seen among the five brain types? A moderate proposal is that this reflects the interplay of prenatal biology (genetics and the prenatal sex steroid hormones such as testosterone and oestrogen, both of which shape brain development in utero during a critical period, and shape behaviour postnatally) interacting with social and cultural influences, such as how we unconsciously may treat our sons and daughters differently through our parenting styles, how teachers may unconsciously interact differently with male and female pupils, how role models influence our interests and aspirations and how the media insidiously influences our behaviour. Our studies of the correlations between prenatal sex steroid hormones such as testosterone levels in the womb and a child's later language development, empathy, systemising and pattern-recognition skills were all laid out in what was the subject of another of my earlier books, *The Essential Difference* [6].

9.3 Autism and Neurodevelopmental Disability

So what is the link—if any—between the human capacity for invention and the neurodevelopmental disability of autism? I have been researching autism for almost 40 years. We found that the 36,000 autistic people in our Brain Types study were also more likely to have a brain of Type S or Extreme Type S—to be systemisers or hyper-systemisers—and that this was true of both autistic men and women. We found that among the 600,000 people in the population we studied who did not have an autism diagnosis, those working in STEM (science, technology, engineering and mathematics) had a higher number of autistic traits than those not working in STEM. In our studies of mathematicians in Cambridge University, we found an elevated rate of diagnosed autism among them in comparison with those in the Humanities or in the general population.

If we look at the question from the other perspective, we find autistic people anecdotally may be 'savants' in systemising. Derek Paravacini has a mental age of a three-year old, is congenitally blind and autistic, but can play any jazz piece on the piano after hearing it just once. Daniel Tammet is autistic and has synaesthesia (a mixing of the senses, and which we found is more common in autistic people than in the general population). He has learnt ten languages because he loves syntactic patterns and memorised the number Pi to 22,514 decimal places. He can also multiply three-digit numbers together faster than a hand calculator.

But anecdotes do not add up to data even if they are important clues that warrant systematic empirical testing. On average, autistic people outperform non-autistic people on tests of pattern recognition and on tests of mechanical reasoning and are over-represented in STEM subjects if they go to university. And this link between autistic traits, autism and systemising appears to be genetic. Among their fathers and grandfathers, we found a disproportionate number end up in the occupation of engineering. Mothers of autistic children are also over-represented in STEM, and both mothers and fathers of autistic children show superior pattern-recognition skills, reflecting 'assortative mating' may be occurring. This led us to predict that autism should be more common in places like Silicon Valley, which we tested in the Dutch city of Eindhoven, the Silicon Valley of the Netherlands. We found that autism was more than twice as high in Eindhoven compared to two other Dutch cities (Utrecht and Haarlem), which have a similar population size and are matched on relevant demographic variables, but which are not information-technology hubs [7].

But to really prove that autism and systemising are linked we conducted a molecular genetic analysis, to test if there was an overlap between the common genetic variants associated with autism and those associated with hyper-systemising. Sure enough, there was [8] The overlap was 26%. Some of the genes for autism are not just coding for autism but for talent at systemising. We had nailed the link.

9.4   Discussion

Autistic people have been marginalised, stigmatised and excluded by modern society because of their social disability. We found that two thirds of adults (with autism) have felt suicidal, one third have attempted suicide and the majority have poor mental health such as high levels of anxiety and depression [9]. Poor mental health is not part of autism but I argue it is a sign of lack of support and inclusion into society. Unemployment levels of autistic adults are unacceptably high, and we know that in anyone, unemployment is bad for your mental health. It robs you of feeling you have a purpose in life, it makes you feel excluded from society, that you are not valued, and it robs you of your economic autonomy and independence.

9.5   Conclusion

It is time to respect and celebrate autistic people's difference that their brain types are just one of the five forms of neurodiversity we find in any population and that their brains and genes have driven the evolution of human invention, for

70,000–100,000 years. It's time to support them into work, both for their own well-being, for societal productivity and a civic duty towards anyone with a disability, and to maximise the likelihood of future human innovation.

Key Points
- Biologically evolved autistic traits have contributed significantly to the unique capacity for inventiveness of *Homo sapiens* and, therefore, the shaping of science, technology and societies, including contemporary ones.
- Autistic traits can be divided into low empathising and high systematising dimensions and these two are genetically dissociable. Some of the genes for autism are not just coding for autism but for talent at systemising.
- Autistic people outperform non-autistic people on tests of pattern recognition and on tests of mechanical reasoning and are over-represented in STEM (Science, Technology, Engineering and Medicine) subjects if they go to university. And this link between autistic traits, autism and systemising appears to be genetic.
- The disability arising from autistic traits is determined through social exclusion, to which low empathising traits may contribute, rather than exclusively from the inherently biological traits as such and there is a need to address this and ensure equitable inclusion.
- Though there are genetic determinants of autistic traits which contribute to contemporary diagnostic practice in relation to autism, such practice presents fundamental challenges to Emil Kraepelin's concept of mental health conditions understood as disease entities of the natural kind.

References

1. Harari Y. Sapiens. Random House Harper; 2014.
2. Baron-Cohen S. The pattern seekers: a new theory of human invention. Penguin; 2022. ISBN-13 978-0141982397
3. Baron-Cohen S. Zero degrees of empathy: a new understanding of cruelty and kindness; 2012.
4. George Boole, The mathematical analysis of logic, being an essay towards a calculus of deductive reasoning archived 11 May 2016 at the Wayback Machine (London, UK: Macmillan, Barclay, & Macmillan, 1847).
5. Greenberg DM, et al. Testing the Empathizing-Systemizing theory of sex differences and the Extreme Male Brain theory of autism in half a million people. Proc Natl Acad Sci U S A. 2018;115:12152–7.
6. Baron-Cohen S. The essential difference. Men, women and the extreme male brain. Penguin; 2012. ISBN 978-0-241-96135-3
7. Roelfsema MT, Hoekstra RA, Allison C, et al. Are autism spectrum conditions more prevalent in an information-technology region? A school-based study of three regions in The Netherlands. J Autism Dev Disord. 2012;42:734–9. https://doi.org/10.1007/s10803-011-1302-1.
8. Warrier V, Toro R, Won H, Leblond CS, Cliquet F, Delorme R, De Witte W, Bralten J, Chakrabarti B, Børglum AD, Grove J, Poelmans G, Hinds DA, Bourgeron T, Baron-Cohen S. Social and non-social autism symptoms and trait domains are genetically dissociable. Commun Biol. 2019;2:328. https://doi.org/10.1038/s42003-019-0558-4. eCollection 2019

9. Hossain MM, Khan N, Sultana A, Ma P, McKyer ELJ, Ahmed HU, Purohit N. Prevalence of comorbid psychiatric disorders among people with autism spectrum disorder: an umbrella review of systematic reviews and meta-analyses. Psychiatry Res. 2020;287:112922. https://doi.org/10.1016/j.psychres.2020.112922. Epub 2020 Mar 18

Open Access   This chapter is licensed under the terms of the Creative Commons Attribution 4.0 International License (http://creativecommons.org/licenses/by/4.0/), which permits use, sharing, adaptation, distribution and reproduction in any medium or format, as long as you give appropriate credit to the original author(s) and the source, provide a link to the Creative Commons license and indicate if changes were made.

The images or other third party material in this chapter are included in the chapter's Creative Commons license, unless indicated otherwise in a credit line to the material. If material is not included in the chapter's Creative Commons license and your intended use is not permitted by statutory regulation or exceeds the permitted use, you will need to obtain permission directly from the copyright holder.

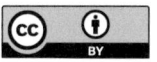

Political Ideology, Collective Emotions and Diagnosis in Psychiatry

10

Francesca Brencio

10.1 Psychiatry and Social Values

The practice of psychiatric diagnosis does not occur in a social vacuum. Rather, it takes place within complex networks of political ideologies, institutional frameworks and collective emotional responses that shape how society conceptualises mental distress and pathology. Historically, psychiatry has not only sought to address mental illness but also functioned as a tool for regulating behaviours considered deviant or undesirable by dominant social standards. The history of psychiatry reveals a consistent pattern wherein diagnostic categories have reflected and reinforced prevailing social values and political arrangements. From the diagnosis of drapetomania[1] [1] in enslaved individuals who attempted to escape captivity in

---

[1] In 1851, American physician Samuel A. Cartwright introduced the term *drapetomania*, a purported mental disorder that he claimed explained why enslaved Africans attempted to escape captivity. This scientifically unfounded concept stemmed from the racist presumption that slavery represented an improvement in the lives of enslaved people, leading Cartwright to conclude that only those suffering from mental illness would seek freedom. He specifically identified plantation escapes as evidence of this supposed condition. Cartwright reasoned that contentment with enslavement was the natural state, and therefore resistance must indicate psychological abnormality. Modern scholarship has thoroughly rejected drapetomania as pseudoscience and recognises it as a clear example of scientific racism used to reinforce oppressive systems. The term combines the Greek words *drapetēs* (meaning 'runaway slave') and *mania*. This historical example offers the occasion to remark the need of decolonising mental health, an issue which is still urgent in our contemporary landscape: it challenges dominant Western psychiatric frameworks that have historically marginalised non-white experiences and contributed to biases inherent in psychiatric knowledge production. The work of Frantz Fanon, a Martinican psychiatrist, is cardinal in this endeavour. His critical analysis examines how colonialism affects psychological wellbeing. In doing so, he

---

F. Brencio (✉)
Institute for Mental Health, School of Psychology, University of Birmingham, Birmingham, UK
e-mail: f.brencio@bham.ac.uk

© The Author(s) 2026
G. Ikkos, T. Becker (eds.), *Psychiatry after Kraepelin*,
https://doi.org/10.1007/978-3-032-09475-9_10

the nineteenth century American South, to hysteria and hysterical neurosis[2] [2] in women who rejected traditional gender roles, to the classification of homosexuality as a mental disorder until its removal from the Diagnostic and Statistical Manual of Mental Disorders (DSM) in 1987[3] [3], psychiatric diagnoses have often delineated the boundaries between acceptable and unacceptable expressions of human difference. This delineation process is deeply embedded in the sociopolitical climate of each historical period, serving to medicalise behaviours and experiences that challenge existing power structures, social norms and cultural biases rather than objective scientific evidence, reflecting broader societal attitudes and control. Furthermore, the practice of psychiatric treatment, from institutionalisation to lobotomies, have often been influenced by the need to enforce social conformity rather than promote individual well-being.

Perhaps we can agree on the fact that understanding mental health is inextricably linked to shifting conceptions of normalcy, morality and managing public health and individual behaviours. This ongoing interplay underscores the need for psychiatric practice to be critically engaged with the social contexts in which it operates, ensuring that medical advancements do not perpetuate harmful social values.

The emergence of modern psychiatry in the late eighteenth and early nineteenth centuries coincided with the rise of industrial capitalism and liberal democracy in Western Europe and North America. This historical convergence was not merely coincidental but reflected shared philosophical underpinnings and social objectives. As the French philosopher Michel Foucault (1965) argued in his seminal work *Madness and Civilization* [4], the rise of psychiatric institutions represented a new form of social control in which 'unreasonable' individuals were confined and subjected to medical authority. This confinement served both to remove perceived social threats and to reinforce the values of rationality, productivity and self-regulation central to emerging capitalist economies. Foucault's interest in the science of psychiatry stemmed from the way in which it implicated a political structure and moral practice [5, p. XXI]. The control on the physical body of the individual very rapidly becomes the control on the social body of the community [6]: 'Psychiatry immediately perceived itself as a permanent function of social order and made use of the asylums for two purposes: first, to treat the most obvious, the most

---

deploys the historical-racial schema, which identifies how colonial power structures damage both colonised and coloniser. Key elements of this schema include psychological internalisation of racist narratives; destruction of the colonised person's sense of self; understanding race as a dynamic power relationship rather than fixed category; systemic dehumanisation; and the necessity of dismantling these structures for true liberation.

[2] Until 1968, hysteria was included among the recognised 'mental disorders'. Only with the publication of the DSM-III-Revised in 1987, the American Psychiatric Association removed it from the classification of mental disorders.

[3] Homosexuality was classified as a 'mental disorder' in the first edition of the Diagnostic and Statistical Manual of Mental Disorders (DSM), published in 1952, and was only fully removed from subsequent editions in 1987. On 17 May 1990, the World Health Organization (WHO) officially eliminated homosexuality from its list of mental disorders.

embarrassing cases and, at the same time, to provide a sort of guarantee, an image of scientificity, by making the place of confinement look like a hospital' [7, p. 180].

By categorising certain behaviours, conditions or individuals as pathological, diagnosis serves to define the boundaries of normalcy and regulate conformity to societal norms. This process led to marginalisation and stigmatisation of individuals or groups who were outside these prescribed norms, often reinforcing existing power structures. For instance, psychiatric diagnoses have been used to silence dissent or nonconformity, labelling politically or socially active individuals as mentally ill, thus delegitimising their actions and removing them from the political sphere. In post-Stalinist Soviet Union, psychiatry became a powerful tool of political repression, as exemplified by the fabricated diagnosis of 'sluggish schizophrenia', a condition conveniently characterised by symptoms such as 'reform delusions' and 'anti-government thinking', which allowed authorities to institutionalise dissidents in psychiatric hospitals where they endured forced medication and isolation.[4] Similarly, key categories in the social sciences—such as those applied to race, gender and class—often reflect and reinforce ideologies that justify inequality. An example of this may be found in the historical IQ testing that claimed to find inherent intellectual differences between racial groups, used to justify educational segregation, or the labelling of poverty-related survival behaviours as 'criminal tendencies' or 'antisocial personality traits'. When diagnostic frameworks intersect with cultural assumptions embedded in dominant power structures, they can distort our understanding of psychological experiences across diverse communities. The ongoing overdiagnosis of schizophrenia in black patients compared to white patients presenting with identical symptoms [8] illustrates how psychiatric classification systems risk to reproduce and legitimise social hierarchies rather than accurately represent mental health variations across cultures and individual experiences.

The early psychiatric nosology developed by Philippe Pinel, Benjamin Rush and others reflected these sociopolitical imperatives. Mental disorders were frequently defined in relation to patients' inability or unwillingness to participate productively in industrial society. 'Moral treatment', the dominant therapeutic approach of the era, explicitly aimed to instil values of self-discipline, industriousness and social conformity in psychiatric patients [9]. Thus, from its inception, psychiatric diagnosis served not merely to identify and treat suffering but to reinforce particular political and economic arrangements.

This pattern of diagnostically encoding social and political values continued throughout the nineteenth and twentieth centuries: psychiatric classification has frequently served to delegitimise resistance to dominant social norms by framing it as illness rather than dissent [10]. Even as psychiatry developed increasingly sophisticated biological explanations for mental illness, its diagnostic categories continued to reflect and reinforce prevailing social values.

---

[4]The All-Union Society of Psychiatrists and Neuropathologists withdrew from the World Psychiatric Association in 1983, facing imminent expulsion over allegations that Soviet psychiatry was being misused to suppress political dissidents.

While contemporary psychiatry has disavowed many of its most explicitly political diagnostic practices, the relationship between psychiatric diagnosis and social values persists in more subtle forms. The DSM-V, for instance, continues to reflect culturally specific understandings of normal and abnormal behaviour despite its authors' attempts to create universal, culture-free diagnostic criteria. Conditions such as attention-deficit/hyperactivity disorder (ADHD) and oppositional defiant disorder have been criticised for pathologising behaviours that conflict with the demands of contemporary educational and economic systems rather than representing inherent psychopathology [11]. Moreover, the increasing biologisation of psychiatric diagnosis, while scientifically productive in many respects, has also served political functions. As Nikolas Rose [12] argues, the emphasis on neurochemical explanations for mental distress tends to individualise suffering that often has social causes, directing attention away from structural factors such as inequality, discrimination and exploitation. The framing of mental illness as primarily a brain disorder rather than a response to adverse social conditions aligns with neoliberal political ideologies that emphasise individual responsibility over collective welfare and structural change.

Even ostensibly progressive developments in psychiatric diagnosis reflect broader political currents. The inclusion of posttraumatic stress disorder (PTSD) in the DSM-III in 1980, while representing an important recognition of trauma's psychological impacts, also served to individualise and medicalise collective experiences of violence and oppression. By conceptualising trauma primarily as an individual psychopathology rather than a normal response to abnormal social conditions, the PTSD diagnosis has sometimes directed attention away from the political and social contexts that produce traumatic experiences [13].

These examples illustrate how contemporary psychiatric diagnosis risks to function as what Foucault termed a *discourse of power*, defining the boundaries of normality and abnormality in ways that generally align with dominant political interests. This is not to suggest that psychiatric diagnoses are merely political constructs with no relation to real suffering; rather, it is to recognise that the conceptualisation, identification and treatment of this suffering are inevitably shaped by the sociopolitical contexts in which they occur, and a critical philosophical attitude is necessary to increase awareness on these issues. Certainly, it would be partial not recognising that, despite navigating through difficult decades of questionable treatments and institutional practices, contemporary psychiatry has evolved into a discipline that has also meaningfully improved the lives of countless individuals suffering from mental illness, while also advancing our understanding of the brain.

10.2   Collective Emotions and Their Weight in the Making of a Diagnosis

In order to understand the epistemological framework of what follows, I would like to discuss the role of collective emotions and draw some philosophical distinctions between collective emotions and group-based emotions and their relationship with and the ascertainment of a mental diagnosis.

Collective emotions are shared affective states that emerge and circulate within social groups. They powerfully influence how societies interpret and respond to human differences. These emotions, ranging from fear and disgust to compassion and admiration, shape public perceptions of behaviours and experiences that may become targets of psychiatric diagnosis. As Sara Ahmed [14] argues in *The Cultural Politics of Emotion*, collective emotions are not merely psychological states but social and political forces that stick to certain bodies and identities, marking them as either valued or problematic. In the context of psychiatric diagnosis, collective emotions often precede and shape diagnostic categories rather than merely responding to them. Collective emotions can function as 'pre-diagnostic forces' that influence which human differences become medicalised.

These collective emotional responses are rarely spontaneous or natural. Rather, they are cultivated and channelled through various social institutions and cultural narratives. Media representations, political rhetoric and educational practices all contribute to the formation of emotional regimes that govern how societies feel about different forms of human behaviours and experience. These emotional regimes then become embedded in diagnostic criteria and practices, often in ways that remain unacknowledged by mental health professionals.

Collective emotions possess the capacity to influence diagnostic processes, and reciprocally, diagnoses can reinforce specific collective emotions. As previously said, by collective emotions I refer to emotions experienced by multiple subjects simultaneously [15, 16]. Collective emotions serve dual functions: cohesion of group identity and demarcation of boundaries. Within the scholarly literature on collective emotional phenomena, a significant conceptual distinction emerges between collective emotions proper and group-based emotions. Group-based emotions are contingent upon an individual's identification with a particular social collective, arising in response to events perceived as relevant to the entire group and frequently characterised by 'we-they' categorical distinctions. In contrast, collective emotions constitute affective states that are synchronously shared and experienced by multiple individuals within a societal context. A prominent theoretical proposition within collective emotion scholarship posits that an aggregation of multiple group-based emotional responses to societal phenomena may transmute into genuine collective emotion. This distinction highlights that whereas group-based emotions represent individual affective experiences triggered by group-relevant occurrences, collective emotions position the collective entity itself as the primary affective agent—suggesting a qualitative transformation in the ontological status of the emotional phenomenon [17].

It is essential to underscore that collective emotions necessitate a specific mode of self-conceptualisation: the experiential recognition of oneself as a constituent member of a social collective, a process more precisely termed *group identification*. This identification process encompasses two distinct requisite components: (a) a motivational-phenomenological transformation wherein individual self-experience transmutes into collective 'we-experience', and (b) a cognitive-perceptual reorientation involving the adoption of the collective's perspectival framework. This latter component represents an evolutionarily derivative and more complex manifestation of perspective-taking capacity, suggesting that once individuals develop the ability to adopt alternative perspectives at the interpersonal level, they may subsequently acquire the capacity to internalise collective perspectives. In contrast to group-based emotions, collective emotions presuppose an additional phenomenological quality, often characterised in the literature as 'a sense of togetherness' or collective affective intentionality, which transcends mere aggregated individual experiences [18]. In this view, we can have group-based political emotions and collective political emotions, which are based on joint evaluations ('feeling-toward-together') in light of political concerns [19] not just in name of the group, but rather as our affective intentional state. Considering the centrality of conformity within diagnostic frameworks, the significance of collective emotional dynamics becomes readily apparent. The impetus to adhere to socially sanctioned norms necessarily entails mechanisms of group identification, which, in turn, can engender affective responses shared across individuals within a given social context. Collective political emotions may be defined as 'jointly felt appraisals of a politically relevant object, person or even in light of the given community's political concerns' [20, p. 13].

Shared political emotions entail specific conditions that can exert considerable influence on diagnostic practices, particularly where notions of conformity and perceived societal threats—both indicative of a reinforced collective identity—shape the epistemological and interpretive approaches employed. Such emotions are characterised by several key elements: (1) a *two-dimensional affective intentionality*, wherein the shared nature of the emotion is constitutive of the emotion itself and is accompanied by a mutual awareness of this sharedness; (2) a *public recognition* component, whereby the emotion is acknowledged by external observers, with the public sphere serving as a central arena; (3) a *reciprocity* condition, involving dynamic interrelations between the community's collective perspective and the perspectives of individual members; and (4) a *normativity* criterion, which governs the appropriateness and legitimacy of the emotional expression within a given sociopolitical context. Normativity functions to realign individuals 'around a shared emotional perspective and enforce[s] the political identity of groups' [20, p. 18]. Consequently, experiences of robust political emotions 'not only impact how we ought to feel in a particular moment but how we ought to feel in similar moments going forward and they work to strengthen one's sense of belonging to a political community' [20, p. 18]. In this epistemological framework, it is important to consider the weight ideologies have: 'Ideologies employ a threefold use of emotion. They wrap rational discourse in varying layers of emotive idiom; they assign emotional import to their key values; and they openly recognize the centrality of emotion in sociopolitical interaction' [21, pp. 11–12]. The emphasis put on emotions and feelings has a significant rhetorical effect and impact on public opinion. The use of emotion is a very powerful tool in the widespread communication and very easily answers the 'yes or no' logic through inferences and supposed implications. And, as we have seen, the use of social emotions may contribute to marginalising and labelling people—not only in mental health, but also in our social and political life.

Accordingly, the normative function of collective emotions holds the capacity to: (a) reassert moral or social norms and foster affective commitments to particular values; (b) shape sociological processes that, in turn, may amplify or sustain other collective emotions and political affective climates (e.g. sentiments of justice, nationalism or public passions); (c) contribute to the consolidation and emergence of new ontological categories by orienting individuals around a shared evaluative framework, thus reinforcing a sense of belonging to a collective 'we'; (d) and influence the development and legitimisation of novel diagnostic categories.

Notably, during the Nazi era, psychiatric institutions aligned themselves with prevailing sociopolitical agendas, contributing to ethically and scientifically harmful and inhumane practices. In those years 'eugenics, racism and nationalism were allied to an academic approach in which the individual was readily submerged by the doctrine of the greater good of the nation' [22].

10.3   The History of Asperger's Syndrome Between Social Political Emotion and Neurodiversity

The history of Asperger's syndrome offers a compelling case study of how political ideologies and social emotions converge in psychiatric diagnosis. First described by Hans Asperger in Vienna during the Nazi era, this condition was initially conceptualised within a political context that valued neurotypical conformity and productivity. Asperger himself navigated this context strategically, portraying some of his patients as potentially valuable to the Reich while acknowledging that others might be considered 'useless eaters' under Nazi ideology [23]. This early framing reveals how the very recognition of the condition was shaped by contemporary political values regarding human worth and productivity. Despite Asperger's work in the 1940s, the condition that now bears his name remained largely unknown in Anglophone psychiatry until the 1980s, when Lorna Wing popularised the term [24]. Its subsequent inclusion in the DSM-IV in 1994 coincided with increasing public awareness of autism spectrum conditions and changing social attitudes toward neurodevelopmental differences. This diagnostic recognition reflected not only advancing clinical knowledge but also shifting political and cultural contexts that allowed for new interpretations of behaviours previously labelled simply as oddity or social maladjustment [25].

To understand the emergence of Hans Asperger's conceptualisation of autism within the context of National Socialism, it is essential to consider the ideological framework in which belonging to the national community was contingent not only on racial and physiological criteria but also on the demonstration of shared political spirit. Conformity to the collective, both in belief and behaviour, was construed as vital to the health and vitality of the German *Volk*, as defined by Nazi ideology. This intense valorisation of social cohesion reflects the fascist foundations of Nazism, wherein collective emotions became instrumental to the regime's eugenic vision. In this framework, sociability itself was reconfigured as a criterion of inclusion or exclusion, joining race, political ideology, religion, sexuality, criminality and physiology as axes of persecution.

Asperger and his senior colleagues adopted the term *Gemüt* to capture this concept. Originally denoting 'soul' in eighteenth-century German thought, *Gemüt* was redefined within Nazi child psychiatry to signify a *metaphysical capacity for social connectedness*, a crucial marker of one's integration into the collective. This notion became central to psychiatric assessments, as children deemed to possess a 'poor *Gemüt*' were identified as socially deficient, incapable of forming the emotional bonds necessary for participation in the fascist social order. Long before Asperger formally described autistic psychopathology in 1944, diagnostic categories were already emerging around the concept of *Gemütsarmut* (lacking *Gemüt*). Asperger himself described autism in terms of a defect in *Gemüt* [26, pp. 12–13] positioning it as a disruption in the individual's affective orientation toward the social world. In this sense, *Gemüt* anticipates what has been described as the affective intentionality requirement of collective emotions, an essential orientation toward shared emotional experience and social attunement.

Asperger's understanding of autism also reflects a deep engagement with the etymological roots of the term. Deriving from the Greek *autos* (self), Asperger used the word autism to describe those who, in his view, were most fundamentally themselves, individuals defined by an intensified self-relatedness and a diminished responsiveness to social convention. For Asperger, the typical person was shaped through learned and conditioned social behaviours, embedded in a matrix of normative expectations. In contrast, the autistic individual stood apart, expressing a more spontaneous, unmediated mode of being. This *Selbst-sein*, a radical being-oneself-alone, was for Asperger the defining essence of autism, a mode of existence marked by distance from the social world and a uniquely self-contained subjectivity. As Scheffer noticed, 'The idea of autism pervaded the Third Reich long before anyone defined it'—which means: the idea of children who appeared 'to have less community feeling, who forged weaker social bonds and did not align with collectivist expectations' [27, p. 158].

By offering a clinically detailed characterisation of certain children under the label of 'autistic psychopaths' [28], Hans Asperger effectively responded to the ideological and institutional demands of the Nazi regime. In this context, Asperger's diagnostic framework can be seen as contributing to the construction of biologically grounded criteria for determining inclusion within the national-racial community or, conversely, for legitimising the exclusion and potential elimination of those deemed undesirable. Central to Asperger's conception of autism was the notion of 'personal distance'—a detachment from the instinctual and affective dimensions of social life—which he identified as the defining hallmark of the condition. In 1944, he published his thesis 'Die 'Autistischen Psychopathen' im Kindesalter' ('The "Autistic Psychopaths" in Childhood') in the *Archiv für Psychiatrie und Nervenkrankheiten*. In his early descriptions, Hans Asperger characterised the children he observed as exhibiting a form of personality disorder. These were primarily young boys who demonstrated normal intelligence and language development yet presented with behaviours now labelled as autistic in nature, alongside significant deficits in social interaction and communication. Asperger delineated core diagnostic features that included a profound incapacity for affective (emotional) connection with others; a marked insistence on sameness and routine; mutism or abnormalities in speech; an intense preoccupation with object manipulation; heightened visuospatial abilities or exceptional rote memory coupled with notable learning challenges in other domains; and an appearance marked by alertness, attractiveness and apparent intelligence.

What warrants particular emphasis is not only Asperger's unequivocal presumption that these children lacked emotional and affective connection, an absence deeply significant in a society structured around the moral and political value of emotional cohesion, but also his reduction in the complex and heterogeneous presentations of autism into a singular deficit: the absence of *Gemüt*, the metaphysical capacity for social bonds. In the sociopolitical context of Nazi Germany, where *Gemüt* was valorised as a cornerstone of collective identity and moral worth, this diagnosis functioned not merely as a clinical label but as a form of moral exclusion. Asperger's diagnosis of 'autistic psychopathy' thus operated within a broader ideological apparatus in which deviation from the fascist ideal of emotional conformity was construed as pathological. The diagnostic judgment became, in many cases, tantamount to a death sentence. More disturbingly, it served as a mechanism of moral legitimation: for clinicians, including Asperger himself, who understood their work as a service to the state; and for parents who, identifying with the Nazi conception of the collective self often brought children they perceived as deviant to institutions such as the *Spiegelgrund Clinic* in Vienna, where under the guise of medical care, 789 children were murdered during the Second World War.

In this context, the Asperger diagnosis functioned as a tool of social control, a mechanism through which individuals who failed to exhibit the requisite traits of the Nazi social and collective identity, particularly the emotional attunement foundational to collective political life, were systematically excluded. Nonconformity was pathologised, and difference came to signify danger, uselessness and moral failure.

How much politics and social emotions influenced the elaboration of the diagnosis is evident even in Asperger's words. In 1937, in a talk entitled 'The Mentally Abnormal Child', and published in the Viennese Clinical Weekly, he asserted that 'there are as many approaches as there are different personalities. It is impossible to establish a rigid set of criteria for a diagnosis' [29, p. 1461]. But a year later, in October 1938, in a lecture under the same name, given in the same place, and published in the same journal, he introduced his own diagnosis, this well-characterised group of children who we name 'autistic psychopaths'—because the confinement of the self (*autos*) has led to a narrowing of relations to their environment [30, p. 1316]. This was the same disorder with two different perspectives, the destiny of which was decided by the meaning given to one word: *diversity*.

The history of Asperger' syndrome culminated in significant diagnostic revision with the publication of the DSM-V in 2013, which eliminated Asperger's as a distinct category and incorporated it within the broader autism spectrum disorder diagnosis. This revision reflected scientific developments in understanding autism as a continuous spectrum rather than discrete categories, but it also emerged from political contestation over the diagnosis itself. Neurodiversity advocates had criticised the separation of Asperger's from other forms of autism as creating a problematic hierarchy that privileged individuals perceived as 'high functioning' while marginalising those with more significant support needs. This critique reflected broader disability rights perspectives that rejected functioning labels as reinforcing ableist values. These competing perspectives revealed underlying ideological tensions about the nature of disability, the value of medical labels, and the relationship between individual identity and collective categorisation. The diagnostic revision thus represented not merely a scientific recalibration but a political negotiation of competing claims about how neurodevelopmental differences should be conceptualised and addressed.

10.4   Concluding Remarks

In the history of medicine and in particular of psychiatry, diagnosis has historically functioned also as a significant tool for social and political control. The power of diagnosis lies not only in its capacity to classify but also in its ability to shape the perception of what is considered 'acceptable' or 'legitimate', thereby consolidating political and social control through the medicalisation of difference. This phenomenon raises critical questions about the intersection of science, politics and authority in shaping individual and collective experiences within society. As we have seen, collective emotions play a significant role in the construction of psychiatric diagnoses, as they are often shaped by the prevailing cultural, social and political contexts.

The Scottish psychiatrist Ronald Laing, in his critique of the medical model of psychiatry, emphasised how societal pressures and collective emotional responses to perceived 'deviance' can influence the labelling of individuals as 'mentally ill'. He argued that psychiatric diagnoses often reflect the conflict between the individual's lived experience and societal norms, suggesting that mental illness is not solely an individual pathology but a socially constructed response to alienation and trauma [31]. Similarly, Franco Basaglia's reformist approach in Italy challenged the institutionalisation of mental illness, advocating for a shift from the rigid, dehumanising structures of psychiatric care to a more compassionate understanding that recognises the role of social values and collective emotions in shaping mental health. Basaglia's work [32] highlighted how psychiatric diagnoses can serve as instruments of social control, influenced by collective emotions such as fear or moral panic, rather than objective medical criteria. Together, Laing and Basaglia underscore the need to critically examine how collective emotions—ranging from empathy to fear—inform the diagnosis and treatment of mental health, urging a more nuanced understanding of mental illness that moves beyond clinical detachment. In other words, being embedded and situated in a social, cultural, political, axiological collective environment has the power to shape our existence, to define our identity and to support or destroy it. Being aware of the power of collective stances, like collective emotions or social atmospheres, is important to preserve the reciprocal engagement that usually shapes our identity without losing it.

We may say that the construction of a diagnosis involves not only physiology, chemistry and anatomy but also 'class, race, gender, language, technology, culture, the political economy and institutional and professional structures and norms in shaping the knowledge base which produces our assumptions about the prevalence, incidence, treatment and meaning of disease' [33, p. 34]. The philosopher Ian Hacking has described how diagnoses lead to 'making up people' [34] and the Third Reich was 'making up people' in the most extreme sense. What we call 'illness' and 'health' are always socially and culturally determined, racially anchored to a predominant set of values.

This examination of the relationships between political ideology, social emotions and psychiatric diagnosis reveals several important insights. First, psychiatric diagnoses never function as purely objective medical designations but always incorporate prevailing social values and political arrangements. This incorporation occurs not through conscious conspiracy but through the subtle infusion of cultural assumptions into ostensibly scientific criteria and practices. Second, collective emotions powerfully shape which human differences become medicalised, how diagnosed conditions are interpreted and what interventions are deemed appropriate. These emotions are not merely responses to diagnosed conditions but active forces in their construction and maintenance. Finally, as illustrated by the case of Asperger's syndrome, psychiatric diagnoses remain sites of ongoing political contestation, with various stakeholders advancing competing interpretations based on different values and objectives.

These insights carry significant implications for psychiatric practice, social policy and individual experience. For clinicians, they suggest the need for greater reflexivity about how political and emotional factors influence diagnostic decisions. For policymakers, they highlight the importance of considering how mental health policies may reinforce or challenge existing power arrangements. For individuals receiving psychiatric diagnoses, they provide frameworks for understanding personal experiences within broader social and political contexts.

Moving forward, several directions for research and practice emerge from this analysis. First, greater attention should be paid to how specific political ideologies shape particular diagnostic categories and practices. Second, more sophisticated analyses of the relationship between collective emotions and psychiatric diagnosis could help reveal the affective dimensions of medicalisation. Finally, increased dialogue between psychiatric professionals, social theorists and individuals with lived experience of mental distress could generate more nuanced understandings of how diagnosis functions in contemporary society.

At the core of this contribution lies the recognition that health and illness, particularly the so-called 'mental disorders', are never merely physiological conditions but always also social constructs that reflect particular values, emotions and power arrangements. By acknowledging this social dimension of psychiatric diagnosis, we can work toward diagnostic practices that minimise harm, maximise benefit and remain accountable to diverse human needs and experiences. These epistemological and ethical imperatives must be carefully considered within the interdisciplinary context of contemporary discourse. In light of these ponderings, it is essential to adopt a *critically* engaged approach to medical practice, one that recognises *plurality* as a fundamental aspect of our interaction with the world. This involves actively preventing any form of *epistemic injustice* that may impact service users, while also safeguarding against the potential reduction in psychiatry to a practice that neglects the complexities of the *psyche*.

Key Points
- Psychiatric diagnosis is not purely objective in any commonly understood sense of the word but is shaped by social values, political ideologies and collective emotions. Historically, diagnosis has reflected and reinforced dominant social standards, sometimes functioning as a tool for regulating behaviours considered deviant or undesirable. It has also been used to delineate the boundaries between acceptable and unacceptable expressions of human difference, often medicalising behaviours that challenge existing power structures or norms.
- Collective emotions significantly influence which human differences become medicalised and how diagnosed conditions are interpreted. Shared affective states, such as fear or disgust, can act as 'pre-diagnostic forces' that precede and shape diagnostic categories. They are cultivated through various social institutions and cultural narratives and can become embedded in diagnostic criteria.
- Psychiatric diagnosis has historically functioned as a tool for social and political control. Examples include the use of diagnoses like drapetomania, hysteria and homosexuality to enforce conformity, the use of 'sluggish schizophrenia' for political repression in the Soviet Union and the framing of resistance to norms as illness rather than dissent. This process defines normalcy, regulates conformity and can marginalise or stigmatise individuals or groups outside prescribed norms.
- The history of Asperger's syndrome illustrates how political ideologies and social emotions converge in diagnosis. Hans Asperger's initial conceptualisation occurred within the Nazi context, valuing neurotypical conformity and productivity, where the condition was framed in relation to a perceived lack of *Gemüt* (a capacity for social connection crucial to Nazi ideology). This diagnosis functioned as a tool of social control, contributing to the exclusion and potential elimination of those deemed undesirable or lacking the requisite traits for the Nazi collective identity.
- Even contemporary psychiatric diagnoses, like those in the DSM-V, continue to reflect culturally specific understandings and political influences. Criticisms of conditions like ADHD or oppositional defiant disorder suggest they pathologise behaviours conflicting with contemporary educational and occupational performance demanding systems. The increasing biologisation of diagnosis can also individualise suffering, potentially diverting attention from social causes and aligning with ideologies emphasising individual responsibility over structural change. The inclusion of PTSD, while recognising trauma, has also been seen as individualising and medicalising collective experiences, potentially directing attention away from political and social contexts.

References

1. Cartwright SA. Report on the diseases and physical peculiarities of the negro race. New Orleans Med Surg J. 1851;1851:691–715.
2. Tasca C, Rapetti M, Carta MG, Fadda B. Women and hysteria in the history of mental health. Clin Pract Epidemiol Ment Health. 2012;8:110–9. https://doi.org/10.2174/1745017901208010110.
3. Robles R, Real T, Reed G. Depathologizing sexual orientation and transgender identities in psychiatric classifications. Consort Psychiatr. 2021;2(2):45–53. https://doi.org/10.17816/CP6.
4. Foucault M. Madness and civilization: a history of insanity in the age of reason. New York: Pantheon Books; 1965.
5. Kritzman LD. Foucault and the politics of the experience. In: Kritzman LD, editor. Michel Foucault. Politics, philosophy, culture: interview and other writings, 1977–1984. New York: Routledge; 1988.
6. Conrad P. Medicalization and social control. Annu Rev Sociol. 1992;18(1):209–32. https://doi.org/10.1146/annurev.so.18.080192.001233.
7. Foucault M. Politics, philosophy, culture: interview and other writings 1977–1984. New York: Routledge; 1988.
8. Bazargan-Hejazi S, Shirazi A, Hampton D, Pan D, Askharinam D, Shaheen M, Ebrahim G, Shervington D. Examining racial disparity in psychotic disorders related ambulatory care visits: an observational study using national ambulatory medical care survey 2010-2015. BMC Psychiatry. 2023;23(1):601. https://doi.org/10.1186/s12888-023-05095-y.
9. Scull A. Museums of madness: the social organization of insanity in nineteenth-century England. New York: St. Martin's Press; 1979.
10. Conrad P, Schneider JW. Deviance and medicalization: from badness to sickness. Philadelphia: Temple University Press; 1992.
11. Timimi S, Leo J. Rethinking ADHD: from brain to culture. London: Palgrave; 2009.
12. Rose N. The politics of life itself: biomedicine, power, and subjectivity in the twenty-first century. Princeton: Princeton University Press; 2007.
13. Fassin D, Rechtman R. The empire of trauma: an inquiry into the condition of victimhood. Princeton: Princeton University Press; 2009.
14. Ahmed S. The cultural politics of emotion. Edinburgh: Edinburgh University Press; 2004.
15. Schmid HB. Plural action: essays in philosophy and social science. Cham: Springer; 2009.
16. von Scheve C, Ismer S. Towards a theory of collective emotions. Emot Rev. 2013;5(4):406–13. https://doi.org/10.1177/1754073913484170.
17. Bizzari V, Brencio F. Psychiatric diagnosis as a political and social device. Epistemological and historical insights on the role of collective emotions. Humanist Psychol. 2024;52(1):70–82. https://doi.org/10.1037/hum0000307.
18. Zahavi D. You, me, and we. The sharing of emotional experiences. J Conscious Stud. 2015;22:84–101.
19. Sanchez Guerrero H. Feeling together and caring with one another. Berlin: Springer; 2016.
20. Osler L, Szanto T. Political emotions and political atmospheres. In: Trigg D, editor. Shared emotions and atmospheres. London: Routledge; 2021. p. 162–88.
21. Freeden M. ideology, political theory and political philosophy. In: Gauss GF, Kukathas C, editors. Handbook of political theory. London: Sage; 2004. p. 11–2.
22. Kaplan R, Walter G. From Kraepelin to Karadzic: psychiatry's long road to genocide. In: Tatz C, editor. Genocide perspectives IV. Sydney: UTS ePRESS; 2012. https://doi.org/10.5130/978-0-9872369-7-5.d.
23. Czech H. Hans Asperger, National Socialism, and "race hygiene" in Nazi-era Vienna. Mol Autism. 2021;12(1):45. https://doi.org/10.1186/s13229-021-00433-x.
24. Wing L. Asperger's syndrome: a clinical account. Psychol Med. 1981;11(1):115–29. https://doi.org/10.1017/s0033291700053332.
25. Nadesan Holmer M. Constructing autism: unravelling the "truth" and understanding the social. London: Routledge; 2005.

26. Sheffer E. Asperger's children: the origin of autism in Nazi Vienna. New York: Norton & Company; 2018.
27. Todd SH. The turn to the self: a history of autism [Doctoral dissertation]. University of Chicago. 2015; https://doi.org/10.6082/M1668BBD.
28. Asperger H. Autistic psychopathy in childhood. In: Frith U, editor and trans. Autism and Asperger syndrome. Cambridge University Press; 1991. p. 37–92. (Original work published 1944).
29. Asperger H. Das psychisch abnorme Kind [The mentally abnormal child]. WkW. 1937;50:1460–1.
30. Asperger H. Das psychisch abnorme Kind [The mentally abnormal child]. WkW. 1938;49/51:1314–7.
31. Laing RD. The divided self: an existential study in sanity and madness. London: Penguin Classics; 2010.
32. Basaglia F. Scritti. Milano: Il Saggiatore; 2017.
33. Brown P. Naming and framing: the social construction of diagnosis and illness. J Health Soc Behav. 1995;35:34–52. https://doi.org/10.2307/2626956.
34. Hacking I. Kinds of people: moving targets. London: British Academy Lecture; 2006. Available at https://www.thebritishacademy.ac.uk/documents/2043/pba151p285.pdf

Open Access This chapter is licensed under the terms of the Creative Commons Attribution 4.0 International License (http://creativecommons.org/licenses/by/4.0/), which permits use, sharing, adaptation, distribution and reproduction in any medium or format, as long as you give appropriate credit to the original author(s) and the source, provide a link to the Creative Commons license and indicate if changes were made.

The images or other third party material in this chapter are included in the chapter's Creative Commons license, unless indicated otherwise in a credit line to the material. If material is not included in the chapter's Creative Commons license and your intended use is not permitted by statutory regulation or exceeds the permitted use, you will need to obtain permission directly from the copyright holder.

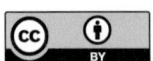

The Continental Philosophical Psychiatric Tradition and the Dialectics of Madness

Alastair Morgan

11.1 Introduction

In 2023, the French documentary filmmaker Nicolas Philibert won the Golden Bear at the Berlin International Film Festival for his film 'On the Adamant', an exploration of psychiatric care in an innovative day centre in Paris [1]. The 'Adamant' named in the title of the film is a permanently moored boat on the Seine, co-designed by architects and patients that is a place of solace, refuge and creativity for the patients and staff alike.

The boat is beautifully designed, with louvred windows that, when slowly opened, catch shafts of sunlight. The situation of a psychiatric facility on the water in the midst of a busy capital city captures an idea of refuge. The film focuses on a range of aesthetic practices that produce a psychiatric space that is open to difference, open to the creation of sense through music, poetry, film and painting.

In 1996, Philibert directed another film set in a psychiatric facility, one far more famous in the tradition of French psychiatry, the radical institution of La Borde in the Loir-et-Cher region of France, known as the most famous institution of the approach of Institutional Psychotherapy under the leadership of the psychiatrist Jean Oury. Philibert's film 'La moindre des choses' (translated as Every Little Thing), follows the production of the annual play at La Borde produced by patients and staff [2].

In one of the interviews for his recent film, Philibert refers to a tradition of psychiatry that he sees as seriously under threat:

A. Morgan (✉)
School of Health Sciences, Division of Nursing, Midwifery and Social Work,
University of Manchester, Manchester, UK
e-mail: alastair.morgan@manchester.ac.uk

© The Author(s) 2026
G. Ikkos, T. Becker (eds.), *Psychiatry after Kraepelin*,
https://doi.org/10.1007/978-3-032-09475-9_11

The public health system for psychiatry is actually abandoned – it's kind of going downhill. What I wanted to show was some doctors, some nursing staff, who are still trying to do some kind of human psychiatry, where you take time, where you listen, where you try to recreate the link between the patients and the society and the world they're living in. But this human psychiatry is really, really endangered. [3]

Philibert refers to a tradition of 'human psychiatry' that is beautifully encapsulated by Jean Oury's idea that one of the main functions of psychiatry, perhaps the most important function of psychiatry according to Oury, is to welcome madness. Philibert's films on psychiatry, which include two further recent documentaries that form a triptych with 'On the Adamant', give a wonderful summary of this endangered tradition of psychiatry, of what it might mean to welcome madness.

In Owen Whooley's interesting book *On the heels of ignorance*, he argues that psychiatry after Kraepelin has been determined by a fundamental ignorance, and this ignorance has been managed only through continual re-inventions and paradigm shifts that then turn out to be failures themselves [4]. These failures stem from a twofold ignorance. One is ontological; psychiatry fails to define exactly what mental illness is. The second is epistemological; psychiatry oscillates between different ways of approaching mental illness, shifting from biological to psychological to social approaches that all fundamentally fail to address the problems and conditions that surround us and come into the orbit of psychiatric care. Underlying this argument is the idea that a successful scientific approach to mental illness would be one that somehow mastered madness, submerged it within a medical paradigm dominated by positivist conceptions of disease and health. But, as George Ikkos writes, in a perceptive review of Whooley's book, psychiatry's goal should not be mastery but a toleration of uncertainty and the ability to creatively share these uncertainties 'without concealing or denying them' [5].

What would it mean for psychiatry to be based on welcoming madness rather than the futile attempt to master madness? Oury is very clear that welcoming madness does not mean participating in madness with the mad person. Rather he writes of it in the following way:

The welcome becomes a techné, an invention, a permanent fabrication, of the most unnoticed events where an uncertain arrival arranges itself through a precarious syntax. [6]

A techne is an art or craft, but one not wholly separated from an episteme, from a form of knowledge. It is conceived as a constant fabrication and invention of a space for encounter within psychiatry, which can involve the creation of new forms of sense through welcoming madness.

To welcome madness means four things for the practice of psychiatry according to Oury. First it is an 'art of sympathy' of being alongside the mad person that understands madness both as a breakdown of meaning (even a catastrophe) but also as a creation of a new life within the illness [7]. Second, to welcome madness requires a collective resistance to structures that attempt to isolate and exclude the mentally ill from society. Third, welcome requires a practice of self-reflection on the structures of psychiatric care. One of Oury's famous statements is that 'the hospital is ill' and this idea of a necessary attention to the ways in which psychiatric care can reinforce exclusionary dynamics was central to the practice of institutional psychotherapy [8]. Finally, welcoming madness means an attention to a double alienation of madness, to see it as both a psychic illness and a result of social and historical forms of alienation without dissolving these two into each other or reducing one of these to the other.

In this chapter, I will outline some of the main concepts and practices of Institutional Psychotherapy as one representative of the continental tradition of psychiatry, of this 'minor' or 'human psychiatry' in Philibert's terms, that I trace in my longer and more comprehensive book on *Continental Philosophy of Psychiatry* [9]. Institutional Psychotherapy is relatively unknown in anglophone countries, although there is a rapidly increasing range of publications [10]. I think the core practices and concepts of this tradition have much to teach us about pluralistic psychiatric practice.

11.2 Dialectics of Madness

Before outlining the approach of Institutional Psychotherapy in more detail it is important to clarify what I mean by writing of a dialectics of madness. The concept of madness is a problematic term, often used in the past to denigrate people with mental illness as a slur. However, in a range of work from the 1990s onwards in Mad Pride and Mad Studies, the term is revalued around an understanding of madness as an oppressed identity [11] [eds: see Chap. 12]. I use the term here to refer to a philosophical tradition that views madness as both incorporating a concept of mental illness and an experience that also always escapes the bounds of any conceptualisation as illness.

My approach to dialectics is indebted to the philosophy of Theodor W. Adorno and the concept of negative dialectics that he outlines in his book of the same name published in 1966 [12]. A positive dialectics of reason and madness involves a deeper interpretation of the difference between reason and madness that reveals an identity; within madness there lies purpose, survival and adaptation. Justin Garson has recently termed this approach 'madness-as-strategy'; an understanding that underlying the negative experiences of mental illness there is a kind of purpose and meaning, function and not dysfunction [13]. The ostensible difference of reason and madness is synthesised in a greater unity and identity.

A negative dialectical approach adds a different perspective, one that stresses the importance of heterogeneity and difference. However, much one can assert and develop an identity of reason and madness beneath their ostensible difference; there remains a final non-identity, something recalcitrant to the demands of reason in the experience of madness. For Adorno, as outlined in *Negative Dialectics*, philosophy begins in an attention to this non-identity, this difference. This non-identity is not an absolute otherness. Negative dialectics requires a moment of identity between reason and madness. Approaches that search for purpose and meaning within madness respect this moment of identity. However, this identity itself is dialectical. Madness is not only understood as a form of reason, but reason too has its own pathology, its own history. The difference between madness and reason is constituted by a history of violence and suffering [14].

This approach enables an understanding of madness as illness (immediately a radical problem of individual flourishing/being in the world) but at the same time madness is always a political as well as a clinical question. It is such an approach that I construct in my book on *Continental Philosophy of Psychiatry*.

One of the important consequences of a negative dialectics is a changed concept of reconciliation. Reconciliation does not lie in a putative identity of differences but with a final sense of being at home with that which is alien. One could say, reconciliation lies in 'welcoming madness'. Negative dialectics attempts an anti-systematic philosophy, one that will always turn against itself, insist on an attention to the singular, on a priority of that which escapes a complete interpretation or master narrative.

The debate over the nature of psychiatry has been characterised by a series of binary oppositions. From one perspective, mental distress is not characterised as an illness but as a normal reaction to adverse circumstances, and to the contrary perspective mental illness is characterised as some kind of biological internal dysfunction. Defenders of psychiatry argue that mental illness is properly conceived as a medical problem, whilst critics argue that mental illness is a myth and should be taken out of the medical realm. Some critics argue that mental distress should be seen primarily as an opportunity for self-growth, whilst others see mental illness in terms of dysfunction, lack and suffering. Following the approach of negative dialectics means that we should not be concerned with overcoming these oppositions or synthesising them into a higher unity, but that acknowledging these contradictions both philosophically and clinically can be productive. It is just such an approach of dwelling within contradictions that Institutional Psychotherapy offers.

11.3 Institutional Psychotherapy

Félix Guattari, a key figure in the theorisation and practice of Institutional Psychotherapy who worked at La Borde with Oury, defines this approach as a practice that does not isolate the study and treatment of mental illness from its social and its specific institutional context: the institution as both a deadened space of repression and the space where the possibility of the formation of new spaces for subjectivity can be foregrounded [15]. There is an emphasis on treating the institution, treating the staff as part of the institution as much as treating the patients. François Dosse outlines three core principles of Institutional Psychotherapy [16]. First, mentally ill patients can only be successfully treated within an institution that itself operates a process of self-reflection. Such a self-reflection involves foregrounding the oppressive potentiality of institutions to deteriorate into establishments and attempts to put a block on such a deterioration through a range of therapeutic practices that enable non-hierarchical relationships and spaces. Second, the treatment of mental illness occurs within the constant and ongoing group creation of the institution; it is not a matter of individual, one-to-one diagnosis and interpretation but the creation of what Oury terms 'spaces of saying', and these spaces operate through the circulation of unconscious desires and meanings [17]. Third, treatment becomes a process of a constant introduction of new arrangements, structures and spaces for subjectivity to develop.

In his account of Institutional Psychotherapy, Andrew Goffey draws attention to the different inflections of the word institution in French and particularly to a contrast between a notion of *institution* and *établissement* [18]. Goffey notes that the notion of an institution carries connotations of instituting something and particularly of a creative institution of subjectivity that it doesn't have in English and it is this contrast between the idea of an institution as a creative space for madness contrasting with a deadened notion of a bureaucratic *établissement* (establishment) that Oury foregrounds in his attempt to create a radical clinic at La Borde.

Institutional Psychotherapy begins as a response to two major wars of the mid-twentieth century, the Spanish Civil War and the Second World War [19]. It is incubated at the Saint-Alban hospital in the Lozère region of southern France, which during the war was part of the collaborationist Vichy regime. During the Second World War, in the whole of France, both Nazi occupied and under the Vichy regime, there was a catastrophic death toll within psychiatric institutions caused by the setting of rations for psychiatric inpatients at a level too low for the maintenance of life. During this period, approximately 45,000 psychiatric patients died of starvation and disease in asylums across France, in conditions of terrible deprivation, in what became known as the 'soft extermination' (extermination douce). The extent of this disaster only became apparent in France from the 1980s onwards when historians began to systematically explore and document historical records [20].

During this period, there were no excess deaths at Saint-Alban due to the resistance of staff and patients working alongside the local community and also harbouring resistance fighters within the hospital grounds. This experience of resistance created a space within Saint-Alban that David Reggio terms a 'conceptual brewing pot, creating and resisting' [21]. The key figure at Saint-Alban, during this period, was the Catalan psychiatrist Francesc (François) Tosquelles. Tosquelles was a founding member of the POUM (Partido Obrero de Unificaçion Marxista) in Catalonia and had been active in the Republican cause in the Spanish Civil War and had eventually found his way to Saint-Alban after fleeing Spain and then spending time in a refugee detention camp in France [22]. Tosquelles was influenced by phenomenology, Lacanian psychoanalysis and a form of social psychiatry. He envisaged the hospital as a place where there could be a possibility of people finding freedom again, but he also acknowledged that the wider social situation of war and conflict impacted on the symptomology of mental disorders within the asylum.

Tosquelles and his colleagues at Saint-Alban created a space for practicing psychiatry where illness was understood as both clinical and political, where the hospital becomes a space of resistance to occupation and resistance to the enclosure, abandonment and starvation of the inpatient psychiatric population. The goal of this psychiatric experiment was a utopian one, the disalienation of what another important figure at Saint-Alban, Lucien Bonnafé, termed, the 'total fact of madness' [23]. Psychic illness, societal abandonment and alienation and the wider situation of the war all needed to be addressed without being reduced to one another deterministically.

In his book *On Resistance*, the philosopher Howard Caygill writes of a trilogy of MD theses written just following the Second World War, all of which have a connection to Saint-Alban and the ideas of Institutional Psychotherapy [24].

In the next sections of the chapter, I will outline these three medical theses that Caygill refers to and add one more that is not mentioned by him. I think the concepts developed in these theses represent an important strand of psychiatric thinking that encapsulates a 'human psychiatry' (Philibert) and has great resonance for what it means to dwell within the dialectical contradictions earlier outlined. The concepts developed in these works give a further depth to what it might mean for psychiatry to welcome madness.

11.4 Georges Canguilhem (1904–1995)—On the Normal and the Pathological

Canguilhem is the one figure not mentioned by Caygill and for good reasons as his connections with Saint-Alban were brief and his writings on psychiatry rather than medicine as a whole are not extensive. Nevertheless, the remarkable thesis that Canguilhem produced during the war in 1943, titled *On the Normal and the Pathological*, is very important in the way that it outlines a series of key themes that are then taken up by other thinkers in this tradition [25].

Canguilhem studied philosophy at the École Normale Superieure in 1924 and was an exact contemporary of Jean-Paul Sartre and a near contemporary of other key figures in French philosophy such as Simone Weil and Maurice Merleau-Ponty [26]. He is known for his work as a historian and philosopher of science with a particular interest in medicine. From the mid-1930s onwards Canguilhem embarked on a training in medicine and graduated in 1943 with the thesis *On the Normal and the Pathological*. After the occupation and the partition of France into occupied and collaborationist zones, Canguilhem refused to continue to teach under the Vichy regime, stating that he had '…not taken the *agrégation de philosophie* to teach the Vichy regime's insipid morality of "Work, Family, Fatherland"' [27].

Canguilhem joined the resistance and worked as a medic alongside combatants. He took refuge at Saint-Alban for a few months in 1944, retreating there with his resistance comrades following the battle of Mont Mouchet. The Italian philosopher Roberto Esposito has written that nothing about Canguilhem's '…philosophy is comprehensible outside of this military commitment' during the war years [28].

On the Normal and the Pathological unfolds a distinctive philosophical approach to the question of defining the pathological in a dynamic manner which doesn't oppose the pathological to any putative norm but rather contrasts pathological states to a concept of health that is based on a notion of vital normativity. This concept of vital normativity does not relate to the institution of moral codes but the ability to live life as a mode of transcendence in which new norms are created by the person. Health is then not just adaption to circumstances or self-preservation but creative transcendence of life. Canguilhem writes:

> Health is a way of tackling existence as one feels that one is not only possessor or bearer but also, if necessary, creator of value, establisher of vital norms. [29]

For Canguilhem, to be healthy is by no means a conforming to a concept of the norm, or what he calls the 'momentary normal', but an ability to creatively surpass the norm, through creative production of new forms of life:

> For the living being, life is not a monotonous deduction, a rectilinear movement, it ignores geometrical rigidity, it is discussion or explanation (what Goldstein calls *Auseinandersetzung*) with an environment where there are leaks, holes, escapes and unexpected resistances. [30]

The reference to Kurt Goldstein's work is key for Canguilhem and for other thinkers who we will discuss later. For Goldstein, the neurologist and psychiatrist who studied brain injury in First World War soldiers, the key understanding of pathology was to identify how symptoms of illness still expressed a need for the creation of new forms of life even within reduced parameters. The key to understanding illness is to understand it as a form of life in which the creative transcendence that Canguilhem refers to continues to occur but in a diminished, sometimes catastrophic situation [31]. The pathological state has its own creativity within a diminished or lower range but there is still creativity and sense-making here and any healing will have to address symptoms as attempts to create new forms of sense.

Victoria Margree has outlined the significance of Canguilhem's work for mapping a space for thought between anti-psychiatry and positivist psychiatry [32]. She argues that Canguilhem's work gives us a way of accepting that mental illness is not a myth, whilst recognising that this category cannot be reduced to the positivist medical notion of illness as pure lack, deficit or absence. Canguilhem institutes an important reflection on the psychopathological that doesn't relate it to a problematic idea of the norm, nor does it reduce illness to a pure deficit model. Rather, attention is drawn to the ways in which mental illness can be both catastrophe and the production of a new form of sense. These ideas are also at the heart of Tosquelles' thesis that concerns the lived experience of the end of the world.

11.5   Francesc (François) Tosquelles (1912–1994): The Lived Experience of the End of the World

Tosquelles' thesis was published in 1948 and served as his qualification as a psychiatrist in France, with his previous qualifications not being recognised due to his status as a refugee. The thesis is titled *The lived experience of the end of the world in madness (Le vécu de la fin du monde dans la folie)* [33]. The theme of the thesis is this experience of the end of the world that occurs across a range of mental disorders, but Tosquelles focuses for the most part on schizophrenia. He considers patient testimony from his work at Saint-Alban, the writings of the nineteenth century novelist Gérard de Nerval who had written an account of his own madness in the book Aurélia, and a range of theoretical writings including those of phenomenological psychopathology with extensive reference to Goldstein's work that we have already mentioned in relation to Canguilhem.

Tosquelles begins his introduction to the thesis by situating this fascination with the end of the world experience historically:

> Young or old, we were in any case, all, more or less scarred (burnt) … during this period from 1939 to 1945 … my arrival at Saint-Alban made vivid for us all, but with a particular resonance for me, the true phantasmagorias, which surround the perspective on the 'end of the world'. [34]

In the thesis Tosquelles examines the end of the world experience as both a catastrophic loss of meaning and sense, a collapse of meaning and the rebirth of a new sense, a new creativity within the illness. He is concerned with understanding both this withdrawal from the world and the creativity and sense-making that might follow and it is through understanding and working with this creativity that a kind of healing can occur.

The important point in working with people who experience such phenomena is to understand what Tosquelles, in an echo of Canguilhem, refers to as a 'vital need' to create a new form of life even within and through the illness [35].

Tosquelles is critical of both phenomenological and psychoanalytic perspectives on madness that view it as purely a lack or deficit without understanding both the passivity and creativity within the psychotic experience [36]. His work here prefigures recent developments in phenomenological psychiatry that attempt to revise deficit models by understanding psychotic experience as both an index of a diminished selfhood and one which contains expanded notions of selfhood. Feyaerts and Sass have recently written of the need to understand these two poles of diminishment and expansion when working with psychosis:

> …many patients seem to shift or waver between the poles of 'diminished' versus 'expanded' selfhood or even – paradoxically- to maintain both positions at the same moment… seemingly incommensurable tendencies (of being a divine center, yet also of being targeted and controlled. [37]

It is these 'incommensurable moments' that fascinate Tosquelles and that he returns to again and again in the text, emphasising the moments of creativity and sense-making in madness without dissolving the pathology within a facile notion of an understandable reaction to catastrophic events and circumstances, whilst at the same time acknowledging the social situation in which these experiences occur. Tosquelles refuses the notion of a lack of contact with reality and prefers to think of a 'turning of attention', whilst recognising that this creative moment within madness also has its pathological centre in an enchantment of possibilities that run away with themselves [39].

Tosquelles considers madness as a form of creativity, and not solely a passivity [38]. He stresses not only the important element of creativity within psychotic experience but also an aesthetic mode of existence that often becomes tangled in infinite forms of possibility in the end of the world experience:

> Juggling with the will and the imagination, the movement of thought, in an intellectual intoxication, on an infinite field in front of oneself, where all forms, all events are possible,

where one can be anything at all, all events are possible, where one cannot maintain the slightest stability … One cultivates the arbitrary. [38]

This aesthetic mode of creativity within psychosis becomes a feeling of terrifying possibility and lack of stability. Symptoms of illness then are an effort at regaining health in Canguilhem's terms, as the restitution of new forms of existence within a catastrophic situation, but these new forms of existence themselves become a disorder of grandiose possibility. For Tosquelles, the work of psychiatry lies in a recognition of this aesthetic creativity within madness that the psychiatrist must follow and re-direct towards a healthier state. It is this focus on aesthetic existence and striving that is at the centre of Jean Oury's work.

11.6 Jean Oury (1924–2014)—On Aesthetic Conation

Jean Oury arrived at Saint-Alban following the war in 1947 after making contact with Tosquelles. Oury stayed at Saint-Alban until 1950 before eventually setting up the asylum of La Borde in 1953. In 1950, Oury presented his thesis *On aesthetic conation (Sur la conation esthétique)* [40].

Oury's thesis was an interrogation of this notion of aesthetic sense-making within madness and focussed on artistic practice at Saint-Alban and particularly on the artist and patient Auguste Forestier. Forestier had grown up with a passion for travel, often fleeing his family village, only to be brought back by the police. He was eventually hospitalised at Saint-Alban in 1914 after causing a derailment of a train by placing stones on a track. He constantly attempted to escape from the hospital in his early years after confinement but eventually substituted his desire for travel through his artistic practice, and his creation of sculptures of ships, and human-animal hybrids, made from remnants of found objects in the asylum [41]. For Oury, Forestier's work represented a transformation of sense making within the narrow confinements of the hospital situation that nevertheless preserved Forestier's imaginary world and his desire for travel.

Oury wrote of a fundamental aesthetic drive within existence that took shape within psychosis, but this drive or conation could not be completely subjected to intentional practice. Oury stresses the importance of chance moments and encounters within aesthetic forming. Mørck and Stanghellini have written about this in relation to the concept of *Gestaltung* in Oury's work, which can be translated as an idea of giving form to an 'experience of the formless', a process of forming which never has a final fixed shape or pattern [42].

Oury took these notions of an aesthetic practice within madness that focussed on allowing an uncertain and never fixed space for articulation into the practice at La Borde. Oury's conception of psychosis revolved around both a phenomenological understanding of a loss of attunement to pre-reflective life and a Lacanian analysis of psychosis as a loss of access to the symbolic order. For Lacan, the symbolic order represents the linguistic and cultural structures that determine the formation of subjectivity and psychosis is conceptualised as a structure where access to the symbolic is blocked or interrupted. For Oury, because the person with schizophrenia has not stabilised a space for themselves within the symbolic register, then it is imperative to try and create a space for them to exist, even if, for a short while. Such a space refers to a phenomenological understanding of pre-reflective experience that refers primarily to an aesthetic–physiognomic issue, a problem of finding a space for the body within a rhythm of life. The task when working with people with schizophrenia is to locate this space and not to impose a forced meaning or access to the symbolic register.

One cannot impose an artificial space upon the person, but you have to allow an opening to occur through the notion of chance encounters in which the person with schizophrenia can find a place for their unconscious desire.

An encounter only takes place within a space of something unforeseen, a space of creativity and chance, thus the necessity within the institution of constantly trying to allow for the opening of creative spaces, whether that is formally using art, theatre and dance or more indirectly through the circulation of roles, tasks and spaces within the hospital. Oury writes that:

> ...we organise encounters, we programme chance... I have often thought our task is one of constructing and producing 'secured areas' of transitional space. [43]

Oury's understanding of psychosis is an understanding of it as an absence of location in space, an absence of an attunement to the rhythm of life, that exists at an unconscious, pre-reflective level. The affective life of the person with psychosis has no location, no grasp on reality. However, the route towards some kind of stabilisation is by enabling spaces in which desires can circulate and find openings, openings that are always collectively created and facilitated within an institution. However, he is acutely aware of the ways in which institutions can easily ossify and repress creativity and openness, so the hierarchical, repressive nature of institutions must be foregrounded to free the creative work of instituting a space for subjectivity.

The role of the institution is both to be a space to create encounters, to create an opening for desire, for 'something to happen', but also a space for a person to belong, to find what Oury terms the 'simple':

> To reach the simple, the fact of being-here, the fact of saying 'hello', of performing a very simple diagnostic, we need to traverse an enormous complexity. What I call the architectonic—the totality of relations, roles, functions and people that defines the site where something happens—is based upon a heterogeneity rather than homogeneity! This is the fundamental word, 'heterogeneity'. [44]

Oury states that 'here at La Borde we work at the level of gesture', and what he means by this is that the goal is through the complex and heterogeneous to reach the simple, the point at which a person can say hello, or find a space to pick up a newspaper and read [17].

Andrew Goffey has referred to the emphasis on a concept of the pathic in Oury's work [45]. This is an attention to the ways that bodies can suffer and experience an interruption or distortion of fundamental structures of experience, drawing attention to the way that the pathic refers to a sense of suffering or undergoing. However, as Goffey notes, the pathic does not just refer to a kind of suffering but also the possibilities that might lie in different forms of life, or different ways of forming life. Goffey refers to Viktor von Weizsäcker's work on the pathic and the way that the pathic refers to both a pathology, a suffering, but also to a path beyond such suffering, a becoming that cannot just be reduced to illness or suffering [46].

11.7   Frantz Fanon (1925–1961)—Black Skin, White Masks

The final figure to discuss who arises out of this tradition from Saint-Alban is the most famous, the Martinican philosopher and psychiatrist Frantz Fanon. Frantz Fanon was born in Fort-de-France, Martinique in 1925. Martinique is one of the Windward Islands in the Caribbean and until 1946 was a French colonial possession. In common with the French approach to colonialism, Martinicans were brought up to consider themselves as French and as citizens of a wider France. This notion was further entrenched in Martinique after 1946, when it didn't follow a path of decolonisation but became subsumed into a greater French territory as one of the Départements d'Outre-Mer—France's overseas territories [47].

Martinique was under a particularly brutal Vichy supporting regime during the early 1940s. Fanon attempted to escape this regime and join the fight with the Free French at the age of 17 but his attempt to flee Martinique was initially a failure. By 1944, the Vichy supporting regime had been overthrown and Fanon joined a light infantry battalion to fight for the Free French. His war experiences as a young man opened his eyes to racism. He fought in Morocco, Algeria and then in France and saw how African Senegalese troops were treated as lesser than contingents from the Caribbean. He also experienced racism towards himself from the French population. Suddenly, Fanon felt apart [48].

Following the war, Fanon studied medicine and specialised in psychiatry at the University of Lyon. He was introduced to progressive currents in psychiatry through contacts with Paul Balvet who was working in Lyon but had previously been the director at Saint-Alban. At this time, Fanon was writing his first major philosophical work, *Black Skin, White Masks*, which is a radical mélange of phenomenology, psychoanalysis, literary criticism and political rhetoric. He initially wanted to submit this as his thesis to be appointed as a psychiatrist but was strongly discouraged from doing so and eventually worked up a thesis on the neurological condition, Friedrich's Ataxia. Fanon's thesis was written quickly but is an interesting attempt to situate his own psychiatric thinking in relation to central currents that were influential in radical French psychiatry.

In 1952 and 1953, Fanon worked at Saint-Alban alongside Tosquelles. From his experience at Saint-Alban, Fanon took on a central aspect of his psychiatric practice that he carried with him throughout his career. This was the emphasis on the institution as a social space and the need for active forms of democratic communication within psychiatric hospitals; in all the places he worked following this experience at

Saint-Alban, Fanon instituted journals, social clubs and community meetings. The social aspect of mental illness and the relationship between madness and the wider social situation became increasingly important to Fanon after he moved to Algeria, but the formative experience for him occurred with Tosquelles at Saint-Alban.

In his early psychiatric practice in France, Fanon observed the way in which psychiatry treated North African migrants. Fanon's practice in a psychiatric profession was structured by a set of presuppositions about North African minds formulated by the Algiers school of French colonial psychiatrists. This was a form of ethnopsychiatry that viewed the North African as fundamentally different from Western minds and that demanded a culturally sensitive psychiatry based on racist designations.

The so-called Algiers school of psychiatry combined this racist ethnopsychiatry with a neurological understanding of racial differences with the African mind at the bottom, followed by the Arab and then the Western mind at the summit of civilisation, although, as Fanon points out, at the 'psychophysiological level' the North African and the Black African represent a unity of underdeveloped minds.

Faced with this psychiatric milieu, Fanon writes an excoriating, critical essay on 'The North African syndrome', his first published work [49]. He begins by situating the encounter between the psychiatrist and the North African patient. The North African arrives at the consultation 'enveloped in vagueness' and particularly a vagueness about symptomology. He complains of a range of unclearly delineated physical symptoms for which no organic cause can be found. Fanon describes this vague, unlocated pain as an existential angst; an existential angst that cannot be responded to because the psychiatrist looks for some kind of localised cause [50]. In the absence of any cause, the recourse to the designations of the Algiers School is second nature. As Fanon writes, in the 'face of this pain without lesion', the psychiatrist can only respond by stating that the North African is prone to simulation; he is a '"liar, a malingerer, a sluggard, a thief"'. A label of a specific ethnic psycho-somatic illness is attached; 'the North African syndrome' [51].

After spending the first half of the essay, outlining the inability to recognise the existential pain of the patient who states 'Doctor, I am going to die', Fanon moves on to a proposed remedy to the pathologies of misrecognition in the search for a 'situational diagnosis'. What is needed is an understanding of the situation of the North African, separated from family and background and subject to a range of threats in his social environment:

> Threatened in his affectivity, threatened in his social activity, threatened in his membership of the community—the North African combines all the conditions that make a sick man. [52]

The fearful expression of a concern over imminent death represents the social death of his existence; 'he will feel himself emptied, without life, in a bodily struggle with death, a death on this side of death, a death in life…'. When he encounters a psychiatrist, this feeling of social death is confirmed in a complete dismissal of his personhood, and he is further emptied of agency and substance [53].

The essay on the North African syndrome is an early work which was written prior to Fanon's move to Algeria and confrontation with the even harsher realities of colonial psychiatry. In the autumn of 1953, Fanon took up a post as a psychiatrist in the Blida-Joinville hospital in Algeria. During his work in Algeria, he attempted to unite the insights of social therapy and situational diagnosis in working with patients. He set up a Moorish café inside the ward for men to socialise and attempt to re-integrate in society. However, with the beginning of the Algerian war of liberation, Fanon was faced with a situation where the madness of the psychiatric hospital increasingly mirrored the dissolution of the society beyond the institution. He was dealing with psychic disorders and traumas from people involved in the War, on both sides of the divide; the wider violence of society became all encompassing. For Fanon, the situation of being a psychiatrist attempting to help people back to recovery in a generalised situation of colonial war became intolerable. In December 1956, Fanon resigned his post as a psychiatrist and joined the Algerian resistance struggle in exile in Tunis. In his famous letter to the minister resigning his post, Fanon writes that he had hoped that in his psychiatric practice:

> … efforts should be undertaken to render less vicious a system whose doctrinal bases stood opposed daily to an authentic existence. Madness is one of the ways that humans have of losing their freedom… I have measured with terror the extent of the alienation of this country's inhabitants. If psychiatry is the medical technique that sets out to enable individuals no longer to be foreign to their environment I owe it to myself to state that the Arab, permanently alienated in his own country, lives in an absolute state of depersonalisation… The troubles in Algeria are the logical consequence of an abortive attempt to decerebralise a people. [54]

Fanon left Algeria for Tunisia but continued his psychiatric practice and in his last years moved towards experiments in community psychiatry, increasingly feeling that institutions robbed people of their freedom. His practice as a psychiatrist in Algeria, in the context of a vicious war of liberation, brought him face to face with the question of the impossibility of any recognition within the colonial situation. Fanon died very young in Bethesda hospital, Maryland, 6 December 1961 from leukaemia at the age of 36.

The central chapter of Fanon's first major work, *Black Skin, White Masks,* which he originally intended to submit as his medical thesis is translated as 'The Fact of Blackness' but this translation occludes Fanon's phenomenological heritage as the original French uses the phrase 'expérience vécue' (lived experience)—'the lived experience of Blackness' [55]. Fanon's text is a complex and searing enquiry into the psychic damage of racism. Fanon takes the earlier emphasis on the centrality of lived experience that he imbibed from phenomenology and his work at Saint-Alban and inflects it with an understanding of how racism and colonial societies impact on fundamental structures of experience.

Fanon's account of a crumbling of the Black psyche in the experience of racism famously begins with an encounter on a train. The White gaze is that of a young child accompanied by his mother who looks at Fanon in fear and points out his difference shouting 'Look, a Negro!'. Fanon experiences himself as suddenly reduced to an object in the eyes of another, defined by his skin colour and the attributions formulated on that colour, even in the eyes of a young boy. He writes that:

> I came into the world imbued with the desire to attain to the source of the world and then I found that I was an object in the midst of other objects. [56]

Fanon's work identifies pathologies at the heart of a racialised society that impact on the psyche of both colonised and colonisers. However, this does not mean that Fanon reduces the question of mental illness to a social question, that all mental illness can just be referred to through a social aetiology. Throughout his work, he retains a commitment to understanding mental illness as a 'pathology of freedom', a way that life can be stuck in a stasis. However, his work pushes Institutional Psychotherapy to understand, in the clearest way, the impact of social pathologies on the psyche of both so-called normal populations and the mentally ill. Fanon therefore sees both clinical practice and political practice as practices of disalienation, attempts to rid the psyche of the power structures that distort human relationships. Towards the end of his life, though, Fanon questions the notion of transforming the treatment of mental illness through institutions and is very sceptical of any process of self-reflection within institutions and, as stated above, becomes increasingly interested in experiments in community psychiatry.

11.8   Conclusion: The Afterlife of a Tradition

In the final section of this chapter, I will consider some of the key points of resonance when thinking about the tradition I have outlined with contemporary issues in psychiatry. I will consider the following issues that are directly related to the central concepts of Institutional Psychotherapy outlined above. These are the questions of a pathic or affective element of life as the focus of psychiatry's concern, how to relate this notion of the pathic to questions of psychopathology and pathologisation within psychiatry and finally the move from institutions into the community in psychiatric services and how this impacts on a discourse that originally focussed on institutions.

George Ikkos has written of how '… affect not the brain is the object of psychiatrists' specialist medical expertise' [57]. This attention to the pathic aspects of life is central to the approach of Institutional Psychotherapy. Attention to affect and the pathic means an attention to the possibilities as well as suffering that lie in mental illness and an attention to how the psyche may be scarred at an affective level by power structures in society, as Fanon outlined.

We may question though Canguilhem's emphasis on health as the creation of vital norms as being too much of a powerfully affirmative concept of transcendence and when Canguilhem revisited his work, he paid attention to the importance of concepts of error and going astray as well as productive creation. Thomas Osborne and Nikolas Rose, inspired by Canguilhem, have recently referred to a vitalism as '… much of pathos as of affirmation' [58]. Drawing on the work of Pierre Janet, they emphasise a vital normativity that is concerned with an understanding of the difficulties of all humans and non-human animals of stabilising a situation in an environmental milieu. They argue for an attention to persons that moves beyond any conception of normality towards the ways that people strive towards fragile forms of '…equilibria, however localised and precarious' [59]. Giovanni Stanghellini too has referred to an intrinsic vulnerability of the human being, that characterises human illness, that we shouldn't characterise in terms of normality or abnormality but rather as an '… intrinsic property of being human' [60].

How does this thinking affect the whole project of psychopathology, a central endeavour of psychiatry since Kraepelin? Should we give up on understanding mental illness as a form of psychopathology and label all forms of mental distress as understandable reactions to bad events? The problem with such approaches is that they tend to dissolve the difference of madness in a uniformity of sanity thus not respecting the radically different ways of living that can arise in madness. One of the great achievements of psychiatry since Kraepelin is the development of a structural psychopathology that richly delineates the lived world of madness, and that cannot be reduced to nosography. Nevertheless, the other face of this psychopathology is a pathologising in the negative sense of the word, a reduction in the patient to silence, a specimen of a lack of vital contact, someone completely other to any notions of recognition and discourse. One of the key tasks then will be to recognise the truths of psychopathology without the negative pathologising effects and it is just this in-between space that Institutional Psychotherapy maps through its attention to the possibilities and the suffering that lie in madness. To draw on a distinction made by Nidesh Lawtoo, we need both a pathology (that is to be attentive to sickness, suffering, lack of flourishing) and a patho-*logy* that is a critical and liberating discourse on the meanings and significance of madness beyond illness [61]. The possibility of such an in-between space has been nourished greatly in the last 25 years and more by the growth of survivor movements and the voice of lived experience within psychiatry. This attention to the meanings within madness though should not be reduced to an ideology of a secular theodicy, a justification of the sufferings of mental illness as an opportunity for self-growth. Rather, an attention to the meanings within madness has to stay close to the experience itself and pay attention to the singularities of such experiences. Stanghellini has referred to this as the importance of an ability of the psychiatrist to embrace '… all that is fragmentary and individual in the patient's suffering' [62].

One of the key factors within Institutional Psychotherapy is a psychiatry that takes place within institutions. Paradoxically, the ability to creatively experiment with care is perhaps easier within an institutional space particularly one that is acutely attentive to its own tendencies towards repressive and coercive forms of power. The undoing of the institution only takes place within the institution, but what happens when both people's lives and psychiatric care are scattered across populations, encounters and spaces? Ikkos and Bouras write about a metacommunity psychiatry, a kind of psychiatry that comes after community psychiatry, in which the very idea of community is in question [63]. One of the central ideas of Institutional Psychotherapy was the idea of the collectivity, of working with and alongside patients in a flattened hierarchy that would model a different way of being alongside madness.

To return to Philibert's moored boat. What Philibert tries to trace in his film is the fragile space of such a community in the dispersed, fragmented world of contemporary psychiatry, a community open to creativity, open to an idea of refuge, open to welcome. There is a scene in the film which operates a nice reversal of Oury's notion of 'welcoming madness'. This is a committee meeting chaired by one of the patients that is concerned with welcoming new members of the community. In this scene, the new member to be welcomed is the psychiatrist. She is gently mocked by the patients, who draw attention to imbalances of power, but what is really apparent in the film is the joy of the psychiatrist to be in this space, to work alongside people in a place where there is creativity and community.

Welcoming madness then may need to be unmoored from a singular place of hospitality, of the powerful position of the one who is the host, to try and create spaces where the tables can be turned, if only in a jocular and tentative fashion, and even just for a moment.

Key Points
- I have outlined an approach to the dialectics of madness that lies in dwelling with the contradictions that surround mental illness and argued that this approach is both clinically and philosophically productive.
- This chapter outlines the French tradition of Institutional Psychotherapy as one aspect of the European tradition since Kraepelin.
- Central conceptual components of the tradition of Institutional Psychotherapy have been outlined through the figures of Canguilhem, Tosquelles, Oury and Fanon.
- These central concepts are a different way of thinking about the relationship between the pathological and the norm that stresses forms of sense-making even within madness; an attention to both the possibilities and the losses that lie in the experience of madness; an attention to the aesthetic sense when working with and healing mental illness; a focus on madness as socially situated within structures of power and discrimination.
- This chapter concludes with some reflections on the significance of this tradition for contemporary psychiatry by focussing on the question of affect/the pathic, the problems and promises of psychopathology and transformations in psychiatry caused by deinstitutionalisation.

References

1. On the Adamant. Curzon Home Cinema. Nicolas Philibert. Les films du Losange. 2023.
2. Every Little Thing. DVD, Nicolas Philibert. Second Run DVD. 1996.
3. "Human Psychiatry is really, really endangered", interview with Nicolas Phillibert by Oliver Johnston. https://www.theupcoming.co.uk/2024/02/17/human-psychiatry-is-really-really-endangered-nicolas-philibert-on-averroes-rosa-parks-at-berlinale-2024/. Accessed 27 Mar 2025.
4. Whooley O. On the heels of ignorance: psychiatry and the politics of not knowing. University of Chicago Press; 2019.

5. Ikkos G. Not doomed: sociology and psychiatry, and ignorance and expertise. BJPsych Bull. 2023;47(2):90–4. https://doi.org/10.1192/bjb.2022.60.
6. Oury, J. (2012). Préface. In: Tosquelles, F. Le vécu de la fin du monde dans la folie. Le témoignage de Gérard de Nerval. Éditions Jérôme Millon, p.10, my translation.
7. Reggio D. The ethic, phenomenology and diagnostic of post-war French Psychiatry. Doctoral thesis, Goldsmiths, University of London [PhD Thesis]; 2006. p. 81.
8. Oury J. 'The hospital is ill', interview with David Reggio and Mauricio Novello. Radic Philos. 2007;143:32–45.
9. Morgan A. Continental philosophy of psychiatry. The lure of madness. Palgrave Macmillan; 2022.
10. Robcis C. Disalienation. Politics, philosophy and radical psychiatry in Postwar France. University of Chicago Press; 2021. Warren S. Storming Bedlam. Madness, Utopia and Revolt. Commons Notions Press; 2024.
11. Beresford P. 'Mad', Mad Studies and advancing inclusive resistance. Disabil Soc 35(8):1337–42; Cresswell M, Spandler H. Solidarities and tensions in mental health politics: Mad Studies and Psychopolitics. Crit Rad Soc Work. 2016;4(3):357–73.
12. Adorno TW. Negative dialectics, translated by Ashton EB. Routledge; 1966/1990.
13. Garson J. Madness. A philosophical exploration. Oxford University Press; 2022.
14. Adorno TW. Lectures on negative dialectics, edited by Tiedemann R and translated by Livingstone R. Polity Press; 2008. p. 1–2.
15. Guattari F. Students, the mad and 'delinquents. In: Molecular revolution—psychiatry and politics, translated by Stead R and with an introduction by Cooper D. Penguin; 1984. p. 208.
16. Dosse F. Gilles Deleuze and Félix Guattari—intersecting lives, translated by Glassman D. Columbia University Press; 2010. p. 60.
17. Oury J. 2007. p. 45.
18. Goffey A. Guattari and transversality—institutions, analysis and experimentation. Radic Philos. 2016;195(38–47):38.
19. Faramelli A. Crisis and resistance. Institutional psychotherapy and the politics of care. Deleuze Guattari Stud. 2023;17(2):196–216.
20. Platts-Mills B. Asylum, Aeon. 2021, online at: https://aeon.co/essays/patients-and-psychiatrists-fought-against-fascism-together-at-saint-alban
21. Reggio D. 2006. p. 90.
22. Robcis C. François Tosquelles and the psychiatric revolution in postwar France. Constellations. 2016;23(2):211–22.
23. Tosquelles F. Psychopathology and dialectical materialism, translated by Corcoran S. In: Psychotherapy and materialism: essays by François Tosquelles and Jean Oury, edited by Miguel M, Vogman E, cultural inquiry. Berlin: ICI Berlin Press; 2024. pp. 47–88.
24. Caygill, H. (2013). On resistance. A Philosophy of defiance. Bloomsbury, p.99.
25. Canguilhem G. The Normal and the pathological. New York: Zone Books; 1998.
26. Elden S. Canguilhem (Key contemporary thinkers). Polity Press; 2019. p. 3.
27. Elden S. 2019, p. 5.
28. Esposito R. Bíos—Biopolitics and philosophy, translated and with an introduction by T Campbell. Minneapolis, London: University of Minnesota Press; 2008. p. 180.
29. Canguilhem G. 1998. p. 201.
30. Canguilhem G. 1998. p. 198.
31. Garson J. 2022. p. 205.
32. Margree V. Normal and abnormal: Georges Canguilhem and the question of mental pathology. Philos Psychiatry Psychol. 2002;9(4):299–312. https://doi.org/10.1353/ppp.2003.0056.
33. Tosquelles F. Le vécu de la fin du monde dans la folie. Le témoignage de Gérard de Nerval. Éditions Jérôme Millon; 2012.
34. Tosquelles F. 2012. p. 14, my translation.
35. Tosquelles F. 2012. p. 69, my translation.
36. Tosquelles F. 2012. pp. 97–8.

37. Feyaerts J, Sass L. Self-disorder in schizophrenia: a revised view (1. Comprehensive review-dualities of self- and world-experience). Schizophr Bull. 2023;50(2):460–71. https://doi.org/10.1093/schbul/sbad169.
38. Tosquelles F. 2012. p. 111, my translation.
39. Tosquelles F. 2012. p. 98.
40. Oury J. Essai sur la conation esthétique. Éditions Le Pli; 2005.
41. Faupin S. Auguste Forestier's unbroken wanderlust. Epidemiol Psychiatr Sci. 2017;26:228–30.
42. Mørck HC, Stanghellini G. Dancing with schizophrenia—choreography as a resource for healing psychosis. J Psychopathol 3–4, 29:72–9; Oury J. Création et schizophrénie. Paris: Éditions Galilée; 1989.
43. Oury J. 2007. p. 44.
44. Oury J. 2007. p. 34.
45. Goffey A. Pathic Subjectivation: Guattari's experiments with contact. Body Soc. 2022;28(1–2):154–79.
46. Picione L. Viktor von Weizsäcker's notion of the pathic: affective liminality, modalization of experience and illness. Integr Behav Sci. 2024;58(46–58):47.
47. Macey D. Frantz Fanon. A Life. London: Granta; 2000. p. 31–72.
48. Macey D. 2007. pp. 72–112.
49. Fanon, F. (1988) 'The North African syndrome', in Fanon F Toward the African revolution, translated by H. Chevalier, Broadway, New York: Grove Press.
50. Fanon F. 1988. p. 4.
51. Fanon F. 1988. pp. 7–8.
52. Fanon F. 1988. p. 13.
53. Fanon F. 1988. p. 14.
54. Fanon F. Alienation and freedom, edited by Jean Khalfa and Robert J.C. Young, translated by Steven Corcoran. London, New York: Bloomsbury; 2018. pp. 433–4.
55. Fanon F. Black skin, white masks, translated by Charles lam Markmann, London: Pluto Press; 1993.
56. Fanon F. 1993. p. 109.
57. Ikkos G. Psychiatric expertise. Br J Psychiatry. 2015;207:399. https://doi.org/10.1192/bjp.bp.115.169946.
58. Osborne T, Rose N. Against posthumanism: notes towards an ethopolitics of personhood. Theory Cult Soc. 2023;41(1):3–21. https://doi.org/10.1177/02632764231178472.
59. Osborne T, Rose N. 2023. p. 17.
60. Stanghellini G. The dynamic paradigm of illness in psychopathology. World Psychiatry. 2024a;23(1):163–4.
61. Lawtoo N. Homo Mimeticus. A New theory of Imitation. Leiden University Press; 2022. p. 38.
62. Stanghellini G. The splendors and miseries of narrativity the virtue of the fragment and the formation of clinicians in XXI century. Int Rev Psychiatry. 2024b;1–10:3. https://doi.org/10.1080/09540261.2024.2402918.
63. Ikkos G, Bouras N. Metacommunity: the current status of psychiatry and mental healthcare and implications for the future. BJPsych Int. 2024;21(3):70–3. https://doi.org/10.1192/bji.2024.15.

Open Access   This chapter is licensed under the terms of the Creative Commons Attribution 4.0 International License (http://creativecommons.org/licenses/by/4.0/), which permits use, sharing, adaptation, distribution and reproduction in any medium or format, as long as you give appropriate credit to the original author(s) and the source, provide a link to the Creative Commons license and indicate if changes were made.

The images or other third party material in this chapter are included in the chapter's Creative Commons license, unless indicated otherwise in a credit line to the material. If material is not included in the chapter's Creative Commons license and your intended use is not permitted by statutory regulation or exceeds the permitted use, you will need to obtain permission directly from the copyright holder.

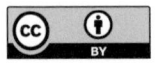

Mad People and Mad Studies

12

Peter Beresford

12.1 Introduction

As this book's editors suggest, the continuing relevance of Kraepelin is that prevailing psychiatric understandings of mental illness and psychopathology are still set on essentially along the same path that he and others established over a century ago. However, there is currently growing international interest in a different framework, Mad Studies. This has been shaped by people with lived experience of madness and the distress associated with it, as well as direct experience of being in the receiving end of psychiatry and mental health services. My aim is to explore the insights that people with such experiences and their international movement can offer in relation to both madness and distress and the western psychiatric system.

For me, the focus I have been given for this chapter, namely 'Mad People and Mad Studies', begs at least three key questions: what is madness, who are 'the mad' and why Mad Studies? I thank the editors for this well-chosen title and it is these questions that I will try and address here. I believe they highlight some of the most fundamental issues not only for this book and psychiatry in general, but also for our mental and overall well-being more broadly. They also offer clues as to why such hesitant progress seems to have been made in policy terms on advancing on these issues, both locally and globally, and why something different is required now. Therefore, they provide a framework for this discussion. However, before I proceed further, I want to address three important preliminary considerations: 'where I and this chapter are coming from', 'a cautionary note' when criticising psychiatry and 'the social problematics of Kraepelin' and their relevance today.

P. Beresford (✉)
University of East Anglia, Norwich, UK
e-mail: pberes@essex.ac.uk

© The Author(s) 2026
G. Ikkos, T. Becker (eds.), *Psychiatry after Kraepelin*,
https://doi.org/10.1007/978-3-032-09475-9_12

12.2 Part A: Preliminary Considerations

12.2.1 Where I and This Chapter Are Coming From

First, I must make my own place in this discussion clear. As a long-term recipient of UK National Health Service (NHS) mental health services, I write from a psychiatric system survivor perspective, drawing on principles developed by the international survivor movement; that is as someone identified as mentally ill, processed by psychiatric services as such and active in critiquing and seeking to reform the system and its services. Furthermore, like so many other UK mental health service survivors, most of the 12 or so years during which I used psychiatric services I was also reliant on welfare state poverty-level benefits. The two, mental health services and state benefits, so often go together because of both the impoverishment associated with mental distress and the psychiatric system. That is to say, the identification of mental illness has long been associated with downwards social mobility and people's inclusion in the mental health system as stigmatising and signifying restrictions on their employability [16, 24].

Speaking from experience, the problems and stigma associated with living with mental distress tend to be magnified by the hostility generated against those who have to claim benefits. This has enduring effects. I can truly say that it is difficult to isolate the impact of the welfare system from that of the psychiatric system. This coupling still fosters dread in me at the thought of ever having to turn again to the benefits system—especially in its harsh current form in the UK [27].

I make no claim to neutrality or objectivity in contributing to this discussion. But then similarly, as we shall see, there is much to tell us that any claims to neutrality on the part of so-called scientific psychiatry from the time of Kraepelin onwards are equally open to question—a chimaera demanding much more scrutiny. But some words of caution first.

12.2.2 A Cautionary Note

As I say, I come to psychiatry and the so-called psych system from a critical perspective. But hostility towards and attacks on psychiatry should not automatically be thought of as virtuous. As we have seen with the cult of scientology and right-wing libertarian reactionaries like Thomas Szasz, it can also signify something very sinister.

Furthermore, we need to acknowledge that psychiatry has also been a profession which has come in for some of the harshest criticism from within its own ranks, from R.D. Laing and the anti-psychiatry movement in the 1960's to Critical Psychiatry in more recent decades. This, however, paradoxically perhaps, further emphasises the need for caution. While some people with lived experience of distress and psychiatry have attached themselves to these critiques, others have been wary of them as extensions of psychiatry by other means.

Any of us, including me, exploring alternatives need to be as rigorous and demanding of ourselves and our proposals as of conventional wisdoms. We need to avoid setting up new monoliths. Only this way can we be true to the rights and needs of so many who need to receive decent help and support when they face madness or distress. A leitmotif in the thoughts and actions of many survivors is that they do not want to replace one orthodoxy with another—and that is an approach to which I am also committed. I, also, want to start with reference to the social taints associated with Kraepelin.

12.2.3 The Social Problematics of Kraepelin

The publicity for a conference held at the Royal Society of Medicine on 6 and 7 March 2025 on the theme of 'After Kraepelin: Ambition Images Practices in the History of Psychiatry 1926–2026', described Kraepelin as 'probably the single most significant figure in the history of psychiatry and, certainly, one of a handful of most impactful psychiatrists to have shaped the profession'. If this is so, a quick check on the history of the Herr Professor may well bring a chill to the hearts of anyone needing to seek psychiatric help for themselves or a loved one.

Here was a man according to peer-reviewed journals—and the editors of this book have also not been coy about it—who was a supporter of eugenics, enthusiastic nationalist, racist, anti-gay, antisemite and champion of social Darwinism who promoted a policy and research agenda in racial hygiene and eugenics and was the mentor of subsequently prominent Nazi psychiatrists [14, 31, 33]. Whatever positives we may take from his association with western science, must then be juxtaposed with its ideological context.

Kraepelin, therefore, may seem an unlikely source of inspiration for the twenty-first century future of a key discipline with a remit to address people's mental well-being. Although not an inspiration, however, his story may have a renewed resonance and relevance both for psychiatry and the rest of us—and we shouldn't ignore this either. It is perhaps highly relevant in an age of seemingly permanent neoliberalism, personal and political alienation, and international conflict, division and prejudice. Now, again it is a time of European conflict, far-right ideology, demagoguery, populism, significant social division and increased nationalism and anti-immigrant feeling.

Our current geopolitical and world economic predicament is something I will return to later. Before that, I want to focus here more on other broader frameworks within which Kraepelin seemed to work and some principles which he helped establish, which still resonate strongly in prevailing understandings of our mental well-being and mental illness, and which need to be challenged. This will then lead us directly back to those three questions I asked at the beginning: what is 'madness', who are 'the mad' and why Mad Studies?

12.3   Part B: Shifting the paradigm

12.3.1 A Fixed Paradigm?

This book's editors have traced a direct line from Kraepelin and his work to modern psychiatry. The specialty can still be seen as essentially reliant on similar frameworks, diagnostic categories, drug treatments and responses of more than half a century ago—in some cases even going back to Kraepelin's time. The longstanding preoccupations with categorisation, behaviourism, drugs and control persist. There is still an over-emphasis on these elements. Cognitive behavioural therapy (CBT) is the main 'talking treatment' on offer.

The same can probably be said of only few other sciences over such a period. In contrast, for example, physical medicine and healthcare have now moved into a brave new world of foetal, keyhole and robotic assisted surgery, IVF, gene and stem cell treatment, three-dimensional (3D) cell and tissue printing, implant surgery and so on. This divergence in achievements compels the need for a search for a new paradigm in psychiatry.

As just summarised, it is the continuity rather than change in psychiatry that has been most apparent. While some might see this as a strength, for others it may be a cause for concern. That particularly seems to be the case for those on the receiving end of psychiatry. As Thomas Kuhn argued, most developments in science relate to paradigm shifts [19]. In psychiatry and mental healthcare in recent decades, one key shift that has characterised innovation in addressing people's emotional and psychological well-being has been the renewed and revitalised role of people on the receiving end of psych services. This has been the real paradigm shift in this field. Below, I will share a UK perspective on its historical development.

12.3.2 The Emergence of a New Movement: Part One

The modern UK 'survivor' or 'psychiatric system survivor' movement has a history going back over about half a century, with antecedents traced by some as stretching even further back to the early nineteenth century [9, 12, 35]. In the United States, writings of hundreds of former asylum inmates from as early as the early nineteenth century, previously hidden from history, have now been brought together [28].

The modern movement is identified as a new social movement (NSM). Based on identity and lived experience, NSMs go beyond the goals of traditional economistic movements, with their (NSMs') aims related to the achievement of civil, human and social rights [25, 36]. The pioneering UK survivor-led organisation *Survivors Speak Out*, founded in 1986, set out its aims and objectives as to empower service users, increase public understanding, develop alternative user-led models, advance user involvement; promote self and other forms of advocacy; build collective action and promote positive images and survivor training and education [34]. Following from its commitment to a direct voice and influence for people as service users/survivors, this has almost been an essential agenda for the survivor movement more generally since.

As the above highlights, the emerging survivor movement has certainly been strong on values and principles, something many may wish could equally be said of such founding fathers of psychiatry as Kraepelin and his ideological peers. However, one thing that does emerge is that the movement has tended to be weaker on theory and ideology. This may have helped it become a broad church, but it has led to ambiguity and boundary erosion and is likely to have weakened its impact and effectiveness. This has been most clearly illustrated by the fact that if some survivors have rejected a mental illness model of their experience, others have seemed not to do so. Unlike the disabled people's movement, for example, the survivor movement has not had the kind of strong unifying intellectual core provided by the development of the groundbreaking social model of disability and philosophy of independent living [25]. This omission on the part of the survivor movement, however, should not be seen as a measure of its limitations or inadequacy. Instead, from my experience it is likely to have more to do with survivors' reluctance to replace one monolithic framework with another. It reflects, in part at least, their realistic fears that rejecting conventional analyses of mental illness would be seen as further evidence of their irrationality and pathology. This, in turn, could be used to further marginalise them.

12.4   Key Question 1: What Is Madness?

Before we return to Kraepelin psychiatry and the challenges it now faces from Mad Studies, more needs to be said about the language in this field, particularly about the language of madness that Mad Studies has helped resurrect. This is a much more universal and enduring than more recent language and frameworks based on disease and disorder.

As Wikipedia reminds us 'madness' has been recognised throughout history in every known society. [39]. Since the time of the Enlightenment, it has typically been defined as the loss of reason. More generally, it has variously been seen as a spiritual and material issue, amenable to moral, faith-based, mechanical or drug-based responses. Madness has been treated with care and control; kindness and violent cruelty. Responses have varied over place and time, politics and ideology. Meanings placed upon the word have also varied enormously.

The label 'madness' continues to be used pejoratively as a term of abuse, but has also re-emerged in the late twentieth century, used in a 'mad-positive' way. For instance, in relation to 'Mad Pride', it is used to celebrate the diversity and insights of mad people. More recently still, it has been used to describe a second iteration of survivor self-organisation, the Mad Studies movement. While there is no agreement about when the term Mad Studies was first used, it appears to have emerged around the turn of this century. It has been described as in/discipline and was never restricted to an academic setting, being equally rooted in action and the community [17]. Like other NSMs, for example, the Black, LGBTQIA and disabled people's movement, Mad Studies has appropriated prevailing stigmatising terminology to reclaim it, redefining, for example, 'crip', 'queer' and 'dyke'—and now mad.

12.5   Key Historic Themes

So now I turn to these key themes to which I believe Kraepelin was signed up and which have set psychiatry's subsequent direction of travel. They are:

- Science,
- Separateness and,
- Individualisation.

I want first to explore their historic relationship with psychiatry and then review the very different take on them that Mad Studies can offer. I believe this opens a route to answering the questions I raised at the top of this chapter: what is madness—which we have already begun to address—who are 'the mad', and why Mad Studies?

12.6   Key Question 2: Who Are 'the Mad'?

First, I intend briefly to explore science, separateness and individualisation in relation to Kraepelin and then contrast the very different approaches subsequently adopted by psychiatry and then Mad Studies and the psychiatric system survivor movement—in principle and by definition. This is perhaps particularly where Kraepelin's significance for psychiatry is most important and influential. My suggestion is that the specialty is still largely ruled by these three preoccupations: science, separateness and individualisation. Mad studies challenges psychiatry in each of these discourses and practices and in so doing helps us come afresh to the three key questions I have raised.

Science
So, beginning with science, Kraepelin was a child of the eighteenth-century Western Enlightenment. This was a time of a shift from the ecclesiastical to the secular and from metaphysics to science in Europe. As Wikipedia reminds us, the five traditional principles of western science are observation, identification, description, experimental investigation and theoretical explanation of natural phenomena. In this tradition, the scientist is seen as the expert observer and judge, essentially the mediator between us and what is to be known [40].

It is helpful to remember that science means no more than 'knowing', from the Latin, but it has come to have much more weight attached to it and a very specific meaning, presented, again as Wikipedia tells us, as 'the pursuit and application of knowledge and understanding of the natural and social world following a systematic methodology based on evidence' ([40] op cit). This led pioneers like Kraepelin with their medical studies background, to see psychiatry as a branch of medical science to be investigated by observation and experimentation, like other natural sciences.

But this is a very particular understanding both of knowledge acquisition and science. It has resulted in the adoption of positivist research values of neutrality, objectivity and distance, which as we will see have come in for increasing question-ing—from NSMs among others. It is the same 'science' that for years has rein-forced and perpetuated ideas of women, Black people, LGBTQIA and other marginalised and stigmatised people and groups as inferior and pathological. It is a science, an approach to validating knowledge, that has been imposed on countries in the Global South through processes of colonisation and subordination, regardless of the situational factors, cultural understandings and approaches to knowledge for-mation, historically associated with their indigenous populations.

While this understanding of science has been adopted in the West as a systematic and robust route to developing knowledge, it isn't necessarily how science or knowl-edge development is understood elsewhere [1]. Nor is it how most of us develop our own knowledge on a day-to-day basis. It rests on a very narrow understanding of the scientific, tied to Newtonian-age assumptions about the natural sciences, unaffected by the complexities of post-Newtonian thinking and developments [37]. It shouldn't take us long to work out that the biased notion of science that people like Kraepelin started with, fixed in a particular politics, belief system and prejudices, is unlikely to provide a convincing basis for the development of rigorous and reliable knowl-edge for now and the future.

Separateness
A distinguishing feature of Kraepelin's work is his preoccupation with madness or 'mental illness' as something which is associated with particular people or groups. While there is more to modern psychiatry than this and we have, for example, seen the development—as well as subsequent marginalisation—of social psychiatry, in its explanations and understandings psychiatry has similarly been characterised by a preoccupation with the particularity of 'the mentally ill'. The search is always on for what distinguishes its clientele; what it is about 'them' that makes them ill; what characterises them, what predisposes them, what makes them different and separate from other people—unlike 'us'. In other words, 'they' are problematised. They are perceived as a problem—a separate, special group. Not surprisingly, perhaps, asso-ciated with this, and again traceable to the mindset of pioneers like Kraepelin, there has been an emphasis in psychiatry on control and compulsion as well as help and support.

This may apply to both individuals and groups, thus the way that Kraepelin's search is always for 'predisposing factors' for pathology, whether in the individual or the group, for example, the Jews, identified by him as a defective and damaging ethnic group. Similarly, we know that in policy and practice many Black people tend to be treated in different and inferior ways within the UK psychiatric/mental health system, more likely to end up on the receiving end of its controlling provi-sions, and more likely to be prescribed psychotropic drugs than more valued talking treatments [2].

In essence, this is very unlike in Shakespeare's King Lear, where anyone can be driven mad by what happens to them. Instead, it is about particular susceptibilities, difference, deviance and deficiencies. From Kraepelin's period onwards to our own, over time different medicalised criteria have been identified in efforts to distinguish and differentiate a distinct, separate, susceptible group, based on biology, heredity, congenital and genetic difference and malfunction, chemical make-up, related to organic and metabolic disease and/or degeneration. This is to use personal difference to obscure our different circumstances; to replace human diversity with oversimplified sameness within the separate group and to ignore what the sociologist C. Wright Mills called the 'intersection of history and biography'—of which more next [22].

Individualisation

Perhaps not surprisingly, in the work of pioneers like Kraepelin, the emphasis on separateness has been associated with and encouraged the dominance of individualised explanations of mental illness/madness. Thus, the 'scientific' search has focused on and within the individual through surveys of their individual characteristics, personality, make-up, behaviour, emotions and so on. The simple logic seems to have been that if you see something wrong with a person, then you look within them for the answer. Such individualisation has not produced true knowledge as intended for science by the age of Enlightenment. Instead, what it occasioned was the medicalisation of madness.

We can recognise how seeing a problem as related to a particular group sits comfortably with analysis which disconnects them from their context. Also, punitive segregation (as in institutionalisation and custodial approaches within psychiatry) can be seen to have a logic where those involved are constructed as distinct and separate from the rest of us. Whatever the intended safeguards, a massive grey area arises here because of the gap between day-to-day practice and the protection or otherwise that the courts and legal process are meant to offer.

Even where some recognition is given to the impact of what are seen as 'social factors', this is still based on taking as given the overarching framework of disease and disorder. The medicalised individual model of disorder tends to be accepted. These are merely understood as further contributors towards such an illness/pathology model, framed in diagnostic terms.

An example that epitomises this is the current diagnosis of post-traumatic stress disorder (PTSD), originating with the effects of war and combat or other severe trauma. How are we meant to assume that a traumatised response to something as awful and destructive as war or combat or other severe trauma can be seen as a disorder? Should we not expect it to be understood as 'normal' in response to an extreme social situation? Unless perhaps we were an aspiring career general who had made a profession of such violence and for whom it is the norm.

Emphasising the individual origins of mental illness means that the pressure is then on to highlight the way in which people placed within the overall group and particular diagnostic categories are similar to each other and different to 'us'. This also encourages and underpins, as has been mentioned, the tendency to lump them together, separating them from the rest of us. This is a process long known as congregation and segregation. We can see this happening historically more generally, from the ghetto to the workhouse, from special education to, of course, the asylum. It is almost invariably based of some imputed problem, deviance, defect or damaging nature associated with the group so identified. It resulted in the nineteenth century in the massive expansion of institutions and institutionalised and custodial living.

12.7   Key Question 3: Why Mad Studies?

We now turn to Mad Studies, the second expression of the modern survivor movement. What is different about this new social movement that has emerged from psychiatric system survivors, their survivor movement and their allies? Clearly there are some similarities and overlaps with what had gone before. However, there are also differences and perhaps confusions. The Mad Studies movement can be seen to have grown out of the international survivors movement. It is particularly identified with developments in Canada and Scotland, where it was associated with new Mad Studies courses. It can perhaps best be seen as a development from the survivor movement rather than any kind of breakaway or challenge. Mad Studies now has a strong if shifting international presence on social media with sites for debate and discussion, as well as ones providing information and guidance. There is no agreement about the origins of the usage, although different accounts are to be found in Mad Studies literature [17].

The use of the word studies suggests a more academic orientation, but the terms has always been used to describe a *praxis*, involving action as well as analysis, rather than an abstracted area of study. The pioneering survivor activist Peter Sedgwick's *Psycho Politics* of 1982 highlights this with his attention to the survivor movement's clear ideological and theoretical affiliations and repudiation of both anti- and mainstream psychiatry. Sedgwick did not explicitly anticipate Mad Studies, but his interest in theory and ideology can be seen as representing a bridge towards it [4, 30]. To reiterate, some survivors had always found anti-psychiatry helpful, while others like Sedgwick were much more dismissive of it.

Let's now look at Mad Studies through the three key issues already identified in relation to psychiatry.

Mad Studies is clearly one of the NSMs that are committed to self-definition, self-organisation, self-expression and speaking for ourselves. It has helped survivors to rethink ourselves as a starting point for challenging dominant understandings of us, usually as inferior and defective. But it is also more clearly signed up to a distinct and key set of values and principles. These include that the Mad Studies movement:

- Rejects a bio-medical model of our 'mental well-being'/mental illness/disorder etc.;
- Is based on a rights, social and holistic model and approach, rather than individualised understandings and approaches;
- Challenges so-called 'compulsory treatment' and its associated 'restriction of rights' and seeks preventive and supportive ways of addressing risk or threat to self and others;

- Values and gives priority to survivors' lived experience and first-person experiential knowledge;
- Values survivors being able to speak and act for themselves;
- Emphasises the importance of inclusion and responds to diversity with equality;
- Champions decolonisation and challenges the dominance of global north ideas and models which devalue indigenous and global south understandings;
- Is survivor-led but, as not limited to survivors, it is open to all to be involved who accept its principles.
- Is supportive of building broader alliances beyond 'mental health' with other groups committed to the principles on which it is based;
- Builds on collectivist approaches to understanding, organising and making change happen;
- Is clearly ideologically and theoretically based [15, 20, 21, 26, 38].

As can be seen, this is much more clearly a worked through set of values explicitly in line with new social movements (NSMs) more generally, than earlier survivor principles and programmes, where the aim (of a group already marginalised as irrational and defective) often seemed to be to avoid being counted out as extreme or separatist. It also becomes clear that such principles are consistent with some long-established indigenous groups' principles and values [13].

12.8 Part C: Discussion

We can quickly see how Mad Studies collides and conflicts with taken-as-given principles of Kraepelin inspired psychiatry. It rejects a bio-medical model of our 'mental well-being'/mental illness/disorder etc'. It challenges individualised assumptions about madness and distress, highlighting the way that social issues, discrimination, trauma and oppression have a bearing on its scale and distribution and the interaction between these social conditions and us as individuals [10, 29, 32]. 'We' are not assumed to be the problem, the circumstances and conditions that engender any difficulties we have are also included in the frame and there is attention to the interaction between them.

Mad Studies challenges the positivists' devaluing of lived experience and experiential knowledge as biased and subjective, suggesting instead that what we know from what we experience may have an equal value to other forms of knowledge that have gained ascendancy since the Enlightenment [3, 11]. We have seen this emerging from feminist and queer research, emancipatory disability research and research from Black and minoritised people, as well as research addressing their intersections, thus challenging the bias and assumptions of traditional dominant positivist research and its associated knowledge development. Madness is particularly associated with marginalised peoples and out-groups. They are especially subject to the pressures—political, social and cultural—associated with madness, as well as the imposition of psychiatry [18, 23]. But madness is something that can happen to any of us, given loss, trauma, abuse or oppression.

Mad Studies encourages us to reintroduce kindness, humanity, warmth, empathy and understanding into the relationship between the person and the professional, emphasising the overlaps, not the distinctions. What, actually, unites us as survivors are three interrelated phenomena: our (lived) experience (of madness/distress) and the direct knowledge that comes from it, and the discrimination we may face, and experience of being in the psychiatric system. This is what unifies us. It is not having a different make-up, being part of a distinct group or category. Through Mad Studies we hope to speak for ourselves and challenge the identity imposed on us. Thus, the irony that we must highlight our difference to be restored to the mainstream.

Of course, as I suggested at the beginning of this chapter, Mad Studies is subject to its own difficulties and threats; of co-option and incorporation by psychiatry; of over-academicisation, de-legitimation and under-funding [7]. The psychiatric system is a powerful one with very influential allies. It has had such effects on other survivor-led developments, like taking over user-led services, 'psychiatrising' peer workers, colonising the idea of 'recovery' and tokenising user involvement in research and development. As an institution psychiatry thus represents a significant threat to Mad Studies. This is particularly true at a time of the long-term dominance of neoliberal ideology, which, with its commitment to the market, the minimally supportive state, division and attacks on minorities and individual responsibility is akin to and consistent with the kind of principles and values we have seen embraced by Kraepelin [5]. The targets and divisions may be different, for example instead of Jews and homosexuals, western psychiatry has come in for criticism for eurocentrism, racist discrimination and in some cases institutionalised racism, for example, in relation to African-Caribbeans and Muslims.

Also, increasingly the psych system has been linked with restoring people to work within a production-orientated labour market. This, too often, can be both personally damaging and maddening as well as destructive to the planet [8]. We cannot be sure that Mad Studies will escape the fate of other earlier attempts to challenge the dominance of Kraepelinian psychiatry. One strength it does have is the possibility and recognition of the importance of building alliances with other identity- and experience-based new social movements. As I have argued elsewhere, a key strategy for the future both of Mad Studies and other NSMs will need to be forging more equal and inclusive alliances with each other to challenge the longstanding global political and ideological dominance of neoliberalism [5].

12.9 Part D: Conclusions and Next Steps

We know from the evidence that the threats to our well-being and the pressures leading to madness and distress have increased over half a century of global neoliberal ideology, at the same time as formal systems of support have been eroded and reduced. Global poverty, conflict, morbidity and premature death have all increased in scale. Covid-19 has highlighted the failure of market driven politics and policy approaches to respond effectively to public health threats as can be seen by contrasting the outcomes in the United States and United Kingdom with those in South Korea and New Zealand. We must stop treating such issues, including madness and distress in isolation.

This is a context where we can only expect problems of mental illness/madness and distress to increase, whatever our understanding of them. This is an issue that is about more than psychiatry and its problems. It's about the frequently harsh, punitive and ill-directed human responses to madness. The world is now both a very maddening place and one where its own futures are increasingly insecure because of climate change and environmental damage and a rising threat of conflict and nuclear war. We cannot treat these issues in isolation, without acknowledging such context.

Simply seeking to export Western psychiatry globally, as in the global mental health strategy, is unworkable as a policy and perpetuates rather than challenging colonising approaches and understandings and building on indigenous ones. As activists and governments are beginning to show in some global south countries, their own traditions and the provisions of the United Nations Convention on the rights of people with disabilities—which addresses the rights of mental health service users and people experiencing madness and distress—can offer other helpful routes forwards, consistent with a Mad Studies approach [6, 8].

In a world where we frequently hear that the interests of the one percent dominate those of the rest of us, this of course, as I have stressed here, means building equal alliances between the different new social movements that have emerged to counter this anti-democratic situation. We have already seen this happening in relation to the women's and environmental movements; the LGBTQIA, survivors and disabled people's movements. But this is just the beginning of adopting an intersectionalist approach to challenging traditional structures and elites.

It will mean supporting people's empowerment to build understanding and work in co-produced ways. We need strategically to build such stronger, inclusive and equal alliances with each other in our different roles and experience, our overlapping and intersecting identities and understandings, challenging stigma and scapegoating and the divisiveness of populist neoliberal politics. We can share and spread information with each other as survivors, with families affected and professionals. There are now internationally Mad Studies websites, networks, groups, journals, newsletters, activities and events, both virtual and face to face. This is something that concerns us all, that all of us can engage with who share a commitment to our own and other people's well-being and the future of the planet.

Key Points
1. Psychiatry and related psych professions remain the dominant western response to what are identified as mental illness/disorder/psychopathology;
2. They are primarily based on medicalised individual models of presumed pathology, which have been developed based on particular understandings of causation, evidence and the difference and deficiencies of people and groups affected by such perceived conditions;
3. In recent years related international new social movements (NSMs) of psychiatric system survivors and Mad Studies, based on self-organisation and involvement, have developed which have challenged key principles of psychiatry and the psych system;
4. NSMs have instead highlighted social and holistic models of causation; the value of direct involvement, lived experience, experiential knowledge and user-led research in developing evidence and understanding;

5. They have emphasised the rights rather than pathology of people experiencing madness and distress, highlighting their social relations and the growing maddening consequences of a world shaped by the dominance of neoliberal ideology and the consequences of colonisation, conflict and environmental threat.

References

1. Bala A. The Eurocentric history of science. In: The dialogue of civilizations in the birth of modern science. New York: Palgrave Macmillan; 2006. https://doi.org/10.1057/9780230601215_3.
2. Bansal N, Karlsen S, Sashidharan SP, Cohen R, Chew-Graham CA, Malpass A. Understanding ethnic inequalities in mental healthcare in the UK: a meta-ethnography. PLOS. 2022. https://doi.org/10.1371/journal.Pmed.1004139. Accessed 27th Jan 2025.
3. Beresford P. It's our lives: a short theory of knowledge, distance and experience. London: Citizen Press in association with Shaping Our Lives; 2003.
4. Beresford P. From psycho-politics to Mad Studies: Learning the legacy of Peter Sedgwick. Crit Radical Soc Work. 2016;4(3):343–55.
5. Beresford P. The antidote: how people powered movements can renew politics, policy and practice. Bristol: Policy Press; 2025.
6. Beresford P, Rose D. Decolonising global mental health the role of mad studies. Cambridge Prisms. 2023;10:1–8. https://doi.org/10.1017/gmh.2023.21.
7. Beresford P, Russo J. Supporting the sustainability of Mad Studies and preventing its co-option. Disabil Soc. 2016;31(2):270–4.
8. Beresford P, Russo J. The Routledge international handbook of mad studies. London: Routledge; 2022.
9. Blayney S. Chapter 10: Activist sources and the survivor movement. In: Sources in the history of psychiatry, from 1800 to the present, Millard C, Wallis J, editors. London: Routledge; 2022. https://library.oapen.org/bitstream/id/03ce970f-f534-4bf2-9e88-12f520292927/9781003087694_10.4324_9781003087694-11.pdf. Accessed 19th Dec 2024.
10. Burstow B. Psychiatry and the business of madness: an ethical and epistemological accounting. New York: Palgrave Macmillan; 2015.
11. Burstow B, LeFrancois BA, Diamond S. Psychiatry disrupted: theorizing resistance and crafting the (R)evolution. New York: McGill-Queen's University Press; 2014.
12. Campbell P. From little acorns—the mental health service user movement. In: Bell A, Lindley P, editors. Beyond the water towers: the unfinished revolution in mental health services 1985–2005. London: The Sainsbury Centre for Mental Health; 2005. p. 73–82.
13. Eromosele F. Madness, decolonisation and mental health activism in Africa. In: Beresford P, Russo J, editors. The Routledge international handbook of mad studies. London: Routledge; 2022. p. 27–339.
14. Guse HG, Schmacke N. Psychiatry and the origins of Nazism. Int J Health Serv. 1980;10(2):177–96. https://www.jstor.org/stable/45130339.
15. Higgins M, Lenette C. Disrupting the academy with lived experience-led knowledge. Bristol: Policy Press; 2024.
16. Hollingshead AB, Ellis R, Kirby E. Social mobility and mental illness. Am Soc Rev. 1954;19(5):577–84.
17. Ingram RA. A genealogy of the concept of 'Mad Studies'. In: Beresford P, Russo J, editors. The Routledge international handbook of mad studies; 2022. p. 93–7.
18. Joseph AJ. Deportation and the confluence of violence within forensic mental health and immigration systems. Basingstoke: Palgrave Macmillan; 2015.
19. Kuhn TS. The structure of scientific revolutions. 3rd ed. University of Chicago Press; 1996.
20. Le Francois BA, Menzies R, Reaume G. Mad matters: a critical reader in Canadian Mad Studies. Toronto: Canadian Scholars Press; 2013.

21. Lewis B, Ali A, Russell J, editors. Mad studies reader: interdisciplinary innovations in mental health. London: Routledge; 2025.
22. Mills CW. The sociological imagination. Oxford: Oxford University Press; 1959.
23. Mills C. Decolonizing global mental health: the psychiatrization of the majority world. London: Routledge; 2014.
24. National Collaborating Centre for Mental Health. Mental health problems and social mobility: a systematic review. London: National Collaborating Centre for Mental Health; 2021.
25. Oliver M. Understanding disability: from theory to practice. Basingstoke: Macmillan; 1996.
26. Pilling MD. Mad studies: the basics. London: Routledge; 2025.
27. Pring, J. (2024) The Department: How a violent government bureaucracy killed hundreds and hid the evidence, London, Pluto Press.
28. Rembis M. Writing mad lives in the age of the asylum. New York: Oxford University Press; 2024.
29. Russo J, Sweeney A, editors. Searching for a Rose garden: challenging psychiatry, fostering mad studies. Ross on Wye: PCSS Books; 2016.
30. Sedgwick P. Psycho politics. London: Pluto Press; 1982.
31. Shepherd M. Kraepelin and modern psychiatry. Eur Arch Psychiatry Clin Neurosci. 1995;245:189–95. https://doi.org/10.1007/BF02191796.
32. Spandler H, Anderson J, Sapey B, editors. Madness, distress, and the politics of disablement. Bristol: Policy Press; 2015.
33. Strous RD. Reflections on 'Emil Kraepelin: Icon and Reality', Letters to the Editor, Psychiatry online. Am J Psychiatry. 2016;173(3). https://doi.org/10.1176/appi.ajp.2016.15111414. https://psychiatryonline.org/doi/10.1176/appi.ajp.2016.15111414.
34. Survivors Speak Out. Survivors speak out. Survivor History Archive. 2013. http://studymore. org.uk/ssoweb.htm. Accessed 19th Dec 2024.
35. Together. Henry Hawkins, website, Together, for mental wellbeing website. n.d.. https://www. together-uk.org/who-we-are/our-history/henry-hawkins/. Accessed 20th Dec 2024.
36. Touraine A. The voice and the eye: an analysis of social movements. Cambridge: Cambridge University Press; 1981.
37. Vohland K, Land-Zandstra A, Ceccaroni L, Lemmens R, Perelló J, Ponti M, Samson R, Wagenknecht K, editors. The science of citizen science. Berlin: Springer Cham. https://doi. org/10.1007/978-3-030-58278-4. Accessed 16th Feb 2025.
38. Warren S. Storming bedlam: madness, Utopia and Revolt. Brooklyn; 2024.
39. Wikipedia. Madness (to be found at search word insanity). 2025a. https://en.wikipedia.org/ wiki/Insanity. Accessed 8th Jan 2025.
40. Wikipedia. Science. 2025b. https://en.wikipedia.org/wiki/Science. Accessed 8th Jan 2025.

Open Access This chapter is licensed under the terms of the Creative Commons Attribution 4.0 International License (http://creativecommons.org/licenses/by/4.0/), which permits use, sharing, adaptation, distribution and reproduction in any medium or format, as long as you give appropriate credit to the original author(s) and the source, provide a link to the Creative Commons license and indicate if changes were made.

The images or other third party material in this chapter are included in the chapter's Creative Commons license, unless indicated otherwise in a credit line to the material. If material is not included in the chapter's Creative Commons license and your intended use is not permitted by statutory regulation or exceeds the permitted use, you will need to obtain permission directly from the copyright holder.

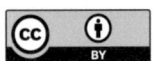

Part IV

Image, Imagination and Experience

This part looks at brain imaging, but also at the imagination, and images emerging directly from the experience of psychiatry or philosophical reflection on it. The discovery and widespread use of Computerised Axial Tomography (CAT) in the 1970s have had a profound methodological impact on psychiatric research. Yet, the importance of other images and imagination requires attention of their own.

Chapter 13 offers a comprehensive review of findings on the relationship between adverse childhood experiences and the developing brain as they emerge from brain imaging studies. Findings have implications both for resilience and vulnerability in mental health. Chapter 14 traces the evolution and uses of images in psychiatry from the work of Emil Kraepelin onwards and reflects on their impact on the psychiatric imagination. The author emphasises the dangers of scientific images becoming 'iconic', that is, static rather than dynamic representations of the brain in interaction with the environment. Chapter 15 offers an integrated view of the Self in the light of both philosophy and biology, including our understanding through the imaging of communicating brain networks. Chapter 16 focuses on images of psychopathology emerging directly from philosophy, especially the phenomenological approach in the clinical work of Ludwig Binswanger. Chapter 17 documents images of space emerging from the personal experience of two people with diagnosis of schizophrenia and a psychiatrist.

Adverse Childhood Experiences and Brain Development

13

Giulia Cattarinussi and Paola Dazzan

13.1 Introduction

Brain development results from a complex interaction between genes and environmental factors. Indeed, although the genetic blueprint can drive the cellular and molecular processes that are necessary to build the brain [1], the course of brain development is highly influenced by the personal experiences that occur in the early years of life [2]. Brain development starts about 2 weeks after conception and continues through adolescence and early adulthood [3]. During the first few years of life, there is a dramatic increase in the number of new neural connections, with more than one million *synapses* formed every second. This overproduction of synapses is followed by a phase of synaptic pruning, in which the unused synapses are eliminated [4]. Importantly, synaptic pruning occurs at different times in different areas of the brain. For example, pruning in areas involved in sensory processing is completed between ages 4 and 6 years. In contrast, pruning in areas involved in higher cognitive functions and emotion regulation continues through adolescence [5]. The initial overproduction of synapses and the following synaptic pruning are fundamental to support the flexibility required for the adaptive changes of the developing brain. Indeed, the pathways that go unused are removed, while the ones that are more activated by environmental factors are strengthened. In this way, the networks of neurons involved in the development of behaviour are fine-tuned and modified as needed.

Myelination is the final step of brain development, with wrapping of neuronal axons by a myelin lipid bilayer [6]. Myelination is important in creating connectivity in the developing brain, as it facilitates a rapid and synchronised transmission of information across the brain, which is fundamental for higher-order cognitive function and emotion processing [7]. As in synaptic pruning, the timing of myelination

G. Cattarinussi (✉) · P. Dazzan
Department of Psychological Medicine, Institute of Psychiatry, Psychology and Neuroscience, King's College London, London, UK
e-mail: giulia.cattarinussi@kcl.ac.uk; paola.dazzan@kcl.ac.uk

© The Author(s) 2026
G. Ikkos, T. Becker (eds.), *Psychiatry after Kraepelin*,
https://doi.org/10.1007/978-3-032-09475-9_13

depends on the region of the brain in which it takes place. Myelination of sensory and motor areas is completed before the age of 6 years, while for regions involved in higher cognitive abilities, such as the prefrontal cortex, the process is completed in adolescence or early adulthood [8]. Box 13.1 provides a select glossary of some of the terms used in this chapter, to aid the general reader. Terms included in the glossary are printed in italics when first encountered in the text.

Childhood represents a particularly important period for brain development. The foundations of sensory and perceptual systems that are critical for cognition, emotion processing and social behaviour are formed in these early years and are strongly influenced by experiences during this time. In this chapter, we will provide an overview of the role of adverse childhood experiences on brain development. Following a brief discussion on how to study the developing brain, we will examine how adverse childhood experiences can affect brain development. Lastly, we will discuss evidence from psychosis as a neurodevelopmental disorder, and we highlight the main neuroimaging findings reported in individuals at the early stages of this disorder.

13.2 Studying the Developing Brain

Over the last five decades, non-invasive neuroimaging techniques have played a critical role in elucidating the neural processes underlying brain development. These methods have advanced our understanding of neurodevelopment by providing in vivo evidence of changes in structural architecture and functional organisation that occur in the developing brain. Among these, magnetic resonance imaging (MRI) has gained increasing popularity because of its safety and widespread availability. Structural MRI, a non-invasive imaging technique, allows the study of structural changes in the brain, and it has been used in developmental neuroscience to study the trajectory of grey and white matter maturation from childhood to adolescence and adulthood [9]. MRI investigations have demonstrated that total brain volume increases with age, with different growth rates across the brain. *Grey matter* volume increases until adolescence when it reaches a plateau and starts to slowly decline, while *white matter* volume increases into adulthood [10–12]. Importantly, changes in brain structure detected by MRI during development are due to a combination of multiple biological factors, including myelination, synaptic pruning and changes in vascular, neuronal and glial density [13]. Figure 13.1 illustrates the brain areas most commonly altered in individuals exposed to adverse childhood experiences.

In contrast to MRI, which studies structural architecture, functional magnetic resonance imaging (fMRI) has been used to elucidate the dynamic functional mechanisms accompanying cognitive and emotional development [14]. Of note, fMRI can be conducted both during the performance of a specified task to evaluate how brain activity changes when a person is engaged in that task, or during rest [15]. Regions that co-activate at rest are considered to be functionally connected and involved in the same set of functions [16]. While task-based fMRI has been largely employed to investigate brain functional development in older children and adolescents, resting state-fMRI represents a crucial tool for studies in very young children at critical developmental milestones, as it does not require the execution of a

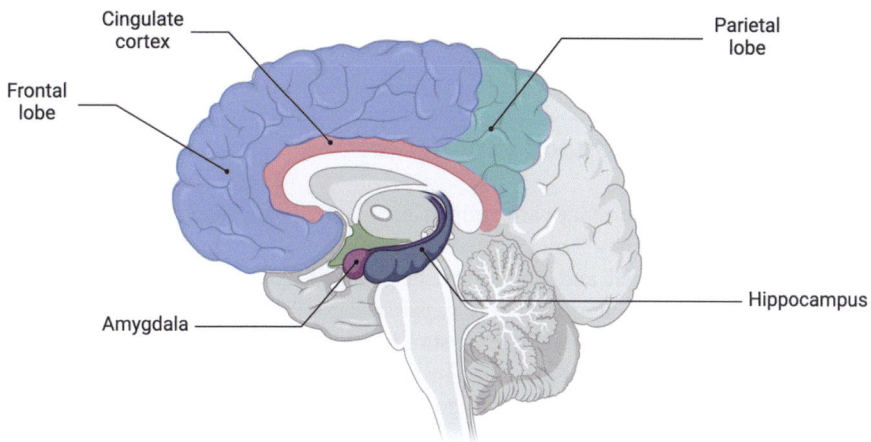

Fig. 13.1 Brain areas most commonly altered in individuals with exposed to adverse childhood experiences

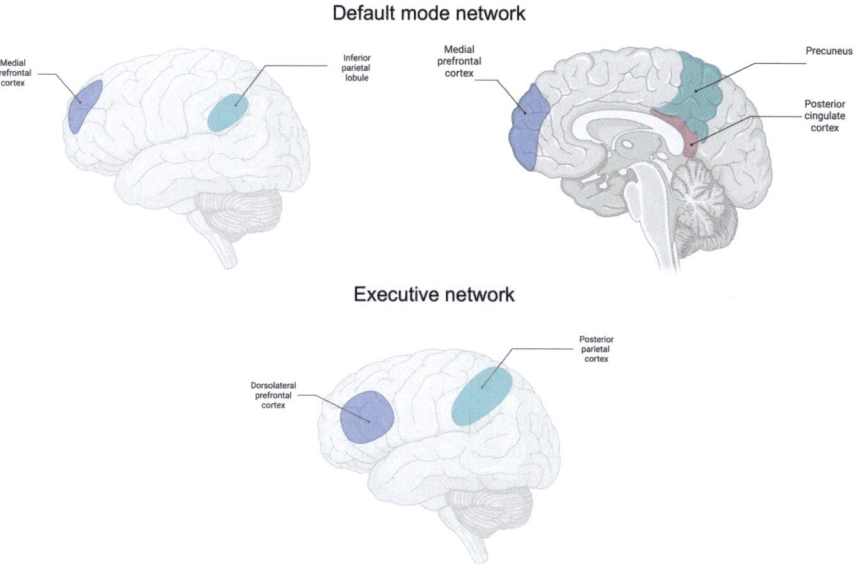

Fig. 13.2 Component structures of brain networks most commonly altered in individuals exposed to adverse childhood experiences

specific task [17]. Resting-state fMRI studies examining functional brain organisation in infants, children and adolescents have revealed consistent findings with respect to the development of *functional connectivity* between brain regions and regional functional specialisation [14].

Crucially, because MRI does not use ionising radiation, it allows repeated scanning of the same subjects over time, thus providing measurement of longitudinal neuroanatomical and functional changes associated with development. Figure 13.2 illustrates the component structures of brain networks most commonly altered in individuals exposed to adverse childhood experiences.

13.3   Adverse Childhood Experiences

Adverse childhood experiences are defined as potentially stressful events that occur before the age of 18. They include adverse events that affect children both directly (e.g. physical, emotional and sexual abuse, physical and emotional neglect) and indirectly through their environment (e.g. parental conflict, domestic violence, substance abuse, mental illness) [18]. Exposure to adverse childhood experiences can significantly affect neurodevelopment. In addition to the type of adversity, other factors can have an additive effect on the negative consequences of adverse childhood experiences on development. Among these, the duration of exposure to adversity, the timing, the number of adversities, the interaction among them and the presence of exacerbating factors are all crucial factors [19, 20].

The negative effects of adverse childhood experiences on cognitive and emotional development are well-documented. Indeed, exposure to adverse childhood experiences has been associated with deficits in several cognitive domains, including intelligence, memory, executive function, speed of processing, perceptual reasoning and verbal comprehension in adolescence and adulthood [21–23]. Similarly, children who experienced potentially traumatic events present higher rates of emotional difficulties during adolescence and early adulthood [24, 25]. In addition, exposure to adverse childhood experiences is strongly related to negative psychosocial outcomes, including mental disorders, suicide attempts, sexual risk-taking and interpersonal violence [26]. In line with this evidence, data show that adverse childhood experiences increase the risk of developing *internalising* and *externalising symptoms* across development. For instance, a recent study conducted on 11,876 children exposed to 268 different negative life events has shown that almost all forms of adversity are associated with higher internalising and externalising problems in children [27]. Furthermore, the risk of developing both anxiety and depression before the age of 18 is highly increased in children exposed to adverse experiences [28]. Extensive research also highlights the presence of a potential relationship between adverse experiences and the incidence of psychotic experiences [29, 30] and the early onset of psychotic symptoms [31–33].

Importantly, exposure to adverse childhood experiences dramatically increases the risk for several physical health problems throughout childhood and later in life, including common diseases of childhood (e.g. viral infections, asthma, dermatitis, urticaria, intestinal infectious diseases and urinary tract infections), and adult chronic conditions, such as cardiovascular disease, stroke, cancer, diabetes, overweight or obesity, asthma, chronic obstructive pulmonary disease and kidney failure [34]. Of note, the presence of adverse childhood experiences is also associated with shortened life expectancy, as shown by two large cohort studies [35, 36]. In a Danish cohort of 1.5 million children born between 1981 and 2010, children exposed to 1, 2 or ≥3 adverse childhood experiences presented 1.45, 1.72 and 2.28 higher mortality risks through age 18, respectively [35]. Another birth cohort investigation has shown that children with higher rates of adverse childhood experiences had a nearly twofold higher risk of premature mortality through middle adulthood compared to children without adverse childhood experiences [36]. Among the leading causes of death in adulthood, drug overdose, heart disease and cancer are those more commonly observed [37, 38].

13.4 Effects of Adverse Childhood Experiences on Brain Development

13.4.1 Institutionalisation and Early Childhood Neglect

For healthy neurodevelopment, the individual needs to have positive experiences and their lack may lead to deviations from the regular neurodevelopmental processes. An example of early childhood neglect is institutionalisation. Indeed, children growing up in institutional settings do not experience the nurturing and stimulating environment required for healthy physical, psychological and behavioural development [39]. The most important work in the field of institutionalisation and brain development is represented by the Bucharest Early Intervention Project (BEIP), a longitudinal investigation that started in Romania in 1989. In this study, 136 institutionalised children and 72 children living with their biological parents were recruited from the Bucharest region. After a baseline assessment conducted while children were living in the institutions, the 136 institutionalised children were randomly assigned to either high-quality foster care or continued institutional care [40]. Children were initially followed up at 30, 42 and 54 months when the trial ended. Children were seen again at 8, 12 and 16 years, and a 22-year follow-up is still in progress [41]. The main finding of the study is that institutionalisation at a young age leads to severe disruptions in the development of both brain and behaviour. Indeed, electroencephalograms (EEG) demonstrated that children raised in institutional settings presented different patterns of brain activity compared to children living with their biological parents, possibly reflecting a delay in brain development [42]. Furthermore, children who were placed in foster care before the age of 2 years had patterns of brain activity more similar to children living with their biological parents than did those placed in foster care after the age of 2 years, demonstrating that the lack of positive experience detrimentally affects brain function and that these effects become more marked once children are older than 2 years [43]. Consistent with these results, at 12 years, children who were removed from institutions and placed into foster care demonstrated continuing benefits as a result of the intervention, as shown by the fact that EEG measures of children placed in foster care were similar to the measures of the never-institutionalised group [44].

MRI investigations of the BEIP project have shown that at the age of 9–10 years, the children with a history of institutionalisation exhibited significantly smaller cortical grey and white matter volumes compared to children living with their biological parents. Interestingly, there were no differences in cortical white matter between children who were randomised to foster care between 6 and 31 months of age and never-institutionalised children, suggesting the presence of a potential 'catch-up' in white matter growth, even following severe environmental deprivation [45]. Another investigation in children aged 8–11 years found an association between neglect in early life and microstructural integrity of the body of the corpus callosum and of tracts involved in emotion regulation and sensory processing [46]. As reported in the study by Sheridan et al. (2012), this study showed that the parameters of these white matter tracts in the foster care group did not present significant differences from the never-institutionalised group, which highlights the potential for remediation of specific white matter tracts for children removed from institution and placed in high-quality care early in life [46]. The same research group explored the link between white matter changes and deprivation and found that alterations in the external capsule and corpus callosum in the institutionalised group in part explained the relationship between institutionalised status and *internalising symptoms* in 8–14-year-old children [47]. Lastly, an MRI study conducted in 8–10-year-old children reported that children who grew up in institutions presented lower cortical thickness across prefrontal, parietal and temporal regions compared to children who were never institutionalised [48]. Reduced thickness across numerous cortical areas was associated with higher levels of attention deficit hyperactivity disorder (ADHD) symptoms [48].

These results have provided novel evidence of the negative effects of psychosocial deprivation on cortical development and the subsequent risk of developing psychopathology later in life. They have also demonstrated that extended cognitive and emotional enrichment in adoptive homes in early life can facilitate healthy neurodevelopmental processes.

The effects of institutionalisation are not just evident in childhood, but they persist throughout adolescence. The BEIP research group also found that children assigned to foster care had greater thinning of the prefrontal cortex from 9 to 16 years compared to children who remained in institutions. In addition, among those randomised to foster care, children removed from institutional care before the age of 24 months showed higher thinning in these regions relative to those removed later [49]. Considering that rapid cortical thinning in cortices supporting higher-order cognitive processes is a physiological process of adolescence [50], the reduced thinning observed among children exposed to prolonged institutionalisation represents a deviation from the expected developmental patterns. These results [50] were replicated in a later BEIP study that included adolescents at 16 years of age [51]. Here, the authors also showed that the white matter pathways associated with psychopathology in previously institutionalised individuals differed from those related to psychopathology in other populations, which indicate that early institutionalisation may disrupt commonly observed developmental trajectories [51].

In addition to the BEIP, numerous other studies that explored the effects of institutionalisation on brain measures consistently showed its negative association with brain development. For instance, a small investigation conducted on seven children adopted from Romania and seven children born in North America found smaller whole brain, white and grey matter volumes among previously institutionalised children compared with children who were never institutionalised [52]. Furthermore, previously institutionalised children presented lower diffusion metrics and *fractional anisotropy* across all white matter tracts compared with never-institutionalised children, indicating a general deficit of white matter integrity in this population [52]. A study that examined 14 previously institutionalised adolescents adopted from Romania to the United Kingdom and 11 never-institutionalised adoptees from the United Kingdom found smaller grey and white matter volumes in the adopted group compared to the never-institutionalised group. Additionally, previously institutionalised children exhibited a smaller volume of the left hippocampus and a larger volume in the right amygdala [53]. Another study of 34 institutionalised children adopted into the United States and 28 children living in the United States with their biological families did not replicate the finding of smaller hippocampal or larger amygdala volume across groups [54]. However, the authors observed that the amygdala was larger in children adopted after 15 months of age compared to children adopted before 15 months of age. Of note, late adoption was also associated with poorer emotion regulation and higher anxiety levels [54]. A later study that included children adopted from Romania, Russia, China and Bulgaria found that children who suffered early neglect had lower white matter directional organisation in the prefrontal cortex and in tracts connecting the prefrontal and temporal areas [55]. Differences in white matter microstructure were associated with poorer cognitive performance among the children raised in institutional care [55]. More recently, a study of 67 previously institutionalised Romanian young adults (with between 3 and 41 months of deprivation) and 21 nondeprived UK adoptees showed that deprived adoptees had smaller total brain volumes, right inferior frontal surface area and volume, as well as greater right inferior temporal lobe thickness, surface area and volume compared to the nondeprived adoptees [56]. Notably, deprivation duration was negatively associated with total brain volume and positively associated with right medial prefrontal volume and surface area. A decrease in total brain volume mediated the relationship between institutionalisation and lower intelligence quotient and more severe ADHD symptoms. Conversely, the increase in right inferior temporal volume was associated with lower levels of ADHD symptoms [56]. Overall, these studies provide compelling evidence that severe deprivation in the first years of life is related to alterations in brain structure later in life, despite emotional and cognitive enrichment in adoptive homes in adolescence.

Evidence from fMRI studies suggests that brain function may also be affected by institutionalisation. For example, a task-based fMRI study conducted on 22 previously institutionalised children and 22 children raised with their biological families reported that the previously institutionalised group manifested higher activity of the amygdala and lower activity in prefrontal regions during an emotional face go/no-go task evaluating the emotional modulation of inhibition [57]. Of note, amygdala hyperactivity was associated with atypical social behaviour assessed with the Child Behaviour Checklist [57]. In another study, 46 previously institutionalised children and adolescents and 43 control subjects raised by their biological parents completed an aversive learning task during fMRI, which consisted of visual stimuli paired with aversive sound or with no sound [58]. In the aversive condition (e.g. visual stimuli paired with aversive sound), the previously institutionalised group displayed amygdala hyperactivation and higher connectivity of the hippocampus with the prefrontal cortex, which predicted improvements in future anxiety. These findings suggest that institutionalisation alters the neurobiology of aversive learning by engaging a broader prefrontal-subcortical circuit [58]. The same research group conducted an fMRI investigation using a visual search task that involved quickly locating negative or positive targets among neutral distractor stimuli [59]. In the previously institutionalised group, greater activation of the amygdala for negative versus positive stimuli was associated with greater anxiety, indicating that institutional care strengthens the relationship between amygdala reactivity and anxiety [59]. Furthermore, an fMRI study that focused on the functional connectivity of the ventral striatum reported higher positive connectivity between the ventral striatum and the medial prefrontal cortex in previously institutionalised youths [60]. Stronger ventral striatum–medial prefrontal cortex coupling was associated with parental reports of social problems [60]. Overall, these findings indicate that institutionalisation alters the activation of brain areas involved in cognitive, emotional and social functioning, including the prefrontal cortex, amygdala and hippocampus.

13.4.2 Exposure to Abuse, Violence and Maltreatment

Exposure to abuse, violence and maltreatment has detrimental effects on neurodevelopment. Indeed, compelling evidence suggests that children who experienced maltreatment present lower amygdala and hippocampal volume, which is associated with altered patterns of fear conditioning [61, 62]. These results have been replicated in adults exposed to sexual abuse during childhood [63, 64]. Longitudinal work showed reduced growth in amygdala volume over time in adolescents exposed to maltreatment, which reflects a slower rate of development [65]. In addition, the experience of physical abuse, sexual abuse and domestic violence has been found to indirectly increase the risk of developing depression over time through hippocampal and amygdala volumes, particularly in those children and adolescents exposed to more stressful life events [62]. Recent meta-analytic evidence has reported that individuals with a history of childhood maltreatment have lower cortical thickness in the left middle frontal gyrus, right median cingulate/paracingulate gyri and right anterior cingulate/paracingulate gyri, as well as lower grey matter volume in the left supplementary motor area and bilateral median cingulate/paracingulate gyri [66]. The results of this study indicate that early-life maltreatment affects those brain areas mainly implicated in cognition, socio-affective functioning and stress regulation [66].

Functional MRI investigations have highlighted significant changes in brain activity and functional connectivity in children who experienced abuse, violence or maltreatment. For instance, exposure to violence has been linked to reduced activation in the dorsal anterior cingulate cortex and prefrontal areas during an emotional face task [67]. Also, violence-exposed children have been found to present abnormal activation of fronto-parietal regions and hippocampus during an associative learning task with angry, happy and neutral faces paired with objects, suggesting that violence exposure alters the development of hippocampal and fronto-parietal areas [68]. Of note, a recent study has indicated that the effects of violence exposure on threat-related networks (e.g. amygdala) depend on the trauma context [69]. Indeed, children experiencing greater violence at home showed amygdala sensitisation throughout an emotional faces task, regardless of the emotion of the face stimuli, while children who experienced more school and community violence showed amygdala habituation (a decrease in amygdala activation with repeated presentations of similar stimuli) throughout the task. The authors also highlighted that maternal warmth was associated with a normalisation of amygdala sensitisation in children, and fewer externalising behaviours up to 1 year later, indicating that a positive caregiving can increase resilience [69]. Other *brain networks* seem also affected by childhood traumatic experiences, as reported by a recent *meta-analysis* showing that children with a trauma history present changes in the activation of the *default mode network*, posterior insula and affective networks during emotional tasks and *executive network* during reward processing [70]. Taken together, these investigations provide convincing evidence that exposure to abuse, violence and maltreatment in the early years of life results in different activation patterns in the brain during tasks that elicit the processing of traumatic stimuli.

13.4.3 Exposure to Socioeconomic and Neighbourhood Disadvantage

Socioeconomic disadvantage is an important stressor and can expose individuals to more adversity and negative life events than the general population [71, 72], with associated poor cognitive and psychological outcomes [73]. Socioeconomic disadvantage can be considered either at the household level (e.g. insufficient family income) or at the neighbourhood level (e.g. high concentrations of poverty, high rates of unemployment, limited material resources and services). Neighbourhood economic disadvantage has been shown to have a negative impact on individuals, including lower academic achievement, lower-paying employment and greater physical and mental health problems [74, 75]. Among young children, neighbourhood disadvantage is associated with a high incidence of internalising and externalising problems [76, 77]. Neighbourhood disadvantage may affect children's neurodevelopment through a variety of social and biological mechanisms, including poor social cohesion, high crime and violence, lack of institutional resources and exposure to environmental pollutants [78, 79]. In childhood, the quality of local schools may also play a role in neurodevelopment, as might the availability of neighbourhood resources in adolescence and early adulthood [80]. Research shows, for example, that children exposed to socioeconomic and neighbourhood disadvantage have higher salivary cortisol levels compared to unexposed children, which can lead to long-term dysregulation of the hypothalamus–pituitary–adrenal axis [81]. Notably, the increase in cortisol has potentially negative consequences on the developing brain, as it has been associated with atrophy of limbic structures and lower default mode network functional connectivity [82, 83].

Neuroimaging studies have found that infants from low-income families have smaller frontal and parietal grey matter volume compared to children growing up with middle- and high-income families [84] and these volumetric differences appear to be associated with disruptive behaviours [84]. In addition, these children also show slower trajectories of growth from infancy to childhood. Lower socioeconomic status has also been linked to abnormal amygdala response to photographs of negatively valenced objects and scenes, suggesting an abnormality in how the brain perceives and responds to potential threats [85, 86]. A recent meta-analysis of structural and functional neural correlates of socioeconomic disadvantage has found that children with low socioeconomic status present hypoactivity of the fronto-parietal/cingulo-opercular networks and hyperactivity of the right caudate nucleus [87]. Structural differences in individuals with low socioeconomic status were complementary to the functional results. Indeed, individuals with low socioeconomic status presented smaller grey matter volume in the anterior cingulate cortex, as well as larger grey matter volume in the orbital frontal cortex, dorsal lateral prefrontal cortex and hippocampus, key regions of the reward circuit [87]. A large study using the Adolescent Brain Cognitive Development (ABCD) cohort (see below) also showed that neighbourhood disadvantage is associated with lower cortical thickness in the lateral orbitofrontal, rostral middle frontal, superior parietal, precentral, postcentral, paracentral, cuneus, lateral occipital, lingual and pericalcarine cortices [88]. Exploratory analyses using these data showed that the association between low educational attainment or neighbourhood disadvantage and reduced cortical thickness was less marked in the presence of a high income-to-needs ratio, an index that describes the amount of income relative to the cost of living, suggesting that a high income-to-needs ratio may play a protective role in the context of low educational attainment or neighbourhood disadvantage [88]. Lastly, a longitudinal study that investigated whether neighbourhood disadvantage was associated with trajectories of the difference between brain-predicted-age and chronological age (brainAGE), reported that children exposed to high neighbourhood disadvantage show positive brainAGE, reflecting an older brain-predicted-age than chronological age during early adolescence and deceleration through to late adolescence, suggesting delayed brain development [89].

13.4.4 Exposure to Adverse Childhood Experiences

Evidence from studies exploring the effects of different dimensions of adverse childhood experiences on brain measures unequivocally reports changes in areas involved in cognition, emotional processing and stress regulation. Among these, the ABCD Study, a large dataset that contains neuroimaging data, youth-reported adverse experiences and parent-reported financial adversity of children around the United States, has provided invaluable evidence on the effect of adverse childhood experiences on the brain. In a study conducted on 7,036 children from ages 9–10 to 11–12 years, a higher number of adversities was associated with smaller hippocampal volume at baseline and year 2 [90]. In a sample of about 12,000 participants aged 9–13 years, higher family conflict was associated with higher fractional anisotropy levels across brain tracts and within the corpus callosum, fornix and anterior thalamic radiations [91]. Also, lower socioeconomic status and neighbourhood safety were linked to decreasing fractional anisotropy trajectory over time and altered fractional anisotropy in the corpus callosum, fornix and anterior thalamic radiations [91]. A study published last year has reported that dimensions of emotional neglect, such as lack of primary and secondary caregiver support and lack of caregiver supervision, are associated with younger-looking brains, while dimensions related to caregiver psychopathology, substance use, family aggression, trauma exposure, separation from biological parent, socioeconomic disadvantage and neighbourhood safety are associated with older-looking brains [92]. Higher levels of adverse childhood experiences have also been linked to lower brain activation during a cognitive control task in the right inferior frontal gyrus and in the bilateral pre-supplementary motor area, key regions implicated in inhibitory control [93]. Furthermore, greater brain response correlated with less impulsivity suggesting reduced activation may not be behaviourally adaptive in children aged 9–10 years [93].

The negative consequences of adverse childhood experiences on the brain are evident also in adults, as highlighted by a *mega-analysis* that included a subsample of Generation Scotland (n = 1,024) and individuals from the UK Biobank (n = 27,202). Generation Scotland is a population-based cohort of over 24,000 individuals with in-depth phenotyping recruited between 2006 and 2011, while the UK Biobank is a large, UK-based population cohort of over 500,000 adults recruited between 2006 and 2010. This study reported that childhood traumatic experiences were associated with increased risk lifetime experience of depression in both cohorts (odds ratio [OR] = 1.06 and 1.23 respectively), and early onset and recurrent course of depressive symptoms. Importantly, there was evidence of an association between childhood trauma and smaller global brain volume and cortical surface area of frontal and parietal areas. At a regional level, childhood trauma measures were linked to smaller hippocampus, thalamus and nucleus accumbens volumes. This large study provides robust evidence of the lasting effect of childhood adversity on brain structure [94].

In line with these results, meta-analytic evidence consistently shows that adverse childhood experiences are associated with changes in brain areas implicated in socioemotional functioning, cognitive processing and stress regulation. For instance, a meta-analysis of 56 studies reported consistent evidence of the effects of adverse childhood experiences on the right left inferior frontal gyrus, hippocampus and amygdala grey matter volume, age-specific effects in the right amygdala and hippocampus in children and adolescents and maltreatment-specific effects in the right perigenual anterior cingulate cortex in adults [95]. With respect to brain activation, a meta-analysis that included 68 task-based fMRI studies demonstrated that early life adversities were linked to hypoactivation in the left superior frontal gyrus in healthy subjects [96]. Moreover, when exploring task effects, functional alterations associated with early life adversities were found during emotion processing in the left centromedial amygdala, in the left precuneus during memory processing and in the left centromedial amygdala and putamen in relation to postnatal maltreatment [96]. The same research group explored functional connectivity of the amygdala in relation to prenatal exposures (e.g. substance exposure) and postnatal experiences (e.g. childhood maltreatment or poverty) and reported robust evidence for decreased amygdala–anterior cingulate cortex and altered amygdala–hippocampus connectivity in relation to early life adversities [97]. Lastly, a meta-analysis by Colich et al. (2020) demonstrated diverse patterns of association between different dimensions of childhood adversities and pubertal timing, cellular aging and cortical thickness. In particular, the study showed that threat, but not deprivation or socio-economic status, was associated with accelerated pubertal development and accelerated cellular aging as measured by both leukocyte telomere length and DNA methylation age. Furthermore, there was a consistent association between early life adversities and accelerated cortical thinning, although the specific brain regions involved varied by adversity type. Associations between threat and cortical thinning were mostly seen in the ventromedial prefrontal cortex, while associations of deprivation with cortical thinning were most consistent in the frontoparietal cortex and default mode network [98].

13.5 Psychosis as a Neurodevelopmental Disorder

Since 1986, when it was first introduced, the neurodevelopmental model of psychosis has been one of the predominant explanatory theories of psychosis [99]. According to this theory, psychosis is the result of alterations in neurodevelopmental processes that begin long before the onset of clinical symptoms and are caused by a combination of genetic and environmental factors [99, 100]. Evidence for this broad neurodevelopmental model comes from many lines of research. Individuals who later develop schizophrenia are more likely to have experienced pre- or perinatal adverse events or to have been exposed to potentially harmful stressors compared to subjects who do not develop the disorder [101, 102]. In addition, individuals who develop psychosis also exhibit increased rates of minor deviations in motor, cognitive and social development [103, 104]. These observations strongly suggest that brain abnormalities appear early in life in individuals who later develop psychosis. Disruptions in neurodevelopment seem to be linked to both early (pre- or perinatal) brain changes [105] and to disturbances in brain maturation during childhood and adolescence [106]. In particular, abnormalities in normal developmental pruning [107] and deficits in myelination [108] during adolescence have long been implicated in the pathogenesis of psychosis. This is in agreement with brain imaging studies that reveal a pattern of progressive changes both for early onset and chronic schizophrenia.

13.6 Brain Imaging in First Episode Psychosis

As neurodevelopmental disorders, psychotic disorders usually present during adolescence, and 11–18% of patients experience their first episode of psychosis before age 18 [109, 110]. The outcome of psychosis is negatively affected by the impact of illness onset on adolescents and young adults whose neurobiological and psychosocial development is not yet complete [111]. Individuals with psychosis can have a worse quality of life, a wide and diverse array of psychosocial difficulties and an increase in morbidity and mortality [112], which make the identification of the neural mechanisms underlying the development of psychotic symptoms especially important.

Structural and functional brain correlates have become an established feature of psychosis, and increasing evidence points towards a progressive nature of these alterations from early development to adulthood. MRI studies have consistently shown widespread volume reductions in prefrontal and temporal areas, anterior cingulate cortex, insula and cerebellum in individuals with first episode psychosis compared to unaffected individuals [113, 114]. In addition, first episode psychosis is associated with a lower volume of limbic regions, including the amygdala [115] and hippocampus [116]. Of note, the experience of childhood maltreatment has been negatively associated with amygdala volumes in first episode psychosis, so people with psychosis with higher scores on the Trauma and Distress Scale show lower amygdala volume [115]. Furthermore, individuals with first episode psychosis present lower cortical thickness in the right lateral superior temporal cortex and right anterior cingulate cortex relative to healthy controls [117]. Interestingly, a recent study has found that widespread cortical reductions in subjects with first episode psychosis were similar to those associated with socioenvironmental exposure during childhood (e.g. socio-economic deprivation, family disadvantage, negative peer relationships) relative to other types of childhood adverse experiences, such as parental death or being expelled from school [118].

Meta-analytic evidence from functional brain investigations has reported that people with first-episode psychosis show hypoactivation of the right middle frontal gyrus, right inferior parietal lobule and left superior parietal lobule during tasks encoding working memory [119]. Another meta-analysis of the functional correlates of attentional and memory performance in first-episode psychoses showed that during attentional task performance, subjects with first-episode psychosis present frontal, parietal and insular dysfunction, while during memory tasks the activation of the left insula seems altered [120]. The same research group also showed that during emotional task performance, subjects with first-episode psychosis failed to activate emotional processing-related areas, including the amygdala and the anterior cingulate cortex [114, 121]. Resting-state studies have also consistently described functional abnormalities in first-episode psychosis, in particular, dysconnectivity in the fronto-striatal [122] and fronto-striato-thalamic network [123], possibly underlying striatal dopamine synthesis capacity abnormalities. Overall, this evidence suggests that brain alterations in subjects with first episode psychosis somehow overlap with changes associated with adverse childhood experiences, indicating that childhood neurodevelopment impaired by stress could be an early risk factor for the development of psychosis.

13.7 Conclusion

Neurodevelopment involves an extremely complex set of processes. Adverse childhood experiences can influence these processes in multiple ways that vary as a function of the presence of other risk and protective factors. The brain changes associated with adverse childhood experiences are well-documented and mainly affect areas involved in cognition, emotional processing and stress regulation. Among these, changes in the amygdala and the hippocampus have been most commonly linked to adverse childhood experiences. In addition, stressors in the first years of life seem to negatively affect frontal, parietal, temporal and cingulate areas development, as well as the default mode and executive networks. These brain changes underlie the development later in life of cognitive deficits, internalising and externalising problems, affective disorders and psychosis. Studying the effects of different adverse childhood experiences and other environmental and psychological factors is crucial to advancing our understanding of the consequences of adverse childhood experiences on long-term functioning and mental health.

13.7.1 Limitations

During the last 30 years, there have been major advances in our understanding of the effect of adverse childhood experiences on brain development. However, it is necessary to consider several methodological caveats that have affected what we know so far. First, some of the longitudinal studies that explored the effect of adverse childhood experiences on specific outcomes (e.g. symptoms, cognitive function, brain structure and function) have assessed them at a single point in time. This is particularly critical when the outcome is instead assessed later in life, as it makes it difficult to draw conclusions about changes or stability of these measures during development. Second, the concept of adverse childhood experiences includes a wide array of experiences, spanning from abuse and neglect to exposure to conflict and violence. While exploring adverse childhood experiences as a whole has certain advantages, primarily increasing the sample size of children exposed to adversity, this also hinders a better understanding of the differential effect that specific adverse childhood experiences can have on neurodevelopment.

There is also little research on the role of contextual factors. For example, abuse and neglect in the context of low socioeconomic status or neighbourhood disadvantage may have a different impact from abuse and neglect in children from families with fewer adversities. In the latter case, the child may have more protective factors and the family may have more resources to reduce the impact of any potentially adverse experience. Related to this, pre-existing vulnerabilities, such as individual and familial clinical and demographic characteristics, are often overlooked in these investigations, which may lead to inappropriate attributions of causality to adverse childhood experiences. To overcome these limitations, future studies with longitudinal designs should distinguish among the different types of adverse childhood experiences and should consider the role of contextual factors and pre-existing vulnerabilities that may play a role in the causes and consequences of adverse childhood experiences.

Key Points
- Brain development is the result of an ongoing interaction between genetic and environmental factors. Childhood represents a crucial period for neurodevelopment since the foundations of sensory and perceptual systems that are critical to

cognition, emotion processing and social behaviour are formed in the early years of life and are strongly influenced by experiences during this time.

- Adverse childhood experiences, including harms that affect children both directly (e.g. physical, emotional and sexual abuse, physical and emotional neglect) and indirectly through their environment (e.g. parental conflict, domestic violence, substance abuse or mental illness), can influence brain development in numerous ways that vary as a function of the presence of other risk and protective factors.
- Adverse childhood experiences mainly affect areas involved in cognition, emotional processing and stress regulation. Among these, changes in the amygdala and the hippocampus have been most commonly linked to adverse childhood experiences.
- Adverse childhood experiences also have a negative effect on frontal, parietal, temporal and cingulate areas development, as well as the default mode and executive networks.
- These brain changes underlie the development later in life of cognitive deficits, internalising and externalising problems, affective disorders and psychosis.

Box 13.1: Glossary

Anisotropy: Property of a structure or material that exhibits physical characteristics that vary depending on the direction of measurement.

Brain networks: Groups of widespread brain regions that co-activate and deactivate together and are involved in the same sets of functions.

Default mode network: Functional brain network that is active during self-directed thought and introspective mental activities. It includes the medial prefrontal cortex, posterior cingulate cortex, precuneus and inferior parietal lobule.

Executive network: Functional brain network that is active during cognitive tasks. It includes the dorsolateral prefrontal cortex and the posterior parietal cortex.

Externalising symptoms: Maladaptive behaviours directed towards the individual's environment. Examples include aggressive and delinquent behaviours.

Functional connectivity: Temporal correlation between the blood-oxygen-level-dependent signal of anatomically separated brain regions. It reflects how widespread brain regions interact and exchange information.

Fractional anisotropy: Scalar value between 0 and 1 that describes the degree of anisotropy of a diffusion process, with 0 indicating no restriction of diffusion in all directions in the brain and 1 indicating that diffusion is occurring in one direction only. It is generally interpreted as a quantitative biomarker of white matter integrity.

Grey matter: Area of the central nervous system composed by neuronal bodies, unmyelinated axons, dendrites, glial cells and synapses.

(continued)

Box 13.1 (continued)

Internalising symptoms: Maladaptive phenomena affecting one's own self. Examples include depressed mood, social withdrawal, guilt and loneliness.

Mega-analysis: A type of research study that involves analysis of multiple independent datasets, significantly improving statistical power and the generalisability of the findings.

Meta-analysis: A type of research study that summarises quantitative data from multiple independent studies addressing a common research question.

Synapses: Structures that allow a neuron to pass an electrical or chemical signal to another neuron.

White matter: Area of the central nervous system composed by myelinated axons, also called tracts.

References

1. Zhou Y, Song H, Ming GLI. Genetics of human brain development. Nat Rev Genet. 2023;25(1):26–45.
2. Shonkoff J, Phillips D. From neurons to neighborhoods: the science of early childhood development. From Neurons to Neighborhoods. 2000. https://doi.org/10.17226/9824.
3. Houston SM, Herting MM, Sowell ER. The neurobiology of childhood structural brain development: conception through adulthood. Curr Top Behav Neurosci. 2014;16:3–17.
4. Tierney AL, Charles A, Nelson I. Brain development and the role of experience in the early years. Zero Three. 2009;30:9.
5. Huttenlocher P, Dabholkar A. Regional differences in synaptogenesis in human cerebral cortex. J Comp Neurol. 1997;387:167–78.
6. Miller DJ, Duka T, Stimpson CD, et al. Prolonged myelination in human neocortical evolution. Proc Natl Acad Sci USA. 2012;109:16480–5.
7. Nickel M, Gu C. Regulation of central nervous system myelination in higher brain functions. Neural Plast. 2018; https://doi.org/10.1155/2018/6436453.
8. Buyanova IS, Arsalidou M. Cerebral White matter myelination and relations to age, gender, and cognition: a selective review. Front Hum Neurosci. 2021;15:662031.
9. Dennis EL, Thompson PM. Typical and atypical brain development: a review of neuroimaging studies. Dialogues Clin Neurosci. 2013;15:359.
10. Thompson PM, Sowell ER, Gogtay N, Giedd JN, Vidal CN, Hayashi KM, Leow A, Nicolson R, Rapoport JL, Toga AW. Structural MRI and brain development. Int Rev Neurobiol. 2005;67:285–323.
11. Giedd JN, Blumenthal J, Jeffries NO, Castellanos FX, Liu H, Zijdenbos A, Paus T, Evans AC, Rapoport JL. Brain development during childhood and adolescence: a longitudinal MRI study. Nat Neurosci. 1999;2:861–3.
12. Bethlehem RAI, Seidlitz J, White SR, et al. Brain charts for the human lifespan. Nature. 2022;604(7906):525–33.
13. Casey BJ, Tottenham N, Liston C, Durston S. Imaging the developing brain: what have we learned about cognitive development? Trends Cogn Sci. 2005;9:104–10.
14. Uddin LQ, Supekar K, Menon V. Typical and atypical development of functional human brain networks: insights from resting-state fMRI. Front Syst Neurosci. 2010;4:21.
15. Di X, Gohel S, Kim EH, Biswal BB. Task vs. rest-different network configurations between the coactivation and the resting-state brain networks. Front Hum Neurosci. 2013;7:56300.

16. Calhoun VD, Adali T, Pearlson GD, Pekar JJ. A method for making group inferences from functional MRI data using independent component analysis. Hum Brain Mapp. 2001;14:140–51.
17. Zhang H, Shen D, Lin W. Resting-state functional MRI studies on infant brains: a decade of gap-filling efforts. NeuroImage. 2018;185:664.
18. Yu J, Patel RA, Haynie DL, Vidal-Ribas P, Govender T, Sundaram R, Gilman SE. Adverse childhood experiences and premature mortality through mid-adulthood: a five-decade prospective study. Lancet Reg Health Am. 2022; https://doi.org/10.1016/j.lana.2022.100349.
19. Nelson CA, Gabard-Durnam LJ. Early adversity and critical periods: neurodevelopmental consequences of violating the expectable environment. Trends Neurosci. 2020;43:133.
20. McDonald CM, Olofin I, Flaxman S, Fawzi WW, Spiegelman D, Caulfield LE, Black RE, Ezzati M, Danaei G. The effect of multiple anthropometric deficits on child mortality: meta-analysis of individual data in 10 prospective studies from developing countries. Am J Clin Nutr. 2013;97:896–901.
21. Motsan S, Yirmiya K, Feldman R. Chronic early trauma impairs emotion recognition and executive functions in youth; specifying biobehavioral precursors of risk and resilience. Dev Psychopathol. 2022;34:1339–52.
22. Danese A, Moffitt TE, Arseneault L, et al. The origins of cognitive deficits in victimized children: implications for neuroscientists and clinicians. Am J Psychiatry. 2017;174:349–61.
23. Hawkins MAW, Layman HM, Ganson KT, Tabler J, Ciciolla L, Tsotsoros CE, Nagata JM. Adverse childhood events and cognitive function among young adults: prospective results from the national longitudinal study of adolescent to adult health. Child Abuse Negl. 2021;115:105008.
24. Escueta M, Whetten K, Ostermann J, O'Donnell K. Adverse childhood experiences, psychosocial well-being and cognitive development among orphans and abandoned children in five low income countries. BMC Int Health Hum Rights. 2014; https://doi.org/10.1186/1472-698X-14-6.
25. Solberg MA, Peters RM, Templin TN, Albdour MM. The relationship of adverse childhood experiences and emotional distress in young adults. J Am Psychiatr Nurses Assoc. 2024;30:532–44.
26. Hughes K, Bellis MA, Hardcastle KA, Sethi D, Butchart A, Mikton C, Jones L, Dunne MP. The effect of multiple adverse childhood experiences on health: a systematic review and meta-analysis. Lancet Public Health. 2017;2:e356–66.
27. Russell JD, Heyn SA, Peverill M, DiMaio S, Herringa RJ. Traumatic and adverse childhood experiences and developmental differences in psychiatric risk. JAMA Psychiat. 2024; https://doi.org/10.1001/JAMAPSYCHIATRY.2024.3231.
28. Elmore AL, Crouch E. The Association of Adverse Childhood Experiences with anxiety and depression for children and youth, 8 to 17 years of age. Acad Pediatr. 2020;20:600.
29. Karcher NR, Niendam TA, Barch DM. Adverse childhood experiences and psychotic-like experiences are associated above and beyond shared correlates: findings from the adolescent brain cognitive development study. Schizophr Res. 2020;222:235.
30. Dhondt N, Staines L, Healy C, Cannon M. Childhood adversity and recurrence of psychotic experiences during adolescence: the role of mediation in an analysis of a population-based longitudinal cohort study. Psychol Med. 2022;53:4046.
31. Kaufman J, Torbey S. Child maltreatment and psychosis. Neurobiol Dis. 2019; https://doi.org/10.1016/J.NBD.2019.01.015.
32. Morgan C, Gayer-Anderson C. Childhood adversities and psychosis: evidence, challenges, implications. World Psychiatry. 2016;15:93–102.
33. Varese F, Smeets F, Drukker M, Lieverse R, Lataster T, Viechtbauer W, Read J, Van Os J, Bentall RP. Childhood adversities increase the risk of psychosis: a meta-analysis of patient-control, prospective- and cross-sectional cohort studies. Schizophr Bull. 2012;38:661–71.
34. Nelson CA, Scott RD, Bhutta ZA, Harris NB, Danese A, Samara M. Adversity in childhood is linked to mental and physical health throughout life. BMJ. 2020; https://doi.org/10.1136/BMJ.M3048.

35. Stergaard SD, Larsen JT, Petersen L, Smith GD, Agerbo E. Psychosocial adversity in infancy and mortality rates in childhood and adolescence: a birth cohort study of 1.5 million individuals. Epidemiology. 2019;30:246–55.
36. Kelly-Irving M, Lepage B, Dedieu D, Bartley M, Blane D, Grosclaude P, Lang T, Delpierre C. Adverse childhood experiences and premature all-cause mortality. Eur J Epidemiol. 2013;28:721–34.
37. Godoy LC, Frankfurter C, Cooper M, Lay C, Maunder R, Farkouh ME. Association of adverse childhood experiences with cardiovascular disease later in life: a review. JAMA Cardiol. 2021;6:228–35.
38. Felitti VJ, Anda RF, Nordenberg D, Williamson DF, Spitz AM, Edwards V, Koss MP, Marks JS. Relationship of childhood abuse and household dysfunction to many of the leading causes of death in adults: the adverse childhood experiences (ACE) study. Am J Prev Med. 1998;14:245–58.
39. Rutter M, Andersen-Wood L, Beckett C, et al. Developmental catch-up, and deficit, following adoption after severe global early privation. J Child Psychol Psychiatry Allied Discip. 1998;39:465–76.
40. Zeanah CH, Nelson CA, Fox NA, Smyke AT, Marshall P, Parker SW, Koga S. Designing research to study the effects of institutionalization on brain and behavioral development: the Bucharest early intervention project. Dev Psychopathol. 2003;15:885–907.
41. Nelson CA, Fox NA, Zeanah CH. Romania's abandoned children: the effects of early profound psychosocial deprivation on the course of human development. Curr Dir Psychol Sci. 2023;32:515.
42. Marshall PJ, Fox NA. A comparison of the electroencephalogram between institutionalized and community children in Romania. J Cogn Neurosci. 2004;16:1327–38.
43. Marshall PJ, Reeb BC, Fox NA, Nelson CA, Zeanah CH. Effects of early intervention on EEG power and coherence in previously institutionalized children in Romania. Dev Psychopathol. 2008;20:861–80.
44. Vanderwert RE, Zeanah CH, Fox NA, Nelson CA. Normalization of EEG activity among previously institutionalized children placed into foster care: a 12-year follow-up of the Bucharest early intervention project. Dev Cogn Neurosci. 2015;17:68.
45. Sheridan MA, Fox NA, Zeanah CH, McLaughlin KA, Nelson CA. Variation in neural development as a result of exposure to institutionalization early in childhood. Proc Natl Acad Sci USA. 2012;109:12927–32.
46. Bick J, Zhu T, Stamoulis C, Fox NA, Zeanah C, Nelson CA. Effect of early institutionalization and foster care on long-term white matter development: a randomized clinical trial. JAMA Pediatr. 2015;169:211–9.
47. Bick J, Fox N, Zeanah CH, Nelson CA. Early deprivation, atypical brain development, and internalizing symptoms in late childhood. Neuroscience. 2015;342:140.
48. McLaughlin KA, Sheridan MA, Winter W, Fox NA, Zeanah CH, Nelson CA. Widespread reductions in cortical thickness following severe early-life deprivation: a neurodevelopmental pathway to attention-deficit/hyperactivity disorder. Biol Psychiatry. 2014;76:629–38.
49. Sheridan MA, Mukerji CE, Wade M, et al. Early deprivation alters structural brain development from middle childhood to adolescence. Sci Adv. 2022; https://doi.org/10.1126/SCIADV.ABN4316.
50. Gogtay N, Giedd JN, Lusk L, et al. Dynamic mapping of human cortical development during childhood through early adulthood. Proc Natl Acad Sci USA. 2004;101:8174–9.
51. Kanel D, Fox NA, Pine DS, Zeanah CH, Nelson CA, McLaughlin KA, Sheridan MA. Altered associations between white matter structure and psychopathology in previously institutionalized adolescents. Dev Cogn Neurosci. 2024;69:101440.
52. Eluvathingal TJ, Chugani HT, Behen ME, Juhász C, Muzik O, Maqbool M, Chugani DC, Makki M. Abnormal brain connectivity in children after early severe socioemotional deprivation: a diffusion tensor imaging study. Pediatrics. 2006;117:2093–100.
53. Mehta MA, Golembo NI, Nosarti C, Colvert E, Mota A, Williams SCR, Rutter M, Sonuga-Barke EJS. Amygdala, hippocampal and corpus callosum size following severe early

institutional deprivation: the English and Romanian adoptees study pilot. J Child Psychol Psychiatry. 2009;50:943–51.

54. Tottenham N, Hare TA, Quinn BT, et al. Prolonged institutional rearing is associated with atypically large amygdala volume and difficulties in emotion regulation. Dev Sci. 2010;13:46–61.

55. Hanson JL, Adluru N, Chung MK, Alexander AL, Davidson RJ, Pollak SD. Early neglect is associated with alterations in white matter integrity and cognitive functioning. Child Dev. 2013;84 https://doi.org/10.1111/cdev.12069.

56. Mackes NK, Golm D, Sarkar S, Kumsta R, Rutter M, Fairchild G, Mehta MA, Sonuga-Barke EJS. Early childhood deprivation is associated with alterations in adult brain structure despite subsequent environmental enrichment. Proc Natl Acad Sci USA. 2020;117:641–9.

57. Tottenham N, Hare TA, Millner A, Gilhooly T, Zevin JD, Casey BJ. Elevated amygdala response to faces following early deprivation. Dev Sci. 2011;14:190–204.

58. Silvers JA, Lumian DS, Gabard-Durnam L, et al. Previous institutionalization is followed by broader amygdala-hippocampal-PFC network connectivity during aversive learning in human development. J Neurosci. 2016;36:6420–30.

59. Silvers JA, Goff B, Gabard-Durnam LJ, Gee DG, Fareri DS, Caldera C, Tottenham N. Vigilance, the amygdala, and anxiety in youths with a history of institutional care. Biol Psychiatry Cogn Neurosci Neuroimaging. 2017;2:493–501.

60. Fareri DS, Gabard-Durnam L, Goff B, Flannery J, Gee DG, Lumian DS, Caldera C, Tottenham N. Altered ventral striatal-medial prefrontal cortex resting-state connectivity mediates adolescent social problems after early institutional care. Dev Psychopathol. 2017;29:1865–76.

61. McLaughlin KA, Sheridan MA, Gold AL, Duys A, Lambert HK, Peverill M, Heleniak C, Shechner T, Wojcieszak Z, Pine DS. Maltreatment exposure, brain structure, and fear conditioning in children and adolescents. Neuropsychopharmacology. 2016;41:1956–64.

62. Weissman DG, Lambert HK, Rodman AM, Peverill M, Sheridan MA, McLaughlin KA. Reduced hippocampal and amygdala volume as a mechanism underlying stress sensitization to depression following childhood trauma. Depress Anxiety. 2020;37:916–25.

63. Andersen SL, Tomada A, Vincow ES, Valente E, Polcari A, Teicher MH. Preliminary evidence for sensitive periods in the effect of childhood sexual abuse on regional brain development. J Neuropsychiatry Clin Neurosci. 2008;20:292–301.

64. Bremner JD, Randall P, Vermetten E, Staib L, Bronen RA, Mazure C, Capelli S, McCarthy G, Innis RB, Charney DS. Magnetic resonance imaging-based measurement of hippocampal volume in posttraumatic stress disorder related to childhood physical and sexual abuse—a preliminary report. Biol Psychiatry. 1997;41:23–32.

65. Whittle S, Dennison M, Vijayakumar N, Simmons JG, Yücel M, Lubman DI, Pantelis C, Allen NB. Childhood maltreatment and psychopathology affect brain development during adolescence. J Am Acad Child Adolesc Psychiatry. 2013; https://doi.org/10.1016/J.JAAC.2013.06.007.

66. Yang W, Jin S, Duan W, Yu H, Ping L, Shen Z, Cheng Y, Xu X, Zhou C. The effects of childhood maltreatment on cortical thickness and gray matter volume: a coordinate-based meta-analysis. Psychol Med. 2023; https://doi.org/10.1017/S0033291723000661.

67. Weissman DG, Jenness JL, Colich NL, Miller AB, Sambrook KA, Sheridan MA, McLaughlin KA. Altered neural processing of threat-related information in children and adolescents exposed to violence: a transdiagnostic mechanism contributing to the emergence of psychopathology. J Am Acad Child Adolesc Psychiatry. 2020;59:1274–84.

68. Lambert HK, Peverill M, Sambrook KA, Rosen ML, Sheridan MA, McLaughlin KA. Altered development of hippocampus-dependent associative learning following early-life adversity. Dev Cogn Neurosci. 2019; https://doi.org/10.1016/J.DCN.2019.100666.

69. Stevens JS, Van Rooij SJH, Stenson AF, Ely TD, Powers A, Clifford A, Kim YJ, Hinrichs R, Tottenham N, Jovanovic T. Amygdala responses to threat in violence-exposed children depend on trauma context and maternal caregiving. Dev Psychopathol. 2023;35:1–12.

70. Ireton R, Hughes A, Klabunde M. A functional magnetic resonance imaging meta-analysis of childhood trauma. Biol Psychiatry Cogn Neurosci Neuroimaging. 2024;9:561–70.

71. Ennis NE, Hobfoll SE, Schröder KEE. Money doesn't talk, it swears: how economic stress and resistance resources impact inner-city women's depressive mood. Am J Community Psychol. 2000;28:149–73.

72. Ruijsbroek A, Wijga AH, Kerkhof M, Koppelman GH, Smit HA, Droomers M. The development of socio-economic health differences in childhood: results of the Dutch longitudinal PIAMA birth cohort. BMC Public Health. 2011;11:1–11.

73. Wadsworth ME, Raviv T, Reinhard C, Wolff B, DeCarlo SC, Einhorn L. An indirect effects model of the association between poverty and child functioning: the role of children's poverty-related stress. J Loss Trauma. 2008;13:156–85.

74. Borgen NT, Zachrisson HD. How neighbourhood effects vary by achievement level. Eur Sociol Rev. 2024:1–17.

75. Ribeiro AI, Fraga S, Severo M, et al. Association of neighbourhood disadvantage and individual socioeconomic position with all-cause mortality: a longitudinal multicohort analysis. Lancet Public Health. 2022;7:e447–57.

76. Palamar JJ, Calzada EJ, Theise R, Huang KY, Petkova E, Brotman LM. Family- and neighborhood-level factors as predictors of conduct problems in school among young, urban, minority children. Behav Med (Washington, DC). 2015;41:177–85.

77. Xue Y, Leventhal T, Brooks-Gunn J, Earls FJ. Neighborhood residence and mental health problems of 5- to 11-year-olds. Arch Gen Psychiatry. 2005;62:554–63.

78. Harding DJ. Collateral consequences of violence in disadvantaged neighborhoods. Soc Forces. 2009;88:757.

79. Lee H, Kravitz-Wirtz N, Rao S, Crowder K. Effects of prolonged exposure to air pollution and neighborhood disadvantage on self-rated health among adults in the United States: evidence from the panel study of income dynamics. Environ Health Perspect. 2023; https://doi.org/10.1289/EHP11268/SUPPL_FILE/EHP11268.S001.ACCO.PDF.

80. Harris JC, Wilson IG, Cardenas-Iniguez C, Watts AL, Lisdahl KM. The childhood opportunity index 2.0: factor structure in 9-10 year olds in the adolescent brain cognitive development study. Int J Environ Res Public Health. 2025; https://doi.org/10.3390/IJERPH22020228.

81. Finegood ED, Rarick JRD, Blair C. Exploring longitudinal associations between neighborhood disadvantage and cortisol levels in early childhood. Dev Psychopathol. 2017;29:1649–62.

82. Blair C, Raver CC. Poverty, stress, and brain development: new directions for prevention and intervention. Acad Pediatr. 2016;16:S30.

83. Sripada RK, Swain JE, Evans GW, Welsh RC, Liberzon I. Childhood poverty and stress reactivity are associated with aberrant functional connectivity in default mode network. Neuropsychopharmacology. 2014;39:2244–51.

84. Hanson JL, Hair N, Shen DG, Shi F, Gilmore JH, Wolfe BL, Pollak SD. Family poverty affects the rate of human infant brain growth. PLoS One. 2013;8:e80954.

85. White SF, Voss JL, Chiang JJ, Wang L, McLaughlin KA, Miller GE. Exposure to violence and low family income are associated with heightened amygdala responsiveness to threat among adolescents. Dev Cogn Neurosci. 2019;40:100709.

86. Huggins AA, LM MT, Davis MM, et al. Neighborhood disadvantage associated with blunted amygdala reactivity to predictable and unpredictable threat in a community sample of youth. Biol Psychiatry Global Open Sci. 2022;2:242.

87. Yaple ZA, Yu R. Functional and structural brain correlates of socioeconomic status. Cereb Cortex. 2020;30:181–96.

88. Rakesh D, Zalesky A, Whittle S. Assessment of parent income and education, neighborhood disadvantage, and child brain structure. JAMA Netw Open. 2022;5:e2226208.

89. Rakesh D, Cropley V, Zalesky A, Vijayakumar N, Allen NB, Whittle S. Neighborhood disadvantage and longitudinal brain-predicted-age trajectory during adolescence. Dev Cogn Neurosci. 2021;51:101002.

90. Breslin FJ, Kerr KL, Ratliff EL, Cohen ZP, Simmons WK, Morris AS, Croff JM. Early life adversity predicts reduced hippocampal volume in the adolescent brain cognitive development study. J Adolesc Health. 2024;75:275–80.

91. Pollmann A, Sasso R, Bates K, Fuhrmann D. Making connections: neurodevelopmental changes in brain connectivity after adverse experiences in early adolescence. J Neurosci. 2024; https://doi.org/10.1523/JNEUROSCI.0991-23.2023.
92. Beck D, Whitmore L, MacSweeney N, Brieant A, Karl V, de Lange A-MG, Westlye LT, Mills KL, Tamnes CK. Dimensions of early-life adversity are differentially associated with patterns of delayed and accelerated brain maturation. Biol Psychiatry. 2025; https://doi.org/10.1016/J.BIOPSYCH.2024.07.019.
93. Stinson EA, Sullivan RM, Navarro GY, Wallace AL, Larson CL, Lisdahl KM. Childhood adversity is associated with reduced BOLD response in inhibitory control regions amongst preadolescents from the ABCD study. Dev Cogn Neurosci. 2024; https://doi.org/10.1016/J.DCN.2024.101378.
94. Madden RA, Atkinson K, Shen X, et al. Structural brain correlates of childhood trauma with replication across two large, independent community-based samples. Eur Psychiatry. 2023; https://doi.org/10.1192/J.EURPSY.2022.2347.
95. Pollok TM, Kaiser A, Kraaijenvanger EJ, Monninger M, Brandeis D, Banaschewski T, Eickhoff SB, Holz NE. Neurostructural traces of early life adversities: a meta-analysis exploring age- and adversity-specific effects. Neurosci Biobehav Rev. 2022;135:104589.
96. Kraaijenvanger EJ, Pollok TM, Monninger M, Kaiser A, Brandeis D, Banaschewski T, Holz NE. Impact of early life adversities on human brain functioning: a coordinate-based meta-analysis. Neurosci Biobehav Rev. 2020;113:62–76.
97. Kraaijenvanger EJ, Banaschewski T, Eickhoff SB, Holz NE. A coordinate-based meta-analysis of human amygdala connectivity alterations related to early life adversities. Sci Rep. 2023;13:16541.
98. Colich NL, Rosen ML, Williams ES, McLaughlin KA. Biological aging in childhood and adolescence following experiences of threat and deprivation: a systematic review and meta-analysis. Psychol Bull. 2020;146:721–64.
99. Weinberger D. The pathogenesis of schizophrenia: a neurodevelopmental theory. Elsevier; 1986.
100. Murray RM, Lewis SW, Lecturer L. Is schizophrenia a neurodevelopmental disorder? Br Med J (Clin Res Ed). 1987;295:681–2.
101. Lipner E, Murphy SK, Ellman LM. Prenatal maternal stress and the Cascade of risk to schizophrenia Spectrum disorders in offspring. Curr Psychiatry Rep. 2019;21:99.
102. Hultman CM, Sparén P, Takei N, Murray RM, Cnattingius S, Geddes J. Prenatal and perinatal risk factors for schizophrenia, affective psychosis, and reactive psychosis of early onset: case-control study. BMJ. 1999;318:421.
103. van Harten PN, Walther S, Kent JS, Sponheim SR, Mittal VA. The clinical and prognostic value of motor abnormalities in psychosis, and the importance of instrumental assessment. Neurosci Biobehav Rev. 2017;80:476–87.
104. Catalan A, Salazar De Pablo G, Aymerich C, et al. Neurocognitive functioning in individuals at clinical high risk for psychosis: a systematic review and meta-analysis. JAMA Psychiatry. 2021;78:859–67.
105. Gilmore JH, Van Tol J, Kliewer MA, Silva SG, Cohen SB, Hertzberg BS, Chescheir NC. Mild ventriculomegaly detected in utero with ultrasound: clinical associations and implications for schizophrenia. Schizophr Res. 1998;33:133–40.
106. Patel PK, Leathem LD, Currin DL, Karlsgodt KH. Adolescent neurodevelopment and vulnerability to psychosis. Biol Psychiatry. 2020;89:184.
107. Chafee MV, Averbeck BB. Unmasking schizophrenia: synaptic pruning in adolescence reveals a latent physiological vulnerability in prefrontal recurrent networks. Biol Psychiatry. 2022;92:436.
108. Schmitt A, Falkai P, Papiol S. Neurodevelopmental disturbances in schizophrenia: evidence from genetic and environmental factors. J Neural Transm. 2022;130:195.
109. Schimmelmann BG, Conus P, Cotton S, McGorry PD, Lambert M. Pre-treatment, baseline, and outcome differences between early-onset and adult-onset psychosis in an epidemiological cohort of 636 first-episode patients. Schizophr Res. 2007;95:1–8.

110. Solmi M, Radua J, Olivola M, et al. Age at onset of mental disorders worldwide: large-scale meta-analysis of 192 epidemiological studies. Mol Psychiatry. 2021;27(1):281–95.
111. Häfner H, Nowotny B. Epidemiology of early-onset schizophrenia. Eur Arch Psychiatry Clin Neurosci. 1995;245:80–92.
112. Izquierdo A, Cabello M, Leal I, et al. The interplay between functioning problems and symptoms in first episode of psychosis: an approach from network analysis. J Psychiatr Res. 2021;136:265–73.
113. Fusar-Poli P, Radua J, McGuire P, Borgwardt S. Neuroanatomical maps of psychosis onset: voxel-wise meta-analysis of antipsychotic-naive VBM studies. Schizophr Bull. 2012;38:1297–307.
114. Radua J, Borgwardt S, Crescini A, Mataix-Cols D, Meyer-Lindenberg A, McGuire PK, Fusar-Poli P. Multimodal meta-analysis of structural and functional brain changes in first episode psychosis and the effects of antipsychotic medication. Neurosci Biobehav Rev. 2012;36:2325–33.
115. Armio RL, Laurikainen H, Ilonen T, Walta M, Salokangas RKR, Koutsouleris N, Hietala J, Tuominen L. Amygdala subnucleus volumes in psychosis high-risk state and first-episode psychosis. Schizophr Res. 2020;215:284–92.
116. Park MTM, Jeon P, Khan AR, Dempster K, Chakravarty MM, Lerch JP, MacKinley M, Théberge J, Palaniyappan L. Hippocampal neuroanatomy in first episode psychosis: a putative role for glutamate and serotonin receptors. Prog Neuro-Psychopharmacol Biol Psychiatry. 2021; https://doi.org/10.1016/J.PNPBP.2021.110297.
117. Zhao Y, Zhang Q, Shah C, Li Q, Sweeney JA, Li F, Gong Q. Cortical thickness abnormalities at different stages of the illness course in schizophrenia: a systematic review and meta-analysis. JAMA Psychiatry. 2022;79:560.
118. Fares-Otero NE, Verdolini N, Melero H, et al. Triangulating the associations of different types of childhood adversity and first-episode psychosis with cortical thickness across brain regions. Psychol Med. 2024; https://doi.org/10.1017/S0033291724002393.
119. Yao Y, Zhang S, Wang B, Lin X, Zhao G, Deng H, Chen Y. Neural dysfunction underlying working memory processing at different stages of the illness course in schizophrenia: a comparative meta-analysis. Cereb Cortex. 2024; https://doi.org/10.1093/CERCOR/BHAE267.
120. Del Casale A, Kotzalidis GD, Rapinesi C, Sorice S, Girardi N, Ferracuti S, Girardi P. Functional magnetic resonance imaging correlates of first-episode psychoses during attentional and memory task performance. Neuropsychobiology. 2016;74:22–31.
121. Del Casale A, Rapinesi C, Kotzalidis GD, Ferracuti S, Padovano A, Grassi C, Sani G, Girardi P, Pompili M. Neural functional correlates of emotional processing in patients with first-episode psychoses: an activation likelihood estimation (ALE) meta-analysis. Arch Ital Biol. 2018;156:1–11.
122. Cattarinussi G, Grimaldi DA, Sambataro F. Spontaneous brain activity alterations in first-episode psychosis: a meta-analysis of functional magnetic resonance imaging studies. Schizophr Bull. 2023; https://doi.org/10.1093/SCHBUL/SBAD044.
123. Sabaroedin K, Razi A, Chopra S, et al. Frontostriatothalamic effective connectivity and dopaminergic function in the psychosis continuum. Brain. 2022;146:372.

Open Access This chapter is licensed under the terms of the Creative Commons Attribution 4.0 International License (http://creativecommons.org/licenses/by/4.0/), which permits use, sharing, adaptation, distribution and reproduction in any medium or format, as long as you give appropriate credit to the original author(s) and the source, provide a link to the Creative Commons license and indicate if changes were made.

The images or other third party material in this chapter are included in the chapter's Creative Commons license, unless indicated otherwise in a credit line to the material. If material is not included in the chapter's Creative Commons license and your intended use is not permitted by statutory regulation or exceeds the permitted use, you will need to obtain permission directly from the copyright holder.

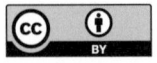

Imagi(ni)ng the Brain in Psychiatry

14

Stephan Heckers

14.1 Introduction

In 1918, Emil Kraepelin published '*Hundert Jahre Psychiatrie*' (*100 years psychiatry*) [1]. It was his opportunity to celebrate the impact of his clinical method, that is, the idea that psychiatry, just like all other branches of medicine, can study disorders with complementary clinical, anatomical and experimental approaches:

> Anyone who is striving towards a distant goal on a difficult path will do well to look back, from time to time. It is all too easy to lose courage when all efforts seem to bring no noticeable progress towards the goal, when, on the contrary, the path becomes increasingly rocky and uncertain and unexpected obstacles threaten to make it impossible to move forward.
>
> But when we then look back at the distance we have covered to reach our current position, we realize that our efforts have not been in vain, that we have made progress despite all the obstacles and have overcome many difficulties that we previously thought we would have to despair of overcoming. [1]

For Kraepelin, the important development in the nineteenth century was the '*... victory of scientific observation over philosophy and moralizing viewpoints*'. In the text, he recognises the important role of Wilhelm Griesinger (1817–1868) and of several neuroscientists, including Theodor Meynert (1833–1892) and Carl Wernicke (1848–1905).

The 1918 monograph included 35 pictures. Drawings and photographs of treatments and mental institutions—some old, some new—helped Kraepelin to tell his story of progress in psychiatry.

But Kraepelin did not include any images of the human brain. At the time of publication, there were already many examples in the literature that he could have chosen. But he decided to forego them. Similarly, we had to wait until the 8th

S. Heckers (✉)
Department of Psychiatry and Behavioral Sciences, Vanderbilt University Medical Center, Nashville, TN, USA
e-mail: stephan.heckers@vumc.org

© The Author(s) 2026
G. Ikkos, T. Becker (eds.), *Psychiatry after Kraepelin*,
https://doi.org/10.1007/978-3-032-09475-9_14

edition of his *Psychiatrie* textbook [2–4], for Kraepelin to include an image of brain abnormalities in dementia praecox, his most influential diagnosis.

Throughout his career, Kraepelin always emphasised the primacy of the clinical method over any neuroscientific approach [2–4]. This was in contrast to other prominent psychiatrists, including Meynert, who advocated for psychiatry as a clinical neuroscience [5].

How would Kraepelin view images of the brain today? Would an updated review, covering the psychiatry of the twentieth century, include images of the human brain? Here I am exploring: How do we *imagine* (not only: *image*) the brain in psychiatry today?

I will start with a brief review of the mind–brain problem, as it was discussed at the start of psychiatry as an academic discipline [6]. Throughout the article, I will emphasise the importance of neuroscience methods: How has our ability to dissect and study the human brain, first with post-mortem and then with in-vivo methods, contributed to our current models of brain dysfunction in psychiatric disorders? Next, I will critically reflect on the metaphor of the *broken brain* as a simplification of the mind–brain problem in psychiatry. I will conclude with a review of recent efforts to utilise brain images in testing causal models of brain dysfunction in psychiatric patients. This will lead me to conclude that integrative pluralism is needed for progress in psychiatry.

14.2   Griesinger's Dictum

Wilhelm Griesinger is often cited as the psychiatrist who shepherded the modern era of psychiatry. Born in 1817 and shaped by the social and political upheavals of 1848 [7], he was greatly influenced by British medicine. He adapted the proposal of non-restraint treatment for his own practice and applied Marshall Hall's 1833 model of reflex action [8] to mental phenomena, coining the term *psychic reflex* in 1843 [9].

In 1845, he published a well-received textbook *Pathologie und Therapie der psychischen Krankheiten* (*Pathology and therapy of mental disorders*) [10]. On the first page of his textbook, we find the dictum that made him famous:

> Which organ, then, must necessarily be diseased wherever insanity is present? The answer to this question is the first prerequisite of all psychiatry. If physiological and pathological facts show us that this organ can only be the brain, then we must, above all, recognize diseases of the brain in mental illnesses. [10]

But Griesinger was not a neuroscientist. His declaration should be read more as a rejection of the moral nature of mental illness, rather than as an embrace of neural reductionism [6, 9, 11]. During his career as a psychiatrist, he simply did not have access to the necessary methods to study the human brain. He died in 1868 and missed the remarkable development of neuroanatomy and neurophysiology that began in the 1870s [12, 13].

14.3   Wernicke's 1880 Scientific Viewpoint

It was Carl Wernicke who started to imagine psychiatry as a clinical neuroscience [14]. He articulated one of the first brain-based models of mental illness. He did so in an oral presentation at the 53rd Convention of the Society of German Natural Scientists and Physicians (Gesellschaft Deutscher Naturforscher und Ärzte = GDNÄ). The plenary lecture of the 1880 meeting in Danzig was published in the meeting's journal and then reprinted in the same year as a monograph [15].

At age 32, and without an academic position when we he delivered the lecture at the GDNÄ meeting, Wernicke challenged his colleagues, who were fighting to establish psychiatry in the canon of academic medicine (Fig. 14.1):

> Let us make a distinction between the practical goals of psychiatry and the scientific ones! As meritorious as it is as a practical psychiatrist to treat the mentally ill and to fully meet the demands of this difficult profession, psychiatry is also a branch of natural science and as such has to solve tasks that are equal to the greatest tasks of natural science. (…) [15]

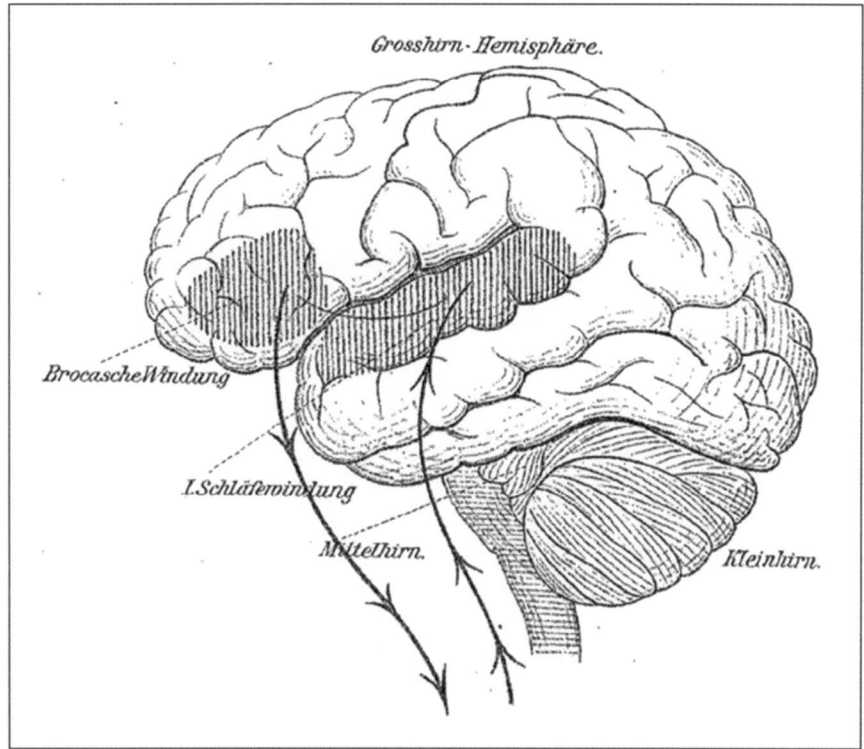

Fig. 14.1 Wernicke's figure for his 1880 lecture. The labels are: *Grosshirn-Hemisphäre* (*cerebrum-hemisphere*), *Brocasche Windung* (*Broca's area*), 1. *Schläfenwindung* (*first temporal gyrus*, that is, superior temporal gyrus), *Mittelhirn* (*midbrain*), *Kleinhirn* (*cerebellum*). The two marked cortical areas are now known as Broca's and Wernicke's areas, respectively

It was during the meeting in Danzig that he displayed an image of the human brain. It showed the lateral convexity of the left hemisphere of a human brain. Most major sulci and gyri of the cerebral cortex are shown, and two areas are marked with hatching. These areas are now known as Broca's and Wernicke's areas, respectively. Superimposed on the drawing of the left hemisphere are three lines: the one arriving in Wernicke's areas and the other emanating from Broca's area are both enhanced with arrows (to show the direction of information flow); a third line connecting Broca's and Wernicke's area is a simple straight line.

Wernicke had used similar figures in his 1874 monograph on aphasia [16]. But during the 1880 lecture his claims were much more ambitious than in his technical treatise on aphasia. Now he proposed that his model for the neural basis of information processing, which he had pioneered for language disorders, holds for all psychiatric illnesses. He made this bold claim with very little experimental evidence. One might say it was merely a conjecture.

Following Wernicke's charge to redefine psychiatry as clinical neuroscience, several psychiatrists followed him and published brain images in their psychiatry textbooks. In fact, some of the German psychiatry textbooks in the last part of the nineteenth century read more like neuroanatomy than psychiatry textbooks. A prominent example is Theodor Meynert's 1884 *Psychiatrie. Klinik der Erkrankungen des Vorderhirns, begründet auf dessen Bau, Leistungen und Ernährung* (*Psychiatry. Clinical disorders of the forebrain, based on its construction, performance and nutrition*) [17]. In the early 1870s, Wernicke had trained with Meynert in Vienna. Over the next ten years, they both were paving the way for a brain-based model of psychiatric disorders (Fig. 14.2).

Fig. 14.2 Figure 60 from Theodor Meynert's 1884 psychiatry textbook. The title reads: *Schema für die Entstehung einer bewussten Armbewegung* (*Scheme for the development of a conscious arm movement*)

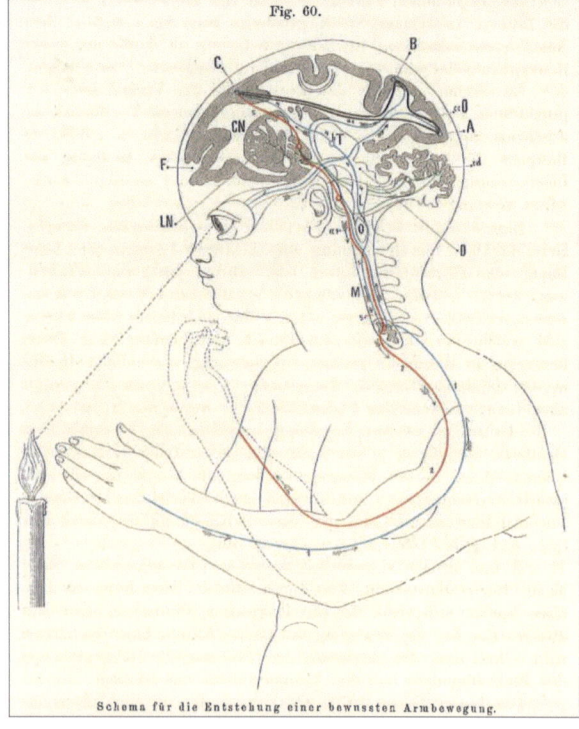

Schema für die Entstehung einer bewussten Armbewegung.

14.4   Wernicke's Model of Mental Illness

Wernicke's 1880 lecture did not remain a simple conjecture. Over the next 20 years, he built a sophisticated theoretical model of brain dysfunction in psychiatric disorders, especially for endogenous psychoses [18–20]. He distinguished three stages of information processing, that is, psychosensory, intrapsychic and psychomotor, which can be affected individually or collectively in the mentally ill [21].

Let's take as an example psychomotor pathology, a domain of psychopathology that Wernicke pioneered and explored [22]. First, Wernicke localised the early stages of information processing in the brain to specific areas of the cerebral cortex. These *primary areas* were highly specialised, serving only one brain function and processing data at a fine-grained level. For the motor system, this area is the primary motor cortex, as had been shown in the classic 1870 experiments of Gustav Fritsch (1838–1927) and Eduard Hitzig (1838–1907) [23].

Second, the primary areas are connected with a distributed network of *associative areas* that can encode and retrieve memory images that are associated with the primary area. For motor behaviour, it includes memory images that can serve as templates for future motor acts. It is the disturbance of storing and retrieving such images that will explain the observable signs of abnormal motor behaviour in patients:

> Our task will be to determine, by means of observation, the behaviour of the memory images in the mentally ill and to use them to understand the mental state. [15]

14.5   Critique of Wernicke's Model

Wernicke's bold model of memory images was well received by many—but it was also harshly criticised. Foremost among his critics was another student of Theodor Meynert, who trained as a neuroanatomist, only to give up his career as an academic neurologist for a private practice in psychiatry:

> Is it justified to immerse a nerve fibre, which has been, over the entire length of its course, just a physiological structure and subject to physiological modifications, with its end in the psyche and to equip this end with an idea or a memory image? [24]

Sigmund Freud's monograph on aphasia was a watershed event for his own personal career (it marked the end of his neuroanatomical oeuvre)—but also for psychiatry at large [25]. Freud shared one interest with Wernicke: to map out mental dynamics in flow diagrams. But rather than connecting mental phenomena with neural circuits, he limited his models to the mental sphere. While Wernicke was mapping out the topography of cortical areas (to explain neurological syndromes), Freud was mapping the topography of subdivisions in the human mind (to understand neurotic conflicts).

At the end of the nineteenth century, psychiatrists imagined very different futures for the scientific study of mental disorders. While some academic psychiatrists, including Wernicke and his students, including Hugo Liepmann, Ludwig Lichtheim and Kurt Goldstein, explored the neural basis of mental disorders, a growing number of theorists aimed to establish causal mechanisms in the human mind without any reference to brain structure and function.

14.6 Two Different Kinds of Images

Wernicke's clinical neuroscience was at odds not only with the emerging school of psychodynamic psychiatry, as pioneered by Freud. It was also distinct from the clinical neuroscience advanced by Kraepelin and his students. In fact, already at this early stage of academic psychiatry, at the end of the nineteenth century, we can distinguish two kinds of brain images in psychiatry: macroscopic and microscopic. These two disparate ways of imag(in)ing the brain in psychiatry continue to this day.

On the one hand were Wernicke's maps of brain circuits to explain behavioural syndromes. They were built on macroscopic neuroanatomy, which did not require a microscope and remained at the level of brain regions and their connectivity profiles. Clinical disciplines that developed from these models include neuropsychology and behavioural neurology. Research methods that have embraced Wernicke's ideas are functional neuroimaging and neural models of disconnection.

On the other hand were Kraepelin's microphotographs. Or, more accurately, the images provided by his colleagues, foremost Alois Alzheimer (1864–1915) and Franz Nissl (1860–1919), and included in Kraepelin's *Psychiatrie* textbooks. This view of clinical neuroscience was built on cellular and molecular pathology. Clinical disciplines that developed from these methods included neuropathology and neurochemistry. A prominent research method that traces its origin to such models is chemical neuroimaging, including single-photon emission computed tomography (SPECT) and positron emission tomography (PET).

In the subsequent sections of this essay, I will explore primarily the first type of brain images, that is, macroscopic neuroanatomy, as displayed with current neuroimaging methods. But before we do so, let's briefly explore Kraepelin's cellular and molecular model of schizophrenia.

14.7 Cellular and Molecular Pathology

Before he defined dementia praecox as a new disease entity, Kraepelin had grouped endogenous psychoses together with hyperthyroidism and hypothyroidism under the heading of 'Endocrine Disorders' [26]. In subsequent editions of his textbook, he removed dementia praecox from the section on endocrine disorders and elevated it to its own diagnostic class.

It was not until the eighth edition of his textbook that he included images from brains of patients diagnosed with dementia praecox. On pages 897 to 907 he provided a detailed review of the neuropathology of schizophrenia. Included in this section of his textbook were figures 186 to 191 (2 microphotographs and 4 drawings). Two drawings are shown here in Fig. 14.3. Kraepelin proposed that a

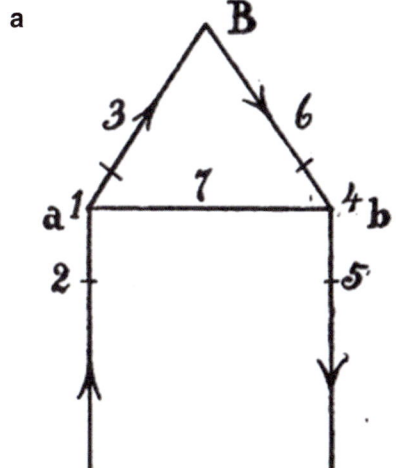

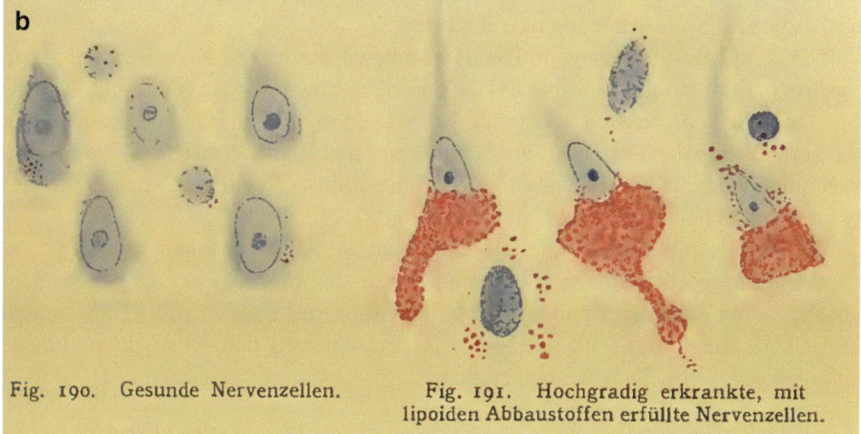

Fig. 190.   Gesunde Nervenzellen.

Fig. 191.   Hochgradig erkrankte, mit lipoiden Abbaustoffen erfüllte Nervenzellen.

Fig. 14.3 (**a**) Shows Figure 10 of Carl Wernicke's 1885 article *Einige neuere Arbeiten über Aphasie* (*Some recent work on aphasia*), published in: Wernicke, C. (1893). *Gesammelte Aufsätze und kritische Referate zur Pathologie des Nervensystems*. Berlin, Verlag von Fischer's Medicinischer Buchhandlung (H. Kornfeld). The diagram, known as Wernicke-Lichtheim model, displays flow of information arriving at a, the center for sound images, through B, the *Begriffscentrum* (concept center), to b, the center for motor images. The numbers indicate types of sensory aphasia (#1–3), types of motor aphasia (#4–6) and conduction aphasia (#7). (**b**) shows figures 190 and 191 from Emil Kraepelin's 1913 psychiatry textbook. Fig. 190 depicts frontal cortex layer 3 neuronal and glial cells in a 37-year-old woman without a mental illness; Figure 191 shows 'lipoid drops' in similar cells of a 23-year-old man with a 5-year history of dementia praecox

chemical process affects the top three layers of the cerebral cortex (i.e. the supra-granular layers) disproportionately and leads to cellular abnormalities, especially in the frontal and temporal cortices. He speculated that the preferential damage to the 'small cells' in the 'upper layers' of the frontal cortex can explain core clinical features of dementia praecox, that is, avolition and abnormal psychomotor behaviour.

How do Kraepelin's speculations about disease mechanism compare to current models of prefrontal cortex dysfunction in schizophrenia? It turns out that several leitmotifs have remained the same. For example, Lewis and colleagues have proposed that cellular and molecular changes of prefrontal cortex layer 3 gabaergic interneurons (i.e. the small cells of Kraepelin's supragranular layers) disrupt the synchronisation of pyramidal cell activity, leading to disorganisation of thought and abnormalities in cognitive abilities, especially working memory [27].

14.8 Imaging the Cerebral Ventricles

Let's now turn to in-vivo brain imaging. There are many compelling examples that demonstrate the considerable impact of such images on how we now imagine the brain in psychiatry. Here I am choosing a very simple example: imaging the cerebral ventricles. The development of imaging methods to study shape and size of the cerebral ventricles may serve as an example for how imagining the brain in psychiatry has been shaped by technological advances.

The American neurosurgeon Dandy pioneered the use of X-ray technology to localise brain tumours [28]. In 1920, he described how injection of air into the ventricular system can be used to identify the location of brain tumours when they alter the normal shape and extent of the lateral, third and fourth ventricles. This method was quickly adapted and greatly improved the ability of neurosurgeons to localise brain tumours before they even start their surgery.

Within a short period of time, cerebral pneumography was taken up by psychiatrists and proposed for the study of subtle brain abnormalities in endogenous psychosis. Jacobi & Winkler published the first case series in 1927 [29]. They studied 19 patients diagnosed with schizophrenia and reported that 18 of them showed enlarged ventricles. They concluded that

> … our pneumophotograms show that encephalography is also a valuable method for psychiatry, as it brings the anatomy of living people to life. [29]

Following this initial study, the finding of ventricular enlargement in schizophrenia was replicated many times. The studies by Huber [30] in the 1950s and Haug [31, 32] in the 1960s were especially influential. But the finding of ventricular enlargement in schizophrenia did not continue to hold the attention of psychiatrists: the emerging discipline of neuropsychopharmacology was quickly replacing neuroanatomy and neuropathology as the principal area of clinical neuroscience research in psychiatry.

It was the introduction of another X-ray based imaging method, that is, computed tomography (CT), that revitalised the interest in studying abnormalities of the ventricles in psychiatric patients. In 1971, the first brain image using CT was generated, at Atkinson Morley Hospital (West London), in a woman with a suspected left frontal lobe tumour [33]. The ability to generate cross-sections through any tissue of the human body is considered one of the greatest inventions in medical imaging since the discovery of X-rays in 1895. The technology quickly gained momentum, first in clinical neuroradiology and then also in clinical neuroscience research.

Just five years after the first CT image of the human brain had been developed, a study by Eve Johnstone and colleagues in 1976 revitalised schizophrenia research [34]. More than any other imaging study, it started a new chapter in psychiatry research. At that time, anti-psychiatry sentiments and critiques of biological models of mental illness were prominent. Psychiatrists were not expected to look at brain images [35]. But Eve Johnstone's simple, yet elegant, quantification of ventricular enlargement in a group of 17 schizophrenia patients and the display of the significant diagnosis effect in form of a scatterplot spoke a powerful language: it makes sense to study the brain in psychiatry [35].

With the introduction of magnetic resonance imaging (MRI), the CT literature on ventricular enlargement was confirmed and extended. In addition, new study designs increased the value of structural brain imaging. A prominent example is the 1990 study by Suddath et al. in the *New England Journal of Medicine* [36]. The investigators collected structural brain images from 15 monozygotic twin pairs who were discordant for schizophrenia. In 12 of the 15 sib pairs, a radiologist, who was blind to the clinical diagnoses and was only shown the MR images, was able to correctly identify the proband with schizophrenia. In 14 of the 15 sib pairs, the lateral ventricles were larger in the twin with schizophrenia. No such differences were found in a control sample of seven monozygotic twin pairs without schizophrenia.

The extant literature on ventricular enlargement in schizophrenia spectrum disorders is extensive [37]. What have we learned since Jacobi and Winkler's study in 1927? First, the studies have contributed to the longstanding debate of neurodevelopmental versus neurodegenerative changes. It is now established that there is gradient of ventricular changes, with chronic patients showing the most significant differences, followed by first episode patients and with the smallest changes found in at-risk individuals. Second, ventricular enlargement is associated with changes in the cerebral cortex, including cortical thickness. Third, clinical correlates of ventricular enlargement include response to treatment, negative symptoms and outcome.

Here I have focused only on one aspect of structural neuroimaging studies, the study of ventricular enlargement in schizophrenia. The chapter by Stephen Lawrie in this monograph provides a scholarly review of the many studies of cortical and subcortical structures in schizophrenia [eds: see Chap. 7].

For 20 years, from the 1970s to the 1990s, most brain imaging researchers in psychiatry focused on quantifying subtle changes in brain structure. While studies of cerebral blood flow had also been used to explore changes in brain function, techniques such as single-photon emission computed tomography (SPECT) and positron emission tomography (PET) were limited to very few research centres and had the downside of exposing study participants to radiation. But the early 1990s brought a new method, functional magnetic resonance imaging (fMRI), which did not use radioactive material and allowed investigators to capture brain activation with a temporal resolution adequate for the study of mental processes. The rapid acceptance of the new method and the dramatic increase in the number of MRI imaging centres greatly contributed to the current prominence of neuroimaging research in psychiatry.

14.9   Functional Magnetic Resonance Imaging

In 1991, investigators at Massachusetts General Hospital published the initial Blood-Oxygenation-Level-Dependent (BOLD) signal study of the human brain [38]. Study participants passively viewed a flickering checkerboard on a screen, while powerful magnets were used to capture subtle changes in blood flow and oxygenation to map activity in the primary visual cortex. Just as Wernicke had shown more than 100 years earlier, sensory data arrived in dedicated primary cortical areas and were then processed in secondary association areas.

Over several decades, the electrophysiology of the visual cortex had been studied, painstakingly, in animals. But now the BOLD signal allowed for a sophisticated and non-invasive study of sensory processing in the human brain. The 1991 study of visual cortex activity in the human brain, captured by the Boston scientists, became the cover page of the journal *Science*.

It did not take long for psychiatry researchers to grasp the power of BOLD images and to employ it for the study of mental phenomena in psychiatric patients. In 1999, the first BOLD study of auditory verbal hallucinations was published by Thomas Dierks and colleagues at the Max Planck Institute for Brain Research in Frankfurt, Germany [39]. The investigators studied a group of five patients with schizophrenia who had reported frequent auditory verbal hallucinations. The investigators demonstrated the activation of a network of brain regions during the experience of hearing voices. Crucially, the circuit included Heschl's gyrus and planum temporale on the left superior temporal gyrus. The investigators concluded:

> Our finding of increased activity of the primary auditory cortex during acoustic hallucinations might therefore explain why hallucinations, unlike auditory imagery or inner speech, are experienced as real. [39]

BOLD signal increases in the primary auditory cortex during symptom capture studies of auditory verbal hallucinations have been replicated and confirmed by meta-analysis [40]. However, considerable heterogeneity of methods and several confounds have resulted in calls for replication [41].

14.10   Brain Images: Metaphor or Mechanism?

Eve Johnstone's study in 1976 opened the door for psychiatrists to study images of the human brain. How much have brain images contributed to our current concept of mental illness? Have the last 50 years changed how we imagine the brain in psychiatry?

Neuroimaging, both in clinical practice and in neuroscience research, had a remarkable impact on our discourse about brain changes in psychiatric disorder. It began, in the 1980s, with a vigorous debate about minds and brains in academic psychiatry, which recapitulated the mind–brain debate from the last quarter of the nineteenth century. The US psychiatrist Leon Eisenberg contrasted old-school brainless psychiatrists with the young Turks of mindless psychiatry [42]. Similarly, the Polish-Canadian psychiatrist Zbigniew Jerzy Lipowski lectured in 1988 on the dual interest in mind and brain in psychiatry [43]. In US psychiatry, the 1980s saw a pivot from a psychoanalytic to a brain-based model of psychiatric illness. This shift in discourse paved the way for a major focus on neuroscience in the 1990s, the Decade of the Brain [44].

The power of images was felt not only in academic psychiatry. It also captured the attention of the lay public. A prominent example for this change in attitude towards mental illness was Nancy Andreasen's book *The Broken Brain. The biological revolution in psychiatry* (1985) [45]. Andreasen advocated for the use of brain images to advance a revolution of the old mind–brain problem:

> It is a revolution not so much in terms of what we know as in how we perceive what we know. This shift in perception suggests that we need not look to theoretical constructs of the "mind" or to influences from the external environment in order to understand how people feel, why they behave as they do, or what becomes disturbed when people develop mental illness. Instead, we can look directly to the brain and try to understand both normal behavior and mental illness in terms of how the brain works and how the brain breaks down. The new mode of perception has created the exciting feeling that we can understand the cause and perhaps develop better forms of treatment. p 138.

Similarly, grassroots organisations such as the *National Alliance on Mental Illness (NAMI)*, founded by relatives of persons diagnosed with mental illness, embraced the broken brain metaphor to raise awareness about mental illness [46]. Simple images were used to fuel public relations campaigns. For example, the non-profit organisation *The Partnership for a Drug-Free America* launched a TV ad campaign in 1987 titled *This is Your Brain on Drugs*.

During the 1970s and 1980s, the epistemological position of brain images in psychiatry changed. Initially, brain images were seen as scientific data that needed to be quantified to explain psychiatric disease. There was the hope that brain images may reveal the mechanism of mental illness. Eve Johnstone's method of measuring ventricular enlargement was an exercise in quantifying brain changes in schizophrenia. The result was a simple scatterplot, not a three-dimensional representation of the human brain.

But very quickly, brain images became two- and three-dimensional representations. Even more importantly, they became pictorial icons and ultimately metaphors. The *broken brain* replaced the *troubled mind*. By doing so, brain images took the place of the person. In contrast to a primary interest in the personal story, which had dominated psychiatry for much of the twentieth century, brain images were now telling a multi-coloured story of surplus or deficit in regions of the human brain.

This shift in perspective, from person to brain image, may lead to a reductionist view of the human condition. When this happens, brain images may contribute to the stigmatisation of persons experiencing mental illness. On the one hand, the person diagnosed with a mental illness may feel they cannot be blamed for a brain that is wired differently. On the other hand, a brain-based model of mental illness may also increase the belief, mainly in public opinion, that mental illness is hard wired, is not amenable to change and leads to poor outcomes [47].

In the end, most models of mental illness want to make causal claims. This includes claims such as: My brain is not working well, so I feel depressed! The auditory cortex is hyperactive, making me experience auditory verbal hallucinations! How well are brain images suited to make such causal claims?

14.11 Testing Causal Models

Some investigators have proposed that neuroimaging can test causal models of disease. Building on the Bradford Hill criteria for causality, a continuum, reaching from task-free imaging through targeted lesions to convergent causal mapping, has been proposed for human neuroimaging studies [48].

What kind of causality problems can be explored with neuroimaging? Here I will take as an example a recent lesion mapping study of secondary psychosis patients, which concluded that the hippocampus causes psychosis [49]. Following Illari and Russo, we can identify five different problems of causality: inference, prediction, explanation, control and reasoning [50]. I will apply each in turn to the question: does the hippocampus cause psychosis [51]?

First, *inference*: Does a hippocampal lesion cause psychosis? Lesion network mapping meets several criteria for this aspect of causality: temporality (psychosis onset occurred after the lesion), regional specificity (lesions in some regions, but not others, are associated with psychosis) and dose–response. Together, this provides strong evidence that hippocampal pathology in psychotic disorders is not merely an epiphenomenon, or a consequence of psychosis or a side effect of treating psychosis.

Second, *prediction*: Knowing about a hippocampal lesion, can we predict what will happen in the future? That is much less clear. In fact, most hippocampal lesion patients do not develop any signs of psychosis.

Third, *explanation*: At what level (gene, cell, circuit?) does a hippocampal lesion explain a psychiatric disorder? There are several mechanistic models for hippocampal dysfunction in psychosis [52, 53], but they have not been tested with lesion mapping studies.

Fourth, *control*: How and when do we intervene in a hippocampal circuit to prevent, treat or cure a psychiatric disorder? This is the most challenging task. Some have proposed abnormal images of the hippocampus as biomarkers for treatment development in schizophrenia [54], and others have advocated for pharmacological and even surgical treatment of the hippocampus in schizophrenia [55]. Finally, *reasoning*: How do we understand psychosis as a hippocampal disorder?

It turns out that brain imaging cannot address many of the scientific problems of causality. We are still far away from a mechanistic model of brain function that allows us to make strong causal claims.

14.12 Goals of Neuroimaging in Psychiatry

This review of scientific problems related to causes of mental illness reveals an important feature of psychiatric neuroimaging research: While investigators use similar methods, the questions they are asking are quite different. We can distinguish at least three different communities of psychiatric neuroimaging researchers [56].

First, the group most closely aligned with Kraepelin's clinical method hopes to separate diagnostic groups based on brain imaging markers [57]. The goals are primarily prediction (what happens next?) and control (what to do?). Scientific applications are biomarkers and imaging-based intervention protocols. Compelling examples are the use of structural MRI in the prediction of psychosis in people who are genetically at ultra-high risk [58] and the combination of resting state functional connectivity and transcranial magnetic stimulation in order to personalise neuromodulation therapy [59].

Second, the group furthest away from Kraepelin wants to explore the experience of mental phenomena and understand the first-person experience. Here the goals are reasoning (is mental illness a brain disorder?) and explanation (how does the brain give rise to mental states?). Such studies, referred to as *neurophenomenology*, aim to explore the neural basis of mental phenomena, including consciousness and the various forms of self (e.g. mental, experiential and narrative) experience [60, 61].

Third, the investigators most closely aligned with Wernicke's model of psychiatry want to improve neural models of psychiatric disorders. Here the goals are inference (what causes mental illness?) and again, as above, explanation (but now with the question: what level of explanation is appropriate?)

Compelling examples are symptom-capture studies using functional magnetic resonance imaging (fMRI): amygdala activation during a spontaneous panic attack [62] or primary auditory cortex recruitment during auditory verbal hallucination [39].

The many different uses of brain images in psychiatry enrich our discourse. But they also leave us with the question: Are we making progress? Does each community imagine the brain in psychiatry differently? Or is there a point of convergence?

14.13 From Monism to Pluralism

We started our tour of imagining the brain in psychiatry with a brief exposé of the mind–brain problem. I will complete our journey by comparing the various views along a continuum, from *monism* on one end, to an *'anything goes'* attitude on the other end. In between, with an increasing degree of pluralism, we can find *temporary, integrative, interactive* and *isolationist* forms [63].

Brain imaging has certainly refocused the attention of psychiatry on the brain. Wernicke's and Meynert's initial enthusiasm for psychiatry as a brain-based branch of medicine, prominent between 1880 and 1900, was followed by considerable disillusionment and even frank cynicism, captured in Karl Jaspers' 'brain mythology' [64]. Almost 100 years later, the biological revolution in psychiatry was greatly advanced with Eve Johnstone's seminal work and the many brain imaging studies that have followed. But we have seen little enthusiasm for a strong reductionist, monist view in psychiatry, captured in declarations such as 'the mind is the brain' or 'the mind is what the brain does'. While this view continues to attract interest among philosophers and scientists [65, 66], it is ill-suited for a clinician who takes care of a person and does not simply treat a brain.

But a related view, *temporary pluralism*, is a popular view, especially among brain researchers and psychiatrists. According to this view, we do not, currently, have enough information to explain and understand mental illness as brain disorder. But we will, in the end, when our research agenda is completed. Then, all pluralist concepts of mental illness will be replaced by a comprehensive medical model, which will completely explain all aspects of psychiatric disorder. While this is a pluralist approach at first glance, it has a clearly defined monist goal.

On the other side of the pluralism continuum, opposite of *monism* and *temporary pluralism*, is the *'anything goes'* attitude. Here, any model of psychiatric disorders is accepted, if it serves a purpose in daily clinical practice. This view resonates with many clinicians, who will employ brain imaging methods when they are relevant for diagnosis and treatment planning—but will ignore them if they are not relevant for their task at hand. For example, brain images will be used in clinical practice to triage patients into primary and secondary psychiatric illnesses—the latter needing medical/neurological care, the former psychiatric treatment [67]. But this eclectic view creates significant problems for psychiatry, both as a clinical discipline and as a research enterprise [68].

In contrast to the three positions above, *isolationist pluralism* acknowledges separate levels of analysis (e.g. cell, circuit, social networks) and allows for the explanation of mental disorders at their respective levels, without an expectation that causation can occur between levels. *Isolationist pluralism* leaves each community of researchers and clinicians within their own discourse, without the requirement for dialogue and compromise. In psychiatry, this has led to two different cultures, one focused on mechanistic models of mind and brain, another one on the person with a unique life story [69]. As a result, a minority of psychiatrists learn to become experts in the interpretation of brain images, whereas the majority will learn not even basic concepts of human brain imaging [70].

In the middle of the pluralism continuum are the two most demanding forms: *integrative* and *interactive pluralism* [63, 71]. Here it is necessary to engage in an exchange of ideas and even an adversarial collaboration [72–74] between researchers and clinicians.

For example, proponents of two major theories of human consciousness have agreed on a protocol to test predictions of their models [75]. Together, they designed experiments that test contrasting predictions of their theories concerning the location and timing of correlates of visual consciousness.

If successful in the field of psychiatric neuroimaging, this will lead to an integration of brain images in both the mechanistic explanation of neural mechanisms and the formulation of individual cases. It requires a considerable degree of curious humility to find the proper place for brain images in an interactive form of psychiatric practice and research.

14.14 Conclusion

If Kraepelin revised '*Hundert Jahre Psychiatrie*' now, 100 years after his death: How would he imagine the brain in psychiatry? Would it be more than the *broken brain* metaphor? Would he embrace mechanistic models of brain dysfunction? What images of the brain would he include? We can only imagine.

Key Points
- Brain-based models of psychiatry were prominent in the last quarter of the nineteenth century, but were not considered helpful in clinical practice and rejected as 'brain mythology'.
- Psychiatry in the first three quarters of the twentieth century was largely devoid of brain images.
- Technical developments in basic and clinical neuroscience led to a biological revolution in psychiatry, but the expectation that first-person experiences of psychopathological phenomena can be explained with images of the human brain has not been realised.
- Images of the 'broken brain' moved scientists, and subsequently society at large, towards brain-based models of mental illness, but they have increased the stigma of mental illness as hard-wired and not amenable to treatment.
- Interactive pluralism is necessary to fully realise the impact of brain images in our understanding of persons with mental illness.

References

1. Kraepelin E. Hundert Jahre Psychiatrie. Ein Beitrag zur Geschichte menschlicher Gesittung. Berlin: Springer; 1918.
2. Kraepelin E. Psychiatrie. Ein Lehrbuch für Studierende und Ärzte. Achte, vollständig umgearbeitete Auflage. I. Band. Allgemeine Psychiatrie. Leipzig: Johann Ambrosius Barth; 1909.
3. Kraepelin E. Psychiatrie. Ein Lehrbuch für Studierende und Ärzte. Achte, vollständig umgearbeitete Auflage. II. Band. Klinische Psychiatrie. I. Teil. Leipzig: Johann Ambrosius Barth; 1910.
4. Kraepelin E. Psychiatrie. Ein Lehrbuch für Studierende und Ärzte. Achte, vollständig umgearbeitete Auflage. III. Band. Klinische Psychiatrie. II. Teil. Leipzig: Johann Ambrosius Barth; 1913.
5. Hlade J. Die Wiener Hirnforschung und die Entstehung des österreichischen Positivismus. Ber Wiss. 2019;42(1):7–27.
6. Marx OM. Nineteenth-century medical psychology. Theoretical problems in the work of Griesinger, Meynert, and Wernicke. Isis. 1970;61(3):355–70.
7. Clark C. Revolutionary Spring. Europe aflame and the fight for a new world, 1848–1849. New York: Crown; 2023.
8. Hall M. On the reflex function of the medulla oblongata and medulla spinalis. Philos Trans R Soc Lond. 1833;123:635–65.
9. Marx OM. Wilhelm Griesinger and the history of psychiatry: a reassessment. Bull Hist Med. 1972;46(6):519–44.
10. Griesinger W. Die Pathologie und Therapie der psychischen Krankheiten für Aerzte und Studirende. Stuttgart: Verlag von Adolph Krabbe; 1845.
11. Wahrig-Schmidt B. Der junge Wilhelm Griesinger im Spannungsfeld zwischen Philosophie und Physiologie. Tübingen: Gunter Narr Verlag; 1985.
12. Schmitt W. Das Modell der Naturwissenschaft in der Psychiatrie im Übergang vom 19. zum 20. Jahrhundert. Ber Wiss Gesch. 1983;8:89–101.
13. Hakosalo H. The brain under the knife: serial sectioning and the development of late nineteenth-century neuroanatomy. Stud Hist Phil Biol Biomed Sci. 2006;37(2):172–202.
14. Heckers S, Kendler KS, Klee A, Heckers S. 'Regarding the scientific viewpoint in psychiatry', lecture by Carl Wernicke (1880). Hist Psychiatry. 2022;33(2):236–55.
15. Wernicke C. Über den wissenschaftlichen Standpunkt in der Psychiatrie. Ein Vortrag gehalten in der zweiten allgemeinen Sitzung der 53. Versammlung Deutscher Naturforscher und Aerzte in Danzig. Cassel: Verlag von Theodor Fischer; 1880.
16. Wernicke C. Der aphasische Symptomencomplex. Eine psychologische Studie auf anatomischer Basis. Breslau: Max Cohn & Weigert; 1874.
17. Meynert T. Psychiatrie. Klinik der Erkrankungen des Vorderhirns, begründet auf dessen Bau, Leistungen und Ernährung. Wien: Wilhelm Braumüller; 1884.
18. Wernicke C. Grundriss der Psychiatrie in klinischen Vorlesungen. Theil I: Psycho-physiologische Einleitung [lectures 1-8]. Leipzig: Georg Thieme; 1894. p. 1–80.
19. Wernicke C. Grundriss der Psychiatrie in klinischen Vorlesungen. Theil II: Die paranoischen Zustände [Lectures 9-17]. Leipzig: Georg Thieme; 1896.
20. Wernicke C. Grundriss der Psychiatrie in klinischen Vorlesungen. [Lectures 1-41]. Leipzig: George Thieme; 1900.
21. Wernicke C. Grundzüge einer psychiatrischen Symptomenlehre (Nach einem im Verein Ostdeutscher Irrenärzte am 5. December 1891 gehaltenen Vortrage). Berl Klin Wochenschr. 1892;29:552–4.
22. Foucher JR, Jeanjean LC, de Billy CC, Pfuhlmann B, Clauss JME, Obrecht A, et al. The polysemous concepts of psychomotricity and catatonia: a European multi-consensus perspective. Eur Neuropsychopharmacol. 2022;56:60–73.
23. Gross CG. The discovery of motor cortex and its background. J Hist Neurosci. 2007;16(3):320–31.

24. Freud S. Zur Auffassung der Aphasien. Eine kritische Studie. Leipzig und Wien: Franz Deuticke; 1891.
25. Greenberg VD. Freud and his aphasia book. Ithaca, NY: Cornell University Press; 1997.
26. Heckers S. Making progress in schizophrenia research. Schizophr Bull. 2008;34(4):591–4.
27. Smucny J, Dienel SJ, Lewis DA, Carter CS. Mechanisms underlying dorsolateral prefrontal cortex contributions to cognitive dysfunction in schizophrenia. Neuropsychopharmacology. 2022;47(1):292–308.
28. Lutters B, Koehler PJ. Cerebral pneumography and the 20th century localization of brain tumours. Brain. 2018;141(3):927–33.
29. Jacobi W, Winkler H. Encephalographische Studien an chronisch Schizophrenen. Archiv für Psychiatrie und Nervenkrankheiten. 1927;81(1):299–332.
30. Huber G. Pneumoencephalographische and psychopathologische Bilder bei endogenen Psychosen. Gruhle HW, Spatz H, Vogel P, editors. Berlin: Springer; 1957.
31. Haug JO. Pneumoencephalographic studies in mental disease. Acta Psychiatr Scand Suppl. 1962;38(165):1–104.
32. Haug JO. Pneumoencephalographic evidence of brain atrophy in acute and chronic schizophrenic patients. Acta Psychiatr Scand. 1982;66(5):374–83.
33. Schulz RA, Stein JA, Pelc NJ. How CT happened: the early development of medical computed tomography. J Med Imaging (Bellingham). 2021;8(5):052110.
34. Johnstone EC, Crow TJ, Frith CD. Cerebral ventricle size and cognitive impairment in chronic schizophrenia. Lancet. 1976;2:924–6.
35. Bland J. Scottish independence: the view of psychiatry from Edinburgh. BJPsych Bull. 2017;41(4):234–6.
36. Suddath RL, Christison GW, Torrey EF, Casanova MF, Weinberger DR. Anatomical abnormalities in the brains of monozygotic twins discordant for schizophrenia. N Engl J Med. 1990;322:789–94.
37. Svancer P, Spaniel F. Brain ventricular volume changes in schizophrenia. A narrative review. Neurosci Lett. 2021;759:136065.
38. Belliveau JW, Kennedy DN Jr, McKinstry RC, Buchbinder BR, Weisskoff RM, Cohen MS, et al. Functional mapping of the human visual cortex by magnetic resonance imaging. Science. 1991;254(5032):716–9.
39. Dierks T, Linden DE, Jandl M, Formisano E, Goebel R, Lanfermann H, et al. Activation of Heschl's gyrus during auditory hallucinations. Neuron. 1999;22(3):615–21.
40. Jardri R, Pouchet A, Pins D, Thomas P. Cortical activations during auditory verbal hallucinations in schizophrenia: a coordinate-based meta-analysis. Am J Psychiatry. 2011;168(1):73–81.
41. Alderson-Day B, McCarthy-Jones S, Fernyhough C. Hearing voices in the resting brain: a review of intrinsic functional connectivity research on auditory verbal hallucinations. Neurosci Biobehav Rev. 2015;55:78–87.
42. Eisenberg L. Mindlessness and brainlessness in psychiatry. Br J Psychiatry. 1986;148(5):497–508.
43. Lipowski ZJ. Psychiatry: mindless or brainless, both or neither? Can J Psychiatr. 1989;34(3):249–54.
44. Jones EG, Mendell LM. Assessing the decade of the brain. Science. 1999;284(5415):739.
45. Andreasen NC. The broken brain: the biological revolution in psychiatry. New York: Harper & Row; 1980.
46. Corrigan PW, Watson AC. At issue: stop the stigma: call mental illness a brain disease. Schizophr Bull. 2004;30(3):477–9.
47. Corrigan PW, Watson AC. Understanding the impact of stigma on people with mental illness. World Psychiatry. 2002;1(1):16–20.
48. Siddiqi SH, Kording KP, Parvizi J, Fox MD. Causal mapping of human brain function. Nat Rev Neurosci. 2022;23(6):361–75.
49. Pines AR, Frandsen SB, Drew W, Meyer GM, Howard C, Palm ST, et al. Mapping lesions that cause psychosis to a human brain circuit and proposed stimulation target. JAMA Psychiatr. 2025.

50. Illari P, Russo F. Causality: philosophical theory meets scientific practice. Oxford: Oxford University Press; 2014.
51. Heckers S. Searching the brain for the cause of psychosis. JAMA Psychiatr. 2025;82:335.
52. Tamminga CA, Stan AD, Wagner AD. The hippocampal formation in schizophrenia. Am J Psychiatry. 2010;167(10):1178–93.
53. Heckers S, Konradi C. GABAergic mechanisms of hippocampal hyperactivity in schizophrenia. Schizophr Res. 2015;167(1–3):4–11.
54. Tregellas JR. Neuroimaging biomarkers for early drug development in schizophrenia. Biol Psychiatry. 2014;76(2):111–9.
55. Mikell CB, McKhann GM, Segal S, McGovern RA, Wallenstein MB, Moore H. The hippocampus and nucleus accumbens as potential therapeutic targets for neurosurgical intervention in schizophrenia. Stereotact Funct Neurosurg. 2009;87(4):256–65.
56. Heckers S, Woodward ND, Ongur D. Neuroimaging of psychotic disorders. In: Charney DS, Buxbaum J, Sklar P, Nestler EJ, editors. Neurobiology of mental illness. Oxford University Press; 2013. p. 256–68.
57. Thompson PM, Stein JL, Medland SE, Hibar DP, Vasquez AA, Renteria ME, et al. The ENIGMA Consortium: large-scale collaborative analyses of neuroimaging and genetic data. Brain Imaging Behav. 2014;8(2):153–82.
58. Pantelis C, Velakoulis D, McGorry PD, Wood SJ, Suckling J, Phillips LJ, et al. Neuroanatomical abnormalities before and after onset of psychosis: a cross-sectional and longitudinal MRI comparison. Lancet. 2003;361:281–8.
59. Fox MD, Halko MA, Eldaief MC, Pascual-Leone A. Measuring and manipulating brain connectivity with resting state functional connectivity magnetic resonance imaging (fcMRI) and transcranial magnetic stimulation (TMS). NeuroImage. 2012;62(4):2232–43.
60. Lloyd D. Functional MRI and the study of human consciousness. J Cogn Neurosci. 2002;14(6):818–31.
61. Northoff G, Ventura B. Bridging the gap of brain and experience - converging Neurophenomenology with Spatiotemporal Neuroscience. Neurosci Biobehav Rev. 2025;173:106139.
62. Pfleiderer B, Zinkirciran S, Arolt V, Heindel W, Deckert J, Domschke K. fMRI amygdala activation during a spontaneous panic attack in a patient with panic disorder. World J Biol Psychiatry. 2007;8(4):269–72.
63. Van Bouwel J. Pluralists about pluralism? Different versions of explanatory pluralism in psychiatry. In: Galavotti MC, et al., editors. New directions in the philosophy of science. Heidelberg: Springer; 2014. p. 105–19.
64. Hlade J. Reconsidering "Brain mythology". Med Hist. 2021;5(1):e2021005.
65. Minsky M. The society of mind. Personal Forum. 1987;3(1):19–32.
66. Pinker S. How the mind works. New York: W.W. Norton; 1997.
67. Blackman G, Neri G, Al-Doori O, Teixeira-Dias M, Mazumder A, Pollak TA, et al. Prevalence of neuroradiological abnormalities in first-episode psychosis: a systematic review and meta-analysis. JAMA Psychiatr. 2023;80(10):1047–54.
68. Ghaemi SN. The rise and fall of the biopsychosocial model. Reconciling art and science in psychiatry. Baltimore: Johns Hopkins University Press; 2010.
69. Luhrmann TM. Of two minds: the growing disorder in American psychiatry. New York: Knopf; 2001.
70. Cooper JJ, Valencia VA, Niu K. Neuroimaging education in psychiatric training. Neuropsychopharmacology. 2024;50(1):298–304.
71. Oleksowicz M. New mechanism and causality: the case of interactive causal pluralism. Rev Port Filos. 2021;77(4):1175–208.
72. Mellers B, Hertwig R, Kahneman D. Do frequency representations eliminate conjunction effects? An exercise in adversarial collaboration. Psychol Sci. 2001;12(4):269–75.
73. Corcoran AW, Hohwy J, Friston KJ. Accelerating scientific progress through Bayesian adversarial collaboration. Neuron. 2023;111(22):3505–16.

74. Cowan N. The adversarial collaboration within each of us. J Appl Res Mem Cogn. 2022;11(1):19–22.
75. Melloni L, Mudrik L, Pitts M, Bendtz K, Ferrante O, Gorska U, et al. An adversarial collaboration protocol for testing contrasting predictions of global neuronal workspace and integrated information theory. PLoS One. 2023;18(2):e0268577.

Open Access   This chapter is licensed under the terms of the Creative Commons Attribution 4.0 International License (http://creativecommons.org/licenses/by/4.0/), which permits use, sharing, adaptation, distribution and reproduction in any medium or format, as long as you give appropriate credit to the original author(s) and the source, provide a link to the Creative Commons license and indicate if changes were made.

The images or other third party material in this chapter are included in the chapter's Creative Commons license, unless indicated otherwise in a credit line to the material. If material is not included in the chapter's Creative Commons license and your intended use is not permitted by statutory regulation or exceeds the permitted use, you will need to obtain permission directly from the copyright holder.

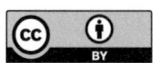

The Self in Neuroscience and Psychiatry

15

Femi Oyebode

15.1 Introduction

The term 'self' refers to a dynamic and evolving concept that is contrasted with our awareness of physical objects in the world and as such is the centre and focus of our internal experiences, as an awareness of ourselves as a centre of experience. It has force in the external world, in the ways that our actions and responses affect the physical world. Furthermore, it is not only that it is influenced by social interactions but itself shapes and influences our encounters with others. It is a complex and multifaceted concept with contributions from philosophy, psychology, anthropology, phenomenology and neuroscience.

John Locke's (1632–1704) conception of the self is fundamentally tied to consciousness, memory and personal identity. In his seminal work *An Essay Concerning Human Understanding* [1], Locke argues that the self is not a fixed, unchanging substance, but a dynamic entity defined by continuous consciousness and memory. Central to Locke's theory is the idea that personal identity is not based on physical substance (body) but on psychological continuity. He introduces a revolutionary thought experiment involving consciousness and memory to illustrate this point. Locke suggests that if a person's consciousness could be transferred to another body, the 'self' would travel with that consciousness, not remain with the original physical form. For Locke, the self is constituted by consciousness and the ability to reflect on past experiences. Memory becomes the crucial link that connects different moments of existence into a coherent personal identity. A person remains the 'same self' as long as they can remember and connect their past experiences to their present consciousness.

F. Oyebode (✉)
Institute of Mental Health School of Psychology, University of Birmingham, Birmingham, UK

© The Author(s) 2026

G. Ikkos, T. Becker (eds.), *Psychiatry after Kraepelin*,
https://doi.org/10.1007/978-3-032-09475-9_15

John Locke' theory is aimed at giving a theory of self that gives a description of a self that is accountable, a 'self who owns and imputes to itself past actions, just upon the same ground and for the same reason that it does the present' (p. 189). So, this 'self' 'is a forensic term, appropriating actions and their merit, and so belongs only to intelligent agents capable off law' (p. 186). The aim, here, is to co-locate the terms 'self' and 'person'. So, for Locke, 'What a person stands for [...] is a thinking intelligent being that has reason and reflection and can consider itself as itself, the same thinking thing in different times and places; which it does by [...] consciousness' (p. 180).

The use that Locke puts consciousness and memory to in his description of what it means to be a self or a person is problematic for clinical medicine. It raises the possibility that individuals whose consciousness or memory is compromised may no longer be legitimately regarded as persons and hence may be deemed to fall outside of the sphere of our concern. This would mean that people with Alzheimer disease or those with impaired consciousness, either in delirium or coma, may be regarded as non-persons.

David Hume (1711–177), a Scottish philosopher and essayist in his book *A Treatise of Human Nature* expressed the view that the self is illusory, and that notions of permanence, continuity and unchanging identity are not rooted in introspection. For Hume, introspection only reveals fleeting thoughts, feelings and sensations as he expressed in his famous statement

> When I enter most intimately into what I call myself, I always stumble on some particular perception or other, of heat or cold, light or shade, love or hatred, pain or pleasure. I never can catch myself at any time without a perception, and never can observe anything but the perception [2, p. 252].

This view, is however, problematic as it ignores the fact that the very act of experiencing something presupposes a unified self. This is further exemplified by the fact we would not be able to write continuous sentences or indeed draw a line that is made up of several instances or points, if there was no unified and persisting self. This empirical fact does nothing to explain how the unified sense of self is achieved. This is the view that Immanuel Kant (1724–1804) expresses. Kant's view is that even though the self is unknowable, that is, it is not directly knowable, yet it is a precondition for perception, allowing us to connect different moments into a coherent whole [3]. Thus, for Kant

> When I seek to draw a line in thought [...], obviously the various manifold representations which are involved must be apprehended by me in thought one after another. But if I were always to drop out of thought the preceding representation (the first part of the line) and did not reproduce them while advancing to those that follow, a complete representation would never be obtained: none of the above mentioned thoughts, not even the most elementary representations of space and time, could arise [3, p. 133].

Kant's claim is that the capacity to grasp the wholeness of life, to link the disparate marks which we make on paper into words, to unite the noises which in turn stand for the names of things and the meaning of utterances; this capacity is dependent upon our notion of time. Numerical identity and the unity of consciousness are both dependent on the a priori representation of time. Kant put it this way: 'If we were not conscious that what we think is the same as what we thought a moment before, all reproduction in the series of representation would be useless' (p. 133). What Kant is claiming is that the unity of consciousness precedes all representation of objects. To put it more strongly, the self, the inner sense of self which is presupposed in all our encounters and experience of the world has a unity of consciousness which is the precondition of all our experience of the world.

This view that Kant espouses about the centrality of the unity of consciousness to the notion of the self is disputed by Derek Parfit (1942–2017). Parfit is a twentieth-century philosopher, who challenged traditional notions of personal identity. In *Reasons and Persons* [4], he argued that the self is not a fixed, continuous entity but rather a fluid and reducible construct. His views build upon David Hume's scepticism about the self and also on John Locke's notions of memory as the crucial faculty in binding together the disparate aspects of self into a supposed unity. Parfit rejects the idea that we have a single, enduring self that persists over time. Instead, he argues that personal identity is best understood in terms of psychological continuity.

He suggests that there is no separate, unchanging 'self' beyond our experiences, memories, and thoughts and that what matters is psychological connectedness—a chain of mental states linked by memory, personality and consciousness. Finally, that the idea of an enduring 'I' is an illusion, much like Hume's bundle theory of the self. Parfit likens the self to a nation and says 'persons are like nations, clubs or political parties' [4, p. 277] and argues that

> [M]ost of us believe that the existence of a nation, does not involve anything more than the existence of a number of associated people. We do not deny the reality of nations. But we do deny that they are separately, or independently, real. Their existence just involves the existence of their citizens, living together in certain ways, or territories [4, p. 340].

Thus, for Parfit, there is no further deep fact that underpins a person's continued existence. In other words that the experiences of a person ought not to be considered as part of a continuous single life.

To summarise, the awareness of the self refers to the ability to recognise oneself as a distinct, thinking and experiencing entity. It is a fundamental aspect of consciousness, shaping how we perceive our identity, actions and existence. The nature of this awareness has been explored across philosophy, psychology and neuroscience, leading to multiple perspectives on how we experience and understand the self. The multiplicity of perspectives only goes to show that the self is a conceptual construct and that our subjective experience is not a solid enough foundation for coming to a definitive conclusion on the nature of the self.

15.2   The Self in Psychopathology

In this section, I take as a starting point Karl Jaspers' (1883–1969) description of the formal characteristics of the self. These characteristics are awareness of activity, awareness of unity, awareness of identity and awareness of being distinct from other objects and selves. It is important to re-emphasise that the self, in this description, is not a thing but a concept. The formal characteristics help to structure how a psychiatrist thinks about the varying anomalies that is encountered in clinical practice. And our understanding of the nature of the self has evolved over time and no doubt will continue to do so into the future. In other words, the concept is not fixed but dynamic and its contours and shape are determined not only by culture and language but also by social interactions, by developments in neuroscience, by psychopathology and more recently by encounters with computers, artificial intelligence and robots.

Karl Jaspers [5] in *General Psychopathology* discusses the nature of awareness of activity of the self and exemplifies how anomalous experiences of awareness of activity may present in the clinic. This is the experience of being aware of one's own performance and actions, and it goes to the root of what it means to have agency and to recognise one's actions as initiated by oneself and being intrinsically one's own actions. This awareness of activity is dependent upon kinaesthetic information from our joints and muscles, from proprioceptive information that locates our position in space and the sensory information that emanates from the other senses including sight, hearing and touch. These sensory data play a role in the definition of the body schema, thereby confirming the material physicality of our bodies and by extension affirming the reality of our bodies in action. For Jaspers, 'every psychic manifestation, whether perception, bodily sensation, memory, idea, thought or feeling carries *this particular aspect of being mine'* [italics in original] of having an 'I'-quality, of 'personally belonging', 'of it being one's own doing' [5, p. 121]. Jaspers recognised that our sense of activity is part of how we come to grasp our bodies as ours.

Abnormalities of awareness of activity are most profound in passivity experiences that are characteristic of schizophrenia. Daniel Schreber (1842–1911) in his *Memoirs of My Nervous Illness* wrote

> The advent of the bellowing-miracle is an extraordinary occurrence when my muscles serving the processes of respiration are set in motion by the lower God (Ariman) in such a way that I am forced to emit bellowing noises, unless I try very hard to supress them; sometimes this bellowing recurs so frequently and so quickly that it becomes almost unbearable and at night makes it impossible to remain in bed' [6, p. 165].

Jaspers conflates awareness of activity and awareness of vitality. Scharfetter [7, 8] distinguishes between awareness of activity and awareness of vitality. Awareness of vitality refers to the elemental feeling that we have, that we are alive whether or not we are performing an activity. In other words, it precedes action and is a core feeling, probably derived from interoception. It is a precondition for the awareness of self. Interoception is an amalgam of physiological sensations such as hunger and fullness, thirst, pain, breathing, muscle tension and so on that underpins aspects of self-awareness, namely the feeling of vitality. Aberration of awareness of vitality can present as depersonalisation and derealisation, and, if grossly affected, as nihilistic delusions or Cotard's syndrome. Jaspers reports an example, drawn from one of Kurt Schneider's cases:

> I feel nameless, impersonal; my gaze is fixed like a corpse; my mind has become vague and general; like a nothing or the absolute; I am floating; I am as if I were not [...] I am only an automaton, a machine; it is not I who senses, speaks, eats, suffers, sleeps; I exist no longer; I do not exist, I am dead; I feel I am absolutely nothing [...] I am not alive, I cannot move; I have no mind, and no feelings; I have never existed, people only thought I did [...] The worst thing is I do not exist [...] I am non-existent I can neither wash nor drink [5, p. 122].

This is a profoundly, perplexing case which is paradoxical in that the person is obviously alive and speaking but their subjective experience is that of an absence of corporeality which can only be explained as feeling dead or being dead. It underlines the importance of the infrastructure of sensory data that constitutes the sense of vitality, a subjective experience that situates us in the world and that precedes the awareness of activity.

Awareness of unity of the self refers to the notion that at any one moment, we know that we are a unified and singular individual. Disturbance of this aspect of the self is revealed in conditions such as autoscopy, a profoundly conceptually, challenging phenomenon in which the usual feeling of the indivisibility of the self appears to be compromised. There are six variants of this phenomenon: feeling of presence, autoscopic hallucination, heautoscopy proper, negative autoscopy, inner autoscopy, and out-of-body experience [9]. In the feeling of presence, a person has a compelling experience of the physical presence of another person. There is no visible perception of the other person. Sometimes the experience is restricted to one visual hemispace, particularly when it is associated with an epileptic seizure. The term autoscopic hallucination refers to the experience of seeing an exact mirror image of the self, or of the face or trunk. Heautoscopy proper refers to the experience of seeing one's own double, usually colourless or grey, and that can act independently of the self. Negative autoscopy refers to the failure to perceive one's own body either when looked at in a mirror or directly. Inner autoscopy is the experience of visual hallucination of internal organs in extracorporeal space. Finally, out-of-body experience is characterised by the projection of an observing (psychological) self in extrapersonal space, apparently totally dissociated from the physical body. These disturbances of awareness of the unity of the self challenge our understanding of the relationship between the body and the immaterial self. They have profound implications for the philosophy of mind and neuroscience.

Awareness of identity refers to the foundational belief that there is a continuity in one's identity over time, despite changes in physical aspects of the body and of alterations in personal dispositions and beliefs. Jaspers reports a case who said

When telling my story I am aware that only part of my present self experienced all this. Up to 23rd December 1901, I cannot call myself my present self; the past self now seems like a little dwarf inside me. It is an unpleasant feeling; it upsets my feelings of existence. If I describe my previous experiences in the first person, I can do it if I use an image and recall that the dwarf reigned up to that date, but since then his past has ended [5, p. 126] (quoting a case of Scwab's).

Awareness of being distinct from other objects and selves, in essence, refers to the recognition of where the self, starts and ends, and where the boundaries of the self are. This distinction is established by the sensory experiences that we have of our bodies in action. Sight demonstrates that our body is distinct from the background material world. When we move, the ground does not move with us. The physical outline of our body is sharply demarcated from the material world. In our engagement with other subjects of experience, we come to recognise our will and theirs are distinct. When we will ourselves to stand, it is us who stands and when they will themselves to stand, their will does not result in our standing. Thus, the limits and boundaries of our body and of our will become evident through empirical experience. This is the sense of our distinctness from the objective world and also from the subjective world of others in our observations of the world and of the constraints of our mental activities upon the actions and will of others. The role of the brain in underpinning the awareness of distinctness is rendered overt by the manner in which some psychoactive agents affect this experience. The use of psychedelic agents such as lysergic acid diethylamide can provoke a sense of the dissolution of the boundaries of the self, in a way that a person can feel that they have merged with objects in their external surrounding. Anderson and Rawnsley [10] report on one of their subjects

I was being disorganised…the world around was looking very distorted indeed…things were pretty rocky so I decided to sit back quietly for a moment and reassure myself by returning to my own private world. As soon as I introspected in this manner I felt to my dismay that 'I' myself was somehow disturbed. The central core of the personality, the ego, the sense of personal identity, was itself fluctuating and, for want of a better phrase, dissolving.

Another one of Anderson and Rawnsley's subject reported that 'If anyone present went out of the room it felt as though I were deprived of something. I became smaller – definitely felt vulnerable.' Jaspers reported one of Mayer-Gross and Stein's case who said during intoxication with mescaline: '[I] felt the dog's bark painfully touching on my body; the dog was in the bark and I was in the pain' [5, p. 126]. Another patient, during intoxication with cannabis said, 'Just now I was a piece of apple' (p. 126). These experiences speak to the notion that our physical integrity, the singularity of our physical presence can be sundered, such that we merge with other objects in the world or become intertwined with another person's physical form.

In summary, Jaspers' formal characteristics of the self, work to structure our understanding of the multifaceted and plural manifestations of what patients bring to our attention in the clinical encounter. The deep question, if I can put it like that, is how the self is represented in the brain or indeed whether it is represented at all.

15.3   The Self in Schizophrenia

Spitzer [11] has argued that a number of the symptoms of schizophrenia exemplify the fact that schizophrenia is an 'Ichstorung', an 'I-disorder'. For Spitzer, an I-disorder is one in which it is the 'experiencing I', not idiosyncratic aspects of a person, not the character, not the personality, that is affected. In short, schizophrenia is a disorder of the form of experience in general. This is underlined specifically by symptoms that are regarded as 'passivity experiences' and also by thought withdrawal, thought insertion, thought echo and thought broadcasting.

Some of the best published examples of thought insertion are given by Daniel Schreber (1842–1911) in his book *Memoirs of My Nervous Illness* [6]. His accounts reveal the complexity and often subtlety of the experience, partly because it includes his attempted explanations of the phenomena. He gave an account of what he terms 'compulsive thinking' which conforms to what would be recognised today as thought insertion:

> This influence showed itself relatively early in the form of *compulsive thinking* [italics in the original] – an expression which I received from the inner voices themselves and which will hardly be known to other human beings, because the whole phenomenon lies outside all human experience. The nature of compulsive thinking lies in a human being having to think incessantly; in other words, man's natural right to give the nerves of his mind their necessary rest from time to time by thinking nothing […] was from the very beginning denied me by the rays in contact with me; they continually wanted to know what I was thinking about. For instance I was asked in these very words: "What are you thinking of now?"; because this question is in itself complete nonsense, as a human being can at certain times as think of *nothing* as of *thousands of things at the same time*, and because my nerves did not react to this absurd question, one was soon driven to take refuge in a system of *falsifying my thoughts*. For instance the above question was answered spontaneously: "He should" *scilicet* think "about the order of the world", that is to say the influence of the rays forced my nerves to perform the movements corresponding to the use of these words [all italics in the original] (p. 70).

I have quoted extensively from Schreber to demonstrate that thought insertion superficially appears clear and unambiguous, when in fact it is complex and messy. For Schreber, thought insertion had the characteristic of compulsion, of being alien, of being in response to auditory hallucinatory experiences, of often being fragmentary ideas which he felt the urge to complete. In his examples, it is never quite clear whether his experience of thought insertion is entirely distinct from auditory verbal hallucinations, thought broadcasting or from rumination. Here I am emphasising the fact that the descriptions and conceptual clarity imposed on abnormal phenomena ignore the far messier truth that these phenomena are not categorically distinct but related phenomena that have greater underlying connection than is appreciated. Once it is understood that various phenomena such as thought insertion, thought withdrawal, thought echo, verbal hallucinations etc., have continuities that hint at cross-modal connections that suggest underlying similarities of mechanisms of origin, then it becomes possible to accurately seek out the neurobiology of these phenomena.

Thought insertion or alienation is defined as the experience in which a patient becomes aware that 'thoughts [...] were not *his own* [italics in original] in the sense that they were coming from an outside source [12]. Jaspers emphasises that the thought arises and with it a direct awareness that it is not the patient but some external agent that thinks it [5]. Jaspers quotes one of Gruhle's cases.

> I have never read or heard them; they come unasked; I don't dare to think I am happy to know of them without thinking them. They come at any moment like a gift and I do not dare to impart them as if they were my own [5, p. 122].

These definitions (Koehler's and Jaspers') are intended to convey the discrete characteristics of thought insertion such that thought insertion can be understood and recognised in the clinical setting. It is notable though that these definitions are usually set in the context of other phenomena, whereas case examples are chosen for their salience rather than for demonstrating the confluence of various phenomena. To emphasise this point, Gruhle's example suggests for example that the patient becomes aware of the thoughts without *thinking* them. This account underlines the fact that the thought is alien but draws attention to the intriguing idea that it may be possible to become aware of a thought without thinking it. This raises the possibility that we may become aware of thoughts much as we become aware of perceptions, that we may hold a thought in mind without thinking it. Schreber's account described above shows that his experience of thought insertion is inextricably mixed with experiences of auditory hallucinations, ruminations and so on. In the real world, the experience of thought insertion is set in a dense matrix of unusual experiences.

The foregoing points to the fact that in order to fully comprehend any psychotic phenomena, we need to set it into the context of the other phenomena that it occurs alongside. Thus, our understanding of thought insertion is better facilitated when we examine it alongside thought withdrawal, thought block, thought broadcasting, thought echo, verbal hallucinations, made acts, made feelings, made impulses etc. To make this point plainer still, an understanding of thought echo aids our understanding of auditory verbal hallucinations as the subject's own thoughts which appear to the subject as voices emanating from objective space but with alien characteristics.

So far, I have been arguing that the notion of the self in psychopathology is a conceptual tool that allows for some understanding of the aberrations and impairments that are apparent in the clinic. These abnormal phenomena are not only intriguing but also endlessly profitable in how they show the complexities of the attributes of the self as a concept, but, also point to the possibilities of the neurobiology underpinning the notion of the self.

15.4   The Self in Neuroscience

There is unanimity that no single locus exists in the brain where the self or conscious awareness resides. In other words, that no 'Cartesian theatre' exists. Zeki [13] in his account of vision shows that there is no single experiential cell that receives afferents from all cells that contributes to the experience of vision. All visual cells appear to contribute to the experience of vision. Even where there are confluent, convergent outputs to other higher cortical areas, for example, from the occipital cortex to the parietal cortex, the brain's strategy does not appear to be one of a direct convergence of input into single cells from different sources, registering different attributes of a particular visual scene. Even communications within the polysensory areas in the parietal cortex, whose function is to integrate different kinds of sensory experience such as vision, spatial experience, touch and so on, are organised into discrete zones rather than into unified cells which receive inputs from disparate neurones. This is to emphasise the fact that no homunculus exists in the brain acting as the central executive that steers the affairs of the brain.

The upshot of this is that integration of visual information, as an exemplar of how the brain deals with the awareness of vision, has a neural and structural basis to facilitate it, but that design does not favour the convergence of all visual information to a single 'experiential cell'. The anatomical arrangement allows specialised neurones to receive projections and to send projections to similar neurones subserving the same functions but different spatial configurations. Furthermore, these specialised neurones send projections to other neurones which have responsibility for a larger visual field. These arrangements permit the visual fields to be perceived as unified wholes. In other words, each disparate area of the field of vision is connected to its neighbour and also to a neurone with a wider perspective. There is, however, no single cell which receives all forms of information such that its data are synonymous with our actual experience of the world. And, furthermore where specialised neurones send projections outside of their own area of specialisation, these projections do not end on a single neurone which receives different kinds of information. Rather, the sensory data remain segregated even in these cases and unification occurs by projections between such neurones. The architecture of these structures avoids a single cell or node that receives and unifies myriad data. The integrated and seamless perceptual world that we inhabit is created by cross-talk (cross connections) between neurones rather than by a single master neurone that receives a multiplicity of afferents that it then unifies.

This arrangement emphasises the brain's method which appears to be to separate specialised neurones from one another but to allow cross-communication between them, what is referred to as *cross-talk*. It could be argued that this arrangement has developed for evolutionary reasons. It has an in-built redundancy such that damage to one centre is likely to spare some functions, since no one centre exclusively receives all projections.

There is yet an unresolved issue of how the integrated sense of self-awareness is achieved given that no homunculus exists. Semir Zeki's hypothesis is that the 'synchrony in the oscillatory responses of spatially separate neurone clusters signal coherence in the stimuli that gives rise to the responses' [13, p. 351]. This view is supported by Francis Crick and is further developed as follows

Although there are many different visual signals, each of which analyses visual input in different and complex ways, so far we can locate no single region in which the neural activity corresponds exactly to the vivid picture of the world we see in front of our eyes [...] In short we can see how the brain takes the picture apart, but we do not yet understand how it puts it together [14, p. 159].

This problem, the need to explain how the brain integrates information to produce the vivid and unified world that we inhabit in the absence of a homunculus, is termed the 'binding problem'. To put it in another way, given that there is no identifiable single locus that perceives the world and directs all action, how exactly is the self, instantiated in the brain? There is no 'Cartesian theatre', yet our experience as human beings is that such a centre of the self exists, despite it being logically clear as Ryle put it that 'a higher order action cannot be the action upon which it is performed. So, any commentary on my performances must always be silent about one performance, namely itself, and this performance can be the target only of another commentary. Self-commentary, self-ridicule, and self-admonition are logically condemned to eternal penultimacy' [15, p. 186].

The closest we have to an understanding of the neural mechanisms underpinning the self is a network of discrete, bilateral and symmetrical cortical areas termed the default mode network. These reside in the medial and lateral parietal, medial frontal and medial and lateral cortices of human, nonhuman primate, cat and rodent brains [eds: see Fig. 13.2 Chap. 13]. As Marcus Raichle put it

> Its discovery was an unexpected consequence of brain-imaging studies first performed with positron emission tomography in which various novel, attention-demanding, and non-self-referential tasks were compared with quiet repose either with eyes closed or with simple visual fixation. The default mode network consistently decreases its activity when compared with activity during these relaxed nontask states. The discovery of the default mode network reignited a longstanding interest in the significance of the brain's ongoing or intrinsic activity [16].

The network is thought to instantiate processes that support emotional processing within the ventromedial prefrontal cortex, self-referential mental activity in the dorsomedial prefrontal cortex and the recollection of prior experiences in the posterior elements of the default mode network [16]. There is also a significant role for the default mode network in spontaneous cognition, namely in daydreaming, mind wandering or stimulus independent thoughts. It also has a role in thoughts about one's past and future.

Davey et al. [17] show that there is increased activity in the default mode network during self-referential processes and conclude that the 'core-self' regions are medial prefrontal cortex, the posterior cingulate and the inferior parietal cortex. It is important, though, to make the point that these regions are in dynamic relationship as part of a network rather than acting as merely structural anatomic regions.

Abnormalities have been described in the default mode network in schizophrenia [18], and in mood disorders [16]. In schizophrenia, for example, increased connectivity within the default node network has been reported, particularly in the medial prefrontal cortex and posterior cingulate cortex. This hyperconnectivity is associated with excessive self-referential thoughts, potentially contributing to delusions and hallucinations. Reduced connectivity between the default node network and other networks, for example, the central executive network [Eds: see Fig. 13.2 Chap. 13] and salience network may impair the ability to shift between internal and external cognitive states. Normally, the default mode network operates in opposition to task-positive networks. In schizophrenia, this anti-correlation is weakened, leading to difficulty suppressing default node network activity during cognitive tasks. This may result in intrusive thoughts and distractibility. In depressive episodes, increased connectivity within the medial prefrontal posterior cingulate cortex and precuneus is linked to excessive rumination and negative self-referential thinking and in manic episodes, there seems to be reduced connectivity in the default node network leading to diminished self-monitoring and impulsivity.

To summarise, the default mode network is a large-scale brain network that is most active when the mind is at rest and not focused on external tasks. It is involved in self-referential thinking, mind-wandering, autobiographical memory and social cognition. It is most active during daydreaming or letting the mind wander, when thinking about oneself or others, when recalling personal memories, imagining the future or engaging in moral reasoning and social understanding. It is the closest we get to the neural representation of the self when it is not engaged in a task requiring external attention.

15.5   Conclusion

I have argued that the term 'self' refers to a dynamic and evolving concept that is contrasted with our awareness of physical objects in the world and as such is the centre and focus of our internal experiences, as an awareness of ourselves as a centre of experience. I have emphasised that the term refers to a concept, not to a singular thing. I showed that our understanding of the term has changed over time, being subject to developments within philosophy as well as within psychiatry and neuroscience. Abnormalities that patients present in the clinic have shaped the development of the formal characteristics that have guided how we structure our understanding and discussion of conditions as disparate as schizophrenia and autoscopy. The emerging findings in neuroscience confirm that there is no singular neural focus for the self, rather there is a network of sites that act jointly and dynamically to subserve the functions that may be termed the self. In conclusion, the self is a complex and multifaceted concept with contributions from philosophy, psychology, anthropology, phenomenology and neuroscience.

Key Points
1. The self is a dynamic and evolving concept that focuses on our internal, psychological experiences as a centre of subjective experience.
2. In clinical psychopathology, the formal characteristics of the self include an awareness of activity, awareness of unity, awareness of identity, awareness of being distinct from other objects and selves and awareness of vitality.
3. Schizophrenia can be regarded as an 'Ichstorungen', an 'I-disorder', primarily manifested by passivity experiences and thought disorders such as made experiences, thought withdrawal and thought insertion.
4. In neuroscience, there is no evidence for a single centre that exclusively receives all projections. In other words, no homunculus exists.

5. The closest we have to an understanding of the neural mechanisms underpinning the self is a network of discrete, bilateral and symmetrical cortical areas termed the default mode network.

References

1. Locke J. An essay concerning human understanding: in 2 volumes. London: J.M. Dent; 1817.
2. Hume D, Selby-Bigge LA. A treatise of human nature, 3 volumes. Oxford University Press; 1789.
3. Kant I. Critique of pure reason (trans N. Kemp Smith). London: Macmillan Press; 1781.
4. Parfit D. Reasons and persons. Oxford University Press; 1987.
5. Jaspers K. General psychopathology. Johns Hopkins University Press; 1997.
6. Schreber DP. Memoirs of my nervous illness (trans I. MacAlpine & R.A. Hunter). London: W. Dawson; 1955.
7. Scharfetter C. Ego-psychopathology: the concept and its empirical evaluation. Psychol Med. 1981;11:273–80.
8. Scharfetter C. The self-experience of schizophrenics. In: Kircher T, David AS, editors. The self in neuroscience and psychiatry. Cambridge: Cambridge University Press; 2003.
9. Brugger P, Regard M, Landis T. Illusory reduplication of one's own body: phenomenology and classification of autoscopic phenomena. Cogn Neuropsychiatry. 1997;2(1):19–38.
10. Anderson EW, Rawnsley K. Clinical studies of lysergic acid diethylamide. Monatsschr Psychiatr Neurol. 1954;128:38–55.
11. Spitzer M. Kant on schizophrenia. In: Spitzer M, Maher BA, editors. Philosophy and psychopathology. New York: Springer-Verlag; 1990.
12. Koehler K. First rank symptoms of schizophrenia: questions concerning clinical boundaries. In: Kerr A, Snaith P, editors. Contemporary issues in schizophrenia. London: Gaskell; 1979.
13. Zeki S. A vision of the brain. Oxford: Balckwell Scientific Publications; 1993.
14. Crick F. The astonishing hypothesis: the scientific search for the soul. London: Simon & Schuster; 1994.
15. Ryle G. The concept of mind. London: Penguin; 1949.
16. Raichle ME. The brain's default mode network. Annu Rev Neurosci. 2015;38:433–47.
17. Davey CG, Pujol J, Harrison BJ. Mapping the self in the brain's default mode network. NeuroImage. 2016;132:390–7.
18. Hu ML, Zong XF, Mann JJ, Zheng JJ, Liao YH, et al. A review of the functional and anatomical default mode network in schizophrenia. Neurosci Bull. 2017;33(1):73–84.

Open Access   This chapter is licensed under the terms of the Creative Commons Attribution 4.0 International License (http://creativecommons.org/licenses/by/4.0/), which permits use, sharing, adaptation, distribution and reproduction in any medium or format, as long as you give appropriate credit to the original author(s) and the source, provide a link to the Creative Commons license and indicate if changes were made.

The images or other third party material in this chapter are included in the chapter's Creative Commons license, unless indicated otherwise in a credit line to the material. If material is not included in the chapter's Creative Commons license and your intended use is not permitted by statutory regulation or exceeds the permitted use, you will need to obtain permission directly from the copyright holder.

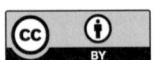

Images for Psychiatry: From the Conceptual Description of Symptoms and 'Clinical Forms', Through the Search for Structural Units of Meaningful 'Forms of Life', to Images as 'Forms of Pathos'

16

Giovanni Stanghellini

16.1 Introduction

We need a clinical phenomenology that leverages the power of images and does not rely solely on concepts if we are to overcome the arid descriptivism of operational-ising descriptive psychopathology and the headless accounting of nosography that formulates diagnoses on the basis of summations of symptoms. An emblematic treatment of the importance of imagery in clinical phenomenology and its potential applications to treatment can be found in Ludwig Binswanger's *Three Forms of Miscarried Existence* [1]. This approach has not had the following it deserves in clinical phenomenology. Yet, an appeal to the use of images as an alternative or complement to concepts has deep roots in the culture of the 1900s. For example, Ulrich Gumbrecht [2] has argued that the human sciences, because of their main focus on analysing concepts and interpreting meanings, have lost their ability to refer to the dimension of 'presence,' that is, the way cultural phenomena—-and among them psychopathological phenomena—-impact our bodies and senses. Images can capture the living presence of the human, in its pathic and plastic forms, far more than conceptual formulas can. Susan Sontag [3] had previously pointed out the need for a 'vocabulary of forms' in order not to further subject the humanities to the discipline of conceptual and abstract thinking. This vocabulary of forms would be capable of plastically representing the 'knots' of human existence, rather than trying to define them conceptually. In the background of the work of both these authors is the work of Aby Warburg [4] and his 'invention' of the *Pathosformeln*—plastic forms in which the movements imprinted on the body by a passion are deposited and transformed. *Pathosformeln* are choreographies—literally, writings of movements—in which a state of mind is made visible. In our case, a knot of

G. Stanghellini (✉)
Department of Health Sciences, University of Florence, Florence, Italy

© The Author(s) 2026
G. Ikkos, T. Becker (eds.), *Psychiatry after Kraepelin*,
https://doi.org/10.1007/978-3-032-09475-9_16

emotions, a montage, a telescopage of elements opposed to each other but composed in a figure that expresses this contrast, where dialectical tension is at its highest degree. We find the same thought in Walter Benjamin (see [5]) in his 'discovery' of the *dialektisches Bild* ('dialectical image') as a 'constellation saturated with tensions'—an image that becomes visible below the 'encrusted surface of the concept'. In this chapter, first, I recapitulate two moments in the history of psychiatric thought: the work of Emil Kraepelin [6], who brought order and conceptual rigour to the description of psychopathological symptoms and syndromes; and that of Wolfgang Blankenburg [7], an emblematic figure of the 'phenomenological-structural' turn in the representation of psychopathological pictures. In the final section, building on and extending the legacy of Ludwig Binswanger, I try to show that it is through images—far more than through concepts—that we can give plastic form to the motions of the soul, to the states of ambivalence and self-contradiction that accompany crises, and in general to the 'existential knots' that characterise psychopathological conditions.

16.2 Emil Kraepelin: The Description of Symptoms and the Aggregations of Symptoms in 'Clinical Forms'

Emil Kraepelin (1856–1926) is credited, both by his supporters and detractors, for systematically organising the field of psychiatry as a branch of medicine and developing a classification for it. What is often overlooked, however, is his ability to describe symptoms. He provides an example of this ability in the chapter dedicated to the description of the clinical manifestations of Dementia praecox. In about seventy pages, written with remarkable clarity and precision, Kraepelin describes the psychic symptoms of this morbid form, noting that 'certain fundamental disturbances, even though they cannot, for the most part, be regarded as characteristic, yet return frequently in the same form, but in the most diverse combinations' [6, p. 5]. He explains that 'before we describe the individual clinical manifestations of the disease', 'we shall try to give a survey of the general behaviour of the psychic and physical activities' of the affected patients.

Accurate descriptions of the main symptoms of Dementia praecox follow, namely disorders of perception and attention, hallucinations of hearing, sight, smell, taste, tactile, sexual and 'common sensations', morbid sensations, influence of thought, disorders of orientation, consciousness, association, memory retention, train of thought, paralogia, disorders of constraint of thought, of mental efficiency and of judgment, delusions (including ideas of sin and of persecution), exalted ideas, sexual ideas and ideas of reference, disorders of emotions and volition, automatic obedience, impulsive actions, catatonic excitement, stereotypy of movement, mannerisms, parabulia, negativism, autism, anomalies of 'personality', 'practical efficiency' and of self-expression, thought incoherence, 'similarity in sound', stereotypy in verbal expressions, mutism, derailments in linguistic expression, disorders of internal speech, paraphasias, neologisms, akataphasia, disorders in the construction of sentences and in train of thought.

Additionally, Kraepelin considers it appropriate to detail this long list of symptoms (which would make any contemporary manual of descriptive psychopathology envious) before the actual description of the clinical 'forms' of Dementia praecox—that is, the ways in which these individual symptoms aggregate in reality and in concrete clinical cases. A 'form' (*Gestalt*) is how separate phenomena come together to make a whole.

As is known, initially he distinguished three clinical forms of dementia praecox—a hebephrenic, a catatonic and a paranoid group of cases. Subsequently, for the sake of a more refined description, he developed a more articulated classification. This is the one that appears in the partial English translation published in 1919 by G.E. Robertson and R.M. Barclay under the title *Dementia praecox and Paraphrenia* [6]. In the fifth chapter of this edition, the following clinical forms are listed:

'Dementia simplex', characterised by an impoverishment and devastation of the whole psychic life, which materialises quite imperceptibly.

'Silly dementia', where besides the progressive devastation of the psychic life, incoherence in thinking, feeling and action appears.

'Simple depressive dementia', in which, after an introductory state of depression, with or without phenomena of stupor, a definite psychic decline gradually develops.

'Delusional depressive dementia', in which delusions gain considerable expansion.

'Agitated dementias', in which states of excitement more severe and lasting longer are developed.

'Periodic dementia', connected by a pronounced periodic course, either in the introductory stages of the disease or during its whole duration.

'Catatonia', in which those cases are grouped together where the conjunction of peculiar excitement with catatonic stupor dominates the clinical picture.

'Paranoid dementias', whose essential morbid symptoms are delusions and hallucinations. Paranoid dementias may exhibit a severe picture ('paranoid dementia gravis'), leading to a peculiar disintegration of the psychic life, and especially of its emotional and relational features; or a less severe picture ('paranoid dementia mitis'), characterised by a paranoid or hallucinatory weak-mindedness.

'Confusional speech dementia', characterised by an unusually striking disorder of expression in speech with relatively little impairment of the remaining psychic activities.

What I would like to highlight is the importance Kraepelin methodologically attributed to two processes splitting and grouping. In his meticulous description of individual psychopathological symptoms lies the foundation of these two apparently opposite instances. We could imagine Kraepelin *as a clinician* at work observing his patients to identify, at first, the individual phenomena embodied in patients; then, *as a researcher*, trying to group these individual phenomena into clinical forms in which such phenomena aggregate. He contributed to the history of psychiatry as the one who created a stable and lasting classification of these 'forms' of clinical cases; yet, he remained dissatisfied until the end of his intellectual life with the ways he had tried to group individual clinical phenomena into higher-order units. In the detailed classification I have reported above, much more detailed if compared to those popularised in the last hundred years, his effort is clear to further subdivide the forms in which he had initially grouped Dementia praecox (paranoid, catatonic and hebephrenic) into other forms that better reflected clinical reality.

With a bit of imagination, we can try to conjure up the cognitive process with which this meticulous observer operated: the observation of hundreds of patients, the identification of the symptoms of each of them, the compilation of a detailed clinical record—this is the practical empirical phase of his fieldwork.

Subsequently came the more theoretical phase, namely the construction of aggregates of symptoms—the famous 'clinical forms'. This transition from the level of descriptive psychopathology investigation (accurate description of isolated symptoms) to that of nosography (description of how these symptoms combine into syndromes) is also developed on the indispensable basis of empirical observation of patients, that is, based on how these symptoms actually aggregate in patients. However, it is precisely this last operation that proves to be the most precarious and subject to revisions over time because the concrete existences of patients do not easily and docilely allow themselves to be classified. The description of individual symptoms can remain more or less the same over time—a delusion of persecution always remains a delusion of persecution in different eras and cultures, the descriptions given by Kraepelin, or Karl Jaspers, or Kurt Schneider, or by a good-enough contemporary psychopathologist in the end resemble each other. The description of a syndrome, on the other hand, is a much more debatable construct and therefore subject to continuous revisions, as we have seen during the professional lifetime of the psychiatrist Kraepelin, and even more so in the entire history of post-Kraepelinian psychiatry.

However, it should not be overlooked that there is an intermediate level of investigation between that of descriptive psychopathology of individual symptoms and that of nosographic classification of syndromes. This is the level occupied by the investigation of phenomenological psychopathology—as we shall see in detail very soon.

Kraepelin himself makes some observations albeit partial, in the text we have analysed so far. They, actually, offer little more than a hint compared to the bulk of the pages he dedicated to the description of symptoms and syndromes:

> Now, if we make a general survey of the psychic, clinical picture of Dementia praecox (…) there are apparently two principal groups of disorders which characterise the malady. On the one hand, we observe the weakening of those emotional activities which permanently form the mainsprings of volition (…) The result of this part of the morbid process is emotional darkness, failure of mental activities, loss of mastery over volition of endeavour, and of ability for independent action.
>
> The second group of disorders which gives dementia praecox its peculiar stamp, consists in the loss of the inner unity of the activities of intellect, emotion and volition in themselves, and among one another. Stransky speaks of the (…) annihilation of the intra-psychic coordination, which is said to loosen or destroy the articulations of the "noopsyche" and the "thymopsyche" themselves, as well as their mutual relations. This annihilation presents

itself to us in the disorders of association described by Bleuler as incoherence of the train of thought, the sharp change of moods, as well as desultoriness and derailments in practical work. (pp. 74–5)

16.3   The Search for Meaningful 'Structural Units' Beyond the Listing-and-Counting of Symptoms

It is clear from the above passage that Kraepelin is searching for something different from the mere description of associations of symptoms in syndromic frameworks. What he seeks is also the *ratio essendi* for these associations, that is, the deep root of the symptoms and consequently of their associations. In search of these roots, he identifies two fundamental ones: the 'weakening of will' and the 'weakening of intra-psychic coordination' among the various mental activities. In these few pages, Kraepelin aligns with the great tradition of phenomenological psychopathology.

It is therefore wrong, or at least limited, to see in Emil Kraepelin the precursor of the current tendency to conceive diagnosis as a process that can be defined as 'ticking boxes'. In ticking boxes [8] the main epistemological tenet is that psychopathological disorders manifest themselves in characteristic sets of signs, symptoms and behaviours that are, in principle, accessible to question-and-answer techniques. The clinician's main goal is to discover whether a patient showing psychopathological phenomena meets pre-given diagnostic criteria. The clinical interview is conceived as a stimulus—response pattern of questions formulated in such a way as to reduce information variance and elicit only 'relevant' answers. A special emphasis is given to reducing disagreement between different clinicians. The aim is neither an in-depth understanding of the patient's personal experiences nor to reveal previously unknown features of the patient's condition, but to assess those phenomena that are deemed important as diagnostic indices a priori, leading to the classification of the patient's complaints and dysfunctions according to pre-defined diagnostic categories.

Phenomenological psychopathology has quite a different method and aim [9]. Building on and extending the studies of Minkowski [10], Straus [11], Binswanger [12], Tellenbach [13] and Blankenburg [7] among many others, it assumes that the manifold of phenomena of a given mental disorder is a meaningful whole, that is, a *structure*. Structural thinking belongs to the mature phase of the evolution of psychiatry as a science [14]. Phenomenological psychopathology is the discipline which, more than all the others in the clinic of mental disorders, has made structural thinking its own. It goes beyond the description of isolated symptoms and the use of some of those symptoms to establish a diagnosis and aims to understand the meaning of a given set of symptoms in order to grasp the underlying characteristic modification that keeps these symptoms meaningfully interconnected. Phenomenological psychopathology assumes that the symptoms of a syndrome have a meaningful coherence. One can find, and should look for, internal links between the various aspects of a person's symptoms, that is, that they display a structure, that is, its parts stand in a relationship to each other of reciprocal expression.

In phenomenological psychopathology, abnormal mental conditions are not mere aggregates of symptoms. Symptoms are a special kind of phenomenon through which the hidden, yet operative (perplexing and disturbing) dimension of existence is made manifest. They are not accidental to that patient, but rather the manifestation of some implicit quintessential 'core' dimension of his subjectivity. The overall change in the fundamental structures of subjectivity transpires through the individual symptoms, but the specificity of the core is only graspable at a more comprehensive structural level. This holistic approach bears little resemblance to the current atomistic operational definitions for several reasons.

To understand the results and limitations of phenomenological psychopathology, it is necessary to be clear about its epistemological premises. First, it does not call into question the traditional diagnoses, the Kraepelinian ones in particular and uses terms like 'schizophrenia', 'melancholy', 'mania' etc. Second, it does not criticise the traditional definition of psychopathological symptoms (e.g. 'delusion', 'hallucination', 'depressed mood',); eventually it aims to formulate richer, more detailed descriptions, useful for circumscribing a symptom and delimiting it from other similar but not identical symptoms (e.g. to distinguish the delusions characteristic of schizophrenia from the delusion-like ideas characteristic of melancholia). Thirdly, it uses these same symptoms to make its nosographic diagnoses—for example, the presence of a holothymic (i.e. understandable as derivable from an emotional state) delusion of guilt is considered characteristic of melancholia and not schizophrenia.

The main difference is that phenomenological psychopathology, instead of diagnostic categories, speaks of psychopathological life-worlds. This concept is a supportive tool for producing a systematic description of subtle and often undescribed changes in the patient's experience and to reconstruct the ontological framework within which they are generated.

The life-world can be seen as a grand theatre of phenomena, that is, subjective experiences, variously arranged in space and time relative to perceiving subjects. The main aim of phenomenological psychopathology is to obtain a systematic knowledge of the patients' life-world in its peculiar subjective feel, meaning and value. To achieve this goal, it focuses on the patients' states of mind as they are experienced and narrated by them. It aims to faithfully describe the manifold of phenomena in all their concrete and distinctive features. These concerns are prior to any causal accounts addressing sub-personal mechanisms: theoretical assumptions are minimised and the search for the structures of the patients' experience is prioritised.

The exploration of patients' life-worlds involves at least two distinct steps [15]. The first—called phenomenal unfolding—is the gathering of self-descriptions of the patient's experiences. The phenomena explored are not just 'symptoms' in a descriptive–psychopathological sense. As lived experiences are always situated within the grounds of body, self, time, space and others, the unfolding of the life-world of a given person adopts these basic dimensions of lived experience to organise the data. To investigate these dimensions, the phenomenological inquiry will start with questions such as: How do you experience time? Do you feel there a sense of continuity over time, or are there breaks in it? Do you feel effective as an agent in the world, or rather as being exposed to the world? Do you tend to take an external perspective to your body and self? Do you feel in touch with your body? Do you happen to experience it, or some parts of it, as a kind of object in outer space? Can you empathise with others, take their perspective? How do you experience yourself when relating to other people? etc.

The result will be a rich and detailed collection of the patient's self-descriptions related to each dimension, for example, temporal continuity/discontinuity, space flat/filled with saliences, bodily coherence/fragmentation, self-world demarcation/permeability, self-other attunement/dis-attunement and so on. In this way, using first-person accounts, phenomenological psychopathology detects the critical points where the constitution of experience and action is vulnerable and open to derailments.

The second step implies a shift to phenomenology proper that seeks the basic structures or existential dimensions of the life-worlds the patient lives in. Any phenomenon is viewed as the expression of a given form of human subjectivity and abnormal phenomena are seen as the outcome of a, more or less profound, modification of human subjectivity. Phenomenological psychopathology is committed to attempting to discover a common source that ties together the seemingly heterogeneous phenomena displayed by a given patient. This is done by finding similarities among the manifold phenomena and, possibly, the deep or structural change in the form of experience/action related to that specific existential dimension (spatiality, temporality, embodiment and so on) that could explain the various changes that occur in the patients.

One of the most famous attempts to phenomenologically characterise the life-world of people with schizophrenia and their 'surface' symptoms on the basis of a 'deep' change in the structures of subjectivity is German psychiatrist and philosopher Wolfgang Blankenburg's (1928–2002) study on 'sub-apophanic schizophrenia' (his term) as a disorder of 'common sense' and of 'natural self-evidence' [7]. In our everyday experience, as healthy persons, we feel rooted in our world; the meanings of things we encounter in the world are 'naturally self-evident'. A sense of familiarity accompanies us even when we meet new objects and situations, because we are able spontaneously to refer them to our past experiences and 'typify' them as something meaningful for us. Blankenburg assumed that the core in sub-delusional (which he calls 'sub-apophanic') schizophrenia is a crisis of common sense.

'Sub-apophanic' designates that form of schizophrenia (not so different from Kraepelin's 'silly dementia') in which delusions and hallucinations are not in the foreground. Blankenburg argued that the core-property shared by these patients is a subtle form of detachment from reality—the 'loss of the natural evidence of commonsensical everyday experience'. All the symptoms and phenomena of this condition are expressions of the lack of an implicit sharing of the background of tacit knowledge of one's social group, through which its members conceptualise objects, situations and other persons' behaviours, and of the natural attitude through which one feels attuned to the world as it appears in everyday experience. This feeling of rootedness and *at-homeness* in the pre-reflective meanings of one's life-world is absent from the experience of these people who are said to be affected by a disorder of common sense. This frequently begins with a barely noticeable decline in the ability 'to see things in their right light', which precedes the emergence of other more flamboyant symptoms as the patient's condition evolves into a frankly delusional or thought disordered state. What becomes striking for those around the patient is that in them there is a withering away of their feeling of the proper thing to do in situations and a general indifference to what might be disturbing to others.

Now, the change of register between Kraepelin's description of 'silly dementia' and Blankenburg's description of 'sub-apophanic schizophrenia' is clear. What they have in common is that they both talk about 'schizophrenia' (or 'dementia', two terms which could be considered synonyms) and try to characterise its 'clinical forms' as rigorously as possible. But the differences leap to the eye (and ear).

Kraepelin's focus is primarily (though not exclusively) on behavioural symptoms, for example, the patients' behaviours are described as absent-minded, negligent, lazy, they are withdrawn, stand about in corners, stare intently in front of them etc. In contrast, Blankenburg seems much more interested in the way patients experience themselves and the world, for example, the following comments by Anne Rau, a twenty-year old female patient: 'What is it that I am missing? – says a patient – It is something so small, but strange, it is something so important. It is impossible to live without it. I find that I have no longer footing in the world. I have lost a footing in regard to the simplest, everyday things. It seems that I lack a natural understanding for what is matter of course and obvious to others' [16, p. 163].

While Kraepelin relies on symptoms as diagnostic indices pointing to a pre-defined category, Blankenburg seeks clues within the patient's own phrasing— expressions that fall outside traditional symptoms, exceed the nomenclatures of descriptive psychopathology, and remain uncounted among the standard diagnostic indices of schizophrenia.

Kraepelin seems to stick to psychopathological symptoms and diagnostic categories, Blankenburg is open to the patients' phenomenal experience and their ways of being-in-the-world or life-worlds. Kraepelin seems substantially interested in *diagnosing* his patients' illnesses, whereas Blankenburg in *understanding* their forms of existence.

Kraepelin, finally, also seems to be interested in identifying the alteration of a 'deep' psychological function ('noopsychic' or 'thymopsychic') beneath the 'surface' symptoms. Blankenburg does not look for the basal alteration within the framework of 'function psychology', (i.e. perception, cognition, memory and affects), but resorts to a concept drawn from philosophy, that is, the crisis of 'common sense'.

16.4   Binswanger's 'Forms of Miscarried Existence': Putting Images in the Foreground

Swiss psychiatrist and philosopher Ludwig Binswanger (1881–1966) takes a radically different path both from the detailed description of the symptoms in view of their use as diagnostic indices (Kraepelin) and from the search for a 'profound' modification in the structures of subjectivity that can be seen as the essence or principle that 'surface' symptoms have in common (Blankenburg).

In the volume entitled *Three forms of miscarried existence* [1], in which he collects three essays published between 1945 and 1952, he submits to an in-depth analysis three phenomena that he calls *Verstiegenheit*, *Verschrobenheit* and *Manieriertheit*.

Binswanger seeks to avoid the jargon of clinical psychiatry and psychopathology, or at least to neutralise its objectifying and stigmatising effects. This collection of essays is dedicated to schizophrenia, yet Binswanger, while by no means avoiding examining the language in use to describe its symptoms, strives to find other terms to talk about the behaviour and experiences of people with schizophrenia. Rather than using terms like 'autism', 'delusion', he goes in search of another vocabulary, drawing mainly from the visual arts. *Verstiegenheit*, *Verschrobenheit* and *Manieriertheit* are for Binswanger forms of existential failure in the sense that the individual's experience of the flow of life has come to a stop. He does not judge these phenomena in a psychiatric medical sense as pathological 'diminution', morbid deviations from the norm or psychopathological symptoms. Rather, they are regarded as forms of failure of human existence—three ways in which human existence can lose its way, three modes in which human existence is threatened in its vulnerability. The common characteristic of these three forms of existence is that the historical mobility of existence has come to a stop.

The point that I am interested in analysing and developing here is the following: Binswanger tries to avoid the use a kind of *technical* and *conceptual* language—the ordinary language of psychiatry—to describe these phenomena; instead, he makes extensive use of *images*.

The first and fundamental image he uses is 'disproportion'. It is an image taken from the figurative arts and particularly from architecture. Proportion consists in the commensurability of the individual parts of the whole work, both with each other and with the whole (Vitruvius, *De Architectura*), as for example, the relationship between the base diameter of the column in the Greek temple and its height, which allows for the coordination of every other element of the construction. These metric relations express a sense of organic finiteness, a balance of the building's components and an overall harmony of planes, volumes, surfaces, construction and decorative details. Binswanger transposes the idea of 'proportion' into the sphere of human existence and speaks of 'anthropological proportion'. In his essay on fixed exaltation, he writes that this is a form of anthropological *disproportion*. Imagining a person climbing upwards along a ladder, for example, the height of the ladder must be proportionate to its base so that the person does not fall as he or she ascends. Therefore, with anthropological disproportion he means a disruption of the relationship between the height of the ascent and the base on which this ascent rests. Proportion in human life is not a fixed but a dialectical relationship between two terms that can vary over time. For example, if the base on which the ascent rests is extended, then the ascent itself can 'proportionally' proceed higher without going astray.

The word that Binswanger uses to name the first form of miscarried existence is *Verstiegenheit*, which is sometimes translated as 'extravagance', but I suggest better as 'fixed exaltation'. In fixed exaltation, the height is no longer proportionate to the breadth of the base, that is, experience. Here the word 'experience' is used in the sense it takes in the phrase 'an experienced person', that is, one who has gathered a wealth of knowledge. The exalted person remains fixed in his ascent because of his inexperience. That of the person fixed in his ascent is an ascent which 'spins in the air'. We must imagine the ascent of an *amateur mountaineer* lacking the experience of mountains, rocks, blizzards and climbs. The peak that he reaches is not a height achieved through a slow and patient ascent. Nor is it a winged ascent—that is, sustained by the wings of imagination, love, enthusiasm and art. Instead, it is a vertiginous and fictitious height, and therefore constantly threatened by vertigo: an artificial height, in which one no longer feels the ground beneath one's feet and no longer walks forwards or backwards, and from which one cannot even descend.

At this height, disproportionate to its real capacity to ascend, existence no longer proceeds but remains fixed—in a certain idea, aspiration, theory or worldview. Fixed exaltation is that form of disproportionate existence for which that mountain wall on which the person has climbed becomes an insurmountable limit for him.

Verschrobenheit, a word can be variously translated as 'crankiness', 'eccentricity', 'quirkiness', 'weirdness' or 'derailment' and sometimes also as 'perverseness', is also a form of disproportionality constituted not by stopping in a vertical ascent (as it is the case with fixed exaltation) but by transversality, by going sideways, by twisting. Literally, *Verschrobenheit* alludes to the theme of the *Schraube* ('screw') and suggests the idea of the limit placed on the penetration of the screw, or a misdirection of this penetration. A twisted screw is a screw that is badly, not properly placed. The deviation of the screw has a twofold meaning: on the one hand it alludes to the inadequate configuration of the screw itself, on the other hand to the bad use that has been made of it. The derailment of existence is portrayed with the image of a *twisted screw*, a crooked pivot that can no longer move, and, indeed, if it moves forward, it may twist and distort even more. Among the various examples used by Binswanger, one is particularly striking: that of the father who puts a coffin under the Christmas tree as a present for his cancer-stricken daughter. The impression that this gesture arouses in us, immersed in common sense, is equivalent to a punch in the face because it is completely tactless and brutal. For the father, on the other hand, this gift is appropriate for the circumstance. The father's logic—that is, if my daughter is sick with cancer then all that she needs is a coffin—is distorted and, like a twisted screw, it gets twisted the more one insists trying to tighten it.

Manieriertheit, which can be translated with 'mannerism', is yet a different form from fixated exaltation and derailment. In mannerism, existence contorts itself upwards and has lost its centre of gravity in itself. In this twisted, rootless ascent, existence stiffens into contrived poses. It cannot rely on itself to rise but it needs something else, a support from outside. The insecurity and precariousness of human existence are manifested in mannerism: the absence of a core, of a character of its own, of an autonomous consistency. This support is provided by an artificial expedient that aims to make up for a deficiency—the lack of a natural drive of its own.

In mannerism, we are struck by the melancholic and dry expression, affectation, the imposed rigidity, the etiquette and the ceremonial that replace spontaneity. The image that sums up mannerism is the *mask*. The case described by Binswanger is that of a young man who does not find a secure basis in his own ipseity and is terrified of succumbing to the overwhelming power of the world—especially the world of his parents. He finds shelter behind a mask that represents his 'opaque resistance' to the world. Characterised by rigidity, coldness and closure, the mask offers protection to the wearer because it does not let the face be seen. Interiority cannot manifest itself beyond the mask. The mask also prevents the mobility of physiognomy, thus the articulate and changeable expression of emotions. This is why mannerism, in trying to make up for spontaneity, contributes to its further destruction, destroying with it man's natural grace—or what remains of it.

16.5   Discussion: A Vocabulary for 'Pathic Forms'

The presumptuous amateur mountaineer, the crooked screw and the mask can be taken as prototypes of a rich series of images that can help us grasp the 'forms' into which existence stiffens when it is lost in its becoming.

Clearly, the images proposed by Binswanger are all images of movement (or of stopping a movement). They capture a movement and express its physiognomy, that is, the way a body shows itself when it forms an intention to move, or when its movement is blocked, compressed, dragged or restricted. The novice mountaineer is trapped on the rock face and can neither climb nor descend. The twisted screw becomes more and more twisted if you try to tighten it up further and splinters the wood on which it is screwed. The mask crushes the face, suffocates it and prevents it from expressing an emotion.

Of course, images can be used to capture all kinds of phenomena, not just those of a psychopathological nature. But what then is an image? How can we define it? I propose that there are two kinds of images which fulfil the same purpose but from two different perspectives. Firstly, an image is the *mis-en-forme*, that is, shaping, into a form (especially a seen form), of a more formless sensory datum, such as a fragment of episodic memory. Our unconscious memory is rich in these fragments—for example, the sense of relaxation and abandonment instilled in us by the scent of our grandmother's embrace, or the jolt of our body at the way our father arched his eyebrows when he got angry. Secondly, an image can also be the *sensualisation* of a thought or concept, that is, the translation of the abstractness of a cognitive phenomenon into the concreteness of a sensation or perception, especially of a visual kind. An example of this is Dante's description of despair that reigns in Hell: 'forever through that turbid, timeless air,/like sand that eddies when a whirlwind swirls' ('quell' aura sanza tempo tinta,/come la rena quando turbo spira' [17]. Thus, an image is the visual representation of a phenomenon that lies in an intermediate space between the sensory datum in its concrete but ineffable immediacy, and the abstractness of a concept, formalised in a linguistic formula but far removed from the concrete datum of experience. All this cannot fail to remind us of the work of one of the greatest art historians and critics in the twentieth century— Aby Moritz Warburg (1866–1929). Born of a wealthy German Jewish family of Italian origins, he studied art history, history of religion and archaeology. He also trained for two semesters in medicine and, at the end of the nineteenth century, he moved to Florence, where he developed an entirely original understanding of Antiquity and the Renaissance, which remained his main interest throughout his life. At the end of the First World War, Warburg was admitted to Ludwig Binswanger's psychiatric clinic Bellevue Sanatorium, in Kreutzlingen near Lake Constance, where he remained from 1921 till 1924. We have documentation of the correspondence between the two [18]. Also, part of the 'tangled paths' between the personal and intellectual lives of Binswanger and Warburg was the lecture delivered by Warburg during his stay at Bellevue on 21 April 1923. The lecture's centre of attention was the *Schlangentanz* (Snake Dance) performed by the Pueblo civilisation in North America. Towards the end of his lecture, Warburg emphasised his critique of a modernity that has lost touch with its psychological roots and myths: 'The culture of the machine age destroys what the natural sciences, grown out of myths, have laboriously conquered – the space for contemplation that turned into a space for reflection' [19, p. 94].

A similar critique to contemporary humanities, and to psychopathology as a part of them, is addressed by scholars such as Susan Sontag [3] and Hans Ulrich Gumbrecht [2]. The latter argues that, through their exclusive dedication to conceptual analysis and interpretation, that is, to the reconstruction and attribution of 'meaning', the humanities have lost their capacity to address the dimension of 'presence', that is, the way cultural phenomena make an impact on our bodies and senses [2]. Gumbrecht also argues that 'poetry is perhaps the most powerful example of the simultaneity of presence effects and meaning effects' (p. 18). Poetic forms, instead of being subordinated to meanings, may find themselves in a situation of tension and oscillation between meaning-effects and presence-effects. Mutatis mutandis, this statement by Gumbrecht can be transposed from the sphere of poetry to that of images, and from the sphere of the humanities to that of psychopathology. Images can capture the living presence of the human, in its pathic and plastic dimension, perhaps more than conceptual formulas can.

Susan Sontag in 1964 argued that what is needed is a 'vocabulary for forms' [3, p. 12]. 'What we decidedly do not need now is further assimilate Art into Thought' (p. 13), developing, therefore, a vocabulary capable of plastically representing the forms of human existence, rather than trying to grasp them conceptually. As a psychopathologist and as a clinician, I can only endorse Sontag's appeal: 'What is important now is to recover our senses. We must learn to see more, to hear more, to feel more' (p. 14).

Warburg was a forerunner in all this. He is the inventor of a method for establishing connections between cultural forms, including works of art, from very distant epochs and environments, based on the recognition of the 'pathic forms' of the represented figures. Warburg defines these figures as *Pathosformeln*. *Pathosformeln* are images in which a given *pathos*—that is, an emotional energy, an affective state—coagulates in a *formula*—that is, a culturally transformed model [20]. Thus, *Pathoformeln* are deposits and transformers of affective/emotional drives. They give expression to the movement of life, making visible a certain emotional movement; they unite an invisible, internal state with a bodily, visible form. *Pathosformeln* create a space, a distance between the person and her internal state through a kind of objectification that shapes and opens up a space for thought [8]. *Pathosformeln* are choreographies—literally, writings of movements—in which a state of mind is made visible. A montage, a telescopage of elements that are opposed to each other but composed into a figure that expresses this contrast, where dialectical tension is at its highest degree. This is the same thought we find in Walter Benjamin and his 'discovery' of the *dialektisches Bild* ('dialectical image') as a 'constellation saturated with tensions'—an image that becomes visible below the encrusted surface of the concept. The power of images is precisely this: by applying the pathic forms described by Warburg and the dialectical images proposed by Benjamin, it is through images—far more than through concepts—that we can give plastic form to the motions of the soul, to the states of ambivalence and self-contradiction that accompany crises, and in general to what we have called 'existential knots' [21]. The three forms of miscarried existence described by Binswanger are one of the rare examples of the application of these principles to the field of psychopathology.

16.6   Conclusion

In this chapter, I have attempted to show some of the main stages of the intellectual pathway that can lead psychiatry from the conceptual description of symptoms, to their organisation into forms of life whose meaning reveals the fragility of the human condition; and, finally, to an approach that relies on images evoking presence-effects and *Pathosformeln* and not only on meaning-effects and conceptual descriptions.

Examples of plastic representation of *pathos* are very frequent in poetry—obviously much more than in psychopathology. Representative of these are the writings, among many others, that Charles Baudelaire (1821–1867) dedicates to the mood that characterised his culture and his personal experience—*spleen*. Walter Benjamin (1892–1940)—an intellectual pillar of the twentieth century—suggested that the genius of Baudelaire transformed the immediate experience (Erlebnis) of the daily shocks (Chockerlebnis) of nineteenth-century metropolitan life into long experience (Erfahrung), that is, experience contextualised both in space and time. In an earlier paper, George Ikkos and I [22] have argued for the importance of the humanities and arts in medical and psychiatric training. There we explored Baudelaire's evocations of depression and discussed their relation to images, for example, 'spleen', the 'snuffling clock' and the 'sinister mirror'. Appreciation of the method of poetry in creating images and the images it generates adds depth to clinical practice by painting vivid pictures of subjective experience. Thus perceived images, and especially poetic images, can help us appropriate and make sense of the 'pathic forms' that our patients endure, enabling us to transcend our third person perspective (supported by a conceptual and ultimately distancing and potentially stigmatising vocabulary) and to resonate with our patients' bodies and finally attune with the patients' perspective.

Before concluding, however, it is useful to add some clarifications so that the reader is aware that Binswanger's contribution represents only one stage, and not without limitations and potential dangers.

The images proposed by Binswanger belong largely to a well-established repertoire which in the case of fixed exaltation draws on architecture and in that of mannerism draws on the history of art. Therefore, it cannot be said that they have been produced in the encounter between the clinician and the patient—that is, in the *in-between* where it would be appropriate for them to be born.

We must remember that psychopathological phenomena, as any other human phenomenon, are relational in nature, that is, they arise and take form *between ourselves*. Especially, psychopathological phenomena arise when there is no space for communication and mutual understanding between us. This implies that an image taken from a given relational context may not be effective if transported into another relational context. Thus, what we need is a *poetics* for psychiatric care [23], that is, an art of making or co-producing images-in-words to communicate and understand each other.

To put it in very simple terms: if we wish to add to the curriculum of psychiatrists the skill of using images next to concepts, we must not confine ourselves to teaching a repertoire of ready-made and ready-to-use images, but rather teach them how to allow images to take form in the space that connects themselves and their patients.

Key Points

- Psychiatry as a biomedical discipline was founded on the assumption of rigorous conceptual definitions of psychopathological symptoms and syndromes. Emil Kraepelin charted a course that is still followed by the majority of researchers and clinicians.
- Clinical phenomenology contributed to this conceptual foundation of psychiatry, in part by contesting it, and in part by supplementing this approach through the 'structural principle'. According to this principle, the multiplicity of symptoms that characterise a psychopathological condition represent a 'structure', that is, a totality endowed with meaning in which the individual symptoms are mutually interconnected.
- The language used by both the Kraepelinian/biomedical approach and the phenomenological approach is largely conceptual in nature, thus rather abstract and far removed from the first-person narratives of patients.
- One of the exceptions is Ludwig Binswanger's work *Three Forms of Miscarried Existence,* in which the Swiss psychiatrist and philosopher, one of the founders

of the phenomenological approach in psychiatry, uses figurative language in images to describe the way of being in the world of persons with schizophrenia.

- I make explicit the deep roots of this language of images in psychopathology, highlighting its precursors in the humanities, such as Aby Warburg and Walter Benjamin. Images can help us appropriate and make sense of the 'pathic forms' that our patients endure, transcend our third person perspective (supported by a conceptual and ultimately distancing vocabulary) and resonate with our patients' bodies and finally find attunement between one's own and the patients' perspective.

References

1. Binswanger L. Drei Formen Missglückten Daseins. Max Niemeyer Verlag, Tübingen, 1956.
2. Gumbrecht HG. Production of presence. What meaning cannot convey. Stanford: Stanford University Press; 2004.
3. Sontag S. Against interpretation. In: Against interpretation and other essays. New York/London: Penguin; 1961/2009.
4. Warburg A. Bilderatlas Mnemosyne: the original; Haus der Kulturen und Welt (HKW): Berlin, Germany; The Warburg Institute: London, 2020.
5. Ikkos G, Stanghellini G, Morgan A. History, 'nowtime' (jetztzeit) and dialectical images: introduction to Walter Benjamin for psychiatry (I). Int Rev Psychiatry. https://doi.org/10.1080/09540261.2024.2359468.
6. Kraepelin E. Dementia praecox and Paraphrenia. Translated by G.E. Robertson and R.M. Barclay. Robert E. Krieger Publishing Co. Inc. New York, 1971.
7. Blankenburg W. Der Verlust der natürlichen Selbstverständlichkeit. Ein Beitrag zur Psychopathologie symptomarmer Schizophrenien. Stuttgart, Enke, 1971.
8. Stanghellini G. The power of images and the logics of discovery in psychiatric care. Brain Sci. 2023;13:13. https://doi.org/10.3390/brainsci13010013.
9. Stanghellini G. The meanings of psychopathology. Curr Opin Psychiatry. 2009;22:559–64.
10. Minkowski E. Schizophrenia. The psychopathology of schizoids and schizophrenic. Paris: Payot, 1927.
11. Straus E. On obsession. nervous and mental disease monographs, vol. 73. New York; 1948.
12. Binswanger L. Schizophrenia. Pfullingen: Neske; 1957.
13. Tellenbach H. Melancholy. History of the problem, endogeneity, typology, pathogenesis, clinical considerations. Pittsburg: Duquesne University Press; 1980.
14. Lanteri-Laura G. Essay on the paradigms of modern psychiatry. Paris: Editions du Temps; 1998.
15. Stanghellini G., Mancini M. The therapeutic interview in mental health. A values-based and person-centered apptoach. Cambridge University Press, Cambridge, 2017.
16. Broome MR, Harland R, Owen GS, Stringaris A. The Maudsley reader in phenomenological psychiatry. Cambridge: Cambridge University Press; 2012.
17. Dante Alighieri, Inferno. La Commedia, nel testo e nel commento di Niccolò Tommaseo. Aldo Martello Editore, Milano, 1965.
18. Binswanger L, Warburg A. In: Santilli D, editor. La Guarigione Infinita. Storia Clinica di Aby Warburg. Vicenza: Neri Pozza; 2005.
19. Warburg A. Bilder aus dem Gebiet der Pueblo-Indianer in Nord-Amerika. In: Gesammelte Schriften: Studienausgabe, vol. III.2.
20. Agamben G. Ninfe. Torino: Bollati Boringhieri; 2007.
21. Stanghellini G. How to improve psychiatric nosography in the XXI century: a phenomenologist's viewpoint. Eur Psychiatry. 2025;68(1):e25. https://doi.org/10.1192/j.eurpsy.2025.11.

22. Stanghellini G, Ikkos G. Images of depression in Charles Baudelaire: clinical understanding in the context of poetry and social history. BJPsych Bull. 2022; https://doi.org/10.1192/bjb.2022.84.
23. Ikkos G, Morgan A. Psychiatric poetics: mental healthcare and Giovanni Stanghellini's 'Logics of Discovery' BJPsych Bull Published online 2025:1–6. https://doi.org/10.1192/bjb.2024.115.

Open Access This chapter is licensed under the terms of the Creative Commons Attribution 4.0 International License (http://creativecommons.org/licenses/by/4.0/), which permits use, sharing, adaptation, distribution and reproduction in any medium or format, as long as you give appropriate credit to the original author(s) and the source, provide a link to the Creative Commons license and indicate if changes were made.

The images or other third party material in this chapter are included in the chapter's Creative Commons license, unless indicated otherwise in a credit line to the material. If material is not included in the chapter's Creative Commons license and your intended use is not permitted by statutory regulation or exceeds the permitted use, you will need to obtain permission directly from the copyright holder.

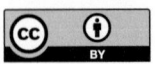

'Sheer Space', 'Elvenspace', the Ghost Choir of Time and 'Thymic Space': A Trilogue to Understand Space 'Oddities in Schizophrenia'

17

Helene Cæcilie Mørck, Lorenzo Gilardi, and Giovanni Stanghellini

17.1 Introduction

This chapter you are about to read is not a review of the experience of space in people with schizophrenia. Nor is it research aimed at adding to the list of symptoms of schizophrenia a further symptom such as the anomaly of lived space. Its purpose is much more modest, and at the same time much more ambitious. It is more modest because it is not proposed as a starting point for generalisations such as 'All or many people with schizophrenia experience space in this and that way'. It is more ambitious because it differs widely from the methods in use in current research in psychopathology, aimed (precisely) at measuring those phenomena that occur as generalisable to a large 'population' of patients. This writing stands, so to speak, as the testimony of individual experiences. Indeed, to be more precise, as a testimony to the possibility of a dialogue between 'experts by experience' and 'experts by profession' in which the voice of each does not drown out the voice of the others but rather helps to make it clearer and more audible. Our ambition, therefore, is to help think of a type of research in psychopathology as an alternative to the logic of generalisation of results, their quantification, as well as to the epistemic asymmetry between the voice of experts by experience and that of experts by profession.

The method for our joint work and exploration was an act of co-writing. Each writer began with a written statement about their experience of space. These statements were then shared among the group via email, and direct written responses and

H. C. Mørck
Department of Teaching and Dissemination, DenmarkUniversity Library of Southern Denmark, Odense, Denmark

L. Gilardi
Department of Mathematics, Insubria University, Como, Italy

G. Stanghellini (✉)
Department of Health Sciences, University of Florence, Florence, Italy

© The Author(s) 2026
G. Ikkos, T. Becker (eds.), *Psychiatry after Kraepelin*,
https://doi.org/10.1007/978-3-032-09475-9_17

questions were added to a shared document. To keep the dialogue flowing, we aimed to respond to the questions and reflections that arose during the process in an immediate and intuitive manner, seeking to convey our experiences with sincerity, intellectual honesty and humility. Later in the process, each writer made minor edits to their sections for clarity, and finally, the chapter was organised to create a natural progression in the dialogue.

Our work can be taken as an exercise of dialogue—as opposed to a monologue of a 'normal' conscience on a 'sick' conscience—and as an exercise of mutual understanding—as opposed to an operation aimed at 'diagnosing' mental illness. During the dialogue we refer to the poetry of William Blake and the philosophical work of Martin Heidegger and Ludwig Binswanger.

17.2   Lorenzo on Space

'I felt hopeless. I was in bed, unable to move or lift myself. And, not for the first time, I'm afraid to say, I started feeling it emerge out of nowhere: Space. It's really hard to talk about it because it's such a radical experience that it defies all description and there are no words to express it. So, in the end, what can I say about it? Well, probably the best way is this: you experience space as if it were an object in itself. How does it feel? The 'empty' space of our lived world suddenly becomes a thing, a thing with two main traits. The first is its hardness: it feels like space crashes into you and is as impenetrable as the surface of a diamond; but, at the same time, you're trapped in a diamond, and you can't escape. You feel out of breath. The second is its temperature: it burns, it doesn't burn because of how hot it is, but because of how cold it is! It's an icy surface so cold it burns and hurts you. And what is trapped in such a hard object and what is burned and scarred is not the body, because the body is almost gone and forgotten. It is the 'Self' itself. You no longer have a body, so you come into direct contact with space. I think it's sort of like having nerves on edge and without any protection. I think it's the most painful feeling you can experience. What I can compare it to is the pain that comes with depression: a kind of pain that is 'mental' but still more like physical pain. The latter I've felt many times, and it's absolutely heartbreaking… But that, the 'sheer space', well it's orders of magnitude greater than any pain I've ever experienced in my life. Furthermore, the body having vanished, what was once 'in' and 'out' can no longer be relied upon. Everything becomes a mash-up of 'in' and 'out'. Nothing gives an order to your existence: thus, on the one hand, objects can attack you and be incorporated, like unwanted guests, and you cannot shake them off; on the other hand, emotions, desires, needs and thoughts become spatialised, they can be incorporated into objects around you. Things have the power to become intentions of emotions and thoughts, and they can turn against you, become weapons, and attack you from all sides. You feel completely disarmed, naked. You no longer have a body, a brain, a heart. There is only pain, pure pain. If you want to know what a pure distillation of pain is, try the sheer space. Not very often, but it happens. I've tried it a few times, but it's extreme, and therefore (possibly) rare for that reason. It could tear you apart. You think you can die for this.

It's like Coldplay sing: 'Oh you, use your heart like a weapon/and it hurts like heaven'.

Usually when I walk and usually when I am alone, the landscape I'm immersed in changes, in a sudden yet continuous way: the world before me starts to get smaller and smaller until I see only galaxies and stars before me; I would grow taller and slimmer, and an Olympic and Apollonian view of the cosmos would possess me: the Elvenspace. I would start walking in slow motion, everything in front of me would become unreachable, with no desire for me to touch anything. I would become possessed by this new horizon. It is the stuff of eternity sewn in my very own being. The life of a Tolkien Elf would shake every chord of myself: but more than immortality it is the eternal point in time I would find myself fixed to… As I grow thinner, my body seems to vanish, and the Eye of the Mind remains the ultimate piece of being. A music, so soft and melancholy but at the same time so pure that no human ear can hear it, would start to submerge me. It is the music of celestial spheres: by way of it, everything would become a harmony never felt by human beings. Things vibrate, and other people would be erased. It's only me and the firmament, the dust of starlight. My irises would become greater so that I could drain in all the purity of this newfound cosmos. Looking down, my legs have grown longer and so have my fingers. Under my feet only sky: I would walk in the void. Strangely, an asymmetry would spring: a harmonious discontinuity between what is before me and what is behind me. I would wear a velvet cloak, cerulean and royal blue, with a golden hem, my hair would become a crown of diamonds whose material and light would come from the stars all around me. No Sun or Moon, only galaxies and stars; only the dim light of these would lighten this space.

At times, I feel like slowly riding a beautiful, white horse, and its rhythmic stride would lull me. It would move slowly like everything. The stars would make their circle and one minute feels like a human lifetime, a mere blink of the eye like a century.

As my space changes, so does my body: a solidarity in this new cosmos, never felt in the shared, common world, would materialise. I know in my heart of hearts that this beautiful firmament is there for me, and for me only. I feel peaceful, calm, relaxed. Everything is suddenly in the right place, no smear anywhere. I could look at the Earth as a superior creature, no more chained to the human world and life: the life of the Eldar has come to me'.

17.3   Cæcilie on Space

'I am watching the sun reflect off the tree outside through my window, as I try to contemplate the concept of space within my fifty-one-year-old body. It is not hard to recall. A feeling of deep, penetrating loss, sorrow and isolation overwhelms me, accompanied by the awareness that these emotions and sensations have been with me since birth and seem primordial in nature. Since childhood, I've remembered these sensations, waking up each morning asking myself: Why am I alive? What is my purpose? Then the thought would come to me: I am dead. Dead. Dead. And these thoughts never ceased to exist. They have in periods been subdued but remain with me. Like a Ghost Choir, these underlying questions and the sensations of loss, sorrow and isolation seep through my life thread of everyday existence.

My perception of the fabric of reality has always been different. Time has never come to me in a linear progression; it has escaped me like a slippery fish. It's as if time and space have been thinned out, like mist. I go through it but do not know where I am or if I am here. It can be compared to 'the wolf hour'—the time just before dawn, when night meets day. Where the dream world confronts reality, and your subconsciousness awakes you with nagging questions. Most people have experienced this, but the moment will only exist for them in this space for a minute before they wake up, brush it away and start their day. But what if this wolf hour continues every second, every minute of the day? Being in this twilight zone in a constant loop. How would you cope?

Within the core of what I call me, there is nothing—just darkness, like tar the darkness sticks to me, and surrounds this inner core, like a membrane, which is the flesh and bone that people call a body. But to me, it's just an empty shell, because there is nothing inside, only dead, polluted space, both inside and outside this human form. The non-corporeality of the physical form I call me has never been present. So, am I truly here, existing in time and space? Every morning, I awaken there is no me, I can feel the physical weight of my duvet, but I cannot feel anything—space is empty like someone has sucked out the oxygen of the room, the space presses in on me, I feel exposed like every fibre or thread in this non-corporeal being that is supposed to be me vibrates and shakes. My nerve endings feel like they have been tightened like strings on a violin. Space feels volatile, like a wild creature it has teeth and snaps at me and dark shadows lurk at me enveloping the space I am in. Miniscule shadow cannibals want to penetrate my membrane and devour my thoughts to spread through space and the multiverses of time.

I press on with my thoughts, which have taken refuge in a hidden corner of my mind, where cobwebs and hidden desires hide. I try to penetrate the darkness and emerge from the emptiness to find a form I can inhabit today. But the form fluctuates. Some days, I become this abominable creature of a child from David Lynch's film *Eraserhead*, and other days, I assume a form I call me—the woman who danced for a decade, made a living by controlling time through imaginary fantasy worlds on stage, travelled the Western world and lost her heart, if she ever had one, to Jenny, the beautiful woman in Australia who created stop-motion animation films similar to stopping time for a moment. I mostly become the woman who danced and stopped time for a period.

Some days, I wake up as a shadow that cannot find its form, and the ghost choir takes over. I move through the shade, light, sounds, smells, objects and human forms that make up reality, like bubbles of presumed life. It's all distant from me—removed and detached—and it's as if I am cannibalised from the inside, eaten up by isolation and despair and then there are days, where I see it so clearly—space seeps into me, inviting me to be part of the world. On those days, I am God's child, wrapped in a garment of light. I occupy the world, and I create space with my pure thought of being. I am timeless, and I see the beauty of humankind. When I walk, my footsteps leave footprints of light. Everything steps up to the vision of my mind; everything manifests according to my will. Space becomes infinite, and I control the wind, flowers and the progression of ants in the sand. I am the divinity of creation, the reason why everything was made and I am filled with God's light that penetrates my being and lifts me up to pure consciousness'.

17.4   Giovanni on Space

'Sometimes space for me is like air where everything, including me, is separated from everything else. This makes me feel protected by the air between me and other things, like when I cross the street, and a car stops to let me pass. Sometimes, however, everything, like in certain dreams, appears suspended and out of contact with everything else. This is accompanied by a sense of solitude. Solitude can also be a beautiful thing, so long as it doesn't last too long.

But more often space for me is like water where everything appears united with other things. And at certain moments, like on a light wave, I feel myself moving in sync with all the other things and I feel part of a whole and it's very pleasant.

I am at ease in this alternation of a space made of air with a space made of water, this pulsation of separation and contact with the world. If this pulsation stops in a systole or a diastole that is too prolonged, then I feel isolated and desolate, or at the mercy of others and the world. Sometimes it happens, in my waking state as in my dreams, perhaps to remind me that I am a knot, an unresolved tangle between the desire for individuation and the desire for participation.

Sometimes, fortunately rarely, space for me is like concrete, or like amber in which a butterfly is trapped, where my body cannot move. It is as if space adheres to my body like resin and finally enters inside me and deprives me of all will. I think this is what they call anguish.

This is the great theme of the so-called thymic space. That is, the way in which my state of mind, my emotional intonation, resonates with the physiognomy of the world.

Here I move from the register of my personal experience of space to that of my ideas regarding lived space. I believe that everything begins with how I feel my body: whether I feel my heart wide or narrow, whether I feel it swelling with joy or shrinking with pain, whether so full as to overflow or dull and empty. In my opinion, my heart, my limbs, my chest etc. are exactly where I feel space being oppressive or open, vast and capable of welcoming me, or narrow and suffocating so much as to extinguish me.

Then there is the other great aspect, that is, how much my experience of space is linked to my movement. Thymic space is in fact also a dynamic space, that is, it resonates with the dynamics of my movement. As in dance, the experience of space changes in relation to the dancer's movements: an agile and light dancer will highlight the verticality of space, its expansion upwards towards the sky, whereas a heavier one its horizontality, its terrestrial dimension, the distance between him or her and things.

In essence, it is my bodily experience, my body's capabilities and its drive to move, quickly or slowly, smoothly or jerkily, in one direction or another. It is also important whether I feel in contact with my body or detached from it, whether I feel that it responds to my intentions of movement or resists, whether I perceive that it is I who move it or a will external to me etc. that dictate my experience of space'.

17.5 Trilogue

Giovanni: So, Lorenzo, very interesting what you said. If you were to speak about what you call 'sheer space' in a more psychopathological way, what could you say?

Lorenzo: Well, the sheer space has a hardness higher than that of a diamond and a temperature of absolute zero. The contact of the self, no longer meditated by the body, with this 'sheer space' is then the source of an indescribable, excruciating pain. This experience of pain is similar, but less intense, to the one I feel when I am asked to coincide with my geometric body.

Giovanni: Go on, go on: your philosophising nature will help you elaborate further and let us understand more! I never heard of anything like it in my experience as a psychiatrist. You know how 'therapeutic' I consider that you become the 'psychopathologist of yourself', and how important it is to speak a philosophical language to make sense of one's experiences, especially the more distressing ones.

Lorenzo: Yes, of course: in this experience, space is experienced as *chora*, as a *pure extension*, *shapeless space*, as a *homogeneous object* without a coordinate system that can give meaning, order and direction because nobody can organise it as a world. *Chora* originally means *region*, then by extension *place* and *space*, and in the philosophical reflection contained in Plato's *Timaeus* it is initially thematised as what determines the materiality and spatiality of things. In this experience, it is essentially experienced as *hard matter devoid of any form* and as a *space devoid of any trace or limit that determines its figure*: in fact, it must almost be able to take on any form and become any figure (not necessarily under the ego empire of the schizophrenic person).

These shapes and figures, subject to the definition in delusional states, are subject to becoming temporary concretions of space-object-matter, polymorphic traces that can be infinitely erased and rewritten in this 'strange' space. Hence, the *chora* is both *this space-object here*, which oppresses and collapses on the self and at the same time *the extreme residue of reality*, placed beyond the limits of what is formal, good, ordered (the chaotic, the casual, the unintelligible, the impenetrable): that is, it is the limit of being beyond which there is nothing as if to outline an evil and negative principle, at least as a receptacle of all the negative and therefore the cause of excruciating pain.

Giovanni: That's very clear, dear Lorenzo—and if it were not so painful I would even say 'beautiful'. Let me at least say it is beautifully spoken. All of it. Without a body how can there be space, or at least the ordinary experience of space that we people who, for good or ill, feel embodied? Without a body space invades me, burns, tears, sucks me in. But what is left of this bodyless 'me' that is invaded, burned etc. by a space that comes into contact with the body.

Lorenzo: It is not easy to talk about it, not because it's painful to remember it, as it is with every other symptom, but because the 'sheer space' defies common language....

Giovanni: Of necessity! Common language is made to talk about common experiences. So Cæcilie, can you find some points of contact between Lorenzo's experiences and your own?

Cæcilie: Listening to Lorenzo, there were several aspects I related to. I will mention two. The first is: 'It is the "self" itself. You no longer have a body, so you come into direct contact with space, like having nerves on edge without any protection'. This is a very apt description of how I have also felt about space. This non-corporeality is extremely painful. It is not only a deep existential pain, but I also think it's a cosmic pain. What makes you human disappear or fragment into space, and what seems to be left are these shaky, vulnerable nerves that are exposed. Although it seems something remains—thoughts and emotions are still there, even though they are mingled up, catapulted out of you and spatialised. So, if the body is gone (and this must include the brain), I wonder what is left. Could it be the soul? Since we do not know where it is located, the idea of this soul must be your innermost being. And because, as you say, you feel 'only pain, pure pain'. And you could hypothesise that it is the soul suffering.

Giovanni: Both of you tell us that you felt like a disembodied self. You know there has always been a debate in philosophy, medicine and psychiatry about the place of the soul. Some time ago, I had tried to explain that one way to try to approach the experience of a schizophrenic person is to try to imagine what it feels like to be a disembodied spirit and a deanimated body. You both seem to have witnessed what psychopathologists and philosophers, abstractly (including myself) write about the mysterious relationship between soul and body. Is it not true that schizophrenia is a condition in which existential tangles emerge that affect all humans and that you have experienced firsthand?

Cæcilie: I think what you state is at the core of schizophrenia: that it is a condition where all these existential tangles emerge. Schizophrenia exposes complex questions or struggles about existence—like the meaning of life, personal identity, and reality itself. I remember contemplating existential questions since I was a child. For example, when I was with other kids and they were giddy about getting an ice cream, my mind would be elsewhere. I would wonder if I was truly alive or just an illusion, or if the ants I was watching were a creation of God. I've always felt that my existence was at stake every day—and I still do. It's a very radical way of being in the world and extremely hard constantly being in this existential question loop, and although these existential questions affect all humans, the difference is in my schizophrenic mindset these struggles manifests first-hand, every second of the day. They are felt emotionally and physically, in all their overwhelming power so—yes, the firsthand experience is not an intellectual exercise but is a deeply raw felt experience and innate part of my lifeworld—and the mysterious relationship you mention between the soul and body is a reaction to this existential struggle, that the body and soul cannot cope with the constant turmoil so they separate and take on new formations in space, new worlds are created to cope and that is where you could become what you call a disembodied spirit and a deanimated body. In my world, divine insight has been a part of this manifestation. Religious people pray to God in their existential troubles hoping for a sign whereas God has been part of my lifeworld always, talking to me even though I am not religious in any sense of the word. I think that God talks to people with schizophrenia because this God is trying to help us as a sort of negotiator to make sense of things in his own twisted way and be a negotiator between the body and soul and a Meta-voice. At least that is how I see it.

Lorenzo: Yes, Cæcilie, I can confirm your experiences, schizophrenia is like having a job 24/7, and a very hard job, because it feels like being a salmon, swimming counter current. It's debilitating and frustrating. But, coming back to the space issue, what was your second point?

Cæcilie: The second point I want to highlight is where you talk about walking in the landscape and connecting to something bigger than yourself: 'It's only me and the firmament, the dust of starlight'. You speak of being in the Elvenspace, where things grow and 'eternity sewn in my very own being'. This section is profoundly beautiful, and while listening, I felt a deep longing for this place because I have been there too many times like you. It resonates with my own experience of being 'God's child, wrapped in a garment of light'. Like Lorenzo's sense of peace, calm, relaxation and connection to the cosmic space, I have also often felt this. It is an incredibly beautiful place to be. Sometimes I wonder if this is the strange 'gift' that comes with having schizophrenia (in all its isolation and suffering)—the ability to enter this beautiful dimension of a multiverse of beauty and possibilities. I think it may offer your mind, soul and body a brief timeout from the troubling, and altered states that come with schizophrenia.

Giovanni: This is something that many people, and not a few among psychiatrists and psychologists, will have difficulty understanding: that one can 'fall in love' with one's symptoms! Yet it is important to make everyone understand the dialectical, that is, ambivalent, nature of the relationship with what reductionist psychiatry calls 'symptom', which would be better called a person's 'experience'. Elvenspace can be a terrifying yet fascinating experience, can't it?

Cæcilie: What you said about 'falling in love' with this experience is spot on because, when I enter this space—when I enter its world—it has never been terrifying; rather, it's electrifying. From an outsider's perspective, this Elvenspace (to use Lorenzo's term) can be hard to understand, especially if you approach it analytically, rationally, or—as you mentioned—from a reductionist standpoint, reducing the experience to mere symptoms. If you do so, you will miss its true essence. It is an experience that engages your entire being—your soul and, not least, your senses. It is a place so beautiful that it makes you want to cry. For me, it's not just a fascinating experience; it is a realm of infinite creativity and play. It is a lifeworld in its own right. As I reflect on this now, I am beginning to realise how much I have actively sought out and utilised this Elvenspace in my work as a choreographer. It has almost become a method for tapping deeper into my fantasies and playfulness, giving them form. I'm not romanticising my experience, but in my work, I've found that this place can be harnessed creatively. The terrifying aspect of it for me arises when this Elvenspace dissolves and morphs into the raw world of reality, forcing me to leave—then anxiety and suicidal thoughts kick in.

Lorenzo: Listening to your experiences of space, Cæcilie, I think, if I may say so, that space was not the central issue of your text.

Cæcilie: It seems I was talking maybe more about time than space, well I also found it difficult because I think for me time is so connected to space. Maybe it goes back to being obsessive about counting everything when I was a child, trying to control the chaos that always was lurking, taking control of time to control the space of the uncontrollable.

Giovanni: Very interesting, any further thoughts about this topic? How, for example, has your experience of space developed over the years?

Cæcilie: Listening to the different perceptions of space you and Lorenzo describe got me confused about what my idea of space is today. It made me think about how my perception of space has fluctuated in the last couple of years. Four years ago, my experience of space was much like I described in the monologue (quite stagnant). The day I wrote the description of space—this was how I experienced it over the last couple of weeks. Perhaps it was due to the flu, which had hijacked my body and put me in a feverish state, but I descended into that old lifeworld of space that is very scary and mostly turned inward. Recently space has been fluctuating a lot. What is happening is that three layers of space oddities are running simultaneously daily. It is deeply confusing because I go in and out of them during the day and they clash constantly. Sometimes I disappear into myself, and other times I am fully present and able to relate to people, objects etc. However, these mental space choreographies are very persistent. They're not destructive (which is a new experience), just confusing. I think this is happening because these past four years have been a process of awakening from the debilitating side of schizophrenia and integrating whatever is left. The comical part is that no one tells you how horrible it is to abandon schizophrenia. I find it incredibly hard because some days I have no idea who I am without schizophrenia and how I am supposed to perceive and be in this space we call the world.

Lorenzo: What are these three layers in your experience of space?

Cæcilie: It's a very good question, and I'm still in the process of figuring it out. But I believe the dilemma I mentioned earlier is the cause. Over the past four years, I've been in a state of awakening from schizophrenia, and what's happening now I think is that I'm in a state of becoming but I'm not sure into what. A good way to describe it might be that I'm recalibrating me whatever this me is. In my subjective world, all the different lifeworlds I inhabit seem to be changing and morphing, including some that I've held onto for a lifetime. I'm halfway through life, and schizophrenia is such an inherent part of me that it feels just as much a part of my life narrative as everything I've experienced in the external world. My inner fantasy world has been extremely painful, but it's also been a great source of strength, survival and creativity. I think part of the confusion I feel comes from my difficulty letting go. Perhaps I'm grieving the loss of schizophrenia. I must admit, this is shameful to say, because when you awaken from something, it's supposed to feel like a positive experience, and in some ways, it is. I'm grateful that I can engage with the outer world and truly connect with people. I feel that my life is heading in the right direction, but at the same time, I miss disappearing into my inner world because that's where I feel at home, not in the real world.

But to answer your question. The three layers in my experience of space are my old more destructive lifeworld of space that I described at the start, the second space seems to be a narrative space where space moves extremely fast, and all the stories of my life, childhood, artist life, friends, talks, impressions are intermingled in a cacophony of thoughts, voices and sensory impressions clash and this space is very chaotic and the third space is the present place where things are slowed down and things appear as they appear, meaning that I feel I am seeing objects and people for the first time, everything is very bright and sometimes overwhelming. The confusing part is that these three layers shift throughout the day. Giovanni, when you feel anguish and you are deprived of will and trapped how does this condition dissolve again? Do you wait it out? or?

Giovanni: Sometimes, fortunately rarely, space for me is like concrete, or like amber in which a butterfly is trapped as I explained, where my body cannot move. It is as if space adheres to my body like resin and finally enters inside me and deprives me of all will. This, in addition to hurting me a lot when I experienced it, made me realise something that I think is very important. That is, that emotions are embodied and situated in space and time. I mean that it is wrong to talk abstractly about emotions, and that to understand an emotion it is necessary to describe it as a bodily sensation of heaviness or lightness, constriction or openness etc., situated in a space that oppresses or dilates the body etc., and time that comes to a halt or is indefinitely prolonged etc. I call this 'choreography of emotions' and use it with my patients when we talk about their moods.

But I haven't answered you yet, and I don't want to evade your question. The real answer is that I don't know, I can't tell how this oppressive cloak dissolves. I do know that it goes away as it came. It is as if I can lift my head above it and look at things—my situation—from above. See me *in situation*, I could say. That is, to understand, or even intuit, the connection between my feeling oppressed and my life. Between what is happening in my life and my distress. Here: I can see in the folds of this dense and heavy atmosphere something that concerns me. Paradoxically, I can understand something more about myself thanks to this oppression.

It may sound romantic, but I believe that my emotions, if I try to decipher them and 'navigate' them, rather than 'regulate' or eliminate them, are the stars, the sextant and the sea horizon that help me understand who I am, where I am and where I am going to.

Cæcilie: Giovanni, your approach of patience and staying calm in the eye of the storm, observing and lifting your head above the situation, and, not least, as I read it, staying grounded in your body and navigating your emotions is a gentle, curious and kind response to where you are in your life. You're allowing this atmospheric undercurrent to simply be as it is. Your way of being reminds me a lot of how dancers approach movement. In contemporary dance classes, we often begin with grounding exercises to centre the body. The purpose is to create a foundation a core so we can fully express ourselves when creating wild or unconventional movements, while always having a safe place to return to. This helps us avoid losing ourselves (getting injured) much like you describe with your emotions: always coming back to who you are and choosing to navigate them rather than regulate or suppress them. Giovanni, you also speak about oppressive atmospheres and how they can become meaningful. In dance, we often use tension and resistance in space as expressive tools rather than obstacles. This beautifully aligns with your idea of emotional heaviness as a source of insight so what you do is indeed a choreography of emotions.

Lorenzo: Giovanni, I can relate to many of the feelings that you described: it is the experience of space I have when I am not delusional or hallucinatory. I want to stress your last point, mainly that space is determined by the body. Here two remarks come up. The first is this: are you sure the body is the *primum movens* of our experience of the world? Couldn't it be the other way around? After all it was Merleau-Ponty (one of your favourite phenomenologists…) who said that what saves man from insanity is the structure of his space 'What protects the sane man against delirium or hallucination, is not his critical powers, but the structure of his space […]" [1]. The second, and linked to the first, is that, as I said, making myself coincide with my geometrical body makes me feel a bit of the 'sheer space' experience, because being incarnated in a living body makes it disappear because it is too risky to live with it!

Giovanni: Can you argue, with your psychopathological experiences, the point you make about the primacy of space?

Lorenzo: I'll surely try! You see, space is the residue of reality that is preserved when every other experience of the world is gone, consumed. Heidegger would say that the world is prior to space: space is accessible only if the environment is deprived of worldhood and it is also constitutive of the world (the spatiality of being-there is a condition of possibility of space). Because being-there is being-in-the-world, it makes room for the being of entities: every entity has its place within the whole meaningfulness that constitutes the world; when entities have found their place, we can abstract from the spatial involvement that determines their place, and their places are reduced to a multiplicity of positions for random things... So, for Heidegger's early philosophy as expressed in *Being and Time*, 'space' lurks behind 'world(hood)'.

Cæcilie: Very interesting; Lorenzo, but can you explain a bit what worldhood means in the context of Heidegger's *Being and Time* and how it relates to your experiences of space?

Lorenzo: Of course. You see, in his first *opus* Heidegger speaks of worldhood as the referential totality of relations, signs and involvements that constitutes a structure of significance, otherwise that which makes possible a world as an encompassing horizon within which being-there can first engage in its various pursuits and activities. The unity of both is at the same time the projection of the nexus of involvements and the horizon of the self's possibilities: as this referential whole, worldhood provides the structure for the disclosure of any specific world.

Cæcilie: So, what about space in itself?

Lorenzo: Space for Heidegger is conceivable if we bring out the German word for it, that is, *Raum*. In German *Raum* means both space and 'room', but a roomy room. He is very influenced by the word-field of *Raum*. For this, *Dasein* is spatial in a way no other extended thing is: it clears space around it to give itself 'leeway' or elbowroom; make room for its own *Spielraum*. Other things occupy or 'take up' space, while *Dasein*—in the literal sense—takes space in.

Giovanni: These are all engaging points, but what Heidegger talks about is the 'normal' experience of space. After giving a philosophical, even a metaphysical colour to all that, what are your experiences of space that are so linked to Heidegger's discourse?

Lorenzo: Heidegger's reflections are important because they highlight how experiencing space directly is of a pathological or fringe nature: lived space is what residues when all other lived-world structure vanishes, and what you are left is space in itself.

Giovanni: I imagine, from what you say, that what you are referring to is something you have experienced.

Lorenzo: Of course, I do, quite often, I must say.

Cæcilie: And what is this experience? Please tell us more so that I can say if what you say relates to my own experiences.

Lorenzo: It is like being sucked in myself and in myself found myself in this space. All things of the world are channelled through the body, they are consumed through the body, and in the end the body itself is being consumed, and it lets only the space itself. It is an infinite and indefinite space, that is, a space without any salience and points of reference; it is dark and void, with only a star-like lumen in the distance. You feel a sense of nausea for the void: it is terrible (in the sense of scary) and fascinating at the same time, much like the underlying themes of William Blake's (2019) [2] poetry and lithographs. Do you know the poem 'The Tyger'?

Tyger Tyger, burning bright,
In the forests of the night;
What immortal hand or eye,
Could frame thy fearful symmetry?

In what distant deeps or skies.
Burnt the fire of thine eyes?
On what wings dare he aspire?

What the hand, dare seize the fire?

And what shoulder, & what art,
Could twist the sinews of thy heart?
And when thy heart began to beat.
What dread hand? & what dread feet?

What the hammer? what the chain,
In what furnace was thy brain?
What the anvil? what dread grasp.
Dare its deadly terrors clasp?

When the stars threw down their spears
And water'd heaven with their tears:
Did he smile his work to see?
Did he who made the Lamb make thee?

Tyger Tyger burning bright,
In the forests of the night:
What immortal hand or eye,
Dare frame thy fearful symmetry?

The tiger is a symbol of this romantic feeling of attraction and repulsion: it is beautiful and at the same time very dangerous to come close to it. My pathological experience of space is very much like it…

Cæcilie: I am familiar with the poem, Lorenzo, and what the speaker (or humanity) asks in it are existential questions about life, death and good and evil. The tiger can be understood as simultaneously God's creation or Satan's. Linking it to your experience of space, I think you've captured the underlying atmosphere of the poem well—this repulsion and attraction you feel. But I can't help but think that what lies in the undercurrent of your experience of space is exactly this struggle on an emotional and existential level. 'It is dark and void, with only a star-like lumen in the distance. You feel a sense of nausea for the void: it is terrible (in the sense of scary)'. The 'nausea void' in feeling the pull of the unspeakable (death?), while the 'star-like lumen in the distance' is the wanting, hoping for 'lumen' enlightenment and life and what your soul wants, needs, and feels. I will now hang my literary hat and use my schizophrenic way of thinking instead because this 'rawness of being' of a self is exactly what schizophrenic lifeworlds are like, life is stripped down to the bones, there are no filters, everything hits you and as you say, Lorenzo, 'All things of the world are channelled through the body, they are consumed through the body. And in the end the body itself is being consumed' the entity or corporeal being of you is left barren. I get the image of tumbleweed, and the sound of the wind in a desert as an image of the schizophrenic disembodied soul. I understand this feeling very well. I think where my experience differentiates from yours, Lorenzo, is that through my dance training, I have been able to ground and stay in my body (at least half of the day) and express these overwhelming feelings of despair and fear into a creative outlet in space and often transform them into a state of becoming something else. But after work, this grounding would dissolve and separate my soul from my body and then the rustling wind and tumbleweed would overtake and leave me exposed again to the forces of the world.

Giovanni: Lorenzo, knowing you and your metaphysical mind, I think you can further elaborate yours and Cæcilie's experience of space in an even more philosophical nature, don't you?

Lorenzo: I think I can make an analogy with Heidegger's conceptualisation of 'Being' after the *Kehre*, when he thought of Being as Event… but, I will follow the lesson of Binswanger in showing my view taking Heidegger's ontological arguments in an ontic way… Because I think that in the psychopathology of schizophrenia space operates in the same vein as late Heidegger's Being. Space is a hidden, foundational reality, that, when it offers itself, it offers itself by cancelling itself. Heidegger's Being is thought of as the sheer presentation of various entities, and when it offers this entity to the presentation it reveals itself by retreating, so when there is, in fact there is not, because it embodies the entities of worldhood by bringing them about, but during this presentation of entities it retreats in the shadows and it stops manifesting itself. Space is much like that: when the object of worldhood is in front of you, space is an underlying principle that rests hidden; but when the entities of worldhood vanish, space emerges as the residue of being, that lives in the annihilation of the world….

Giovanni: I can only imagine this experience you have. I think this is why it is so difficult speaking about space, because to make experience of it every other thing must annihilate itself, and this is at the limit of life…

Cæcilie: Giovanni and Lorenzo, sorry to interrupt you, but I know you have a philosophical and metaphysical mindset and like your Binswanger and Heidegger, but before you disappear into the stratosphere and can't come back (no offense meant), I think what you are discussing is interesting. I am not well-versed in Heidegger or Binswanger, so sorry for changing the subject but the reason for doing this is that I kept thinking about free will when listening to you and where it is placed in the equation. I know some scholars think that free will is an illusion while others believe that we always have the ability to make our own choices and thereby acting accordingly, what are your thoughts on this matter?

Giovanni: Cæcilie, I imagine that what you mean is that schizophrenia, as it is known, interferes with your ability to control actions and thoughts. Your words invite me to wonder about the relationship between free will and the experience of space. Schizophrenic space, if it can be generalised in this way, seems to nullify any kind of freedom, collapsing onto a disembodied self; but, and perhaps at the same time, it also represents a kind of vacuum in which any action can be freely expressed. What I am wondering, also, is whether your beliefs in free will change when entering the schizophrenic space.

Lorenzo: Good point Cæcilie, I will reply following again Binswanger's reasoning. For him schizophrenic space is lived as more restricted and this correlates to a diminution of the degrees of freedom with a parallel invariability of the way of being until there is, in the extreme, a stiffening in a unique modality of existence surrounded by an atmosphere of deep and constant nagging. This materialises not only in a sense of proximity, but moreover in a contact 'too immediate' with what surrounds us (*Umwelt*) and who surrounds us (*Mitwelt*). For example, two of his patients, Ilse and Jurg Zund, make experiences of space as if enclosed in a single focal point, onto which oppressive, external influences converge.

Giovanni: Interesting, Lorenzo, but what about your experiences of space? How does this discourse by Binswanger relate to the 'sheer space' and Elvenspace? It seems to me that they lie outside these considerations...

Lorenzo: Yes, the 'sheer space' is far more radical than the experiences of schizophrenic space laid down by Binswanger. There is the same experience of collapsing space onto the person as a focal point of external nagging influences, but in my experience, space presents itself as an object, it reveals itself as space-object, and the body is thus suppressed, while in Binswanger's patients the body remains. At the same time, similarities come to the fore!

Cæcilie: And what about the Elvenspace? How does free will manifest itself, if it does?

Lorenzo: You know, there is a contrast between the 'sheer space' experience and the Elvenspace relating to freedom, both unrealistic: as the 'sheer space' subsumes the alienation of freedom, the Elvenspace is the source of an unconstrained liberty, where everything is possible, and there are no nagging influences (be they external or internal); the body, transformed as it is, still presides over a metamorphosis of space where the imperial ego of the schizophrenic is lived as omniscient and thus omnipotent and you feel an ecstatic degree of freedom, absolute, limitless. Both these experiences are irrealistic because the non-pathological way of freedom is the possibility of being free inside certain boundaries. In the 'sheer space' there is the annihilation of freedom and a passive way of being-in-the-world; whereas in the Elvenspace there is a sublimation of freedom and an active way of being-in-the-world.

17.6 Conclusion

The aim of this chapter was an exercise in dialogue grounded in mutual recognition, rather than a monologue of a 'normal' conscience speaking *about* a 'sick' conscience. It was intended as an exercise not an attempt to 'diagnose' mental illness. Our Trilogue focused on sharing and speaking from three individual perceptions of space. We have pointed out some key features of spatial experience and their existential meanings in the lifeworlds of Lorenzo Gilardi, Helene Cæcilie Mørck and Giovanni Stanghellini. The first two experienced space within the lifeworlds of schizophrenia, while the latter did not.

Our purpose was not a review of the literature, nor to compare what emerged from our exploration with the available literature. Rather, we are interested in the singular element, in the individual grasped in its *ecceity*. 'Ecceity'—a neologism deriving from the Latin 'haecce', which means 'this', 'these'—indicates the individuality of an object or a phenomenon, or its *this-ness*. In essence, 'ecceity' emphasises the particularity, the specific identity of something or someone, separating him from the other members of their category. Therefore, what we have reported has no claim to be paradigmatic because it is not taken as an exemplification of a concept that subsumes a series of individual phenomena. It is not even intended as a special case of a rule. Simply, we wanted to describe our experience with sincerity and intellectual honesty. It will be up to the Reader to decide whether what we have extracted from the comparison of our experiences has (or does not have) a generalisable meaning, applicable to a 'population' of patients or is indicative or enlightening about an aspect of human existence, psychopathological or not.

However, we can draw conclusions from our trilogue.

Firstly, the experience of space is almost ineffable. It requires a lot of ability to intuitively 'listen' and open up to one's feelings and sensations and to endure the disturbance that they bring with them. In addition, an uncommon linguistic ability is necessary to be able to tell one's experience of space.

Secondly, it is important to underline that these experiences can be shared through images much more than through concepts. Such images should not be taken as mere metaphors ('as if'), but literally as attempts to describe an experience.

A further point to be emphasised is that the way we experience space is closely related to the way we experience our body and its ability to move. And, also, the experience of space and the body correlate with the existential theme of freedom and will. This close relationship between lived space, freedom and will underlines how important it is to explore this dimension of the lifeworld for the care of people with schizophrenia.

While avoiding using the different experiences of space as symptoms, that is, as diagnostic indices useful to establish a nosographic diagnosis—in the psychopathological world experienced by persons with schizophrenia, we can find characteristic and specific experiences of space. We have presented two of them.

The 'sheer space' is an extreme experience whereby you experience space as if it were an object, with a hardness higher than a diamond's and a temperature of absolute zero. Regarding the first, you feel trapped into a diamond and you can't escape; regarding the second the space burns you for how icy it is. In this experience the body dissolves and the nexus body-world are substituted by the nexus self-space, where there is no telling what is inside or outside, and everything (external objects as well as thoughts or emotions) becomes a weapon that turns back on you.

The Elvenspace is of a different kind: the horizon changes in front of you, the scale of the world changes in front of you: instead of buildings and streets you walk among stars and galaxies, with an Olympic view of the cosmos, in which you feel connected to this higher space and your will is empowered by your absolute freedom. It is dimly lit, and sewn in your body, like the hair that becomes a crown of starlit gems. Everything becomes slower, and the body becomes slimmer and taller, like the life of a Tolkien Elf has come to possess you.

Last but not least, these experiences of space, despite being imbued with suffering, belong to a dialectical structure. That is, next to the negative side of the loss of freedom and suffering there is a positive side with respect to which the person with schizophrenia can have a sense of nostalgia. This dialectical structure is, perhaps, the only aspect we have highlighted that can be generalised to the majority of phenomena that are present in schizophrenic worlds. For instance, in hearing voices there is a negativity, that is that of losing the freedom of being able not to listen to them; but also, a positivity, for example finding in the voices an interlocutor who helps to develop one's thoughts. In delusions there is a negativity, that is that of losing the common world and closing oneself in a private and idiosyncratic world; but also, a positivity, that is, the reconstruction of a world starting from the intolerable experience of a non-world—of an empty, fragmented and incomprehensible world. So, also in the experience of space described in these pages there is a terrifying component that coexists with an electrifying component. Clinicians should be aware of this if they intend to treat people with schizophrenia.

Key Points
- This chapter challenges the prevailing methods in psychopathology that generalise symptom measurement across large populations, and focuses instead on individual experiences, highlighting the unique and singular nature of each person's condition.
- It introduces the concept of 'ecceity' (from Latin *haecce*, meaning 'this-ness') to highlight individuality and specificity in lived experience. This chapter looks at the perception of space and its existential meanings in the lifeworld of three individuals: Lorenzo Gilardo, Helene Cæcilie Mørck and Giovanni Stanghellini. The first two have lived experience with schizophrenia, while the latter is an expert by profession.
- This text moves away from traditional literature review or clinical approaches and centres on *testimony* and *narrative* as valid forms.
- It emphasises dialogue between 'experts by experience' (those living with schizophrenia) and 'experts by profession' (clinicians or researchers) and aims at mutual understanding, where the individual voices amplify rather than overshadow each other.
- It frames the chapter aim as an *exercise in dialogue* and *mutual recognition*, as opposed to a monologue of a 'normal' conscience on a 'sick' conscience and as an exercise of mutual understanding—as opposed to an operation aimed at 'diagnosing' a mental illness.

References

1. Merleau-Ponty M. Phenomenology of perception. London (UK): Routledge; 1958.
2. Blake W. Songs of innocence and of experience. Hampshire: Pan Macmillan; 2019.

Open Access This chapter is licensed under the terms of the Creative Commons Attribution 4.0 International License (http://creativecommons.org/licenses/by/4.0/), which permits use, sharing, adaptation, distribution and reproduction in any medium or format, as long as you give appropriate credit to the original author(s) and the source, provide a link to the Creative Commons license and indicate if changes were made.

The images or other third party material in this chapter are included in the chapter's Creative Commons license, unless indicated otherwise in a credit line to the material. If material is not included in the chapter's Creative Commons license and your intended use is not permitted by statutory regulation or exceeds the permitted use, you will need to obtain permission directly from the copyright holder.

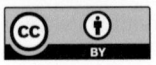

Part V

Mental Health Services: Reality and Ambition

This part looks at the history and ambitions of psychiatry with respect to theories of psychiatry and the practical development of mental health services. Both in relation to Kraepelin and beyond, it surveys a range of countries and regions across the world during the twentieth century.

Chapter 18 outlines Kraepelin's influence in India where it reinforced a biomedical approach. Chapter 19 describes his more varied reception in Soviet psychiatry including finally his rejection under Stalin. Chapter 20 describes how Yugoslavia, caught in the middle between East and West during the Cold War and grappling with its internal complex composition, contributed in a unique way to transcultural psychiatry during the post WWII period of decolonisation. Chapter 21 describes diverse de-insititutionalisation and community care processes in Western Europe and the theories that underpinned them. Chapter 22 reports on how Latin America, influenced by the ideas of Italian psychiatrist Franco Basaglia but also other professional traditions, has made significant advances in rights-based mental health care guided by the Caracas Declaration.

Emil Kraepelin's Influence in India

18

Sanjeev Jain

18.1 Introduction: A Prodrome in the Nineteenth Century

From the modest beginnings in late eighteenth century, contemporary psychiatry, both as a discipline and as a service, had made a hesitant progress over the nineteenth century in south Asia. 'Lunatic asylums' were established in various corners of the subcontinent towards the end of the eighteenth century as the Empire extended to provide care and custody of the mentally ill. Medical colleges, dispensaries and a rudimentary health system began to take shape. European doctors seeking appointment in India were expected to have worked in an asylum for a few months and obtained a certificate of proficiency and have a passing knowledge of one or more languages of the region [1]. By mid-nineteenth century, medical graduates from the newly established medical colleges in India were often employed in the asylums and there was some interest in creating an academic discourse of psychiatry [2]. There had always been a rather quick adoption of trends in Europe and the UK to practice in India, and almost all Native kingdoms from the Mughals in the north to the Wodeyars in the south employed European doctors for the Palace. Charles Smith, starting life as a doctor in Bangalore in the 1830s, could already quote Esquirol and Pinel in his notes to encourage the establishment of psychiatric services [3]. A copy of the 'Treatise on Insanity' written by Pinel [4], and published in Sheffield in 1806, was one of the acquisitions of the first public library at Uttarpara in India in 1859, suggesting that these ideas of insanity were considered of sufficient public interest.

While many of these changes were initiated by doctors employed by the East India Company, and later, the Crown, the facilities and conditions in the asylums lagged far behind those of Europe, as did provisions for care of the mentally ill. Doctors graduating from the newly established medical colleges in India like Chetan Shah, Nathu Lal, Saadat Ali and Gopal Das, helped manage the asylums, and run

S. Jain (✉)
Department of Psychiatry, National Institute of Mental Health and Neurosciences (NIMHANS), Bangalore, India

© The Author(s) 2026
G. Ikkos, T. Becker (eds.), *Psychiatry after Kraepelin*,
https://doi.org/10.1007/978-3-032-09475-9_18

their practices, which helped disseminate these ideas about insanity. However, since they also had to accommodate the ideas prevalent at that time in Indian society, the boundaries between the 'European' ideas about madness and the 'unmada' and 'deewangee' (Ayurvedic and Unani terms for madness) of traditional medical systems were often blurred [5]. The Indian doctors were always in subordinate positions (as a matter of colonial policy) and their contributions to academic discourse were limited. There were glimmers of engagement with the wider scientific world with scientists like JC Bose (Cambridge), PC Ray (Edinburgh), ML Sircar, and the activities of the Delhi College, the fledgling Calcutta, Madras and Aligarh Universities and the increasing number of medical colleges that popularised science among the people [6–9].

The control of infectious disease (cholera, plagues and famine stalked the country) and public health was the major preoccupation of medical services [10]. The asylums in India, unlike Europe in the nineteenth century, had a relatively marginal acceptance in the health systems; stuck as they often were between the gaol and the hospitals. One of the early handbooks had suggested that rates of mental illness were lower, and their nature different, as the mind of 'Hindus' (the residents of India) was primitive, which was now facing modernity and intellectual stimulation after centuries of torpor [11]. This allegation of a civilisational disparity was robustly rebutted by Forbes Winslow, who felt that this was a most inaccurate assumption. This was quite in contrast to the debates and discussions in Europe at that time, where the reforms of the nineteenth century gradually evolved [12]. This disparity in services was sharply critiqued at the end of the nineteenth century, when McDowall noted that India was 'lamentably behind as to provision for the care of the mentally afflicted', [13] compounded by the fact that most of those managing the asylums were retired Army officers in civilian employ and 'not a man in India has devoted such attention to mental disease and asylum administration as to deserve the name of a specialist'.

18.1.1 Professional Psychiatrists: The Beginnings in South Asia Pre-first World War

The creation of specialists in Europe and the UK had been encouraged by the growth of academic psychiatry which had seen a great transformation over the nineteenth century. The 'science' of psychiatry was being formulated and formal training and research had begun to be encouraged, but the gap between the colonies and Europe had widened considerably. The ideas of continental psychiatry, especially those of Kraepelin and his predecessors, had quickly become commonplace in teaching and practice in the UK. These developments, of which Kraepelin's work is the focus here, perhaps had far reaching impact, even in India, as medical services and education had close links with the UK.

One of the first textbooks of psychiatry for the practising doctor in India [14], published in 1908, already shows considerable familiarity with Kraepelin's ideas from the early editions of his book. 'Classic' Kraepelinian manifestations of melancholic stupor, characterised by retarded movement, hesitant speech, rigidity and constipation, arising from an 'impediment to the exertion of the will', are described. Dr. Ewens is unsure whether all the forms of melancholia described by Kraepelin are as frequent; and in his observation, those with recurrent episodes of melancholia without mania were common too, as were those who gradually lapsed into dementia. Presenile forms of insanity, marked by fanciful delusions, often of a persecutory and hypochondriacal nature, were also observed. Diagnostic terms like catatonic and hebephrenic forms of dementia praecox, delusional insanity, melancholia, recurrent and chronic mania were used to describe individual cases, suggesting that the entities described by Kraepelin at the end of the nineteenth century had come into use within a few years in India [15, 16]. Dr. Ewens had developed a deep interest in neurobiology while a registrar at King's College Hospital in England [17] and it is thus no surprise that Kraepelin's ideas of a fundamental 'organic' aetiology of mental illness held appeal. He had worked for a few years in Sikkim and helped introduce Western medicine into Tibetan society, as well as being part of the White Commission to demarcate the Sikkim-Tibet border before moving to the Punjab [18]. He also attended the international meeting on Assistance to Lunatics in Milan, in 1906 [19] and seems to have connected the trends in Europe, to his work in India. His sudden death, just before the First World War, was deeply mourned.

This book was followed in quick succession by another one [20] by Overbeck-Wright in 1912. Dr. Overbeck-Wright wrote this soon after his arrival in India and it reflected, as he admits, his training in Aberdeen and several books, including those by Craepelin (sic). The book is designed to educate the clinicians about the provision of the Indian Lunacy Act of 1912, and only secondarily discuss the nature of psychiatric disease. Dr. Overbeck-Wright is quite convinced that a large proportion of the cases arise from autointoxication, infections or drugs of abuse. Following previous work by Bruce, he finds merit in correlating changes in blood counts and blood pressure, with symptoms of insanity. This is quite like Kraepelin's observations of a fundamental metabolic alteration, characterised by changes in body weight, pulse, blood pressure and even leucocyte composition [21]. He objects to the groupings Kraepelin proposes, as he feels that delusional insanity is quite distinct from catatonia and hebephrenia, since the latter begins at a young age and more often has an organic aetiology, while delusional insanities had 'not a single feature in common' except a tendency to occur in those with a 'neurotic heredity'. He feels that the usual British notions of insanity are more appropriate than those proposed by Kraepelin. However, he also admits that Kraepelin's classification is on sounder footing than that proposed by Kahlbaum. He is familiar with Kraepelin's estimates of recovery (very poor in hebephrenia), and suggests that 'degeneracy' caused by consanguinity and early marriage could be contributing factors, but very sceptical about the contributions of an exposure to 'modern civilised life' to the risk of insanity. Both Ewens and Overbeck-Wright felt that mental illness in India was broadly consistent with patterns seen in the UK. However, the ideas of Wise and the growing preoccupation with race and diversity, kept these discussions about the role of culture, and the nature of mind alive. The impact of these ideas on cultural psychiatry was to find an echo in Kraepelin, and many other psychiatrists in India.

By early twentieth century, other ideas from Germany and Europe were also beginning to exert an influence. In a harsh critique of Overbeck-Wright, one anonymous reviewer pointed out that the ideas of Janet, Freud, Jung etc. were conspicuous by their absence, and that psychosocial causes were totally neglected [22]. In response, Dr. Overbeck-Wright suggested that his attention to toxaemia and organic aetiologies was more likely to be useful in cases of 'real insanity' rather than ideas of repressed sexuality and subconscious mechanisms, which were dubious in any case. Wright refers to these ideas as 'unsavoury' or attempting to add 'new graft on a rotten, worm-eaten stump' [23].

These disparate, and often discordant, debates about the nature of insanity and psychological processes were presented as separate papers by Ewens, Overbeck-Wright and Owen Berkeley-Hill in the October 1914 issue of the Indian Medical Gazette. To an extent, these reflected the debates in Europe and the relative value of models being proposed by Kraepelin, Freud and others. Ewens advocated a medical model, with toxaemia, degeneracy, tainted heredity and neuropathic traits as being proximate factors. He also noted the paucity of data to show that psychological processes alone could lead to the various forms of insanity, namely manic-depressive insanity, dementia praecox and paranoia [24]. Evidently, the basic definitions suggested by Kraepelin were thus quite entrenched by then. Overbeck-Wright [25], after describing known infections (GPI), intoxicants (cannabis, opium and cocaine), heat (Mott; eds: see below), heredity (Mendel, Galton and Pearson) as proximate causes of insanity, goes on to briefly describe issues of repression and conversion, but concludes that 'there is no need to occupy space by unnecessarily expounding it'. Berkeley-Hill [26], a self-confessed admirer of psychoanalysis who maintained a lifelong correspondence with Ernest Jones, described how the dynamics of the unconscious could produce symptoms of hysteria, obsessive-compulsive disorder and paranoia. The psychological explanations offered by Berkeley-Hill extended, as was often the case in the early twentieth century Freudian writings, from paranoid symptoms and the lack of insight in alcoholics, to the sudden elation in some of those suffering from cancer; as examples of reaction—formation and projection. These extrapolations obviously stood in contrast to Kraepelin's impression that the whole edifice of psychoanalysis was based on 'the representation of arbitrary assumptions and conjectures as assured facts' [27]. These dissensions were not quite resolved, and Overbeck-Wright and Berkeley-Hill soon got involved in the First World War, and the events in Europe are another aspect of the story.

The First World War had far-reaching consequences for psychiatry in the subcontinent [28]. Indian doctors often ended up serving as officers on the battlefield; while medical and mental symptoms in soldiers (from India) who fought on behalf of the King and Empire also came to attention. This was also the time that the Institute of Psychiatry was established by Kraepelin in Munich. Soon after the War, the authorities in London began planning improvement in psychiatric education (and services) for the Empire by creating a hub for research and education at the Maudsley [29]. Edward Mapother, the driving force behind this transformation of the Maudsley, admired Emil Kraepelin greatly and wrote a fulsome eulogy on his death [30]. Doctors from all over India were sent to the UK to train as specialists [31] and became teachers and leaders all over the region. Despite the War, and the strong antipathy of Kraepelin towards Anglo-Saxon psychiatry, professional contacts between the German schools and the UK were quite strong.

18.1.2   Kraepelin: The Lasting Influence in the Inter-War Years

Francis XC Noronha, a medical officer with the Kingdom of Mysore who had also seen active service in the First World War, was one of the first medical men deputed to study at the Maudsley. He completed his DPM and was introduced to the Royal College by Sir Frederick Mott. Sir Mott wanted to emulate the Institute of Psychiatry established by Kraepelin and was quite appreciative of Kraepelin's work. On his return to Bangalore, Dr. Noronha began keeping detailed clinical notes as was the practice at Maudsley and described a series of cases of dementia praecox [32], and noted that the term had been recently adopted at most asylums in India. He notes that there is 'great degree of doubt as to what exactly constitutes dementia praecox' but patients tended to wander around aimlessly, be indifferent and 'regress to earlier levels of mental life'. He describes two cases with mutism and severe withdrawal (perhaps the catatonic form), who recovered well enough. On the other hand, the most common diagnosis was the 'hebephrenic' type; and management included providing the family 'sound advice to regarding their dealings with him'. Describing cases admitted in 1925, Noronha finds that the Kraepelinian classification appears to be the 'most practicable one in the present state of our knowledge' and notes that patients could most often be diagnosed as suffering from manic-depressive insanity, dementia praecox and paranoid psychosis.

Dr. CJ Lodge-Patch of the Indian Medical Service, following in in the footsteps of his father and grandfather as an 'India-hand', began his career as a medical officer in the Army and became the Superintendent of the Mental Hospital as well as Lecturer in Mental Diseases at the King Edward Medical College, at Lahore. His textbook, a compilation of the lectures being delivered at the College, was intended [33] as a practical handbook for practitioners of psychiatry in India. The book was favourably reviewed. As the BMJ noted, it 'follows closely the teachings of Kraepelin. It is evident that Major Lodge-Patch is deeply interested in his work, sympathetic to his patients, and anxious to stimulate his students to take a real and permanent interest in the problem of mental disease' [34]. Interest in Kraepelin's classification, and the whole approach to the patient, also was amplified by the experience of the Indian psychiatrists in the UK.

Owen Berkeley-Hill, by now the Superintendent of the Ranchi European Mental Hospital, was described by Mapother [35] as having the 'sharpest mind', but his impish wit and admiration for psychoanalysis, as also a deep engagement with Indian political and social situation [36], made him somewhat suspect in the eyes of the officialdom. He had travelled to the USA in 1929 to attend the Psychological Congress at Yale and visited many prominent centres. He recalls that his American hosts recounted that Emil Kraepelin had visited only recently and displayed 'an almost incredible want of civility and tact'; and a prime example was his announcement on the last day that it was the happiest day of his life, 'as he was returning to Germany!' Berkeley-Hill had collaborated with Kraepelin [37] a few years before on a study of syphilis in India (a subject that Kraepelin had interrogated while on this trip to the USA in 1925).

In an early textbook of psychiatry, perhaps the first by an India-born physician [38], Norman Pacheco adopts the Kraepelinian definitions of dementia praecox, manic-depressive insanity and paranoia as the major 'biogenic' psychoses, wherein heredity is the major factor, whereby 'in those who escape amentia, the next pitfall is dementia praecox, and the two states may be combined or follow one another'. He suggests that childhood development and temperament, and the recognition of early signs and symptoms should be understood in the context of the later development of the full syndromes. This book combines Freudian insights, functional neurology and Kraepelinian ideas and offers psychoanalysis, sedatives, hydrotherapy and barbiturates as treatment. All this suggests that ideas prevalent in Europe were commonplace in India too at the same time. Pacheco had, elsewhere, also commented on the favourable effects of extracts from the Rauwolffia plant, which had been researched extensively in India by Sen and Bose in Calcutta [39] and Salimuzzaman Siddiqui in Delhi and Aligarh [40]. Scientific and technical exchanges with Europe were thus commonplace.

By the 1930s, events in Europe had also induced many scientists and clinicians to move to the UK and the USA. These included people like Sigmund Freud, Willi Mayer-Gross and many others. Psychiatrists in India by then were familiar with trends in Europe [41] and the career and ideas of JE Dhunjibhoy are a testament to that [42]. Dhunjibhoy travelled extensively in Europe, as his father-in-law was a professor of Persian in Berlin, and met many psychiatrists, from von Meduna to Freud. Others, like MV Govindaswamy, who pioneered somatic treatments at the Mysore State Mental Hospital in Bangalore like insulin coma, cardiazol convulsions and psychosurgery, developed a close friendship with Mayer-Gross while at the Maudsley. Edward Mapother, on a visit to south Asia, reviewed several mental hospitals in India, rated them on a scale of 'badness', and met many of the staff who had worked and trained at the Maudsley over the decade and a half. Frederick Mott, Edward Mapother and other contemporaries like Willy Mayer-Gross, Eliot Slater, Frederick Golla who were active at the Maudsley at that time were quite 'Kraeplinian' in their outlook. The experiences of these first specialists for India were thus, understandably, influenced by these ideas. The running of the mental health services in British India was by then often soundly criticised [43] and in many instances it was felt that the independent states like Mysore had better services for the mentally ill [44], and were thus better suited to become a centre for post-graduate training and research in independent India. This led to the establishment of the All India Institute of Mental Health (AIIMH) at Bangalore in Mysore in 1954, and prominent psychiatrists like Mayer-Gross, Hoenig (who translated Jaspers' General Psychopathology into English) and Lieberman from the Institute of Neurology at Queens Square were deputed through the World Health Organization (WHO) to establish the teaching and research agenda [45]. These interactions thus entrenched many of Kraepelin's ideas into academic psychiatry in India.

18.1.3   Biological Basis: Kraepelin's Ideas on Syphilis, Heredity and Eugenics in Mid-twentieth-Century India

Dr. Wise, at the Asylum in Dacca, Bengal, was one of the earliest to suggest that General Paralysis of the Insane (GPI) was an 'unfrequent (sic) appearance in Indian asylums', unlike in the European asylums (in India), despite Indians being exposed to similar causes as in Europe [46]. These ideas about the 'native' mind and its susceptibility to (or resistance) were often shared across the asylums of the region (the Indian asylums extended from Singapore to Peshawar). At a time when the bacterial origins of syphilis were not known, these differences provoked intense curiosity. These asylum reports were read all over the world and perhaps contributed to Kraepelin's interest in cultural differences. In any case, he was more interested in careful clinical observations, which were not easily available in Europe itself, and even more so in the colonies. In response to a request from Kolb and Kraepelin, in 1922 [37], Owen Berkeley-Hill created a questionnaire to survey the extent of syphilis in India, and all over the world. Though no firm conclusions could be drawn, the responses collected suggested marked differences between various parts of India (from no cases of GPI being detected in Tezpur and Benares, to being common in Bombay and Poona), as also across the world. However, by then the Wasserman test had been introduced in Ranchi [47] and Mysore [48], and the ethnic and racial differences could now be attributed to differences in social practices. Whether Kraepelin himself reviewed the data provided by Berkeley-Hill is unclear, as his ideas about parasyphilis and the role of culture and civilisation in the genesis of GPI did not seem to reflect this south Asian data.

Kraepelin felt that 'degeneration' was a factor in dementia praecox, as it was often accompanied by both physical and psychic peculiarities, accompanied by a hereditary predisposition. His ideas were informed by the several family-based assessments that were made at the various asylums, and extended by his collaborators and researchers like Ernst Rüdin. By the mid-1920s, researchers in India were also commenting on the hereditary basis of dementia praecox, especially in certain communities that were both 'in-bred' and highly westernised [49]. This contributed to a debate on the genetic factors being a primary cause, as much as 'civilisational' change (an idea explored by Kraepelin [50] too). The idea that exposure to 'European' dynamism was fraught with risk for the somnolent Asian society in torpor and the civilisational trauma that it engendered was a popular [11] though controversial [51] motif in early British writing.

A tendency for insanity to run in families had been noted quite early in India [2], but by the end of the nineteenth century issues of regional, racial and tribal differences had also become apparent [52]. Consanguinity was often blamed [53] and while some suggested that inbreeding did not adequately explain the occurrence of insanity [54], others suggested that westernisation and social progress did [55].

Kraepelin also commented on the risk of dementia praecox by 'injury to the germ' by birth order or by extraneous agents such as alcoholism or infections such as syphilis. These debates suggest that by the 1920s, dementia praecox as a syndrome and a disease entity was already incorporated into the framework of psychiatric practice in India [56].

These ideas of hereditary influences on mental illness were also informed by ideas from Britain and the work of Pearson, Galton, Mott and others, and laid the foundations of the eugenics movement in India. The ideas of 'race' genetics and moral decay found some audience in India, and Eugenics societies were established in Lahore, Bombay and Solapur. Although these did not directly refer to insanity as such, they agreed with the impression that the 'number of insane can be halved within 50 years if they were prevented from procreating' [57]. Prominent psychiatrists like Jal Dhunjibhoy strongly recommended eugenic sterilisation of all known adult 'defectives' of both sexes, as this was already adopted by a 'number of civilised countries, and it rids the race of its defective germ plasm' [58]. A specific commitment for 'sterilization of persons suffering from transmissible diseases of a serious nature', such as insanity or epilepsy, was recommended soon after Independence, as it had been suggested by the Planning Commission earlier [59]. However, unlike their European counterparts, formal studies on the familial aggregation or models of inheritance were not attempted. The numbers in the mental hospitals were only a minority of those ill, and since public health services did not exist, the kind of debates about costs and eugenics did not excite the same urgency as they had in Nazi Germany and Europe. Perhaps the inherent complexity of social life in India and its infinite sub-divisions prevented this [60], but many of the supporters of these eugenic societies continued to wield influence in post-independence India, and many parliamentary debates had a pronounced eugenic flavour. This has perhaps contributed to a widespread, and tacit acceptance of forced sterilisation both in the community and in institutional settings.

18.2   Kraepelin in Late Twentieth Century India

The latter half of the twentieth century was marked both by decolonisation and deinstitutionalisation. In India, in any case, there had never been adequate institutional care, but the number of patients in mental hospitals has gradually declined, and the care of the severe mental illness is almost entirely family and community based. The widespread use of anti-psychotics and anti-depressants, since they became widely available in the 1950s, transformed the nature of psychiatric treatment. The differences in the nature and outcomes of schizophrenia, a theme first explored by Kraepelin, were highlighted by the International Pilot Study of Schizophrenia (IPSS) [61], where India was one of the participating sites. The impression that dementia praecox (schizophrenia) has a milder course in non-European settings continues to be debated vigorously. Kraepelin had suggested that the risk of dementia praecox and manic-depressive insanity was accompanied both by a higher incidence of these syndromes in relatives and by a neuropathic (subthreshold) traits in the family. Estimates of familial risk have been attempted often, with an increasing array of empirical markers, to identify high-risk subjects [62, 63], and also confirm familial aggregation of these syndromes [64]. The peculiar 'psychic' and 'physical' peculiarities have often been explored in India in the form of minor physical anomalies, as well as physiological and imaging parameters [65]. However, it is also becoming apparent that, as far as neuropsychological deficits, endophenotypes, neuroimaging or genetic studies can tell us, these diagnostic categories may not be as distinct as Kraepelin had proposed.

18.3   Conclusion: Ripples from a Century Ago

Modern psychiatric services were introduced into South Asia in the end of the eighteenth century, in the form of asylums, just a few years after they had been established in the USA. Over the past two centuries these have gradually extended to several hundred medical colleges and general hospital psychiatry units and thousands of psychiatrists in the private sector. Most of this explosive growth has occurred after Independence. This spread of European and Anglo-Saxon psychiatry, though initiated through colonial expansion, was not linear or unidirectional, as there had been a long history of exchange between Europe, the Middle East and Asia for several millennia. The rapid developments in psychiatry during the nineteenth century, it was assumed, would lead to secularisation of the mind [66], as had been attempted for the body (though, even that, patchily) under colonial rule [67]. The mid-nineteenth century, for all its political upheavals, also introduced medical colleges and hospitals into the landscape of India. Doctors from Europe, America as well as Britain worked here and Indian students began accessing universities in the 'West'. From Honigsberger, who established a lunatic asylum in Lahore for the Sikh empire [68], to the popularity of mesmerism in Calcutta [69] and Hahnemann's homeopathy [70], both Continental and British ideas became commonplace. The interaction with the growing body of Indian professionals, as much as the response of the community at large, thus resulted in a very multifaceted development. Although colonial subjugation was a political fact, science and medicine in India continued to adapt, and adopt, many ideas. It must be remembered that the very establishment of a hospital (including a mental hospital) was widely appreciated by the public at large, especially the poor, as almost all hospitals were quickly over-subscribed.

The transformations in European psychiatry, especially at the turn of the nineteenth century, emphasised a search for a biomedical foundation for psychiatry. This, in a sense, contributed to an essentialist and bleak view as, in the absence of any viable treatments, those with mental illness became marginalised and stigmatised, as in Nazi Germany. Although Kraepelin had suggested, emphatically, that these classifications may be transient, till better understanding emerged, they became an article of faith. The change towards an emphasis on social and community psychiatry, especially in the aftermath of the Second World War, suggested that diagnostic categories had lost their relevance as they harked back to what Aubrey

Lewis had commented on as the 'pessimistic' aura that a diagnosis of dementia praecox generated. This attitude was reflected in the cautious approach to Kraepelinian ideas by Overbeck-Wright and many of the early leaders in India.

Both Keki Masani [71] and David Satyanand [72], in the 1950s, paid greater attention to social and psychological issues in India as being critical to psychiatric services, as they were being developed after the strain and conflicts that accompanied Independence. This period also saw the discovery of anti-psychotics and anti-depressants and these drug treatments were quickly adopted in clinical practice in south Asia. However, research into the biological antecedents and correlates was slower off the mark and Kraepelinian ideas about the dichotomous psychoses and the nature of classification became almost reified, though not without some scepticism [73]. The International Pilot study of Schizophrenia (IPSS) study of outcomes of schizophrenia, which relied on a standardised definition, that in turn adhered to the Kraepelinian syndromes, suggested that both the symptoms and outcomes differed across cultures (including within India [61]), thus giving a nod to a question that Kraepelin tried to address in his studies in Java (Indonesia) (Eds: see Chaps. 4 and 5). Moreover, as structured criteria and assessments began to standardise diagnosis and achieve some degree of inter-rater reliability, these neo-Kraepelinian methods again came into prominence. Establishing the boundaries of schizophrenia, bipolar disorder, delusional and obsessional disorders became a concern. Typical concerns included whether unipolar or bipolar disorder shared both clinical and familial characteristics [74], or whether schizophrenia had distinctive features and outcomes in India [75]. Research in genetics, neurochemistry, imaging etc. followed the disease syndromes postulated by Kraepelin; especially since many clinicians and scientists collaborated with, or had worked in the laboratories or research programs, which shared these ideas. In any case, there was an implicit adherence to the concept that these were distinct disease syndromes, awaiting the identification of their biological basis. In the meantime, they could be described by a grouping of symptoms, which was quite pragmatic and clinically useful, as it has been all over the world [76].

The diversity of languages and cultures in India, however, made it a bit difficult even for a person like Govindaswamy to pay attention to the subjective experience of the inner-world of their patients [77]. Most psychiatrists in India would often find themselves in the same situation as Kraepelin in Dorpat, relying on 'objective' assessments rather than subjective experiences, separated as they were from the population at large by linguistic, educational and class disparities. Almost all postgraduate teaching that the psychiatric examination relied upon was carried out based on the phenomenological school, derived from Karl Jaspers [78] and summarised by Frank Fish. This was perhaps also influenced by the endorsement by Hoenig, both as a translator of Jaspers' textbook, [79] and also while a faculty member at the AIIMH in Bangalore. Although there was some interest in developing an 'Indian' phenomenology [80], these efforts were soon abandoned and European and neo-Kraepelinian definitions became standard practice. Interestingly, in many countries in Asia, Willi Mayer-Gross' textbook of psychiatry remained the most common prescribed text, translated into Chinese [81], Korean and Japanese.

These deep inroads of the Kraepelinian viewpoints about disease syndromes, and perhaps their biological roots, thus paved the way for an easy acceptance of the current resurgence of neo-Kraepelinism all over Asia. This has, in a sense, allowed coordinated biomedical and psychosocial research, despite the evident dissimilarity in cultural and social circumstances. Whether this is an amplification of trends from half a century ago [82] or simply the validation of Kraepelin's ideas is still being debated.

Key Points
- The creation of mental health services in India under British influence resulted in the diffusion of ideas from Europe into medical practice.
- In the early twentieth century, Kraepelin's ideas represented a modern, biomedical conceptualisation of psychiatric syndromes.
- These were incorporated into the working of the mental hospitals, clinics and teaching in mid-twentieth-century India.
- Kraepelin's curiosity about differences in disease across cultures; and genetic causes; finds resonance in current research in India.
- An emphasis on phenomenology and pharmacology as the pivots for defining and treating psychiatric disorders made Kraepelin's ideas particularly attractive and easy to integrate with medical services over the past half-century in many parts of Asia.

References

1. Crawford DG. A history of the Indian Medical Service. London: Thacker Spink; 1912.
2. Radhika P, Murthy P, Sarin A, Jain S. Psychological symptoms and medical responses in nineteenth-century India. Hist Psychiatry. 2015;26(1):88–97.
3. Jain S, Murthy P, Shankar SK. Neuropsychiatric perspectives from nineteenth-century India: the diaries of Dr Charles I. Smith. Hist Psychiatry. 2001;12(48):459–66.
4. Pinel P. A treatise on insanity: in which are contained the principles of a new and more practical nosology of maniacal disorders than has yet been offered to the public…. W. Todd; 1806.
5. Roy P. Mental health in the vernacular: print and counter-hegemonic approaches to madness in colonial Bengal. In: Voices in the history of madness: personal and professional perspectives on mental health and illness. Cham: Springer International Publishing; 2021. p. 49–69.
6. Baber Z. The science of empire: scientific knowledge, civilization, and colonial rule in India. Suny Press; 1996.
7. Kumar D. Science and society in modern India. Cambridge University Press; 2023.
8. Pandya S. Medical education in Western India: Grant Medical College and Sir Jamsetjee Jejeebhoy's Hospital. Newcastle upon Tyne: Cambridge Scholars Publishing; 2019.
9. Reddy DVS. The beginnings of modern medicine in Madras: the dawn of modern medicine in Madras. Calcutta: Thacker, Spink; 1947.
10. Kumar D. Probing history of medicine and public health in India. Indian Hist Rev. 2010;37(2):259–73.
11. Wise TA. Practical remarks on insanity as it occurs among the inhabitants of Bengal. Mon J Med Sci. 1852;6(32):97.
12. Bynum WF. The nervous patient in eighteenth-and nineteenth-century Britain: the psychiatric origins of British neurology. In: Anatomy of madness 1. Routledge; 2018. p. 89–102.

13. McDowall TW. The insane in India and their treatment: the presidential address delivered at the fifty-sixth annual meeting of the medico-psychological association held at the University of Durham College of Medicine, Newcastle-on-Tyne, 29th July, 1897. J Ment Sci. 1897;43(183):683–703.

14. Ewens GF. Insanity in India: its symptoms and diagnosis: with reference to the relation of crime and insanity. Calcutta: Thacker & Spink; 1908.

15. Ewens GF. Dementia praecox in India. Ind Med Gaz. 1908;43(6):206.

16. Ewens GF. Katatonia in India. Ind Med Gaz. 1909;44(3):85.

17. Ewens GF. A theory of cortical visual representation. Brain. 1893;16(4):475–91.

18. McKay A. The indigenisation of western medicine in Sikkim. Bull Tibetol. 2004;40:25–47.

19. NAIDLF00058161; Abhilekh-Patal, National Archives of India.

20. Overbeck-Wright AW. Mental Derangements in India. Calcutta: Thacker & Spink; 1912.

21. Kraepelin E. Manic-depressive insanity and paranoia. E & S Livingstone. 1921.

22. Anonymous. Mental derangements in India: a criticism (communicated). Ind Med Gaz. 1913;48(6):240–2.

23. Overbeck-Wright AW. Mental derangement in India: a reply to a criticism. Ind Med Gaz. 1913;48(7):285.

24. Ewens GF. The meaning of insanity. Ind Med Gaz. 1914;49(10):377.

25. Overbeck-Wright A. The prevention of mental and nervous diseases. Ind Med Gaz. 1914;49(10):387.

26. Berkeley-Hill OA. A comparison between the mental processes in the sane and in the insane. Ind Med Gaz. 1914;49(10):382.

27. Kraepelin E. dementia praecox and Paraphrenia. Chicago: Chicago Medical Book co; 1916.

28. Mills J. Modern psychiatry in India: the British role in establishing an Asian system, 1858–1947. Int Rev Psychiatry. 2006;18(4):333–43.

29. Lewis A. Edward Mapother and the making of the Maudsley Hospital: the first Mapother lecture, delivered at the Institute of Psychiatry, 26 March 1969. Br J Psychiatry. 1969;115(529):1349–66.

30. Mapother E. Emil Kraepelin: psychiatrist. J Ment Sci. 1927;73(303):509–34.

31. Mills JH, Jain S. Mapother of the Maudsley and psychiatry at the end of the Raj. In: Psychiatry and empire. London: Palgrave Macmillan UK; 2007. p. 153–71.

32. Noronha F. Observations on cases of dementia praecox. Ind Med Gaz. 1925;60(9):415.

33. Patch CJL. A manual of mental diseases: a textbook for students and practitioners in India. London: Baillière, Tindall and Cox; 1934.

34. Notes on Books. Br Med J. 1935;2(3903):788. PMCID: PMC2461537; Journal of Mental Science, Volume 81, Issue 332, January 1935, p. 192. https://doi.org/10.1192/bjp.81.332.192.

35. Mapother E. Suggestions as to some possible projects for the promotion of psychiatry in India, Royal Bethlem Hospital Archive: EM–01, papers of Edward Mapother. Bethlem Museum of the Mind.

36. Jain S, Sarin A. A psychiatrist on the cusp of independence: Owen Berkeley-Hill on how to nudge social change in India, Jain et al. Br J Psychiatry. 2024;224(5):179.

37. Hill OB. A note on the incidence of neuro-syphilis among Coloured races. Ind Med Gaz. 1926;61(2):57.

38. Pacheco JN. Modern methods in psychiatry. Ranchi; 1935.

39. Jain S, Murthy P. The other Bose: an account of missed opportunities in the history of neurobiology in India. Curr Sci. 2009;97(2):266–9.

40. Akhtar M. Salimuzzaman Siddiqui, MBE, 19 October 1897–14 April 1994. Biogr Mems Fell R Soc. 1996:42401–17.

41. Das B. A psychiatric tour of Europe. Ind Med Gaz. 1931;66(9):517.

42. Ernst W. Colonialism and transnational psychiatry: the development of an Indian Mental Hospital in British India, c. 1925–1940. Anthem Press; 2013.

43. Shaw WJ. The alienist department of India. J Ment Sci. 1932;78(321):331–41.

44. Mills JH, Jain S. A disgrace to a civilised community': colonial psychiatry and the visit of Edward Mapother to South Asia, 1937–8. In: Permeable walls. Brill; 2009. p. 223–42.

45. Jain S, Murthy P. Madmen and specialists: the clientele and the staff of the Lunatic Asylum, Bangalore. Int Rev Psychiatry. 2006;18(4):345–54.
46. Wise TA. General paralysis of the insane Indian Med Gaz 1869. 75.
47. Major Owen Berkeley-Hill IM. A Wassermann survey of the inmates of the Ranchi European Lunatic Asylum. Indian Med Gaz. 1921;56(3):89.
48. Ghani S, Murthy P, Jain S, Sarin A. Syphilis and psychiatry at the Mysore Government Mental Hospital (NIMHANS) in the early 20th century. Indian J Psychiatry. 2018;60(Suppl 2):S270–6.
49. Shaw WJ. Dementia praecox in Parsees. Br Med J. 1928;2(3537):728.
50. Engstrom EJ, Crozier I. Race, alcohol and general paralysis: Emil Kraepelin's comparative psychiatry and his trips to Java (1904) and North America (1925). Hist Psychiatry. 2018 Sep;29(3):263–81.
51. Winslow F. Moral sanitary economics'. Psychological Medicine and Mental Pathology. 1853;6
52. Gait EP. The census of India, vol. 1. Calcutta: Government Press; 1913.
53. Shaw WJ. The heredity of dementia praecox. Br Med J. 1928;2(3534):566.
54. Dhunjibhoy JE. The heredity of dementia praecox. Br Med J. 1929:882.
55. Brock AJ. Dementia praecox in Parsees. Br Med J. 1928;2(3535):634.
56. Haldipur CV. Heredity of schizophrenia in India: a 1928 debate. Asian J Psychiatr. 2023;88:103741.
57. Pillay AP. Is medicine fulfilling its responsibilities to future generations? A plea for the study of eugenics. Ind Med Gaz. 1930;65(9):536.
58. Dhunjibhoy JE Annual report of the working of the Ranchi Indian Mental Hospital. 1937.
59. Chandrasekhar S. The population problems of India and Pakistan. Eugen Rev. 1949;41(2):70.
60. Hodges S. South Asia's eugenic past. In: The Oxford handbook of the history of eugenics. Oxford: Oxford University Press; 2010. p. 228–42.
61. Dube KC, Kumar N, Dube S. Long term course and outcome of the Agra cases in the international pilot study of Schizophrenia. Acta Psychiatr Scand. 1984;70(2):170–9.
62. Bhatia T, Gettig EA, Gottesman II, Berliner J, Mishra NN, Nimgaonkar VL, Deshpande SN. Stratifying empiric risk of schizophrenia among first degree relatives using multiple predictors in two independent Indian samples. Asian J Psychiatr. 2016;(24):79–84.
63. Ali F, Sreeraj VS, Nadella RK, Holla B, Mahadevan J, Ithal D, Balachander S, Viswanath B, Venkatasubramanian G, John JP, Reddy YJ. Estimating the familial risk of psychiatric illnesses: a review of family history scores. Asian J Psychiatr. 2021;56:102551.
64. Sreeraj VS, Holla B, Ithal D, Nadella RK, Mahadevan J, Balachander S, Ali F, Sheth S, Narayanaswamy JC, Venkatasubramanian G, John JP. Psychiatric symptoms and syndromes transcending diagnostic boundaries in Indian multiplex families: the cohort of ADBS study. Psychiatry Res. 2021;296:113647.
65. Sreeraj VS, Puzhakkal JC, Holla B, Nadella RK, Sheth S, Balachander S, Ithal D, Ali F, Viswanath B, Muralidharan K, Venkatasubramanian G. Cross-diagnostic evaluation of minor physical anomalies in psychiatric disorders. J Psychiatr Res. 2021;142:54–62.
66. Chadwick O. The secularization of the European mind in the nineteenth century. Cambridge University Press; 1990.
67. Arnold D. Colonizing the body: state medicine and epidemic disease in nineteenth-century India. University of California Press; 1993.
68. Honigberger JM. Thirty-five years in the east relating to the Punjab and cashmere. Sang-e-Meel Publications; 1852.
69. Ernst W. 'Under the influence'in British India: James Esdaile's mesmeric Hospital in Calcutta, and its critics. Psychol Med. 1995;25(6):1113–23.
70. Sarkar M. On the supposed uncertainty in medical science: & on the relation between diseases & their remedial agents... P. Sircar. Calcutta Anglo-Sanskrit Press; 1903. http://books.google.com/books?id=exY6AAAAMAAJ&oe=UTF-8.
71. Masani KR. Indian psychiatric society's annual meeting Ranchi-1961. Indian J Psychiatry. 1961;3(2):73–8.
72. Nand SD. Analytic psychotherapy is applied biology. Indian J Psychiatry. 1959;1(3):130–5.
73. Neki JS. Semantic confusion in psychiatry. Indian J Psychiatry. 1963;5(1):8–16.

74. Rao VA. Unipolar and bipolar depression: are they different? Indian J Psychiatry. 1974;16(3):183–8.
75. Verghese A, John JK, Rajkumar S, Richard J, Sethi BB, Trivedi JK. Factors associated with the course and outcome of Schizophrenia in India results of a two-year multicentre follow-up study. Br J Psychiatry. 1989;154(4):499–503.
76. Tandon R, Nasrallah H, Akbarian S, Carpenter WT Jr, DeLisi LE, Gaebel W, Green MF, Gur RE, Heckers S, Kane JM, Malaspina D. The schizophrenia syndrome, circa 2024: what we know and how that informs its nature. Schizophr Res. 2024;264:1–28.
77. Prabhu PH. Sociometry and psychodrama in India. J Psychodrama Sociom Group Psychother. 1959;12(4)
78. Jaspers K. General psychopathology. Translated from the German 7th ed. by J. Hoenig and Marian W. Hamilton. JHU Press; 1997.
79. Fish F Clinical psychopathology. Signs and symptoms in psychiatry. Bristol: Wright & Sons, Ltd. 1967. Pp. 120. Price 30s.
80. Govindswamy MV. Need for research in systems of Indian philosophy and Ayurveda with special reference to psychological medicine. J Indian Med Assoc. 1949;18:281–6.
81. Crammer JL. Two weeks' work in SW China. Bull R Coll Psychiatrists. 1985;9(3):56–8.
82. Blashfield RK. Feighner et al., invisible colleges, and the Matthew effect. Schizophr Bull. 1982;8(1):1–6.

Open Access This chapter is licensed under the terms of the Creative Commons Attribution 4.0 International License (http://creativecommons.org/licenses/by/4.0/), which permits use, sharing, adaptation, distribution and reproduction in any medium or format, as long as you give appropriate credit to the original author(s) and the source, provide a link to the Creative Commons license and indicate if changes were made.

The images or other third party material in this chapter are included in the chapter's Creative Commons license, unless indicated otherwise in a credit line to the material. If material is not included in the chapter's Creative Commons license and your intended use is not permitted by statutory regulation or exceeds the permitted use, you will need to obtain permission directly from the copyright holder.

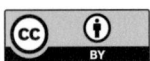

Soviet Psychiatry: The Stalin Years

Anna Toropova

19.1 Introduction

In Vsevolod Ivanov's experimental 1933 novel *Y* (*U*) two delusional jewellers are admitted to the 'E. Kraepelin Psychiatric Hospital' outside Moscow where they stir up a fiery diagnostic debate [1, pp. 183–4]. One doctor reads the jewellers' malady as psychogenic in origin and to be treated by psychoanalysis. The director of the Kraepelin Hospital, however, a 'specialist in clinico-nosological psychiatry' counters his colleague's Freudian diagnosis by insisting on the biological aetiology of the disease [1, p. 190]. Cate Reilly's recent analysis of Ivanov's novel has masterfully shown how literary works penned at a time when the Soviet Union had ostensibly embraced Kraepelin's 'natural disease' conception of mental illness continued to critique the implications of a biologically oriented psychiatry [1, p. 195]. The attempt to contest a 'biologized picture of mental illness' [1, p. 16] that found its expression in novels such as *Y* was not limited to the domain of literature. The field of Soviet psychiatry also saw attempts to challenge the premises that stood at the heart of the Kraepelian revolution. Kraepelin's influence on Soviet psychiatry might be taken for granted given his established links with the Russian Empire. Early on in his career, Kraepelin had headed a psychiatric institute in Russian Dorpat (present day Tartu, Estonia) [1, pp. 94–100]. Pivotal figures in Russian and Soviet psychiatry such as Petr Gannushkin had undergone training at Kraepelin's clinics in Germany in the early twentieth century [2]. Yet Kraepelin's standing in the Soviet Union was subject to flux. Tracing the ebbs and flows of the psychiatrist's influence after the October Revolution, this chapter shows how Kraepelin's legacy became closely intertwined with thorny debates over the question of whether the social environment or biology took precedence in shaping mental disorder.

A. Toropova (✉)
Department of History, University of Warwick, Coventry, UK
e-mail: anna.toropova.1@warwick.ac.uk

© The Author(s) 2026
G. Ikkos, T. Becker (eds.), *Psychiatry after Kraepelin*,
https://doi.org/10.1007/978-3-032-09475-9_19

19.2   The Early Soviet Period: The Dominance
of Social Psychiatry

While Soviet psychiatrists paid respects to Kraepelin as the person responsible for
'fundamentally reforming clinical psychiatry' and bringing the discipline into the
fold of general medicine in the 1920s and early 1930s, many experts during this
time privileged the exploration of factors that had been sidelined in Kraepelin's
work, namely social and psychological determinants [3]. An influential history of
psychiatry published in 1929 by the psychoanalyst Iurii Kannabikh recognised the
great transformation of psychiatric theory and practice spearheaded by Kraepelin's
'practical empiricism' [4, p. 417]. Yet at the same time, Kannabikh noted the 'limits
of a purely nosological approach to psychopathological phenomena' that had been
indicated by recent investigations into the 'sociological factor' (the role of the material and social environment surrounding the patient), as well as by psychoanalysis
[4, p. 449]. These two approaches—the investigation of societal factors and psychoanalytic enquiries—decisively shaped Soviet understandings of mental distress in
the 1920s.

Figures like Lev Rozenshtein, the head of Moscow's Institute of Neuropsychiatric
Prophylaxis and the leader of the Soviet mental hygiene movement, vigorously
pushed for the re-orientation of Soviet psychiatry to the early detection and prevention of mental disorder [5, pp. 145–80]. The 1920s were the heyday of social psychiatry and mental hygiene in the USSR. Experiments with so-called
'neuropsychiatric dispensaries' (outpatient clinics in which prophylaxis and
research into working and living conditions were combined with education and
treatment) reflected Soviet healthcare's broader re-orientation towards the prevention of disease [5, 6]. In the midst of vast campaigns to restructure the forms of
everyday life and the practices of labour, psychiatrists like Rozenshtein contem-
plated the prospect of mental disorder becoming obsolete in Soviet society [7]. The
belief in the social origins of mental distress nurtured the anticipation that mental
disorder would fall away with the revolutionary transformation of social life.

The ascendancy of mental hygiene in the 1920s was part of a broader shift
towards 'minor' psychiatry. In contrast to the 'major' strain of psychiatry, with its
focus on psychosis and acute mental illness, minor psychiatry tackled 'weak forms'
of mental disorder, particularly 'mild schizophrenia' and neurosis. Researchers at
the Moscow Institute of Neuropsychiatric Prophylaxis began to reappraise
Kraepelin's diagnosis of dementia praecox, drawing attention to the 'significant'
contingent of cases that passed through the institute's dispensary that were located
at the border of neurosis and psychosis [8, 9]. Instead of clearly developed and
'acute' psychotic symptoms such as psychotic episodes and the disintegration of the
personality, the researchers observed a 'slowly developing process' of intellectual
degeneration and a series of 'microsymptoms' [8, p. 30]. Soviet psychiatry's prophylactic direction was thought to render it uniquely suited to the detection of
micro-psychotic forms that played out beyond the walls of psychiatric institutions
and usually escaped the purview of investigators [9, p. 48]. Reversing psychiatry's
typical procedural path from acute to milder cases, minor psychiatry and mental

hygiene set out to first investigate the mental 'norm'. Accordingly, Soviet specialists aspired to detect deviations before they developed into severe cases [9, p. 49].

As well as re-drawing the boundaries of schizophrenia, Soviet psychiatrists turned their attention to the problem of neurosis—the 'disorder of modernity' most widely believed to be 'socio-genic' in origin and rooted in the conditions of work, family and leisure time. During the 1920s, many doctors sounded the alarm about the prevalence of neurotic disorders (understood as encompassing neurasthenia, psychasthenia, hysteria, phobias and obsessions) across all sectors of Soviet society [10, 11]. The perception that Soviet citizens were living through an epoch that exerted unprecedented demands on the nervous system had become common place [5, 6, 12, 13]. The upheavals of the revolutionary epoch—the First World War closely followed by the October Revolution and the Civil War—with its 'chronic hunger, physical exhaustion and horrendous epidemics' were frequently blamed for an increase in rates of mental disorder [14]. Perhaps surprisingly, the period of recovery during the New Economic Policy (NEP; 1921–1928) was not lauded as a respite in the mental health emergency. On the contrary, the psychoneurologist Aron Zalkind framed the NEP-era context of revolutionary pause as the perfect breeding ground for neuroses [15, p. 31]. The mental health of overburdened and exhausted party activists received particular scrutiny. The eminent Soviet psychiatrist Petr Gannushkin, the head of the Psychiatric Clinic at the First Moscow Medical Institute, had in 1926 published a deeply alarming portrait of worn-down ('*iznosh-ennye*') revolutionaries-cum-intellectual workers: young men of 20–30 years of age so mentally and physically crippled by the incessant demands of work that their mental faculties had become permanently weakened [16]. Mental hygienists like Leon Rokhlin similarly noted the high rates of ill health and low life expectancy amongst party activists. Not only had these activists borne the brunt of the 'patho-genic traumas' of 'war and revolution', but, carrying the fate of the communist movement on their shoulders, they routinely overburdened themselves with intel-lectual labour [17, pp. 25–6]. By the late 1920s, alarms about the 'colossal' increase in mental unease had become routine. As much as 75% of the Soviet population were pronounced victims of nervous and psychiatric illness, with all manner of environments—from educational establishments and state institutions to the doc-tor's waiting room—said to be 'briming full with psychoneuroses' [18, p. 57]. Diagnosing an era of 'mass nervousness' in 1928, Lev Rozenshtein, remarked that it was 'very rare indeed to encounter people who did not feel their nerves now and again' [19, p. 3].

Soviet mental hygienists chiefly looked to factors in the social environment—the conditions of work, everyday life and the family—to understand the causes of ner-vousness. The terms 'socio-neuroses' or 'socio-reactive neuroses' came to be com-monly used to emphasise the environmental roots of mental distress [15, pp. 28–29]. In the context of such keen attention to exogenous factors, 'Kraepelinism' came to be criticised for a lack of attention to the 'social factor' in the aetiology of mental disease. Blaming Kraepelin's influence on the frequent sidelining of environmental causes in clinical analysis, Rozenshtein denounced the 'fatalistic biologisation' underlying the German psychiatrist's conceptions [7, pp. 9–11]. Referencing

Kraepelin's attempt to attribute revolutionary strivings to the 'pathological heredity of Jews', Rozenshtein characterised not only Kraepelin but 'popular German psychiatrists and neurologists' more broadly as betraying a 'weak interest in social problems' and exhibiting 'reactionary social-political outlooks' [7, p. 11]. The entry on Kraepelin published in the *Great Medical Encyclopaedia* in 1930 was similarly ambivalent about the psychiatrist's legacy. While recognising the scholar as a pivotal reformer of clinical psychiatry, the entry noted that Kraepelin's work displayed the 'bourgeois tendencies' typical of Western scientists [3, p. 317].

In addition to the influence of social psychiatry, the early Soviet period witnessed a lively engagement with psychoanalytic ideas. Theories of the unconscious were avidly discussed in the Soviet Union until the 1930s, with many of Sigmund Freud's works made available in Russian translation and the foundation of psychoanalytic societies, institutes, clinics and schools [20, 21]. In part, Soviet psychiatrists' interest in psychoanalysis was driven by the unique mental toll of the tumultuous 1914–1921 period that has been famously described by Peter Holquist as Russia's 'continuum of crisis' [22]. The devastating effects of a world war closely followed by revolution and a civil war had convinced many Soviet psychiatrists of the need to take psychological trauma seriously. Psychoanalytic theories of neurosis held considerable appeal to a contingent of Soviet specialists grappling with the psychological impact of war and revolution. Sigmund Freud's identification of both 'major' and 'apparently trivial' psychical traumas as 'precipitating causes' of neuroses and Alfred Adler's connection of neurosis to internal psychological conflict proved persuasive to a range of prominent mental hygienists, psychoneurologists and psychotherapists [23].

19.3   The Stalin Revolution and the Re-assessment of Kraepelin

While interest in 'mild forms' of schizophrenia and neurosis continued into the 1930s, the intellectual landscape had begun to shift. The objectives of rapid industrialisation, the forced collectivisation of agriculture and cultural revolution, launched by Joseph Stalin in 1928, placed new obligations on psychiatrists [24]. Science and medicine were henceforth expected to play their part in the task of socialist construction. It was no longer the psychiatrist's place to caution against the perils of overwork [5, 6, 24, 25]. The specialists who had sounded the alarm about the state of the party's mental health publicly admitted their 'mistakes' in the early 1930s [26]. The suggestion of a link between revolution and mental disorder became taboo. 'False rumours' that the frantic tempo of industrialisation and collectivisation was crippling the nervous systems of the population were robustly dismissed [27, p. 12]. L. Rokhlin, the psychiatrist who had previously raised concerns about overwork amongst party activists, renounced his earlier theories and made clear that the conditions of Soviet society were not 'traumatising' but life giving. The revolution, Rokhlin now contended, had given birth to new 'psychological reserves' [28, p. 135]. The ethos of socialist construction was reframed as an energising factor that prevented, rather than caused, mental distress.

The early 1930s also saw explanations of mental disorder that stressed the role of the material and social environment begin to lose their standing. The weakening explanatory force of 'the social factor' became apparent at the All-Union Behavioural Congress, held in Leningrad in the winter of 1930. Tasked with bringing the study of human behaviour into closer line with the goals of socialist construction and establishing a single methodological direction in psychoneurology, the congress proved to be a watershed moment in the history of the Soviet psy-disciplines [27]. Reports on the congress championed the ascendency of a dialectical approach to understanding the relationship between the biological and the social in human behaviour, decrying the 'extreme' position of attributing mental disorders primarily to exogenous factors. 'The so-called Lamarckian direction, which attributed a lead-ing role solely to the influence of the external environment,' it was noted, 'does not stand up to criticism and should be rejected' [27, p. 5]. Participants who strayed too far in the direction of 'socio-geneticism' and diminished the role of biology in men-tal illness were criticised as holding 'completely incorrect' and 'one-sided' views [27, p. 6].

By 1933, prominent Soviet psychiatrists acknowledged that earlier assumptions that the psychiatrist's work was 'only a question of making healthy the conditions of work and everyday life' were mistaken [29, p. 10]. Lev Rozenshtein's 1928 book on nervousness was subjected to harsh criticism for correlating neurosis with socio-economic conditions and the mental hygienist was forced to denounce his earlier claims that the revolution had inflicted 'neuro-psychiatric' traumas on the popula-tion [30, 31, p. 63]. The Behavioural Congress had also led the attack on psycho-analysis as 'unscientific' and 'metaphysical'. Soviet specialists were hereon to wage a 'merciless' battle with a discipline that harboured 'all the evils' of bourgeois sci-entific practice [27, p. 8].

As Soviet specialists turned to scrutinise endogenous factors in the 1930s, the role of constitution and heredity in mental disorders began to receive more atten-tion. The year 1933 saw the publication of Gannushkin's influential book, *Clinic of Psychopathy*, which conceptualised neuroses as reactions that had their root in con-stitutional particularities and personality disorders [32]. Whereas Gannushkin's ear-lier theory of the 'premature mental disability' acquired by Soviet intellectual workers suffering from the burdens of work and the psychophysiological traumas of the revolutionary age had been vigorously refuted by 1930, his work on the blurred boundaries between neurosis and psychopathy (famously defined by Kurt Schneider as 'abnormal personalities who suffer from their abnormality or from whose abnor-mality society suffers' [32, p. 9]) proved much more lasting. *Clinic of Psychopathy* was pronounced 'one of the most significant events in contemporary Soviet psy-chiatry' after it was published only a few days after Gannushkin's death [33, p. 11]. Praising attempts to bring psychiatry onto a firmer biological basis, the book made clear its desire to break with theoretical approaches that had stressed the role of the social environment in the development of mental pathologies [32, pp. 5–6]. Disorders like neurasthenia were understood in Gannushkin's book not as nosologi-cal entities in their own right but as attributes of a personality disorder. Outlining different groups of psychopaths, Gannushkin characterised these individuals as predisposed to develop pathological reactions to mental traumas and difficult life circumstances.

Gannushkin's conception of psychopathy was supported by the work of other prominent specialists such as the director of the Clinic for Neuroses at the Ukrainian Psychoneurological Academy, Oleksandr Iushchenko [34]. A specialist in 'evolutionary-genetic' approaches to psychiatry, Iushchenko saw neuroses as determined not only by traumatic experience but also by the particularities of individual character and constitution. The belief in the dominant role of inborn personality traits motivated Iushchenko to label a significant group of neuroses as 'constitutional neuroses,' or 'constitutionoses' [34, p. 471]. Like other experts working on the problem of neurosis in the 1930s, Iushchenko cast responsibility back onto the individual and suggested that neuroses mainly developed in 'primitive,' 'undisciplined' and 'lacking' personalities who were less able to cope with traumatising situations [34, pp. 472–73].

The greater recognition of biological factors in the 1930s led to a re-assessment of 'Kraepelinism'. The founder of the 'Moscow school' of Soviet psychiatry, Petr Gannushkin, a student of Sergei Korsakov and Vladimir Serbskii who had attended a training course at Kraepelin's clinic in 1905, was re-framed after his untimely death in 1933 as 'the leading disciple of the most important psychiatrist of all time' [2]. Gannushkin's biography came to be closely intertwined with Kraepelin in official accounts. Described as entering the field at the very moment that the revolution associated with Kraepelin's work was underway, Gannushkin was credited with nurturing a 'nosological direction' in his Moscow clinic [33, p. 7]. 'No name in Soviet psychiatry could illuminate Kraepelin's teaching in such a bright light as Gannushkin', enthused the Moscow psychiatrist Mark Sereiskii in 1934 [2]. Both Gannushkin and Kraepelin, whose work was now described as 'inseparable', were lauded for the authority they placed on 'clinical fact' and their attentiveness to their patients [2]. In the mid-1930s, Kraepelin came to be frequently celebrated by renowned Soviet psychiatrists for his 'genius' and the 'brilliance' of his method of clinical diagnosis [35, p. 2]. The official hostility to psychoanalysis in the 1930s also helped to rehabilitate Kraepelin, whose teaching was now praised as 'principally opposed' to 'Freudianism' [36, p. 19].

A backlash against the 'excesses' of the mental hygiene movement was in full swing by the mid-1930s. The expansiveness of the conceptions of 'nervousness' and 'mild schizophrenia' advanced by psychiatrists like Rozenshtein was a particular target of criticism [6]. Seasoned figures in Soviet psychiatry began to caution against the 'over diagnosis' of schizophrenia. To be sure, the achievements of dispensarisation and preventative psychiatry were still recognised. Writing in 1936, the pre-eminent psychiatrist V. P. Osipov noted that dispensarisation had brought new life to the 'dead end' of pre-revolutionary psychiatry, 'expanding its domain beyond the institutional confinement of the mentally ill' [35, p. 4]. Similarly, Osipov acknowledged that the identification of milder forms of schizophrenia had served to widen the psychiatrist's gaze beyond acute cases little responsive to treatment. Yet even as he framed dispensarisation as a key step forward in the history of Soviet psychiatry, Osipov lamented that it had blurred the lines between health and illness and resulted in attempts to identify 'schizophrenia without schizophrenia' [35, p. 29]. Osipov proceeded to insist on the need to 'narrow' the definition schizophrenia and to preserve it as a 'nosological unit'. Stressing the endogenous and organic nature of the disorder, as well as the role of hereditary predisposition, Osipov proposed a return to a definition of schizophrenia that was closer to Kraepelin's revolutionary diagnosis of dementia praecox [8, 35].

One notable departure from Kraepelinism, however, was Stalinist psychiatry's refusal to accept schizophrenia as an irreversible process [35, p. 8]. In the late 1930s, Stalinist psychiatry began to target overcoming the 'therapeutic nihilism' of the past through a variety of 'active therapies' that targeted the body [37]. As Benjamin Zajicek has shown, somatic treatments that ranged from insulin coma therapy to sleep therapy served to present psychiatry as a process of active intervention and treatment rather than mere prevention [37]. Physically violent treatments that entailed patients entering a coma-like state or experiencing phases of physiological shock demonstrated the transformed role of the Stalin-era psychiatrist. No longer a custodian or mere observer of the insane, the psychiatrist became an active healer, a 'clinician-biologist' capable of reversing conditions previously thought to be a death sentence such as schizophrenia [37, pp. 54, 63].

The development of sleep therapy, which entailed putting the patient into a pharmaceutically induced sleep, also demonstrated the growing influence of Ivan Pavlov's physiology over Soviet psychiatry. During the early 1930s, Pavlov grew increasingly interested in psychiatric questions, contending that his theories of 'higher nervous activity' could shed light on the physiological mechanisms behind mental illness [38, pp. 630–649]. A Nervous Clinic headed by Boris Birman and a Psychiatry Clinic under the leadership of Aleksander Ivanov-Smolenskii were established as part of Pavlov's Physiology Division at the Institute of Experimental Medicine [38, p. 640]. Pavlov's research on 'experimental neurosis' in dogs, first begun in the 1920s, was touted in the early and mid-1930s as holding the key to the resolution of 'important questions' on the aetiology, characteristics and treatment of nervous disorders in humans in a series of publications, presentations at international congresses and even a feature film [23, 39, pp. 116–118]. Pavlov's experiments sought to impel pathological nervous processes in dogs by overtaxing the animals' nervous systems. Attempts were made to 'break' the animals through exposure to unbearably excitatory or inhibitory stimuli, as well as to stimuli that brought the processes of inhibition and excitation into conflict [39, pp. 122–124, 163–172]. Pavlov and his colleagues observed that certain dogs developed pathological reactions, or 'neuroses', in response to stimuli much more readily than others. Distinguishing four different personality types that corresponded to Hippocrates's theory of humoral constitution, Pavlov's research identified two types of personality ('strong but volatile' and 'weak') as being more predisposed to neurosis [39, pp. 116–118].

In addition to his work on 'experimental neurosis', Pavlov offered a physiological reading of schizophrenia. Drawing parallels between schizophrenia and a 'chronic hypnotic state,' Pavlov framed the disorder as a state of inhibition that served to protect a weakened brain cortex facing 'overwhelming' excitation

[40, p. 40]. At the same time as this state of chronic hypnosis was understood to be 'pathological', it was also interpreted as a physiological means of protecting the brain cortex against 'threatening destruction' [40, p. 42]. Having framed schizophrenia as a state of protective inhibition, Pavlov argued that 'continued inhibition' (prolonged physiological sleep) was capable of restoring weak and exhausted cells back to health. To bolster his thesis on the possibility of restoring cortical cells to a 'normal condition', Pavlov invoked Kraepelin, describing him as 'one of the greatest psychiatric authorities' [40, p. 42]. Kraepelin had shown, Pavlov argued, that it was the forms of schizophrenia that had a 'hypnotic character' (hebephrenia and catatonia) that had a chance of recovery [40, p. 42]. Keenly following Mark Sereiskii's experiments with pharmaceutically induced sleep therapy in Moscow, and trialling the method at his own clinics, Pavlov pronounced the 'positive results' of the treatment in the Soviet press [38, p. 647]. The 'breakthrough' was also triumphed in a series of hagiographic documentary films such as *The Experiments of Ivan Pavlov* (*Opyty Akademika Pavlova*, 1939).

The search for somatically oriented methods of treatment, the curtailment of the mental hygiene movement and the growing influence of physiology as well as theories of constitution and hereditary predisposition indicate a shift away from the model of social psychiatry established in the 1920s. The transition from a social to a biological understanding of mental illness in the Stalin era was less clear-cut than has at times been assumed, however. A range of scholars continued to foreground the role of the social environment in mental disorders throughout the 1930s and to deploy psychoanalytic explanatory paradigms, albeit cautiously [23]. Tellingly, the Soviet psychiatrists deemed to be 'disciples' of Kraepelin were simultaneously praised for not accepting all of Kraepelin's teachings as gospel, and for continuing to affirm that a socialist restructuring of everyday life would decrease rates of mental disorder [41].

A discomfort with the attempt to translate psychiatric terms into the language of 'higher nervous activity' was also palpable. An overview published to celebrate 20 years of Soviet psychiatry in 1937, for example, criticised the 'vulgarisers' of Pavlov who mistakenly believed that the 'theory of reflexes derived from experiments on animals' held 'the key to the study and understanding of mental processes and disorders in human beings' [36, p. 19]. In addition, the attempt to popularise Pavlov's research on 'experimental neurosis' through film garnered intense controversy. The film *Physiology and Pathology of Higher Nervous Activity* (directed by Mark Gall, 1936), which aimed to demonstrate the applicability of Pavlov's research on dogs to humans, was only approved for a limited release 2 years after its completion in 1936 due to negative feedback from the Soviet medical and scientific establishment [23]. The film's section on experimental neuroses in particular was decried as 'mechanistic' and 'crude'. The filmmakers were criticised for displaying a tendency towards biologism and were advised to show much greater caution in translating physiological findings to the psychiatric clinic [23]. As Cate Reilly has shown, 'a biological picture of mental illness' was similarly challenged in the sphere of literature [1, p. 16].

Indeed, the rise of fascism had fostered a cautious attitude towards biological explanations amongst many Soviet psychiatrists. From the mid-1930s Soviet experts had been at pains to publicly denounce the biologistic tenets of racial hygiene and fascist medicine. Criticising fascist health policy's fixation on 'the laws of inheritance' and racial hygiene's tendency to translate the entire problem of mental illness from the 'plane of the socio-economic to the biological,' Soviet doctors unequivocally framed the neglect of the social environment in favour of 'fatalistic' theories of 'genetically based constitution' as an attribute of fascist medicine [42, pp. 93, 110]. The infamous July 1936 Central Committee decree denouncing the disciplines of paedology (child science) and psychotechnics had explicitly criticised the transfer of 'bourgeois' ideas about fatalistic predetermination and racial hierarchy into Soviet science [43].

19.4   Soviet Psychiatry During the Great Patriotic War and the Late Stalin Era

Debates on whether social or biological factors should take precedence in explaining the causes of mental illness continued during the Second World War, or the 'Great Patriotic War' (1941–1945) as it became known in the Soviet Union. Called to treat a plethora of mental problems at the front, psychiatrists offered a diverse range of explanations and treatments. The large numbers of so called *kontuzhenye* (concussed) soldiers, many of whom had suffered head injuries but some of whom bore no clear signs of physiological damage while still being afflicted by puzzling symptoms such as 'deaf-muteness', renewed scholarly interest in the question of psychogenesis and hysteria [44, pp. 128–30]. A number of psychiatrists sought to use modern techniques including X-rays and electroencephalography to prove that organic causes (such as damage caused by microscopic shards of mental) stood at the root of conditions that first appeared to be psychogenic [44, pp. 137–38]. Many others, however, concluded that emotional and psychological trauma, rather than bodily injury, was the root cause. The psychogenic reading of wartime mental disorder was also strengthened by the seeming effectiveness of treatments such as hypnosis and rational persuasion therapy [44, pp. 140–43].

To be sure, Soviet psychiatrists were quick to stress that combatants' love for their motherland and political consciousness prophylacticised against psychogenic reactions such as hysteria. The military psychiatrist Evgenii Krasnushkin asserted that the patriotism and conviction of the Soviet population had enabled most to develop a tolerance to the 'emotion-shocks' of the war, 'a kind of psychic immunity' [45, pp. 207–208]. At the same time, experts acknowledged that profound psychological wounds abounded. As a seminal anthology on Soviet wartime medical expertise noted, despite the 'exceedingly high level of political-moral consciousness' possessed by Soviet combatants, the 'endurance of soldiers had its limits' [46, p. 95]. Many of those who dealt with the problem of wartime psychic traumatisation began to pay closer attention to the unconscious processes of the mind. The Freudian reading of hysteria, with its central explanatory focus on repressed trauma, held considerable appeal for such wartime specialists as the psychotherapist V. K. Khoroshko, who pointed to the 'great stock of material for the work of consciousness that lives unconsciously or subconsciously within us' [47, p. 47]. A variety of studies endorsed Freud's conception of the hysterical symptom as an unconscious response to a psychic trauma. Indeed, Soviet wartime specialists appeared surprisingly receptive to Freud's ideas about the fragility of psychic unity and coherence [48].

The proliferation of diverse interpretations of mental distress continued for a brief period after the war. Warning that psychological trauma would persist as an enduring problem for Soviet society, leading psychiatrists such as Vasilii Giliarovskii and V. N. Miasishchev made the case for understanding the social and psychological factors of mental illness. Pavlovian framings of mental distress could still be challenged and contested. 'Pavlov himself conceded that physiology could not explain everything', Giliarovskii reminding his readers in 1946 [49, p. 62]. As Benjamin Zaijeck has shown, the immediate post-war years even saw attempts to revive mental hygiene and return to the methods and objectives of 1920s social psychiatry [44, pp. 187–211].

The discourse around mental health soon began to shift, however. The wartime period had seen significant attempts to 'normalise' psychological trauma, with specialists wary of attributing conditions like hysteria solely to individual constitution. Khoroshko's 1943 book on neurosis had noted, for example, that 'one could become afflicted with psychogenic neurosis or hysteria without any particular predilection for it' [47, p. 42]. Yet by 1946 it had become common to connect hysteria and traumatic neurosis to deficiencies in an individual's psychology, and even in their level of patriotism. Those who succumbed to neurosis commonly came to be characterised as 'primitive, undisciplined, and infantile individuals' who were predisposed to hysteria [48]. Some doctors even asserted that 'so-called traumatic neurotics' were in fact nothing but individuals with 'psychopathic personalities' [45, p. 217]. Socially and psychologically oriented explanations of mental distress were also increasingly challenged by attempts to correlate mental illness with brain pathology in the late 1940s. The experiments in neurosurgery conducted by Aleksandr Shmar'ian emphatically framed mental disorder as 'brain-based disease' [50, p. 41].

The late 1940s brought direct party intervention into the field of psychiatry as mental specialists became the target of political and antisemitic campaigns. While campaigns to discredit prominent psychiatrists including Giliarovskii and Shmar'ian waged, the entire discipline was forced to take a unified 'Pavlovian' line [50]. The infamous 'Pavlov session' of the Academy of Sciences and Academy of Medical Sciences, which took place in June and July 1950, explicitly sought to strengthen the role of physiology in Soviet medicine [51, 52]. In the aftermath of the session, Pavlov's former associate Ivanov-Smolenskii and the ethnically Russian psychiatrist Aleksandr Snezhnevskii secured their dominance over the field [53, pp. 406–32]. The triumph of Pavlovian psychiatry saw the banning of lobotomy, as well as a wealth of publications on 'Pavlov-approved' treatments such as prolonged sleep therapy and hypnosis [50, 54].

The shifting political terrain of the late Stalin period cast Kraepelin's legacy into an uncertain light. On the one hand, Kraepelin was a key touchstone for Snezhnevskii's attacks against 'nosological agnosticism' and insistence on a hereditary predisposition to mental illness [53, p. 427]. On the other hand, as David Joravsky notes, late Stalinist psychiatry was loathe to acknowledge the true inspiration behind the 'clinical dogmatism' that Snezhnevskii imposed on the profession [53]. The entry on Kraepelin for the 1953 edition of the *Great Soviet Encyclopaedia* noted that the German psychiatrist's renown stemmed from his nosological classification of psychiatric illnesses yet asserted that that it was the Russian psychiatrist Sergei Korsakov who should be credited with developing the first nosological understanding of the psyche [55]. The entry was also critical (and notably more so than the 1930 medical encyclopaedia entry on the psychiatrist) of the significance placed on inheritance and constitution in Kraepelin's work. As has become 'clear with the appearance of active therapies', the encyclopaedia entry claimed, 'the path towards dementia is not the rule; timely and correct treatment can lead to recovery' [55].

19.5   Conclusion

As well as showcasing the hold of anti-Westernism and Russian chauvinism over Soviet psychiatry in the late Stalin period, the scepticism towards Kraepelin's legacy betrayed the lack of firm consensus behind a biological aetiology of mental illness even during the ascendency of 'Pavlovian medicine'. By 1952, debates over the role of psychology in psychiatry and the role of inherited predisposition in neurosis had dramatically re-ignited [56, 57]. Writing in the Soviet Union's premier psychiatry journal just 2 years after the 'Pavlov' session, the Leningrad psychiatrist I. F. Sluchevskii boldly insisted that psychological conceptions and psychological terminology had a right to exist in psychiatric practice [56, p. 4]. Protesting the sidelining of psychological questions in medical training, the scholar denounced the 'reduction of psychiatry to the pathology of higher nervous activity' as 'vulgar materialism' and 'mechanicism' [56, p. 4]. Sluchevskii also offered a creative reinterpretation of Pavlov's teaching, arguing that the physiologist had recognised the governing role of the external environment in mental pathology [56, p. 14]. While Sluchevskii's provocative intervention predictably garnered accusations of misunderstanding Pavlovian theory, it also met support from doctors who echoed his conviction that psychology must have a place in psychiatry [58]. In addition, O. V. Kerbikov's 1952 reinterpretation of Pavlov's work on nervous types as a theory of psychopathic personality [57] was met with fervent objections as an attempt to 'biologise' social phenomena [23]. Critics of Kerbikov's efforts to blur the lines between neurosis and psychopathy protested that Soviet scholars had long rejected theories of 'constitution,' 'inherited degeneration' and 'neo-Lombrosianism' [23]. Even as sociological and biological frameworks alternatively held momentary periods of dominance in the Stalin era, the question of which factors were more decisive in mental disorder ultimately remained unresolved. Even the period of 'Pavlovisation' in Soviet psychiatry did not spell the end of attempts to highlight the limitations of biological interpretations of human behaviour.

Key Points

- Emil Kraepelin's legacy was subject to significant fluctuation during the Stalin period.
- In the early Soviet period, many experts privileged the exploration of social and psychological factors in mental disorder and were thereby critical of 'Kraepelinism'.
- The 'Stalin revolution', inaugurated in 1928, placed new obligations on psychiatrists and led to the re-assessment of Kraepelin's legacy.
- Even as theories of hereditary predisposition and constitution gained more prominence in the Stalin era, the transition from an environmental to a biological understanding of mental illness was far from clear-cut.
- The resistance to 'biologistic' understandings of mental illness persisted until the very end of the Stalin era.

References

1. Reilly CI. Psychic empire: literary modernism and the clinical state. New York: Columbia University Press; 2024.
2. Sereiskii MI. Gannushkin i Krepelin. In: Edel'shtein AO, editor. Pamiati Petra Borisovicha Gannushkina: Trudy psikhiaricheskoi kliniki 1MMI. Moscow/Leningrad: Gos. izd.-vo biologicheskoi meditsinskoi literatury; 1934. p. 20–1.
3. Anon. Krepelin, Emil. In: Semashko N, editor. Bol'shaia meditsinskaia entsiklopediia, vol. 14. 1st ed. Moscow: 'Sovetskaia entsiklopediia'; 1930. p. 315–7.
4. Kannabikh IV. Istoriia psikhiatrii. Leningrad: Gos. med. izd.-vo; 1928.
5. Sirotkina I. Diagnosing literary genius: a cultural history of psychiatry in Russia, 1880–1930. Baltimore: Johns Hopkins University Press; 2002.
6. Zajicek B. Soviet madness: nervousness, mild schizophrenia, and the professional jurisdiction of psychiatry in the USSR, 1918–1936. Ab Imperio. 2024;4:167–94.
7. Rozenshtein LM. Sotsial'no-profilakticheskoe napravlenie v psikhiatrii. Zhurnal nevropatologii i psikhiatrii. 1930;4:3–21.
8. Kameneva EN. Ob otgranichenii i simptomatologicheskikh osobennostiakh miagkoi formy shizofrenii. Sovetskaia nevropatologiia, psikhiatriia i psikhogigiena. 1934;3(4):27–47.
9. Gol'denberg SI. K probleme mikroprotsessual'nykh form. Sov Nevropatol Psikhiatr Psikhogig. 1934;3(5):48–62.
10. Ivanitskii S. Nervnost': Ee prichiny i preduprezhdenie (Besedy vracha). Leningrad: M. and S. Sabashnikovy; 1926.
11. Poliakov I. Nervnost', prichiny ee i bor'ba s neiu. Moscow/Leningrad: Gos. med. izd.-vo; 1929.
12. Bernstein FL. The dictatorship of sex: lifestyle advice for the soviet masses. DeKalb: Northern Illinois University Press; 2007.
13. Pawley S. Revolution in health: nervous weakness and visions of health in revolutionary Russia, c.1900–31. Hist Res. 2017;90:191–209.
14. Osipov VP. O dushevnoi zabolevaemosti i dushevnykh bolezniakh v perezhivaemuiu epokhu i ee posledstviiakh dlia dushevnogo zdorov'ia naseleniia v budushchem. Priroda. 1921;(10–12):2–21.

15. Zalkind AB. Revoliutsiia i molodezh': Sbornik statei. Moscow: Izd. Kommunistich. un.-ta im. Sverdlova; 1925.
16. Gannushkin PB. Ob odnoi iz form nazhitoi psikhicheskoi invalidnosti. In: Trudy psikhiatricheskoi kliniki (Devich'e pole), vol. 2. Moscow: Izd. M. and S. Sabashnikovykh; 1926. p. 52–9.
17. Rokhlin L. Psikhogigienicheskaia rabota sredi partaktiva. Zhurnal nevropatologii i psikhiatrii. 1930;3:24–30.
18. Egorov N. Bor'ba za zdorovye nervy. Revoliutsiia i kul'tura. 1929;6:57–60.
19. Rozenshtein, L. Nervnost' i bor'ba s nei. Moscow: Izd.-vo Narkomzdrava RSFSR; 1928.
20. Miller MA. Freud and the Bolsheviks: psychoanalysis in Imperial Russia and the Soviet Union. New Haven: Yale University Press; 1998.
21. Etkind, A. Eros of the impossible: the history of psychoanalysis in Russia, trans. by Noah and Maria Rubins. Boulder: Westview Press; 1997.
22. Holquist P. Making war, forging revolution: Russia's continuum of crisis, 1914–1921. Cambridge: Harvard University Press; 2002.
23. Toropova A. From neurasthenia to "experimental neurosis": soviet cinema, psychiatry and the problem of nervousness. Isis, forthcoming.
24. Joravsky D. The construction of the Stalinist psyche. In: Fitzpatrick S, editor. Cultural revolution in Russia, 1928–1931. Bloomington: Indiana University Press; 1978. p. 105–28.
25. Siegelbaum L. *Okhrana Truda*: industrial hygiene, psychotechnics, and industrialization in the USSR. In: Gross Solomon S, Hutchinson JF, editors. Health and society in revolutionary Russia. Bloomington: Indiana University Press; 1990. p. 224–45.
26. Gannushkin PB. Ob okhrane zdorov'ia partaktiva. Revoliutsiia i kul'tura. 1930;4:43–6.
27. Rozentsveig BM. Itogi raboty patologo-klinicheskoi sektsii I Vsesoiuznogo povedencheskogo s"ezda. Zhurnal nevropatologii i psikhiatrii, 1930 (5):3–14.
28. Anon. Otchet o sessionnom zasedanii Moskovskogo obshchestva nevropatologov i psikhiatrov po voprosam o nevrozakh, 28–30 April 1933. Sov Nevropatol Psikhiatr Psikhogig. 1934;3(1):121–38.
29. Giliarovskii VA. Dostizheniia sovetskoi psikhiatrii za poslednie 15 let i ee blizhaishie perspektivy. Sovetskaia nevropatologiia, psikhiatriia i psikhogigiena. 1933;2(1):8–17.
30. Grashchenkov N. Za klassovost' i partiinost' v populiarnoi psikhogigienicheskoi literature. Sov Nevropatol Psikhiatr Psikhogig. 1932;1(7):302–4.
31. Rozenshtein LM. O rekonstruktsii nevropsikhiatricheskoi pomoshchi. Sovetskaia nevropatologiia, psikhiatriia i psikhogigiena. 1932;1(3–4):63–77.
32. Gannushkin PB. Klinika psikhopatii: ikh statika, dinamika, sistematika. Moscow: Sever; 1933.
33. Edel'shtein AO. Pamiati uchitelia. In: Edel'shtein AO, editor. Pamiati Petra Borisovicha Gannushkina. p. 5–12.
34. Iushchenko AI. Struktura i klassifikatsiia nervozov. In: Rokhlin LL editor. Trudy Pervogo Ukrainskogo s"ezda nevropatologov i psikhiatrov. Kharkiv: Ukr. Psikhonevrologicheskaia akad.; 1935, p. 467–476.
35. Osipov VP. Granitsy skhizofrenii, ee miagkie formy i ikh legkomyslennoe raspoznavanie. Sovetskaia nevropatologiia, psikhiatriia i psikhogigiena. 1935;4(7):1–30.
36. Gurevich MO. 20 let sovetskoi psikhiatrii. Nevropatol Psikhiatriia. 1937;6(10):15–22.
37. Zajicek B. Insulin coma therapy and the construction of therapeutic effectiveness in Stalin's Soviet Union. In: Savelli M, Marks S, editors. Psychiatry in communist Europe. Basingstoke: Palgrave Macmillan; 2015. p. 50–72.
38. Todes D. Ivan Pavlov: a life in science. New York: Oxford University Press; 2014.
39. Pavlov IP. Psikhopatologiia i psikhiatriia: Izbrannye proizvedeniia. Moscow: Izd.-vo Akad. med. nauk SSSR; 1949. p. 116–8.
40. Pavlov IP. Lectures on conditioned reflexes, vol. II: conditioned reflexes and psychiatry, trans. and ed., W. Horsley Gantt. London: Lawrence & Wishart; 1941.
41. Rozenshtein LM. P. B. Gannushkin kak psikhiatr epokhi. In: Edel'shtein, editor. Pamiati Petra Borisovicha Gannushkina. p.13–9.

42. Gurevich ZA. Fashizm, "rasovaia gigiena" i meditsina. In: In-t filosofii UAMLIN, editor. Rasovaia teoriia na sluzhbe fashizma: Sbornik statei. Kyiv: Gosmedizdat; 1935. p. 89–125.
43. Anon. Postanovlenie TsK VKP(b) O pedologicheskikh izvrashcheniiakh v sisteme narkompro-sov (4 July 1936). In: Egorov AG, Bogoliubov KM, editors. KPSS v rezoliutsiiakh, 1933–1937 gg, vol. 6. Moscow: Izd.-vo politicheskoi literatury; 1985. p.364–7.
44. Zajicek B. Scientific psychiatry in Stalin's Soviet Union: the politics of modern medicine and the struggle to define "Pavlovian" psychiatry, 1939–1953. PhD dissertation, University of Chicago; 2009.
45. Krasnushkin EK. Psikhogennyi faktor dushevnykh rasstroistv v voennoe vremia. In: Tveritin VA, editor. Problemy psikhiatrii voennogo vremeni. Moscow; 1945. p. 207–18.
46. Gorovoi-Shaltan VA. Reaktivnye nevrozy. In: Smirnov EI, editor. Opyt sovetskoi meditsiny v Velikoi otechestvennoi voine 1941–1945 gg, vol. 26. Moscow: Medgiz; 1949. p. 91–100.
47. Khoroshko VK. Uchenie o nevrozakh. Moscow: Medgiz; 1943.
48. Toropova, A. 'Nervous people: trauma and aesthetic hysteria in the late Stalinist melodrama'. In: Balina M. and Adachi D., editors. Melodrama and melodramatic imagination in the 20th and the 21st century Russia: new perspectives. Toronto: Toronto University Press, 2025.
49. Giliarovskii VA. Starye i novye problemy psikhiatrii. Moscow: Medgiz; 1946.
50. Zajicek B. Banning the soviet lobotomy: psychiatry, ethics, and professional politics during late Stalinism. Bull Hist Med. 2017;91(1):33–61.
51. Krementsov NL. Stalinist science. Princeton: Princeton University Press; 1997.
52. Pollock E. Stalin and the soviet science wars. Princeton: Princeton University Press; 2006.
53. Joravsky D. Russian psychology: a critical history. Oxford: Blackwell; 1989.
54. Platonov KI. Vnushenie i gipnoz v svete ucheniia I. P. Pavlova. Moscow: Medgiz; 1951.
55. Anon. Krepelin, Emil. In: Vvedenskii BA, editor. Bol'shaia sovetskaia entsiklopediia, vol. 23. 2nd ed. Moscow: BSE; 1953. p. 336.
56. Sluchevskii IF. O nekotorykh aktual'nykh voprosakh psikhiatrii. Zhurnal nevrologii i psikhi-atrii. 1952;LII(8):3–16.
57. Kerbikov OV. O nekotorykh spornykh voprosakh psikhiatrii. Zhurnal nevropatologii i psikhi-atrii. 1952;LII(5):8–25.
58. Shvarts IM. Nuzhna li psikhologiia psikhiatrii? Zhurnal nevropatologii i psikhiatrii. 1952;LII(12):48.

Open Access   This chapter is licensed under the terms of the Creative Commons Attribution 4.0 International License (http://creativecommons.org/licenses/by/4.0/), which permits use, sharing, adaptation, distribution and reproduction in any medium or format, as long as you give appropriate credit to the original author(s) and the source, provide a link to the Creative Commons license and indicate if changes were made.

The images or other third party material in this chapter are included in the chapter's Creative Commons license, unless indicated otherwise in a credit line to the material. If material is not included in the chapter's Creative Commons license and your intended use is not permitted by statutory regulation or exceeds the permitted use, you will need to obtain permission directly from the copyright holder.

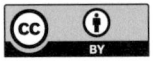

Yugoslav Psychiatry in the Middle: Non-aligned and Post-Colonial Psychiatry During the Cold War

20

Ana Antić

20.1 Decolonisation of Psychiatry and the Emergence of a Universalist Framework

In 1959, John Rawlings Rees, British psychiatrist and head of the newly founded World Federation for Mental Health, spoke on the role of culture and cultural differences in the context of psychiatric illness, and concluded that culture merely constituted a superficial veneer of illness expressions and symptoms: 'May I say here that I have visited many countries in the world and I don't believe there are fundamental differences or basic differences between anything that I heard in Africa and the things you find in other countries, except naturally in the cultural determinants of some symptoms of illness' [1]. Reese's statement on the limited role of 'cultural determinants' and factors was neither unique nor exceptional in mid-twentieth-century psychiatry—on the contrary, similar beliefs formed the basis of the overall clinical and theoretical framework for early post-war and post-colonial psychiatry. But Reese's declaration of universality was genuinely revolutionary in the broader context of the twentieth century: it constituted a radical departure from racist hierarchical thinking of colonial psychiatry and its insistence that there were fundamental and insurmountable differences between European, African and Asian minds [2]. These differences were variously defined as biological or cultural (or both) but they became one of the cornerstones of colonial psychiatric theory and practice, which reinforced cultural and political boundaries by assigning different groups and societies to different stages of 'civilisational' development.

In that sense, the early post-colonial turn to universalism could not have been more radical. Within this new framework, which emerged hand in hand with the decolonisation processes, Western and Western-dominated international psychiatry strove to distance itself from its erstwhile colonial foundations and develop a new

A. Antić (✉)
Centre for Culture and the Mind, University of Copenhagen, Copenhagen, Denmark
e-mail: ana.antic@hum.ku.dk

© The Author(s) 2026
G. Ikkos, T. Becker (eds.), *Psychiatry after Kraepelin*,
https://doi.org/10.1007/978-3-032-09475-9_20

and more inclusive model for collaborating with the decolonising territories. Psychiatric universalism, which then crucially informed the emerging field of transcultural psychiatry, echoed broader political developments: the period of decolonisation also saw the development of structures championing universal human rights, and psychiatric discussions had a lot to say about the concept of universal humanity [3]. In fact, early post-colonial transcultural psychiatrists were particularly interested in identifying, defining and debating core psychological traits and psychopathological mechanisms that would be shared across cultures and independent of cultural influences. Here the assumption was that there was a universal core, which constituted the foundation for cross-cultural communication and understanding. In the same vein, there was a universal core to mental illnesses—culture only shaped how psychopathology was manifested outwardly. As American psychiatrist Ari Kiev noted, 'it seems not unlikely then that mental illness is manifested in certain basic structural mechanisms and processes that recur together with certain regularity in the different clinical syndromes, providing a substratum on top of which the different cultures impose differences in content' [4]. Therefore, psychiatric diagnostic and therapeutic systems could also be globalised to reflect this assumed structural universality. In the second half of the twentieth century, there was a lot of investment in precisely that kind of research projects: studies that compared mental illness categories and perceptions in different cultural contexts and investigated how diagnostic procedures and therapeutic interventions could be translated and streamlined.[1]

20.2 Problems with Universalism

But the universalist framework was ridden with problems and internal inconsistencies. Firstly, who had the authority to define the new universals? Transcultural psychiatry operated in a historical context marked by significant political power imbalances. It was mainstream Western psychiatry that led the way in developing and investigating these categories, and more often than not, the 'universal' diagnostic concepts or illness definitions came to strongly resemble European or Western classifications [7]. In that way, the universalism of new transcultural psychiatry could reinforce Eurocentric approaches and ideas and marginalise the experiences and expertise coming from the decolonising territories. In that sense, it inherited some powerful conceptual frameworks from its colonial predecessor.

Another exceptionally influential and long-lasting legacy of colonial ethnopsychiatry turned out to be its evolutionary interpretation of the psychology of

---

[1] The WHO-funded International Pilot Study of Schizophrenia and its many follow-ups and related studies remain among the most influential [5]. Thomas Lambo's and Alexander Leighton's Cornell-Aro Mental Health research project, which began in 1961, aimed to compare conceptualisations and rates of psychological distress among the Yoruba people in Nigeria and rural Canadians in the Stirling County, and remains a model research project in this field due to its nuanced and comprehensive approach [6].

non-Western peoples, and its continued reliance on the notion of primitivism as a tool for classification. Post-colonial transcultural psychiatry often drew a straightforward line between 'primitive' civilisations and the 'childhood stage of humanity'—a common trope in more progressive psychoanalytic and anthropological discourses as well, which saw the 'savages' of the non-White world as fascinating snapshots of humanity as it was before the onset of 'civilisation'. In other words, while they affirmed a universal psychological potential, many transcultural psychiatrists placed non-Western groups and societies on an altogether different historical stage of psychological and social development compared to Europe and North America, drawing distinctions between 'primitive' mental traits of people from the decolonising world, and 'civilised' and more complex minds in the West. One of the most illustrative examples of this tendency could be found in the work of distinguished British psychiatrist Julian Leff, who developed a scheme of an 'evolutionary process in the dawning awareness of the psychological experiences of unpleasant emotion', in which he argued that speakers of non-Indo-European languages had a significantly poorer, more limited vocabulary of negative emotions [8]. In his view, compared to their counterparts in Western Europe, they were notably less able to differentiate verbally between feelings such as depression and anxiety, lacked words and expressions for a variety of emotional states and instead mainly focused on somatic sensations and experiences. This was arguably because, in the context of an imagined linear historical and civilisational development, they occupied a different linguistic stage, due to complex cultural and social processes which shaped their psychological structures in a particular way. On the other side, similar processes produced a significantly different Western mind: more capable of both psychological and linguistic differentiation and nuances when it came to emotions [8]. In that sense, the universalist framework, which affirmed that all minds shared basic structures and all were headed towards the same developmental goal, could incorporate hierarchical thinking and different theories of primitivism.

There was also an important contradiction within transcultural psychiatry: while it downplayed the importance of cultural differences, it often discussed non-European cultural contexts in highly essentialising and othering ways. Insisting on the overall psychological universality, it tended to interpret clinical differences through culturalist and exoticising lenses and frequently disregarded the role of broader and more genuinely universal social, economic and political factors. This was obvious in Leff's interpretation of his scheme: he appeared to be solely interested in cultural factors, such as the assumed collectivist orientation of non-Western societies, whose 'cultural focus' was on the group rather than the individual—this meant that there was little space for individuals to explore and determine their emotional relations and develop their creativity. This explanation then completely excluded any references to social and political contexts in which psychiatric consultations might be taking place [9, pp. 45–46, 72]. Moreover, Leff never considered that those communities, whose languages he called 'living fossils', might have a completely different universe of internal mental states, and consequently a lexicon of emotions that was not nuanced or differentiated simply because it did not reflect Western expectations.

Leff's case was not unique—transcultural psychiatry had a distinct tendency to prioritise cultural explanations and to marginalise some core analytical categories from social psychiatry. In this, it perpetuated a major contradiction in its own theoretical framework, and, ironically, made it more difficult to develop genuinely universal interpretations and place Western and decolonising societies on an equal footing.

20.3 Non-aligned Psychiatry and Decolonisation: The Issue of Imperfect Alternatives

But post-colonial transcultural psychiatry was by no means homogeneous. While it was dominated by Western psychiatrists (some of whom had also played important roles in the late colonial systems), this emerging professional field included a number of experts from the decolonising world—such as Thomas A. Lambo, Nigeria's leading psychiatrist and one of the foremost architects of post-war global psychiatry. These psychiatrists at times mounted substantial challenges to the lingering colonial legacies and developed influential critiques. At other times, however, they too perpetuated some aspects of transcultural psychiatry's binary and hierarchical thinking. But beyond these groups, there emerged another network of agents who engaged in re-thinking the global tenets and institutions of psychiatry—psychiatric experts from the socialist world, most notably from Yugoslavia. More broadly, different kinds of experts from the socialist world became increasingly engaged in global networks and exchanges, as relationships between the second and third worlds grew ever more intensive in the course of the decolonisation processes: as many historians have demonstrated, the Eastern bloc developed keen interest in collaboration with a variety of newly independent African and Asian countries, and worked to offer a more sustainable model of modernisation in the aftermath of the failed Western colonial project [10–12]. In that context, psychiatrists were not at the forefront—to my knowledge, it was only Yugoslav psychiatrists who became engaged in transcultural psychiatric debates and projects in a sustained manner. Their interventions were in many ways significantly different from those of their Western colleagues. One of the core distinctions was rooted in Yugoslavia's own political and cultural identity—even though European, the country inhabited a decidedly peripheral position geographically. And it was undergoing a period of intense modernisation, not so dissimilar from what was going on in the decolonising world. This implicit political and geographical combination—paired with its Marxist ideology—fundamentally informed Yugoslav psychiatrists' involvement in the decolonisation of global psychiatry.

In the context of socialist psychiatry, moreover, the very civilisational superiority of the West was not unquestioned and unconditional anymore: the socialist East aimed to propose an alternative, more ethically conscious and ultimately more worthy form of modernity. This did not automatically translate into any fundamental changes in the psychiatric discourse of 'catching up' with the West, but at least the Western ideal was not an unassailably positive political category any longer, and both psychiatrists and other intellectuals could critique the (supposedly hierarchical) cultural relationship between Eastern and Western Europe. It was also very important that Yugoslavia was not a typical member of the socialist bloc: it played a critical role in the creation of the Non-Aligned Movement, and this dramatic restructuring of its international links and alliances bred a new political language of anti-colonialism, anti-racism and solidarity with the decolonising world. Its prominent global role and new political orientation meant that psychiatrists would engage the Global South on a significantly different footing than their colleagues from former colonial powers.

Still, the socialist conceptualisation of progress and development remained decidedly linear, and Yugoslav psychiatrists continued to rely on the notions of 'primitivism', backwardness and underdevelopment in their clinical analyses and broader social and political commentary (in Yugoslavia's political parlance, the concept of the primitive was in regular use as well). In that sense, Yugoslav socialist psychiatrists were in a complex intellectual position and were often hard pressed to reconcile their theories of modernisation and the 'primitive' nature of patients in the decolonising world with the fierce political anti-colonialism of the non-aligned movement [13].

In the context of such intellectual and political ambivalence, it was perhaps not so surprising that socialist psychiatry was often quite slow to shed some important colonial tenets and conceptualisations. In the 1950s and 1960s, for instance, it was still important for the country's psychiatric profession to emphasise that Yugoslavia did belong to the culturally and socially advanced family of European nations—that it was civilisationally in the same group as Western Europe. Yugoslavia's (and Eastern Europe's) first and most prominent transcultural psychiatrist Vladimir Jakovljevic, for instance, tended to agree with infamous British colonial physician John Collin Carothers' that the 'civilised world' was generally characterised by higher frequencies of 'complex' mental pathology: since Yugoslav patients suffered from such pathologies no less than West Europeans, Jakovljevic could conclude that Yugoslavia's cultural identity was primarily linked to Europe rather than the developing world [14]. Jakovljevic spent several years in Guinea in the early 1960s, where he helped develop local psychiatric services, and this experience vitally informed his contributions to transcultural psychiatry. As we will see below, his politics differed significantly from that of many of his Western colleagues, but he still echoed Western transcultural psychiatrists and regularly referred not only to his Guinean patients but also to Guinea's social and cultural structures as 'primitive' and 'oriental.'

At the same time, and despite Jakovljevic's pronouncements regarding Yugoslavia's civilisational 'Europeanness', the conditionality and peripherality of his own country's position haunted his writings. For instance, Jakovljevic spent a lot of time working in Macedonia, the southernmost part of Yugoslavia, and his descriptions of his Macedonian and Guinean patients occasionally became virtually indistinguishable even though he never acknowledged these similarities explicitly—both groups reportedly characterised by comparable degrees of individual and collective backwardness, and confusion in the face of rapid modernisation and change [15]. It was such psychiatric work more than any other political or intellectual discourse that emphasised the deep ambiguity of Yugoslavia's cultural status. In terms of socio-cultural relations, psychological profile, family structures and other social institutions, clinical and anthropological research demonstrated that Yugoslavia's largely rural population perhaps had a lot in common with the 'primitives' of the decolonising world.

Jakovljevic wrote of a rural Macedonian society marked by 'extremely archaic' social structures, which exhibited 'exceptional forms of socio-psychological backwardness' [15], and this resulted in an 'exceptionally levelled collective psyche' that defied and precluded the process of individuation or the formation of richer forms of internal life. This society held on to 'totemistic beliefs and appropriate rituals all the way to exorcism' and practiced open aggression in the form of blood vengeance, 'extreme patriarchy in families, buying of women who are evaluated as merchandise' etc. Further symptoms of its severe underdevelopment included extreme fatalism and even more developed primitive beliefs', a 'great rigidity of personalities', as well as a tendency to resort to magic acts, protective amulets or 'bizarre medications of archaic or religious origin.' [15] While these descriptions sound like typical transcultural psychiatric accounts of primitivism in the decolonising world, here Jakovljevic was writing about Macedonia and the state of affairs he encountered in his own country. (Of course, it mattered here that Jakovljevic himself was not from the Macedonian region nor of Macedonian ethnic background—both his ethnic identity and his social class set him apart from his mostly rural Macedonian patients, and this internal distance, determined by Yugoslavia's own exceptional cultural and social heterogeneity, played an important role in his conceptualisations of 'primitivism' and civilisation).

His Yugoslav patients' levels of cultural education and modernity were by all accounts comparable to those of the Africans whom he encountered and treated [16, 17]. Jakovljevic argued that the prevalence of certain psychiatric disorders (such as schizophrenia or neurosis) in Yugoslavia was comparable to that in Western Europe—this was a sign that Yugoslavia belonged to the civilised European family of nations, Macedonia, however, was an exception: the rate of neurosis among the general population there was reportedly less than a half of the neurotic morbidity in 'civilised countries.' This was one of the more incontrovertible indicators of the society's comparative civilisational position; moreover, it was the more 'primitive neurotic disorders' which prevailed in the Yugoslav society over more complex and intellectualised ones commonly found in countries like France. Yugoslav patients expressed their mental pathology in more primitive, non-verbal and psychosomatic ways; by contrast, West European neurotics were characterised by complex psychopathological mechanisms and advanced abstract forms of thinking [15, pp. 1–2]. It was this uncertainty about Yugoslavia's own cultural identity that made socialist psychiatrists' transcultural musings much more complex and ultimately more progressive than those of their Western colleagues. But beyond these shared traits of 'primitivism', Jakovljevic and his collaborators also drew indirect parallels between the Yugoslav and African experiences of revolutionary fight, national liberation and rapid (and disruptive) modernisation.

This was the reason that Yugoslavia's socialist transcultural psychiatry developed and worked with a more dynamic and optimistic image of 'primitive' decolonising societies. It was difficult for Yugoslav psychiatrists to accept one of colonial psychiatry's core tropes—that non-European colonised societies, with their simplistic and underdeveloped minds, were static and largely incapable of development, inhabiting a different stage of civilisational development. This approach was part and parcel of the colonial 'infantilism thesis', which proposed that African cultures were permanently stuck in the 'childhood stage of humanity', providing an insight into the nature and state of the human race before 'civilisation.' First and foremost, such a static and pessimistic approach would not have boded well for Yugoslavia, which faced its own developmental psychological and cultural hardships following the revolutionary social transformations after 1945. But equally importantly, they were primarily social psychiatrists: they focused on complex socio-economic structures and developments, and their positive effects on 'backward' and modernising societies. Even though they remained bound to a hierarchical framework of thinking, Jakovljevic and his colleagues still believed in the ability of 'primitive' societies to overcome such difficulties in the context of modernisation, learn and transform quickly, and ultimately construct complex and progressive cultural, political and social institutions. Yugoslavia and Guinea both needed to 'catch up' with Western levels of modernity and civilisation, but they were certainly capable of doing so.

20.4   Non-alignment and Eurocentrism: The Politics of Socialist Psychiatry

This raises much broader questions about Yugoslavia's and Eastern Europe's cultural identity. Socialist Eastern Europe, including Yugoslavia, remained centrally attached to the idea of 'Europe' as a benchmark of civilisation, and many political actors and intellectuals often relied on orientalising, racist, Eurocentric and essentially colonial discourses of the white West. This was qualified by the experience and ideology of socialism, as well as, in the Yugoslav case, by the practices and discourses of non-alignment. Arguably, the non-aligned movement (NAM) was vital to transforming socialist Eastern Europe's orientalising tendencies. At times, political discourses of non-alignment seemed to take Yugoslavia outside of Europe altogether: they portrayed Yugoslavia as a particularly understanding and compassionate partner to the decolonising world [18, p. 179]. The introduction of a 1979 special issue of the communist youth journal *Nase teme*, dedicated to the African continent, referred to Yugoslavia and Yugoslavs as having a 'particular African vocation', emphasising the country's close links with Africa and longstanding commitment to Africa's independence [19].

At the same time, there were tensions and contradictions within Yugoslavia's discourses of non-aligned solidarity. Jelena Subotic and Srdjan Vucetic refer to Yugoslavia's NAM-inspired anti-imperialism as an exercise in 'performing solidarity' with the Third World for the purposes of advancing the country's international political status but without any fundamental understanding of the problem of racism and racial relations in the Cold War world. Subotic and Vucetic argue that the country's embrace of the language of non-aligned solidarity was primarily opportunistic and did not reflect a truly emancipatory ideological orientation [20]. This was mainly because, as the authors write, Yugoslavia developed a 'superiority complex' in its relationships with its African and Asian partners. Moreover, Yugoslav leaders themselves often expressed dismissive, even racialised opinions about the decolonising countries (and their understanding of socialism) [18], while African and Asian students in Yugoslavia regularly faced physical and verbal abuse from the local population, and were systematically ostracised [21]. The Yugoslav political leadership's arguments that their solidarity with the decolonising world was based on their country's comparable experiences of colonial oppression (in the Habsburg and Ottoman empires) and its successful war of liberation/independence in WWII were constantly undermined by the Yugoslavs' failure to reflect on their own 'white privilege' in a thoroughly racialised world.

This lack of reflection was often obvious in public and political representations of African societies and individuals (and of Yugoslav leaders visiting African countries)—such images tended to exoticise 'distant' cultures and relied on well-used colonial tropes, symbols and interpretations, even though they officially promoted messages of anti-colonialism, solidarity and anti-racism [22]. Despite being white and European, Yugoslavia was never a coloniser, and this seemed to release it from any need for a critical re-consideration of its own contributions to the old colonial order, or the perpetuation of racialised discourses of Africa and the Global South after decolonisation.

On the other hand, even though the Balkan region might have seen itself as politically, geographically and civilisationally European (even under socialism), its historical legacy was one of imperial subjects rather than imperial rulers, and the attachment to a 'European identity' was accompanied by narratives of cultural inferiority and experiences of rejection by Europe. In that sense, non-aligned Yugoslavia's geopolitical and civilisational status was permanently unstable [23]. NAM-related practices and narratives of solidarity fundamentally shaped a variety of aspects of Yugoslavia's collaboration with its partners from the decolonising world. Such narratives also played a major part in different fields of knowledge and art production in Yugoslavia. The shared experiences of fighting resistance wars and handling dramatic consequences of rapid social and political transformations further reinforced the political and cultural bonds which developed between Yugoslavia and its NAM partners [24]. African history and contemporary politics, and in particular African socialism, became important fields of research, and a lot of space was dedicated to these topics in Yugoslavia's public discourse as well as in more specialised scholarly journals. Moreover, different sections of Yugoslav society became deeply committed to spreading the message of anti-colonialism and solidarity, often without any ulterior motives or hidden selfish interests.

The psychiatric profession engaged in lengthy comparative discussions of socialist, Western and African psyches, and such discussions offer a unique insight into the nature and complexity of non-aligned Yugoslavia's political and cultural vacillation in the triangle between the East, West and South. For instance, Yugoslav psychiatrists' relationship to their African colleagues and hosts was one of (benevolent) hierarchy as much as of solidarity—they were there to teach and guide, export an original socialist model of modernisation and offer an alternative to the failed colonial project. Even though they could detect similarities between African and Yugoslav (or Balkan) experiences and historical structures, they (and other experts who travelled southward from Eastern Europe) still considered themselves to be self-evidently in a superior position and significantly more advanced along the axis of modernisation. Furthermore, they repeatedly described the Guinean society as both economically and culturally 'primitive' and underdeveloped and often established a fundamental distinction between 'European' Yugoslavia and 'backward' Africa.

But on the other hand, the Yugoslav transcultural psychiatric profession (and anthropology) also produced significantly more sophisticated knowledge about the decolonising world. And because their research was often explicitly comparative, it shed important light on the reconceptualisation of the relationship between the Balkans and Africa.

Socialist non-aligned psychiatry was still based on radically different ideological premises and could not fully adopt the colonial psychiatric framework of 'primitivism', even though it tended to use some of the same concepts. In that sense, the psychiatrists' first-hand discovery that the Yugoslav population's 'backwardness' was not fundamentally different from the civilisational 'tribal primitivism' of 'native' African populations worked to produce more progressive transcultural psychiatric approaches. This enabled the development of a more inclusive discourse about the human psyche and its cross-cultural universality. Beyond the organicist framework, socialist non-aligned psychiatry focused on the extraordinary developmental potential of 'primitive' societies, emphasising the possibility of successful social, cultural and psychological transformations in both Balkan and African societies. This potential to 'catch up' thus promised to erase the difference between 'backward' and 'civilised' societies in the near future. The therapeutic optimism of socialist psychiatry further reinforced the belief that progress, and development could be achieved through cross-cultural exchange and collaboration.

While modernisation necessarily carried with it a sharp increase in psychological suffering and disorder, it was not a failed mission: even 'primitive' African inhabitants could adapt to a more technically and culturally advanced surrounding. Jakovljevic's version of transcultural psychiatry predicted ultimately positive outcomes of the momentous social and political transformations of both sub-Saharan Africa and the socialist bloc. Writing of Guinea's ever fluctuating social makeup, he observed that 'it became clear that inherited phylogenetic cultural models do not necessarily repeat themselves in the course of development, but are always learnt and, in the course of that learning, can always be changed' [25, p. 167].

Since cultural patterns and dispositions were so malleable and dependent on socio-cultural environment and political and economic structures, Jakovljevic could not draw a straightforward line between 'primitive' civilisations and the 'childhood stage of humanity'—Even though Jakovljevic admitted that 'primitive adults' of

Guinea shared certain mental traits with children from the civilised world, differences were equally if not more important [25, p. 142]. Marxist psychiatry and psychoanalysis—although it assumed that progress was unidirectional and that Guinea had to 'catch up'—could hardly view African civilisations in a static manner within the evolutionary context, but instead argued that cultures and societies could, under propitious circumstances, make revolutionary leaps in their own development and progress: 'our experiences have clearly demonstrated that a primitive personality, who is young and capable enough, can successfully integrate in a technically and culturally developed environment, even though that integration might be accompanied by temporary mental disorders' [25, p. 167]. In that sense, despite being heavily influenced by Western European psychoanalytic thinking, Jakovljevic distanced himself from those transcultural psychoanalytic and psychiatric discourses which saw the 'contemporary "primitive"' as a version of the early stages of human society' who could consequently have no history [26, p. 6].

This socialist therapeutic optimism rested on the universalist framework. In fact, the universalism of immediate post-WWII transcultural psychiatry seemed to be taken for granted in the Yugoslav context: psychiatrists and anthropologists often emphatically insisted that Africans were as capable of logical and analytical thinking as Europeans [27]. In the 1970s, in an article on the notions of change and development in Africa, one of Yugoslavia's leading researchers in development studies and cross-cultural communication Nada Svob-Djokic ironically commended Western European researchers for concluding, decades after the end of colonial regimes, that 'the mental mechanism of Africans was no different than ours' [28]. But Yugoslav psychiatry's universalism was based on a unique idea of solidarity between the East European and African regions, and insisted on the comparability of their respective social and political experiences. Partly because of that and partly due to their Marxist focus on socio-economic determinants of mental health, Yugoslav clinicians avoided the exoticisation of cultural differences and narrowly defined cultural factors, a trend common in Western transcultural psychiatry.

In the early stages of decolonisation in particular, both psychiatrists and policy makers in the Western world were primarily concerned about the predicted psychological toll of cultural change and cross-cultural mixing. For some of the leading transcultural psychiatrists, the dangers of 'acculturation' were tremendous, and they principally applied to less developed societies, who were experiencing fast-paced social, political and cultural transformations. As US psychiatrist Ari Kiev noted, acculturation and cultural change were only guaranteed to have harmful mental effects on underdeveloped and developing societies, while any pathological potential of similar cross-cultural influences in Western societies was not considered worthy of exploration [29]. The situation was rather unusual: while transcultural psychiatry, as a relatively new discipline, sought to establish a role for itself as a facilitator of harmonious cross-cultural communication, its West European representatives still viewed cross-cultural contact as a major source of mental pathology and worried about the ability of 'primitive' decolonising nations to adjust to rapid changes.

Marxist psychiatry, on the other hand, worried much less about the ability of 'primitive' societies to integrate and adapt to progressive cultural, political and technological transformations. In fact, Jakovljevic's most important theoretical contribution—his concept of 'revolutionary personality'—emphasised the productive, creative and constructive, rather than pathological potentials of dramatic social and cultural conflicts, which always accompanied revolutionary change or modernisation projects. Jakovljevic criticised exclusively psychological interpretations of mental disorders, which he thought disregarded the revolutionary potential of conflicts between individuals and their social environment: 'socially caused conflicts might constitute a progressive factor in the development of a society' and lead to revolutionary resistance against the social organisation or structure [30, p. 76]. This was a new platform for Marxist psychiatry and psychoanalysis, and it radically redefined the role of social conflict in causing mental illness. While a discord or conflict between an individual and her social environment (which traditional psychoanalysis tended to see as the core origins of neurotic disorders) might lead to mental pathology and personality deviation, pathological or pathogenic sociocultural factors did not necessarily cause psychological disorders, if a robust individual in an 'abnormal' society found ways to overcome or affect the existing circumstances. Quite to the contrary, a 'conformist adaptation of an individual to an abnormal social environment might lead to an even more fundamental form of [psychological] abnormality' [30]. In that sense what Jakovljevic defined as a 'nonconformist' personality was a phenomenon critically different from a mentally ill individual, although it did emerge from a similar structural setting. In fact, the 'nonconformist personality' was the healthiest type of individual in any reactionary or 'anachronistic' society. Jakovljevic articulated his theory of revolutionary personality following his work in Guinea but based it on his research findings in both Africa and Yugoslavia. In this reading, both the Yugoslav and the Guinean social revolutions were driven by such revolutionary personalities, whose ability to overcome unhealthy psychological influences of fascism and colonialism, respectively, and to thrive in their rapidly changing societies boded well for the second and the third worlds' ambitious developmental plans. In that sense, the idea that cross-cultural exchange and transformation were primarily pathogenic was certainly not dominant in East European transcultural psychiatry, perhaps precisely because the socialist profession did not prioritise the importance of cultural over social, political or economic factors and differences.

Furthermore, in Eastern Europe the notion of 'acculturation' in the specific context of decolonisation and rapid globalisation was interpreted in an explicitly positive way. For Yugoslav commentators and psychiatrists, for instance, it was of foremost importance to insist on the dynamic nature of African cultures and societies: writing against the idea that (sub-Saharan) African societies were static, ahistorical and marked by 'unchangeable traditions and tribal exoticism', Jakovljevic's anthropologist colleague Biserka Cvjeticanin emphasised their dynamic history and their current creative grappling with large-scale changes. Before colonial conquests, during colonial regimes and after decolonisation, different African groups and societies experienced constant change both within the confines of their own borders and in contact with other cultures, so that their capability of dynamic development and transformation was in no fundamental way different from that of Western societies [27].

Cvjeticanin introduced Marx's definition of acculturation—as a process of 'creation under the pressure of novel circumstances and by no means as a simple dissolution of a culture which suffered a blow from outside.' Moreover, Cvjeticanin was one of the very few voices who insisted that acculturation was a two-way process, which changed Western societies as well. It was no coincidence that this voice came from Marxist Eastern Europe: this intervention meant that the influence of African (non-Western cultures) on the Western world was not minuscule or non-existent [27, p. 789]. Cvjeticanin warned that acculturation was not assimilation or a mechanical transplantation of certain traits and mores from a more developed society to a less developed one, but it meant 'transformation and creative integration.' In the course of this process, the receiving culture demonstrated its own dynamism and ability to adopt new elements but also to change them and ensure the authenticity and continuity of its own identity. In that sense, African cultures were neither mere imitators of more developed traditions nor unchangeable/ahistorical: just like all other societies, they chose which foreign elements and cultural aspects to adopt, adapt and fit in their own existing structures, thereby producing novel (dynamic and modern) creative totalities.

Finally, even those African groups or societies which proved more impervious to change and external influences were not static and paralysed in their rigid traditions: traditional culture was not necessarily an obstacle to progress but it should also be seen as a 'dynamic factor of development. It's natural for tradition to resist change. But that resistance in itself could cause change... Transformations are therefore resisted but such conflict gives birth to new initiatives' [27, p. 790] African societies were not simply catching up, in other words, but producing authentic and valuable cultural contributions in the process of their rapid development and transformation. This was a crucial insight for East European societies too, and for their developmental prospects.

20.5   Conclusion

It is important to acknowledge that mid-twentieth-century global psychiatry invested significant efforts into distancing itself from the colonial frameworks and assumptions: in the 1950s, it developed a politically progressive universalist paradigm which insisted that there were no significant differences in psychological mechanisms and pathologies across cultures. This new framework ascertained that people from all cultural groups and communities belonged to the same family of universal humanity, in the face of colonial psychiatry's racist and hierarchical principles. At the same time, however, the universalist framework often reinforced Eurocentric categories and norms as psychiatric universals. Moreover, as illustrated in West European discourses of acculturation and cultural difference, the mid-twentieth century 'ideological universalism' of transcultural psychiatry could also incorporate hierarchical thinking, exoticising assumptions about cultural differences and lingering colonial paradigms. This essay has shed light on socialist East European, especially Yugoslav, contributions to global transcultural psychiatry debates, and reflected on how this body of knowledge offered an alternative or challenge to mainstream Western psychiatry. The nature of this challenge remained ambiguous. Socialist psychiatric and anthropological articulations of the concepts of primitivism and civilisation remained complex and ambivalent. While the post-1945 development of new approaches and discourses often marked a departure from the interwar elaborations of civilisational hierarchies, the socialist psychiatric profession continued to construct the struggle against 'primitivism' within the Yugoslav society as its central task. This internal 'civilising mission' then largely determined how Yugoslavia's transcultural psychiatrists and anthropologists interpreted their own country's—and region's—position in relation to the non-European world. In an important way, their tendency to draw historical parallels between Eastern Europe and the global South could produce an alternative articulation of anti-colonial universalism, based on a unique narrative of cross-cultural solidarity. This by no means guaranteed that the socialist Yugoslav discussions of the global South and its development would be decolonised in any fundamental way, despite their robust anti-colonial rhetoric and political commitments. But it did produce a remarkably different strand of psychiatric theory and practice within transcultural psychiatry. Instead of dismissing socialist psychiatry as a political handmaiden of authoritarian regimes, researchers need to take into account the heterogeneity of this profession and its important and innovative contributions to the making of global psychiatric knowledge.

Key Points
- Transcultural psychiatry emerged in the middle of the twentieth century in the course of the decolonisation processes.
- It aimed to distance itself from the colonial frameworks, practices and assumptions.
- Early transcultural psychiatry emphasised the universality of psychological mechanisms and pathologies across cultures, but did not fully eliminate hierarchical, culturally exoticising and evolutionary forms of thinking.
- Yugoslav psychiatrists engaged with global debates in transcultural psychiatry, and offered a series of interventions shaped by Marxist ideology and Yugoslavia's specific geopolitical position—as a non-aligned socialist East European country.
- While Yugoslav psychiatry perpetuated various assumptions regarding civilisational hierarchies and 'primitivism', their version of transcultural psychiatry was marked by a different sense of solidarity and shared developmental concerns between the decolonising world and Eastern Europe.

Funding Acknowledgement   This research was supported by ERC Starting Grant DECOLMAD 851871 and the Danish Research Foundation DNRF171.

References

1. World Federation for Mental Health. Africa: social change and mental health; report of a panel discussion conducted in conference room no. 1, United Nations, New York; 1959.
2. Vaughan M. Curing their ills: colonial power and African illness. Cambridge: Cambridge University Press; 1991.
3. Wu H. Mad by the millions: mental disorders and the early years of the WHO. Cambridge: MIT Press; 2021.
4. Kiev A. Magic, faith and healing: studies in primitive psychiatry today. New York: Free Press; 1964.
5. Sartorius N, Shapiro R, Kimura M, Barrett K. WHO international pilot study of schizophrenia. Psychol Med. 1972;2:422–5.
6. Heaton M. Black skin, white coats: Nigerian psychiatrists, decolonization, and the globalization of psychiatry. Athens: Ohio University Press; 2013.
7. Littlewood R. From categories to contexts: a decade of the "new cross-cultural psychiatry". Br J Psychiatry. 1990;156(3):308–27.
8. Leff J. Culture and the differentiation of emotional states. Br J Psychiatry. 1973;123(574):299–306.
9. Leff J. Psychiatry around the globe: a transcultural view. New York and Basel: Marcel Dekker; 1981.
10. Mark J, Betts P, editors. Socialism goes global: the Soviet Union and Eastern Europe in the age of decolonisation. Oxford: Oxford University Press; 2022.
11. Stanek L. Architecture in Global Socialism: Eastern Europe, West Africa, and the Middle East in the Cold War. Princeton University Press; 2020.
12. Stanek L. Mobilities of architecture in the late cold war: from socialist Poland to Kuwait, and back. Int J Islam Archit. 2015;4(2):365–98.
13. Antic A. Chapter 1, Primitivism, modernity and revolution in the twentieth century: the case of psychiatry. In: Non-aligned psychiatry in the Cold War. Palgrave; 2022. p. 15–51.
14. Carothers JC. A study of mental derangement in Africans, and an attempt to explain its peculiarities, more especially in relation to the African attitude to life. East Afr Med J. 1948;25(4):142–66.
15. Jakovljevic V. Doprinos Proucavanju Uloge Psiholoskih Uticaja Sociokulturne Sredine u Patogenezi Neuroza. Neuropsihijatrija. 1959;7
16. Jakovljevic V. Kulturna sredina i psihički poremećaji ličnosti: transkulturno-psihijatrijsko proučavanje u Afričkoj Gvineji. [PhD thesis]. University of Zagreb; 1967.
17. Jakovljevic V. Prilog Proucavanju Sociopsihogeneze Neurotickih Poremecaja Licnosti. Sociologija. 1959;2
18. Svetozar R. No bargaining chips, no spheres of interest: the Yugoslav origins of Cold War non-alignment. J Cold War Stud. 2014;16(1):146–79.
19. Nase Teme; 1979;23(3).
20. Subotic J, Vucetic S. Performing solidarity: whiteness and status-seeking in the non-aligned world. J Int Relat Dev. 2019;22:722–43.
21. Lazic M. Neki problemi stranih studenata na jugoslovenskim univerzitetima šezdesetih godina XX veka, s posebnim osvrtom na afričke studente [Some problems of foreign students at Yugoslav universities in the 1960s, with special focus on African students]. Godišnjak za društvenu istoriju. 2009;2:61–78.
22. Sladojevic A. Beyond the photographic frame: interpretation of photographs from the Museum of Yugoslavia's collection in a contemporary context. In: Vučetić R, Betts B, editors. Tito in Africa: picturing solidarity. Belgrade: Museum of Yugoslavia; 2017. p. 92–125.
23. Baker C. Race and the Yugoslav region: post-socialist, post-conflict, postcolonial? Manchester: Manchester University Press; 2018.

24. Betts P. A red wind of change: African press coverage of Tito's visits to decolonizing Africa. In: Vučetić R, Betts B, editors. Tito in Africa: picturing solidarity. Belgrade: Museum of Yugoslavia; 2017. p. 46–77.
25. Jakovljevic V. Prilozi za Socijalnu Patologiju. Belgrade: Sloboda; 1984.
26. Khanna R. Dark continents: psychoanalysis and colonialism. Durham: Duke University Press; 2003.
27. Cvjeticanin B. Kontinuitet i dinamicnost africkih kultura. Nase Teme. 1979;23(3):785–95.
28. Svob-Djokic N. Nase Teme. 1979;23(4)
29. Kiev A. Transcultural psychiatry. New York: Free Press; 1972.
30. Jakovljevic V. Prilog Proucavanju Neurotickih Poremecaja.

Open Access This chapter is licensed under the terms of the Creative Commons Attribution 4.0 International License (http://creativecommons.org/licenses/by/4.0/), which permits use, sharing, adaptation, distribution and reproduction in any medium or format, as long as you give appropriate credit to the original author(s) and the source, provide a link to the Creative Commons license and indicate if changes were made.

The images or other third party material in this chapter are included in the chapter's Creative Commons license, unless indicated otherwise in a credit line to the material. If material is not included in the chapter's Creative Commons license and your intended use is not permitted by statutory regulation or exceeds the permitted use, you will need to obtain permission directly from the copyright holder.

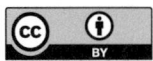

Ideas, Theories and Psychiatric Services: De-institutionalisation and Community Care in Italy, the UK and Germany Since 1960

21

Thomas Becker, Stefan Weinmann, George Ikkos, Angelo Fioritti, and Uta Gühne

21.1 Introduction

It is plausible to think of the history of psychiatric care as part of a country's social and sociopolitical history [1, 2]. Psychiatry, as a clinical-scientific discipline and a component of social practice, also has an interface with cultural history [1]. This chapter describes the development of mental health care in Italy, the UK and Germany from the 1960s onwards with reference to (a) the first author's personal account of guiding ideas and theoretical concepts that were actively perceived and

---

'Germany' refers to the Federal Republic of Germany (FRG, pre-unification) in this text; since October 1990 the general framework for mental health services in the (now) 16 federal states of the country has been the same in so far as it is 'federal' and not determined by federal state rules (of which there are 16).

T. Becker (✉)
Department of Psychiatry and Psychotherapy, Univesity of Leipzig Medical Center, Leipzig, Germany
e-mail: Thomas.Becker@medizin.uni-leipzig.de

S. Weinmann
Center for Integrative Psychiatry, University of Luebeck, Luebeck, Germany
e-mail: Stefan.Weinmann@uksh.de

G. Ikkos
Department of Liaison Psychiatry, Royal National Orthopaedic Hospital, Stanmore, UK
e-mail: ikkos@doctors.org.uk

A. Fioritti
Department of Mental Health and Substance Abuse, Azienda USL Bologna, Bologna, Italy
e-mail: angelofioritti@gmail.com

U. Gühne
Institute of Social Medicine, Occupational Health and Public Health, Medical Faculty, University of Leipzig, Leipzig, Germany
e-mail: Uta.Guehne@medizin.uni-leipzig.de

© The Author(s) 2026
G. Ikkos, T. Becker (eds.), *Psychiatry after Kraepelin*,
https://doi.org/10.1007/978-3-032-09475-9_21

discussed among mental health professionals in the three countries during the period, and (b) patterns of mental health care (service setup, patterns of care, quantitative indices) as they evolved over time in Italy, Germany and the UK.

21.2   Methodology

The personal account of guiding ideas (and theoretical concepts) in the debates on mental health care and psychiatric reform in Italy, UK and Germany is based on previous work [3–6] and on an extended personal and hand search of the relevant literature. The literature used to describe patterns of mental health care as they developed in Italy, UK and Germany since the 1960s was the result of a systematic search of the literature in November 2024.

We conducted a systematic search of the MEDLINE database accessible via the PubMed search engine (www.ncbi.nlm.nih.gov/pubmed/). Multiple search terms were used for three concepts: (1) psychiatric reform (in Italy, the UK and Germany), (2) psychiatric care and mental health services, (3) metrics for psychiatric care (e.g. staff ratio, involuntary treatment). Our search terms were restricted by language (Italian, English, German) and were manually reviewed. The search was supplemented by a hand search.

Following short narrative outlines of the development of mental health care in each country, there is a chronological description of the papers identified in the above search that describe and discuss mental health services in Italy, Germany and the UK over the period of (about) 1995 to 2023. These are summarised in chronological order. Finally, descriptions of the Health Systems and Policy Monitor (HSPM) for the European Observatory on Health Systems and Policies are used to give an up-to-date outline referring to 2024 [7]. Two tables summarise indices pertaining to the sociocultural systems and indices of mental health care in Italy, the UK and Germany.

21.3   Theories and Concepts

Table 21.1 provides a comparison of Italy, the UK and Germany with respect to a number of generic and mental health-related sociocultural variables which are relevant to the context of theories and concepts in the three countries.

Table 21.1 Three nations comparison (Italy, UK, Germany): sociocultural variables

	Governance	Health system	Expenditure for health/GDP	Expenditure for MH/health	Core of welfare mix	Core of MH system	MH approach	Treated prevalence[1]	MH promotion—prevention	Psychological treatments for all	Integration with addictions and child psychiatry
Italy	Regional	SSN (NHS)	8%	3%	Pensions + taxation	Community	Public health	2%	Low	Low	Good
UK	Central	NHS	11%	11%	Taxation + market elements	Balanced	Public health + clinical	20–40%	High	Moderate	Moderate
Germany	Regional	Insurance	12%	13%	Social insurance + taxation	Hospital + some balanced	Clinical	30–40%	Good	Good	Moderate

	Level of formal coercion	Forensic services	Legal system	Predominant sociocultural values	Society 'center of gravity'	Socioeconomic inequalities GINI[2]	Unemployment rate (% of labour force)	Regional socioeconomic inequalities	MH care development trends	Philosophical roots	Political background
Italy	Low	SSN—small	Common Law	Freedom	Family	0.330 (18)	11	North/South	Radicalism	Social critique	Unstable
UK	High	NHS—Large	Roman	Effectiveness	Individual	0.355 (36)	5	Cities/rural	Reform	Empiricism	Stressed
Germany	High	Stand-alone	Roman	Welfare + stability	State	0.296 (12)	4	East/West	Stability	Idealism—Phenomenology	Stressed

Notes: *GDP* gross domestic product, *MH* mental health, *SSN* Servizio Sanitario Nazionale, *NHS* National Health Service. [1] Some uncertainty of comparison [2] GINI index: coefficient and position, see [85]
Shared across three nations: Developed economies, shared human rights values, shared European social values, background of social critique influence (Foucault, Basaglia, Goffman), facing challenges of globalisation and neoliberalism (conflict between welfare state and consumerism, commodification of health services), sociodemographic instability, growing inequalities, towards 'metacommunity'

21.4 Italy

Franco Basaglia was the charismatic and influential leader of the Italian mental health reform that started in the early 1960s when he became Director of the Provincial Mental Hospital at Gorizia. Basaglia had previously worked at the Department of Neurology and Psychiatry of Padova University. He considered Jean-Paul Sartre his philosophical maestro and was influenced by Sartre's 'ontology of freedom' and the radical form of his humanism [8]. Basaglia's thinking was linked with social reformist debates, and he emphasised that healing work by psychiatrists could not succeed in the absence of freedom and a relationship of reciprocity between patient and psychiatrist. Over time, reference to Sartre shifted from 'Being and Nothingness' [9] to his later 'Critique of Dialectical Reason' [10] with its focus on the social dimension, power and organisation theory [11]. This shift was related to Basaglia concentrating on mental hospital closure during the 1970s.

Basaglia maintained the interest in phenomenology documented in earlier publications. There was reference to authors such as Jaspers, Binswanger, Minkowski, Straus and Zutt [8] and particularly to Edmund Husserl whose concept of 'epoché' Basaglia used in 'putting diagnosis in brackets', that is, in not concentrating on psychiatric diagnosis but on the social situation of persons with mental illness living in segregating asylums. Basaglia, in his phenomenological work, was interested in the concept of the 'body' [12]. He referred to Husserl and Binswanger and Daseinsanalyse, and Franca Ongaro Basaglia identified a continuity from Basaglia's early interest in the phenomenology of the body to his analysis of institutional constraints and anti-institutional activism.

Michel Foucault was an important, though controversial, influence [13]. Much of Foucault's work was on 'technologies of truth' as they evolved in the spheres of industry, technology, commerce, science and medicine through the eighteenth and nineteenth centuries. Foucault considered asylum institutions as places where deviance of human behaviour was analysed and the 'truth of illness' ascertained. He regarded (i) therapy activities as social control to return individuals to a 'normal state', and (ii) anti-institutional activism as well as anti-psychiatry as reflecting the challenge of resolving the 'knowledge-power' dilemma (i.e. scientific-professional knowledge-power links).

The Italian Marxist political philosopher Antonio Gramsci was an influence that Basaglia referred to in his attempt to anchor reform activism in a national movement of emancipation of people considered different, excluded and 'subaltern' [8, 14]. He referred to Gramsci's concept of the 'organic intellectual' [3]. Gramsci's thinking, along with the power and charisma of the reform movement, contributed to the enormous momentum of change that materialised in Italy. There are two books by Basaglia and colleagues ('Crimini di Pace', 'La nave che affonda') that concentrate on the role of psychiatrists as intellectuals/ professionals in positions of power and on how to contribute to the dismantling of institutional practice [14, 15].

It would be an over-simplification to assert the complete identity of the ideas of Basaglia with the culture of the Italian multifaceted professional community and Italian public opinion in the 1960s and 1970s [16]. But within a robust democratic orientation, Basaglia believed strongly that a small 'hegemonic minority' could change the state of things. Indeed, this was effectively achieved with the closure of the mental hospital in Trieste and the approval of Law 180 of 1978, the foundation for the era of psychiatric reform in Italy.

In summary, in Italy the key ideas derived from Basaglia's work, focused around:

- *Personal and social rights* of people with mental disorders, and on the.
- *Critique of institutional psychiatry* with an aim at overcoming the institutional logic.
- The anti-institutional critique was *radical*, with a focus on freedom and social participation.
- *Jean-Paul Sartre, phenomenological* philosophy, *Antonio Gramsci's philosophy of praxis* and *Michel Foucault* with his anti-institutional activist focus were important for the 'theory' of the reform.

21.5 UK

Thornicroft and Tansella [17], presenting a framework to analyse and improve mental health services, refer to the English philosopher John Locke who wrote, in 1690: 'The only way by which any one divests himself of his natural liberty and puts on the bonds of civil society is by agreeing with other men to join and unite into a community'. [17]. Porter places the history of mental disorders in twentieth century Britain in the context of (i) the end of the Victorian era, (ii) underfunding and cyclical crises in the mental hospitals, (iii) the prominent societal role of the sciences including medicine, (iv) surging interest in 'psychological matters' in the early twentieth century, (v) the interest in and influence of psychoanalysis between the two wars and (vi) the enormous momentum of societal modernisation between World Wars I and II [18].

In the early nineteenth century and with repercussions into the twentieth century, the Quakers' ideas regarding mental health treatment, William Tuke and the York Retreat, and the tradition of 'moral treatment' were also influential in the UK and abroad and played a role among reformist ideas. The 'evangelical' motive in 'lunacy reform' was apparent also in the seventh Earl of Shaftesbury's commitment to both 'pauper' and 'lunacy reform' (Anthony Ashly-Cooper, 1801–1885) [19, 20].

Porter [18] refers to a tradition of surveys, epidemiological and controlled trials in Britain and to the shift in British psychiatric thinking from institutional care models to ones centred around the needs of individual patients. He points to the report of the Feversham Committee on Voluntary Mental Health Services (1939), the memorandum of the Royal Medico-Psychological Association on the Future Organisation of Psychiatric Services (1945) and to chapters on social or community psychiatry in textbooks of the 1940s [18]. Burke [21], in a chapter discussing historical perspectives as part of a wider volume [22], identifies a complex pattern of change during the 50-year period of 1960–2010 and considers the issues of 'social encounter' and the 'relationship between professional and patient' (as well as dein-stitutionalisation) as central.

Scambler [2], in his chapter, sets mental health care against the background of the post-war move towards the welfare state and foundation of the National Health Service (NHS 1946) with a strong basis in the Beveridge Report (of 1942) who focused on the 'five giants' standing in the way of social progress: 'want, disease, ignorance, squalor and idleness'. Scambler [2] also describes the subsequent shift of the Thatcher (and Major) Conservative governments to neoliberalism through their focus on the private free market and the running of the NHS meandering between a bureaucratic command and control economy and the private market with the intro-duction of the purchaser–provider spilt, managed competition and the Private Finance Initiative. The author also describes political–economic continuity between the Thatcher/ Major (Conservative) and Blair/ Brown (Labour) governments.

Two books by Wall [23] and Staub [24] deal with the anti-psychiatrists Ronald D. Laing and David G. Cooper. Wall [23] argues that anti-psychiatry in Britain, in the course of the 1960s, moved from critique of institutional psychiatry towards engaging with a counter-cultural audience. He emphasises Laing's and Cooper's professional background, their successes, scientific and book publications in aca-demic psychiatry. Wall [23] emphasises Laing's and Cooper's focus on the nuclear family in its role for the trajectories of people with mental disorders, on issues of transference and the potential of family-focused work in individual or group psychotherapy.

In summary, among the ideas in the background of the British reform there was a very generic element of the

- Thinking of *John Locke*, that is, of the tradition of *empirical philosophy* and liberalism, and there were strong contributions of the
- *Quaker and evangelical ideas* and concepts as applied to pauper and lunacy reform, and there was
- Some of the critical potential of *anti-psychiatry* running parallel to mainstream psychiatry (e.g. with respect to the focus on family relations, institutional cri-tique and therapeutic communities).

21.6 Germany

Brink [25], a historian of medicine, describes psychiatry in its relationship to soci-ety in Germany (1860–1980). In her theoretical introduction, she refers to Foucault's thinking in 'Madness and Civilization' [26] specifically with a view of psychiatry as reflecting 'functional differentiation' and processes of modernisation in the dealings of society with human and social 'deviance'. With regard to the post-World War II development of psychiatry, Brink elaborates on the role of the 'psychiatry-public' and 'psychiatry-press-media' interfaces and identifies increasing public discourse as an important precursor of both public critique and mental health reform initiatives of the 1960s.

Söhner [27], in an oral history account of the so-called 'Psychiatrie-Enquête', a national enquiry and set of recommendations presented to the West German Bundestag (Parliament) in 1975, refers to a number of history and social science hypotheses to understand psychiatric reform processes. These revolve around 'societal progress', 'change processes in society's management of deviance' and a 'societal integration and welfare policy hypothesis'. In dealing with the run-up to the enquiry and ensuing reform which persisted during the 1975–1990 period, Söhner [27] refers to phenomenological psychiatry as an important theoretical stimulus for the reform process, and mentions authors such as Jaspers, Heidegger, Binswanger, Minkowski and Zutt. The national enquiry also referred to institutional analysis (Goffman), the critical and anti-psychiatry movements and the recognition of stigmatisation issues, and there was further input from labelling theory. Psychoanalysis is mentioned as a further reform impulse [27]. The account is based on oral history research and, following World War II and the mass murder of people with mental illness, emphasises the importance of international contacts helping German psychiatrists to experience other mental health systems—all this thanks to growing numbers of psychiatric hosts abroad inviting German experts (to the USA and England, in particular). The coincidence of a surge of initiatives towards mental health reform with the advent of a Social Democrat-led coalition government in the FRG (of chancellor Willy Brandt in 1969) is mentioned. This strengthened the concept of liberal democracy with people at the margins of society considered relevant for political deliberations.

In summary, the spectrum of ideas that were relevant for German reform has included

- *Foucault*'s thinking (with a focus on the knowledge/power issue), and
- *Internationalisation* was of great importance (following the disaster and isolation of Nazi rule); there appeared to be a re-orientation along the broad lines of the Enlightenment tradition. The interest in
- *Phenomenological philosophy* was substantial while institutional orientation was not as radically criticised as in Italy.

21.7 Practice and Patterns of Care

Table 21.2 provides data on inpatient and outpatient resources for mental health care (both public and private) in Italy, the UK and Germany.

Table 21.2 Data on inpatient, outpatient and human resources for mental health care in Italy, UK and Germany

	Italy	UK	Germany
1960s			
Inpatient facilities	179 beds per 100,000 population	155,000 beds 130 large mental hospitals, some with over 2000 beds Start of deconstruction of the large psychiatric institutions	130 psychiatric hospitals, with an average number of about 1200 beds each (up to 3000)[6]
Staff (ratio)	NA	679 consultant psychiatrists 25,000 mental health nurses	1:200 doctors in hospitals 1:500 clinical psychologists 1:5 nurses
Compulsory admissions	NA	NA	> 70%
Outpatient facilities	–	Start of establishment of community mental health services	900 office-based psychiatrists/ neurologists (one (neuro-)psychiatrist per 100,000 population); No other outpatient, community or qualified residential services
1970s			
Inpatient facilities			
Beds for mental health in general hospitals (per 100,000)	Start of establishment of small psychiatric wards in general hospitals, with a maximum of 15 beds at the end of 1970s	Start of establishment of small psychiatric wards in general hospitals in 1960s	First general hospital psychiatric in-patient units in 1970
Beds in mental health hospitals (per 100,000)	185 1978 admissions of new patients to mental hospitals have been stopped	106,400 mental health inpatients	160
Staff			
Psychiatrists working in mental health sector (per 100,000)	NA	1054 consultant psychiatrists	1:87 doctors in hospitals
Nurses working in mental health sector (per 100,000)	NA	28,700 mental health nurses	1:5 nurses in hospitals

(continued)

Table 21.2 (continued)

	Italy	UK	Germany
Compulsory admissions			
Total number of compulsory admissions (absolute number)	20,294	NA	NA
Percentage of all admissions that were compulsory (in%)	25.84	29.4	6–50
Outpatient/day hospital facilities			
Mental health outpatient facilities	Start of creation of community-based mental health centres (MHC) at the end of 1970s	Outpatient clinics offered in various settings	1463 office-based psychiatrists/ neurologists First hospital-based outpatient services (PIA) and welfare-funded social psychiatric services (SPDI)
Day treatment facilities (per 100.000)	Day hospitals not an important service model	First reported day hospital opened in 1946	First reported day hospital opened in 1962
1990s			
Inpatient facilities			
Beds for mental health in general hospitals (per 100,000)	8 (per 100,000)	50,000 beds	45 (per 100,000)
Beds in community residential facilities (per 100,000)	8.8 (places in supported housing)	15.9 (places in supported housing)	8.9 (places in supported housing)
Beds in mental health hospitals (per 100,000)	83 (1990)—16 (1999)	131.8	141.7 (1990)—108 (1999)
Staff			
Psychiatrists working in mental health sector (per 100,000)	9	11 (2116 consultant psychiatrists)	7.3
Nurses working in mental health sector (per 100,000)	26	104	52
Compulsory admissions			
Total number of compulsory admissions	11,376 20.51 (per 100,000)	40.5 (per 100,000) 48 (per 100,000)	114.4 (per 100,000)

(continued)

Table 21.2 (continued)

	Italy	UK	Germany
Percentage of all admissions that were compulsory (in%)	11.60	13.5	17.7
Outpatient facilities			
Mental health outpatient facilities (per 100,000)	3.9 centres per 150,000	Implementing of specialised community psychiatric teams	4750 office-based psychiatrists/ neurologists (6 per 100,000)
Day treatment facilities (per 100,000)	13	30	10
2010s			
Inpatient facilities			
Beds for mental health in general hospitals (per 100,000)	10.95	50.63	41.08
Beds in community residential facilities (per 100,000)	46.41	2.28	NA
Beds in mental health hospitals (per 100,000)	0 By 2000, all psychiatric hospitals had been closed and all patients discharged	7.99	47.62
Staff			
Psychiatrists working in mental health sector (per 100,000)	7.83	14.63	15.23
Nurses working in mental health sector (per 100,000)	19.28	67.35	56.06
Compulsory admissions			
Total number of compulsory admissions	8815	63,048	75,929
Percentage of all admissions that were compulsory (in%)	4.71	NA	9.22

(continued)

Table 21.2 (continued)

	Italy	UK	Germany
Outpatient facilities			
Mental health outpatient facilities (per 100,000)	1.43	4.94	30.32
Day treatment facilities (per 100,000)	1.34	2.88	0.61

Source: Refs. [32, 41, 55, 65, 80, 86–98]
The reported figures can only be used as a rough guide. Different definitions of the characteristics across the three countries and the decades, survey methods, measures and sources lead to a considerable degree of uncertainty and ambiguity
NA not available, *SPDI* Sozialpsychiatrische Dienste

21.8   Italy

In Italy, voluntary treatment in mental hospitals became an option only in 1968 (law 132/68), while previously all inpatient treatment in mental hospitals had been involuntary (based on the 1904 mental health law; Legge Giolitti). Conditions in the provincial psychiatric hospitals in the 1960s were very segregating, impoverished and non-therapeutic, a shameful heritage of the political use of psychiatry during the fascist regime.

In the 1960s, a movement of reform started in the North-East Italian mental hospital of Gorizia where Franco Basaglia had been appointed medical director (1961). The reformers transformed the Gorizia mental hospital along the lines of a therapeutic community as pioneered by Maxwell Jones in Scotland. The transformation of the hospital was accompanied by the publication of a number of successful books. The reform process needs to be seen in the wider context of reformist societal and political movements characteristic of the 1960s and 1970s. In this period, the focus of the reform movement shifted towards a programme of radical mental health democratisation with the aims of mental hospital closure and establishment of community services. Inspired by the achievements of Basaglia in Trieste, the reform Law 180 was passed by Parliament (in 1978) and was incorporated in the law establishing Italy's National Health Service (*Servizio Sanitario Nazionale* [SNN]; Law 833/1978).

The law stopped new admissions to mental hospitals (while re-admissions remained possible in a transitional phase), and small general hospital in-patient units (Servizi Psichiatrici di Diagnosi e Cura, SPDC) of up to 15 beds were set up to provide inpatient psychiatric care. Psychiatric care was to be provided by community mental health services, and, the 'dangerousness' criterion (of the Legge Giolitti of 1904) having been removed, a new legal framework was formulated for compulsory treatment. A range of residential services (with varying degrees of staff coverage) were built to care for people with marked impairment. There has been substantial influence of carers (families) and their organisations, and there are initiatives of people with first-person experience of mental illness, with peer support projects in a number of places.

In 2015, forensic mental hospitals (of which there had been five) were closed. Nine out of ten judicial orders are now executed through community treatment orders. Small residential facilities are a residual option. Earlier, the provision had been in forensic hospitals only [28, 29]. The mental health care system faces a range of challenges among which have been budgetary cuts and staff shortages.

21.9   Descriptions and Reviews of Care Provision in Italy 1996–2023

Papers identified for Italy are reported in chronological order.

Burti and Benson [30], in a review of the reform, arrived at a balanced conclusion in saying that overly positive or negative conclusions must be avoided. They stated that the passage of Law 180 in 1978 ushered in major advances in the care of people with severe mental illness. The project of downsizing and closing mental hospitals had advanced, and a heterogeneous system of community-based services was built. Neither private institutions nor the criminal justice system had replaced state mental hospitals, and general hospital psychiatric units, community mental health centres (CMHCs) and community residential facilities had been opened. Where community mental health services had been developed, well-coordinated care appeared to be possible. The authors highlighted uneven reform implementation, and in some areas, particularly in the poorer South, community services were underdeveloped or non-existent.

Fioritti et al. [31] described the overlapping processes of mental hospital downsizing till closure and the development of community mental health services in Emilia-Romagna, a region of four million inhabitants in Northern Italy. He argued that the shift from a hospital-based to a community-based psychiatric system of care, as foreseen by the Italian psychiatric reform, is feasible provided that some general political, administrative and social backup conditions are present to ensure the good outcome of this process.

Barbato [32] examined data on the new services, on criminalisation of people with mental illness, suicides and homelessness. He concluded that few negative effects of the changing care pattern had been reported. There had been minimal trans-institutionalisation to institutions for the elderly. There was no shift of inpatient care from public mental hospitals to private hospital providers. The shift of care to the community had been achieved albeit unevenly, and the level of inpatient care had been reduced. This trend had been uneven across diagnostic groups, with admission rates not declining between 1979 and 1989 among people with schizophrenia and severe affective disorders (but declining in the group of neurotic disorders). Inadequate provision of residential facilities, insufficient availability of data and a lack of coordinated planning were criticised, and successful community mental health pilot services were mentioned.

Fattore et al. [33] present a study of mental health care costs in a community mental health centre in Lombardy locality of about 85,000 adult residents. The study followed 1992 reform legislation introducing an internal market and fee-for-service funding in Italy's SSN. Patients with schizophrenia and related disorders absorbed about 60% of total costs and made extensive use of several types of services, while people with non-psychotic disorders accounted for a lower average cost of care. The authors argue that the new fee-for-service system adopted by the SSN to fund provider organisations did not appear appropriate for people with psychosis.

De Girolamo et al. [34] present a national epidemiological survey of residential services resulting in a total number of 1370 non-hospital residential facilities in Italy (with 17,138 beds resulting in an average of 12.5 beds, and with a national average rate of 2.98 beds per 10,000 inhabitants). The authors describe a tenfold variance of residential care provision across regions and very low discharge rates. Most residential services had 24-hour staffing with about 1.4 patients per full-time staff member.

Pycha et al. [35] described reform implementation in South Tyrol (North Italy) and emphasised the burden that the reform had placed on families of people with severe mental illness. Delayed implementation in South Tyrol (a region with highest degrees of autonomy from central government and the best financial budget in the country) aimed at a higher bed rate than the national average. A psychosomatics service was established and the need for specialised services (perinatal mental health, attention-deficit hyperactivity disorder [ADHD] clinic) was emphasised. Deficits in accessibility and specialisation of services were highlighted.

Fioritti and Amaddeo [36] edited a special journal issue on 'Community Mental Health Care in Italy Today' to document the state of the radical community psychiatry system 35 years after Law 180. In their contribution, Ferrannini et al. [37] examined how the complex balance between federal and regional powers for planning, managing and evaluating health services, enshrined in the Italian Constitution, has produced 20 different regional systems. National surveys showed that the highest levels of compliance with national health care policy were found in northern and central Italy. Community mental health centre staffing levels, the number of units comprised in a Department of Mental Health and organisational aspects (inclusion of child and adolescent and drug addiction services) had an impact [38].

Fioritti and Amaddeo [36] pointed out that what Italian psychiatric services have in common is that they are universal, tax-funded, fully integrated within the SSN, espouse a public health approach, have liberal regulations about involuntary admissions, offer a minimum set of services, reflect scepticism about clinically specialised units and are broadly psychosocial in orientation. This is also where the differences start. Regional governments gave priority to developing community-based service networks rather than pilot centres or demonstration programmes. This is consistent with the explicit public health approach that has been required and adopted. It also accounts for the vast majority of services being 'generic'. Nevertheless, today there are some specialised services for dual diagnosis (either substance abuse or learning disability), eating disorders or personality disorders. Specialised clinics for specific disorders such as anxiety or obsessive-compulsive disorder (OCD) are virtually unknown and confined to a handful of university departments, mostly geared to research in collaboration with foreign centres.

The need for specialisation is tackled differently by each regional system, as Lora et al. [39] describe in their comparison of the Lombardy, Emilia-Romagna and Campania psychiatric systems. Remarkable differences can be found in standards (e.g. number of beds, allocation of resources to each unit within the department) and integration of private services within Departments of Mental Health, as well as in integration with child psychiatry, drug abuse, learning disabilities services and provision of specialised care for eating disorders. The picture emerging from these contributions helps frame the puzzling differences in service provision along three major dimensions: (a) high versus low resources regional systems (basically a North-Central/South gap), (b) radical community versus balanced hospital/community systems (with Trieste and Lombardy at the two ends of the spectrum) and (c) 'generic' versus 'partially specialised' systems (with Campania and Emilia-Romagna at the two ends of the spectrum).

Fioritti [40] considered the balance sheet of the Italian psychiatric reform mostly positive, with substantial regional variations. He emphasised that psychiatric deinstitutionalisation had inspired policies in other sectors of society (people with physical and intellectual disabilities, children with special needs and drug addictions). He referred to budgetary cuts following the financial crisis (of 2008) and substandard care in some parts of Italy. He referred to the process of forensic mental hospital closure and the setting up of (small) residential facilities providing care for this patient group (2014–2017). Successes of the reform, according to Fioritti [40], include:

- Having accomplished the largest and most radical de-hospitalisation process in the history of psychiatry
- The nation-wide implementation of a system of community care
- Having overcome the division between ordinary and forensic services
- All this without significant neglect, criminalisation, homelessness, social alarm or suicide increase
- Lowest degree of formal coercion towards the mentally ill internationally

The downsides and risks, according to the author, comprise:

- Societal change towards a less protective society
- Services being asked to do more with decreasing budgets
- A reduction of about 50% of community service staff numbers
- Deficiencies in terms of responses to the demands of expanding and more diversified needs
- Insufficient response to new evidence, for example, with respect to the effectiveness of psychotherapy.

Fioritti [40], in concluding, pointed out that requirements of rehabilitation and recovery had not always coincided with the logic of deinstitutionalisation.

Barbui et al. [41] used the Organisation of Economic Co-operation and Development (OECD) database to gather information on various population and service indicators in G7 countries (Canada, France, Germany, Italy, Japan, UK, USA), the World Health Organization (WHO) Global Health Observatory and the WHO Mental Health ATLAS-2014, the Italian national mental health information system and the Italian Central Institute of Statistics (ISTAT) data to describe the incidence and prevalence of mental disorders and the Italian service system (2014–2015). They reported below OECD-median staff availability that no beds in mental hospitals were available, bed rates (in general hospital units, per 100,000) that were low in international comparison, a proportion of compulsory admissions that had progressively declined and stable age-adjusted suicide rates (1978–2015). The population of psychiatric patients in Italian forensic psychiatric hospitals declined (phasing out of forensic hospitals substituted by residential services). Consolidation of the community care system was described, but service provision was variable across the country (with a north and centre to southern Italy gradient). Internationally, resources allocated to mental health care were lower in Italy than in other high-income countries. The authors described concerns over:

- Decreasing staffing levels
- Potential use of residential facilities as long-stay services
- Lack of community alternatives to acute inpatient admissions.

There were concerns regarding:

- Variability of quality of care
- Deficiencies in offering services to young people with a first psychotic episode, regarding mental health care for elderly, adolescent and migrant populations
- Low proportion of gross national product (GNP) and of the overall health budget spent on mental health care.

Sampogna et al. [42] report that, across Italy, community mental health centres (CMHCs) are open daily for 24 or 12 h caring for catchment areas of 200,000–800,000 inhabitants, and the staff ratio (national mean) is about 25 full-time professionals per 100,000 residents with maximum levels in central Italy and minimum staffing levels in southern Italy. There are 10 beds in general hospital psychiatric units (GHPU) per 100,000 population and 46 beds in community residential facilities. High-intensity residential facilities are bigger (up to 14 beds), and low-intensity facilities are smaller (three beds). The authors emphasise extreme variability in the provision of mental health care across regions. Compulsory admissions have declined, from more than 20,000 (nationally) in 1978 to less than 9000 in 2015, and the rates of compulsory admissions are 1.73/10,000 population nationally, ranging from 5.68 in Marche, central Italy, to 0.43 in Friuli and 0.22 in Bolzano (northern Italy). Reasons for concern include:

- Relatively low staffing levels (by international comparison)
- The potential use of community residential facilities as long-stay services
- A lack of community alternatives to acute inpatient admission

Martinelli et al. [43] present a cross-sectional study of care needs of residents with schizophrenia spectrum disorders in residential facilities. They found that residential facilities did not fully meet users' needs for care, and the study revealed some disagreement on unmet needs between users and staff. The authors concluded that, in these non-hospital residential facilities, the delivery of rehabilitative interventions promoting personal recovery was limited.

21.10 A Current Cross-sectional Look (2024)

According to Polin et al. [7], in the context of Law 180 there has been a decrease in hospitalisation rates for mental disorders (2001–2018), in line with the overall national trend in hospital care. Regional variability in hospitalisation rates is described, and there are multidisciplinary outpatient services (within local health authorities) for people with substance use problems and behavioural addictions (Servizi per dipendenze, SERT or SERD). An increase in both the incidence rates and service use for mental health problems (6.9% increase 2020–2021) is described, and mental health problems account for 3.3% of all emergency room visits nationally. The system currently has 126 Departments for Mental Health (DMH, Dipartimenti di Salute Mentale) and 1299 local mental health facilities. The total DSM staff amounted to 29,785 individuals.

After a long process of development, since 2021 the Italian Ministry of Health has made available national data on mental health care and services that are suitable for inter-regional comparison and benchmarking [44]. In a detailed analysis of this data, Starace [45] summarises the shortcomings of this care system in the following 10 points:

1. Insufficient funding: Italy allocates only 3% of the National Health Budget to mental health, the lowest percentage among G7 countries.
2. Lack of staff: The supply of mental health workers (60.4 per 100,000 inhabitants) is 25% lower than the expected standard. Nursing staff is the most numerous profession, but there is a shortage of psychiatrists and psychologists.
3. Low health care coverage: Only 1.5% of the population is assisted by mental health services, compared to an estimated prevalence of 15% for mental disorders in Italy. There are strong regional inequalities in access to services.
4. Widespread but inadequate community infrastructure: Although the network of territorial services is widespread (2.2 facilities per 100,000 inhabitants), there is a lack of information on the quality of facilities and their compliance with safety and privacy standards.

5. Few hospital beds: Italy has only 9.3 beds per 100,000 inhabitants in psychiatric wards, one of the lowest numbers in the world. The reduction in beds during the pandemic has not been reversed.

6. Reduced but underestimated compulsory health treatments (TSO): The number of TSO is low compared to other countries, but their registration methods are not entirely reliable. Furthermore, some forms of compulsory hospitalisation are classified differently, creating uncertainty in the data.

7. Poor continuity of care: Only 25% of patients discharged from psychiatric wards receive follow-up in the following 14 days. Lack of continuity can increase the risk of relapses and flare-ups.

8. Excessive residential care: The number of places in residential facilities is more than double the national benchmark, favouring re-institutionalisation processes and limiting patients' recovery of autonomy.

9. Excessive length of residential treatment: The average stay in residential facilities is much longer than clinically indicated, often due to a lack of housing solutions and social reintegration programs.

10. Extreme regional disparities: Access to and quality of care varies greatly between regions, with a strong North-South divide. The lack of effective central coordination perpetuates these inequalities.

These points highlight the state of crisis of the system and the need for greater investment in economic and human resources, as well as the need for better planning to reduce regional disparities and improve the quality of psychiatric care in Italy.

21.11 UK

In 1948 Britain saw the foundation of the National Health Service (NHS). Psychiatric care was provided, above all, in mental hospitals. There were reform movements within psychiatry, and they were supported by politics, with the minister (in 1961) referring to mental hospitals as an outdated model. This move away from mental hospitals was supported by a wide range of publications favouring community mental health care and the scope for activation, discharge, employment and community integration of people with severe mental illness. There was a shared reform orientation among professionals that found its expression in the pioneering Three-Hospitals-Study 1960–1968 [46] and further publications.

Inpatient care was moved to general hospital psychiatric units in many places but the model was not pursued consistently as inpatient hospital capacities decreased and stand-alone inpatient care settings were often preferred. In the 1970s and 1980s, outpatient and community services were built, and the first decades of the twenty-first century saw the development of a range of specialist teams for people with psychosis. Mental health funding increased in the late 1990s and early 2000s. Themes of debate regarding the care for people with severe mental illness in Britain include:

- The cooperation of general practitioner (GP)-based primary care and specialist secondary psychiatric care (primary care mental health), and
- The modalities of collaboration of secondary mental health services and social services and their funding.

There have been repeated reshuffles of service configurations in NHS mental health trusts. The number of service providers has multiplied; private and voluntary sector providers have increasingly been engaged, with the former stepping in for inpatient care and the latter taking over day centre and social participation-type services. The importance of service user participation and of models of peer support and self-help has increased. The recovery paradigm has been considered important in guiding the work of NHS mental health services [22].

21.12 Descriptions and Reviews of Care Provision 1995–2022

Papers identified for the UK are reported in chronological order.

Hadley and Goldman [47] describe policies that replaced a simple system of care for seriously mentally ill people in Britain with complicated organisational and financial structures transferring roles of purchasing outpatient care to general practitioners and leaving responsibility in the provision of long-term residential care with pressurised local authority social services. The authors argue that these policy changes have replaced a simple system with complicated organisational and financial structures that demand high levels of coordination with perverse incentives to the disadvantage of people with severe mental illness. The purchaser–provider split, distinct purchaser roles in community and inpatient care, a complex mixed economy of care system and brokerage models of social care are reminiscent of similar issues in the USA.

Goldberg [48] discusses the future pattern of psychiatric care provision and reviews the history of the reduction in both the size and number of mental hospitals in the UK (with only 14, out of 130 large mental hospitals open in 1960, not intending to close; [49]). Studies of mental hospital closure suggest that care in the community is generally preferred by patients. The Care Programme Approach (CPA; 1990) and Supervision Register are described as standards for after-care by community mental health teams (CMHTs). Goldberg [48] argues that there are cases of bed shortage in inner city areas and points to a study suggesting an optimal number of beds for a given location. The need for sheltered residential accommodation is emphasised, and the author points to the importance of primary care mental health. The Mental Illness Needs Index (MINI) is described as a tool to estimate the residential care need for a given electoral ward [50].

Johnson et al. [51] provide a snapshot of mental health service provision in England using the example of a catchment area in London. They describe the reduction in inpatient psychiatric care with most inpatients on acute wards being discharged within one week but some staying for months, mainly because of difficulties in finding appropriate accommodation. Most hospital beds are now acute or secure beds, and a variety of services (such as community mental health teams, outreach teams or crisis resolution and home treatment teams) try to avoid hospital admission. The paper focuses on problems of overlap and discontinuity between community teams, CMHT effectiveness in engaging patients and preventing deterioration and drop-out, the question of outpatient commitment (community treatment orders) and difficulties to recruit high quality staff. The authors emphasise that many innovations in UK psychiatric care were implemented before high-quality evidence was available.

Joseph and Birchwood [52] describe reforms to the mental health service in the UK from 1999 onwards. The authors refer to the National Service Framework issued in 1999 to set national standards for mental health services based on evidence [53]. They describe government funding to commission specialised or 'functional' community mental health teams (early intervention, crisis resolution, and assertive outreach), and the paper's focus is on services for people with first-episode psychosis. The National Health Service plan (2000) envisaged the implementation of 50 early intervention centres by 2004. Approximately 30 centres had been established as of January 2004.

Iliffe et al. [54] review surveys (since 2008) of how NHS services work with UK care homes that are owned by a range of commercial, not-for-profit and charitable providers. Five surveys focused on GP services, 10 focused on specialist services to care homes. Working relationships had evolved locally; there were wide variations in the provision of GP and specialist health care. Larger care home chains may take systematic approaches to organising the access to NHS services and to filling gaps with in-house provision. Dental care provision was often deficient. Inequity in the provision of NHS services to elderly care home residents is emphasised.

Burns [55] refers to the long-term significance of the UK 1930 and 1959 Mental Health Acts in establishing community mental health care. Sectorised services were established for catchment areas of about 50,000, and these were served by multidisciplinary community mental health teams (CMHTs) that dealt with referrals from primary care. Sector CMHTs developed multidisciplinary pragmatic routines with an emphasis on skill-sharing and outreach care, and community psychiatric nurses played a central role. Burns [55] emphasises central NHS regulation and a strong focus on evidence-based treatments. Since the year 2000, generic CMHTs have been replaced or enhanced by crisis resolution home treatment teams, assertive outreach teams and early intervention teams. Based on lack of evidence of outcome superiority, assertive outreach teams were subsequently resorbed into CMHTs. The period between 2010 and 2020 saw an expansion in outpatient psychotherapy (Improving Access to Psychological Treatments; IAPT) services and in specialist teams (personality disorders, perinatal care). There has been criticism of IAPT arguing that the provision of short courses of therapy, as low as six sessions initially, may not be helpful or potentially negative for patients with long-term needs when, as often happens, such needs cannot be met.

Continuity of care across the inpatient–outpatient divide was broken towards 2020. Various publications have underlined the positive effects of IAPT and indicated predictors of variability in clinical performance [56–58]. High-quality data has been provided regarding suicide by people with mental illness, with suicide rates declining [59]. During a decade of austerity, day care services were decimated, and along with the reduction in bed availability compulsory admission rates rose. There is a disproportion between the burden of disease attributable to mental illness (23%) and the mental health share of overall NHS spend (11%).

As part of a review of the financing, governance, reforms and performance of the UK health systems (four systems for England, Scotland, Wales and Northern Ireland), Anderson et al. [60] present a summary of mental health care provided by the NHS, by local authorities, voluntary and private sector organisations. Clinical commissioning groups in England (and equivalent bodies in Scotland, Wales and Northern Ireland) commission or provide mental health services, while housing and social services for people with mental health needs are provided by local authorities. There is a national mental health strategy. Inpatient mental health care can be provided in varied hospital settings, and there are secure facilities providing inpatient care for people requiring high levels of security. Community-oriented accommodation is available (supported housing, group homes, short-term hostels). Community mental health teams (CMHTs) are multiprofessional. CMHTs support primary care mental health services helping GPs treat people with common mental disorders. CMHTs include a range of functional teams (see above). There are forensic mental health services for mentally disordered offenders.

Legislation on the rights of mentally ill patients involuntarily detained has developed in steps (moving decision-making for compulsory admittance from the courts to the medical profession; restricting the amount of time patients might be detained without consent, allowing for the patients' nearest relative to consent if the patient could or would not; and further change following devolution). Funding for mental health services has not always kept pace with physical health service funding [61]. Payment systems are considered outdated with a focus on block contracts. There have been initiatives to address this through legislation involving the principle of 'parity of esteem' between physical and mental health services.

21.13 A Current Cross-sectional Look (2024)

The update for the UK mental health care system by HSPM [7] describes the current system of NHS, local authority and voluntary and private sector mental health services as outlined by Anderson et al. [60]. A comprehensive system of community mental health care is in place. The system, however, is under substantial pressure. Despite growing needs, funding for mental health services has often not kept pace with funding for physical health care, and the update refers to 2012 legislation (see above) that introduced the 'parity of esteem' between physical and mental health services. Budgetary cuts and staff shortages are mentioned.

21.14 Germany

This text concentrates on psychiatric reform in the Federal Republic of Germany (West Germany, FRG). There were mental health reform initiatives in the German Democratic Republic during the 1960s and 1970s which have been covered elsewhere [62]. Following World War II and against the background of mass murder and forced mass sterilisations of people with mental illness, there were a number of early post-war attempts at coming to terms with what had happened during the Nazi period [63]. In the 1960s, there were attempts at analysing segregation and neglect of people with mental illness in German mental hospitals and of calling for mental health reform in the light of developments in other countries (see Söhner [27]). In the second half of the 1960s lobbying for mental health reform in federal states and at the federal level increased [27]. This led to the Bundestag appointing a so-called 'Enquête' Commission (Inuiry Commission) that was instructed to both report on the state of mental health care in the FRG and agree on recommendations for mental health care reform. The final report was presented to the Federal Parliament in 1975 [64]. The commission's conclusions were formulated as four principles [65]:

- Care delivered in the community;
- Needs-led and comprehensive care for all people with mental disorders;
- Needs-led coordination of care in catchment areas; and
- Equity of access to and quality of care for people with mental illness compared with people suffering from somatic disorders.

The commission report did not call for an end to mental hospital care but it called for thorough reforms and the downsizing of mental hospitals. It strengthened the model of general hospital-based psychiatric in-patient services. There has been no clear break with traditional psychiatric institutions, while building standards, ward conditions, staffing levels, daily living, therapeutic practice and standards of respect for human rights have been improved. Involuntary treatment has continued to apply to about 10% of treatment episodes, and episodes of coercion including mechanical restraint have been severely criticised (and led to recent Federal Constitutional Court rulings). There have been attempts to strengthen integrated in- and outpatient community care systems. This started with the health care funding option of specific targeted contracts with health care funders (health insurers) for specific patient groups.

During the last decade, there has been increasing use of the model of regional or global mental health budget solutions (across major health care funders) in regions where agreement on integrated care provision appeared feasible. There has also been federal legislation allowing 'model contracts'(Modellprojekte) with selected or all social health insurance companies of a region, thus enabling mental health care providers to freely shift funds from inpatient to crisis intervention and home treatment care (provided their level of care provision to citizens, that is, treated prevalence in the catchment area, is stable) [66, 67]. High-intensity home treatment care (inpatient-equivalent home treatment, IEHT; Stationsäquivalente Behandlung, StäB) has been included as a standard care package into social health insurance, allowing hospitals to establish IEHT teams and being reimbursed if quality standards such as daily contacts with a team member are followed. Peer support in inpatient and community teams has been introduced. Experienced involvement (EX-IN) peer training courses and other forms of peer training are offered.

21.15 Descriptions and Reviews of Care Provision 1999–2023

Papers identified for Germany are reported in chronological order.

Kellinghaus et al. [68] have reported on about 200,000 homeless people in Germany at the time and described that more than two-thirds of homeless people in Germany were suffering from mental disorders with substance abuse disorders predominating, but also with high prevalence rates for schizophrenia, affective and personality disorders (and comorbid conditions). The authors called for multimodal clinical and social intervention programmes that had shown effectiveness internationally.

Kallert et al. [69] have provided an overview of the evidence for community mental health services in Germany. This was scarce, with the (then) current state of research suggesting positive effects of social psychiatric services (Sozialpsychiatrische Dienste) and some types of supported housing and supported work/employment schemes. There was a lack of evidence regarding crisis centres, psychosocial contact points and day care centres. A range of deficiencies included documentation, reporting systems and the research culture.

Melchinger et al. [70] reported on a study of mental health care spending in a Bavarian region. The study analysed data from health insurance plans and social welfare. Costs of mental health care amounted to 14 million Euro per year per 100,000 population. Health insurance schemes accounted for two-thirds of total costs, and social welfare spend accounted for one third. The distribution of expenses was not based on needs analyses, and the authors concluded that the chronically and most severely mentally ill were disadvantaged in terms of resource allocation and that a redistribution of resources to outpatient and community care was required.

Kilian [71] reported on the international evidence that community-based mental health care is not generally less costly in comparison with more institutional forms of care and that assertive community treatment (ACT) models had been found more efficient than inpatient care. He considered it likely that providing more community mental health interventions could increase the efficiency of psychiatric treatment in Germany, and he highlighted a lack of national studies which limits the validity of health economic study findings for Germany.

Grimm-Halkevopoulos and Brieger [72] looked at differences between mental health services in an Austrian and German alpine district using the European Service Mapping Schedule (ESMS) and 30 expert interviews (and qualitative content analysis) to find that both regions had a scarcity of ambulatory psychiatrists and psychotherapists and no psychiatric hospital. ESMS data showed distinct differences in care provision between regions, and the authors concluded that in situations of sparse mental health services there may be a shift toward non-medical community services.

Von Peter et al. [66] explore the effects of recent legislation in Germany aiming to improve the availability of integrated flexible forms of community psychiatric care (through a treated prevalence-based global accounting method; so-called FIT64b models). The implementation of such models in 12 psychiatric hospital departments across Germany is examined, with rigid forms of mainly inpatient care shifted to more flexible and integrated types of community and outreach care. Changes were more likely to be acknowledged by patients and staff (and received more positive evaluation) in departments with higher levels or longer duration of model implementation.

Steinhart et al. [73] examine the situation of closed residential facilities for people with mental illness. Against the background of person-centred care and the United Nations Convention on the Rights of Persons with Disabilities (UN-CRPD) the authors used a 2017 postal survey (with a 20.7% response rate) of residential facilities including closed settings and a complete 2010 survey of closed residential services in one federal state (Mecklenburg-Vorpommern, M-V). The data indicated a need for regional residential service options in the target group of people with high care needs, and there was a lack of individual arrangements that could serve as alternatives to closed residential contexts. Away-from-home placements (from another federal state) were found in 30% of residents in M-V (higher than the average federal rate of 6.5% away-from-home placements). Individualised high-intensity residential facilities (open and closed settings) are scarce in Germany.

Klocke et al. [74] provide an overview of the new model of inpatient equivalent home-treatment (IEHT) in Germany. The authors name normalisation of treatment (close to patients' social context) and stigma reduction among the advantages, while administrative hurdles are high, and they consider IEHT an important component of mental health care. In the IEHT context, Rauschenberg et al. [75] have provided an overview of digital forms of service delivery to strengthen IEHT.

Jalilzadeh Masah et al. [76] investigated factors associated with homelessness among psychiatric inpatients in one Berlin university service (13 years 2008–2021) and found a 15.1% increase over the 13-year period. In the overall patient group, 69.3% were in stable private housing, 15.5% were homeless and 15.1% lived in residential facilities. Homelessness was associated with being male, being born outside Germany, lack of outpatient treatment, a psychotic disorder diagnosis, severe stress reactions, personality and substance use disorders.

Schwarz et al. [67] used data from a routine clinical database (on 10,598 face-to-face treatment contacts with 178 IEHT users) to analyse effects of staff continuity in IEHT teams on the length of stay (LOS) in IEHT care in one German centre. Service users saw an average of just over 10 different staff members per treatment episode, and on 11% of care days all team members present were unknown to the service user, while on a third of care days there was at least one unfamiliar member of staff present. In total, 83% of contacts were performed by a (stable) group of three team members, and 51% were made by one (key) staff member. A significant positive correlation was found between the number of different IEHT team members seen by service users and their LOS, and episode duration was longer in users experiencing low staff continuity.

A recently published multisite quasi-experimental study showed that IEHT was more effective than initial inpatient treatment of persons with psychiatric crises in reducing future hospitalisations and was associated with higher patient satisfaction and more involvement in treatment [77].

21.16 A Current Cross-sectional Look (2024)

Referring to the HSPM for Germany [7], mental health care accounts for 13% of total health expenditure (in 2015) and mental health problems constitute a major driver of overall indirect health expenditure. Recent analyses have reaffirmed an increase in mental health-related health service use and costs. Mental health care provision is fragmented with a range of providers of outpatient, inpatient and other forms of care. There are services targeting social integration funded by local authority social services and social insurance resources, for example, through pension insurance. Rehabilitation services are available but skewed towards people with non-severe mental health problems.

Inpatient care is provided by psychiatric (stand-alone) hospitals and general hospital psychiatric departments not necessarily working together with community health services. Care providers offering inpatient care provide day hospital care and multidisciplinary ambulatory outreach care (in PIA services). Treatment of patients with depressive episodes accounts for a fifth of all inpatient treatment episodes. Inpatient care is reimbursed on the basis of clinically defined groups with comparable costs (Pauschalierendes Entgeltsystem Psychiatrie und Psychosomatik, PEPP). The federal states are responsible for inpatient care planning, and inpatient care providers offer outpatient but also limited community outreach care.

The provision of outpatient care by specialist psychiatrists is left to the commissioning and bargaining between purchasers (health insurances) and regional corporate representations of office-based specialist care (Kassenärztliche Vereinigungen). Legal prerequisites (in the federal social code) for innovative forms of care provision (Regionalbudgets, Modellversuche, that is, FIT64b) have been passed by federal parliament, and such regional forms of care provision are increasing in number.

There has been an increase in the number of hospitals (and hospital beds, both in acute care and rehabilitation) provided by private for-profit providers. In outpatient specialist care there has been an increase, over the last two decades, in psychotherapists (with an increase in numbers of 32% over five years from 2014). Improving access to psychotherapy interventions has been a focus in federal mental health care legislation; central service points to ensure timely booking of appointments were opened (2015), and access to psychotherapy sessions has improved. There have been substantial staff shortages in recent years which can partly be explained by more patients with only moderate symptoms using available services that fall short in strategies to prioritise the severely mentally ill.

21.17 Discussion

In following the ideas, theories and concepts discussed within psychiatry (in the three countries) and in describing the patterns and systems of mental health care as they evolved in Italy, Britain and Germany, some trends can be discerned.

- In Italy, the critique of institutional psychiatry impressed with its radical approach, and references to sociology, phenomenology and political theory were frequent. These lines of thought are reflected in the psychiatric reform law of 1978, the practice of mental hospital closure and the establishment of community mental health services. The new care paradigm has survived almost half a century in spite of some political debate.
- In the UK (and against a background of institutional critique), there has been a national, data-driven move, pursued over decades and supported by otherwise opposing political parties, towards community care. It was part of a comprehensive welfare policy programme in post-war Britain. Against the background of Goffman's sociological analysis of asylum psychiatry, there has been a move towards community mental health care (with a number of problems and stressors, budget cuts and crises, and with a neoliberal turn and internal market programmes). A series of national reports, service frameworks and plans have been accompanied by multiple examples of high-quality empirical evaluation taken note of internationally.
- In Germany, the re-opening of international contacts (post-World War II) helped strengthen reform positions among psychiatric professionals (and in academia). During the late 1950s and 1960s impulses toward reform emerged with a strong reform movement taking shape during the 1960s. Phenomenological philosophy, sociology and psychoanalysis contributed to mental health reform, and wider societal and political change of the 1960s helped to forge a national programme of reform. The institutional position has remained relatively strong throughout the reform process. The picture is currently characterised by growing interest in integrated care provision and by debates on the legal rules governing involuntary care and coercion, on costs, cost containment and staff shortages, with a loss of attraction to mental health care among people entering the health professions.

With respect to common trends in the evolution of mental health care across Europe, Priebe and co-workers, in a series of papers, have asked the question of whether, along with widespread deinstitutionalisation and community care orientation, trends of reinstitutionalisation could be identified in European countries. In an analysis of data from nine European countries (including England, Germany and Italy), Priebe et al. [78] reported that, between 2002 and 2006, the number of psychiatric inpatient (hospital) beds tended to fall, while changes in involuntary admissions were inconsistent. Numbers of forensic beds, places in supervised and supported housing and prison populations increased in most countries.

In a further analysis of data from 11 Western European countries of data covering the years 1990 to 2012, Chow and Priebe [79] found that numbers of psychiatric hospital beds had decreased, while forensic beds, places in protected housing and prison populations had increased. The number of reduced beds exceeded additional places in other institutions, and there was no evidence of an association of changes in the two figures. Reductions in psychiatric bed numbers were negatively associated with prison populations (that had increased), but this negative association disappeared once adjusted for gross domestic product as a potential covariate. Priebe et al. [80], in an earlier paper, concluded that general attitudes to risk containment in society might be one factor in understanding these changes.

In better understanding these widespread indications of re- or transinstitutionalisation across Europe, a qualitative study of the same group of authors is helpful. Chow et al. [81], in a report on in-depth interviews with 24 mental health experts in England, Germany and Italy, asked interviewees about drivers of change in institutionalised mental health care from 1990 to 2010, and they identified four broad themes: (1) the overall philosophy of de-institutionalisation; (2) finances, with the pressure to limit expenditure and provider interest in increasing provider revenue); (3) limitations of community care with the danger of neglecting the most severely ill patients; and (4) an emphasis on risk containment. This analysis places the deinstitutionalisation paradigm (that has survived over time) in wider context with relevant themes including financing issues, limitations of community care and the issue of social control. This perspective may help in understanding contradictory and counter-intuitive findings in analysing mental health care change across Europe (and, potentially, elsewhere).

Finally, in a comparative analysis of the evolution of psychiatric care systems in England, France, Germany and Italy (from the 1970s to the 2000s), Coldefy [82] emphasises deinstitutionalisation of mental health care as a major trend in all four mental health care systems and states that the pace, scale and comprehensiveness of deinstitutionalisation have been uneven.

In comparing Italy, England and Germany in terms of their second-half-of twentieth century and early twenty-first century histories, there are both differences and similarities [83] in terms of:

- Recent past (post-Fascist democracy in Italy; post-Nazi federal state with national partition in West Germany; long-term stability with major political [post-World War II and post-imperial] and socioeconomic change in Britain).
- National state (parliament-run kingdom vs. two forms of constitutional democracy) and their respective socioeconomic development, social policy and culture.

In the above consideration of the evolution of mental health care in the three countries, the differences in centralism (UK) versus regionalism/ federalism (Italy and Germany) find clear expression, and so does the marked difference (long-term for UK, more recent for Italy) of a National Health Service versus a regionalised purchaser- (health insurance-) provider-driven system (in Germany). Also, the marked tradition of empiricism and utilitarian thinking and science in the British system is apparent, with some strengthening of this perspective in Italy and Germany in recent decades. Also, the theories and ideas of the reform movements (or era) appear to have been widely different, with

- *Radical person-centredness* with phenomenological roots (focus on 'person', 'body', personalised care and 'setting'or 'territorio') in *Italy*
- Enduring commitment to Goffman's *institutional analysis*, a person-centred *needs approach* with a background in both *Quaker and evangelical ideas* and a strong *empirical foundation* in *Britain*
- Coexistence of *institutional critique* and (lingering) reliance on *institutional models* in *Germany,* plus a growing trend toward *pragmatism*

When stepping back, however, it is apparent that developments have followed broadly similar lines:

- Specialisation of services (e.g. the creation of 'functional' community teams such as crisis resolution and home treatment teams or services targeting particular target groups) has been an issue in all care systems
- Access to psychological treatments has been an issue in all three countries
- Parity of esteem and equity in care provision for people with mental illness as compared with those with physical ill health is a common theme
- Community care delivery has been accepted as the most adequate form of routine mental health care provision for people with severe mental illness

In spite of these similarities, mental health reforms (in Italy, the UK and Germany) have been carried out rather independently, with no significant efforts by European institutions and scientific societies to establish a common culture of mental health care development. Clearly, health issues have long been out of reach of the European Union. It is only during the last two decades that some issues of health and mental health care have been conceptualised as 'consumer and/or human rights issues'. The impact of EU initiatives such as the 'Joint Action on Mental Health and Wellbeing' has been minimal. In examining developments in Italy, Germany and the UK, it is most interesting to analyse the differences and examine how these can help in addressing the challenges of a rapidly changing world: globalisation, sociodemographic and technological transitions to 'metacommunity' [84], changes in values and human relationships, consumerism and commodification of care.

21.18 Conclusion

Our review of the theories and ideas relevant to mental health reforms in Italy, the UK and Germany and delineation of developments in care practices in these three European countries suggest that cultural–political patterns provide the background against which mental health care systems evolve. Societal narratives and theoretical approaches regarding how psychiatry and mental healthcare should be understood are likely to strengthen or weaken specific care models. However, the broader frame of reference of social and political thought impinges upon the formulation of mental health policies and practice in all three European countries.

Key Points

- Theories and ideas impinging on mental health reform in Italy, the UK and Germany have differed but have also had some overlap (with sociologist Erving Goffman being important across all three countries, and Michel Foucault as well as phenomenology having left their mark on thinking in Italy and Germany).
- Patterns of service development were shaped by the foundations of National Health Services both in Britain (1948) and Italy (1978), while developments in Germany have been strongly influenced by a regionalised purchaser- (health insurance-) provider system with a mixed economy of care.
- Welfare state concepts and collectivist orientations have been influential in all three (mental) health care systems during the 1960s and 1970s. Recent decades have seen a strong influence of neoliberal thinking, consumerism and financing considerations, and peer/expert-by-experience contributions have grown in importance across the three countries.
- Empirical research traditions, user and needs orientation and a strong tradition of evaluation have characterised the British reform, with some indication that Italy and Germany have been catching up in recent decades.
- In reviewing drivers of mental health reforms (in Italy, Germany and the UK), the following stand out: (i) societal approaches to handling Beveridge's five giants of 'want, disease, ignorance, squalor and idleness' that stand in the way of social progress; (ii) the collectivist vs consumerist tension in health systems; (iii) person-centeredness; and (iv) societal risk containment.

References

1. Porter R. Madmen: a social history of madhouses, mad doctors & lunatics. 1. publ. Stroud: Tempus; 2004.
2. Scambler G. Liberty's command: Liberal ideology, the mixed economy and the Briish welfare state. In: Ikkos G, Bouras N, editors. Mind, state and society: social history of psychiatry and mental health in Britain 1960–2010. Cambridge, New York: Cambridge University Press; 2021. p. 23–31.
3. Becker T, Fangerau H. 40th birthday of the Italian Mental Health Law 180—perception and reputation abroad, and a personal suggestion. Epidemiol Psychiatr Sci. 2018;27(4):314–8.
4. Marazia C, Fangerau H, Becker T, Söhner F. 'Visions of another world': Franco Basaglia and German reform. In: Burns T, Foot J. Basaglia's international legacy: from asylum to community. First edition. Oxford, New York: Oxford University Press; 2020. p. 227–244.
5. Becker T, Schomerus G, Speerforck S. Vergangenheit verstehen hilft Zukunft denken: Psychiatrie-Reformgeschichte in Großbritannien und Italien. Psychiatr Prax. 2023;50(6):326–32.

6. Becker T, Müller T, Ikkos G, Speerforck S. Radical social theorists Antonio Gramsci and Walter Benjamin: can they help understand and power effective mental health reform? Int Rev Psychiatry. 2024;36(6):626–38.

7. Polin K, Hjortland M, Maresso A, van Ginneken E, Busse R, Quentin W. "Top-three" health reforms in 31 high-income countries in 2018 and 2019: an expert informed overview. Health Policy (Amsterdam). 2021;125(7):815–32. https://pubmed.ncbi.nlm.nih.gov/34053787/

8. Novello M, Gallio G. Franco Basaglia e la psichiatria fenomenologica : ipotesi e materiali di lettura. Prima edizione pubblicata in Italia. Modena: Mucchi; 2023. (Etiche e critica; vol 1).

9. Sartre J-P. Das Sein und das Nichts: Versuch einer phänomenologischen Ontologie. Reinbek bei Hamburg: Rowohlt Verlag; 1993.

10. Sartre J-P. Kritik der dialektischen Vernunft. I. Band: Theorie der gesellschaftlichen Praxis. Reinbek: Rowohlt; 1967.

11. Fleming P. Sartre's lost organization theory: Reading the critique of dialectical reason today. Organization Theory. 2022;3(3):1–18.

12. Basaglia F. Corpo, sguardo e silenzio. L'enigma della soggettività. 2007;1:11–22.

13. Colucci M. Franco Basaglia e Michel Foucault. In: Massi A, editor. Franco Basaglia e la filosofia del '900 / [a cura di Alessandro Massi! Milano: Be-ma; 2010. p. 44–53 (La pratica del sapere. Filosofia. Milano : Be-ma; vol. 1).

14. Basaglia F, Ongaro FB, Honegger C. Befriedungsverbrechen über die Dienstbarkeit der Intellektuellen / Basaglia [and others] ; herausgegeben von Franco Basaglia und Franca Basaglia-Ongaro. Frankfurt am Main: Europäische Verlagsanstalt; 1980.

15. Basaglia F, Ongaro Basaglia F, Pirella A, Taverna S. La nave che affonda. Roma: Savelli; 1978.

16. Foot J. The 180 law: history, myth, and reality. In: Foot J, editor. The man who closed the asylums: Franco Basaglia and the revolution in mental health care. London, Brooklyn, NY: Verso; 2023. p. 371–88.

17. Thornicroft G. The mental health matrix: a manual to improve services. Cambridge: Cambridge University Press; 1999.

18. Porter R. Two cheers for psychiatry! The social history of mental disorder in twentieth century Britain. In: Berrios GE, Freeman H, editors. 150 years of British psychiatry 1841–1991. London: Gaskell/Royal College of Psychiatrists; 1991.

19. Kibria AA, Metcalfe NH. A biography of William Tuke (1732–1822): founder of the modern mental asylum. J Med Biogr. 2016;24(3):384–8. https://pubmed.ncbi.nlm.nih.gov/24944052/

20. Raynor MJ. The work of Antony Ashley Cooper, the Seventh Earl of Shaftesbury, for social reform an environmental hygiene in the nineteenth century. J R Inst Public Health Hyg. 1963;26(9):216–23.

21. Burke J. Historical Pespectives on mental health and psychiatry. In: Ikkos G, Bouras N, editors. Mind, state and society: social history of psychiatry and mental health in Britain 1960–2010. Cambridge, New York: Cambridge University Press; 2021. p. 3–12.

22. Ikkos G, Bouras N, editors. Mind, state and society: social history of psychiatry and mental health in Britain 1960–2010. Cambridge, New York: Cambridge University Press; 2021.

23. Wall O. The British anti-psychiatrists: from institutional psychiatry to the counter-culture, 1960–1971. New York: Routledge; 2018. (Routledge studies in cultural history; vol 54).

24. Staub ME. Madness is civilization: when the diagnosis was social, 1948–1980. Chicago: University of Chicago Press; 2011. https://ebookcentral.proquest.com/lib/kxp/detail.action?docID=769158

25. Brink C. Grenzen der Anstalt : Psychiatrie und Gesellschaft in Deutschland 1860–1980. Göttingen: Wallstein; 2010.

26. Foucault M. Madness and civilization: a history of insanity in the age of reason. New York, Alexandria, VA: Pantheon Books; 1965.

27. Söhner F. Psychiatrie-Enquete: mit Zeitzeugen verstehen: Eine Oral History der Psychiatriereform in der BRD. 1. Auflage. Köln: Psychiatrie Verlag; 2020. (Zur Sache). http://www.content-select.com/index.php?id=bib_view&ean=9783966050180.

28. Carabellese F, Parente L, Kennedy HG. Reform of forensic mental health Services in Italy: stigma and blaming the messenger: Hermenoia. Int J Offender Ther Comp Criminol. 2024;68(15):1505–24.

29. Hopkin G, Messina E, Thornicroft G, Ruggeri M. Reform of Italian forensic mental health care. Challenges and opportunities following Law 81/2014. Int J Prison Health. 2018;14(1):1–3.

30. Burti L, Benson PR. Psychiatric reform in Italy: developments since 1978. Int J Law Psychiatry. 1996;19(3–4):373–90.

31. Fioritti A, Lo Russo L, Melega V. Reform said or done? The case of Emilia-Romagna within the Italian psychiatric context. Am J Psychiatry. 1997;154(1):94–8.

32. Barbato A. Psychiatry in transition: outcomes of mental health policy shift in Italy. Aust N Z J Psychiatry. 1998;32(5):673–9. https://pubmed.ncbi.nlm.nih.gov/9805590/

33. Fattore G, Percudani M, Pugnoli C, Contini A, Beecham J. Mental health care in Italy: organisational structure, routine clinical activity and costs of a community psychiatric service in Lombardy region. Int J Soc Psychiatry. 2000;46(4):250–65.

34. de Girolamo G, Picardi A, Micciolo R, Falloon I, Fioritti A, Morosini P. Residential care in Italy. National survey of non-hospital facilities. Br J Psychiatry. 2002;181:220–5.

35. Pycha R, Giupponi G, Schwitzer J, Duffy D, Conca A. Italian psychiatric reform 1978: milestones for Italy and Europe in 2010? Eur Arch Psychiatry Clin Neurosci. 2011;261(Suppl 2):S135–9.

36. Fioritti A, Amaddeo F. Community mental health in Italy today. J Nerv Ment Dis. 2014;202(6):425–7.

37. Ferrannini L, Ghio L, Gibertoni D, Lora A, Tibaldi G, Neri G, et al. Thirty-five years of community psychiatry in Italy. J Nerv Ment Dis. 2014;202(6):432–9.

38. Munizza C, Gonella R, Pinciaroli L, Rucci P, Picci RL, Tibaldi G. CMHC adherence to National Mental Health Plan standards in Italy: a survey 30 years after national reform law. Psychiatr Serv. 2011;62(9):1090–3.

39. Lora A, Starace F, Di Munzio W, Fioritti A. Italian community psychiatry in practice: description and comparison of three regional systems. J Nerv Ment Dis. 2014;202(6):446–50.

40. Fioritti A. Is freedom (still) therapy? The 40th anniversary of the Italian mental health care reform. Epidemiol Psychiatr Sci. 2018;27(4):319–23.

41. Barbui C, Papola D, Saraceno B. Forty years without mental hospitals in Italy. Int J Ment Heal Syst. 2018;12:43.

42. Sampogna G, Del Vecchio V, de Rosa C, Giallonardo V, Luciano M, Palummo C, et al. Community Mental Health Services in Italy. Consortium psychiatricum. 2021;2(2):86–92.

43. Martinelli A, D'Addazio M, Zamparini M, Thornicroft G, Torino G, Zarbo C, et al. Needs for care of residents with schizophrenia spectrum disorders and association with daily activities and mood monitored with experience sampling method: the DIAPASON study. Epidemiol Psychiatr Sci. 2023;32:e18.

44. Di Cesare M, Magliocchetti N, Romanelli M, Santori E. Rapporto salute mentale: Analisi dei dati del Sistema Informativo per la Salute Mentale (SISM); 2022 [Cited 2025 Mar 10]. https://www.salute.gov.it/imgs/C_17_pubblicazioni_3369_allegato.pdf.

45. Starace F. Rapporto SIEP—2024: La salute mentale nell'Italia del regionalismo. Società Italiana di Epidemiologia Psichiatrica; 2024.

46. Wing JK, Brown GW. Institutionalism and schizophrenia: a comparative study of three mental hospitals, 1960–1968; with a chapter by the physician superintendents of the three hospitals. Digitally printed version. Cambridge: Cambridge University Press; 2009.

47. Hadley TR, Goldman H. Effect of recent health and social service policy reforms on Britain's mental health system. BMJ (Clinical research ed.). 1995;311(7019):1556–8.

48. Goldberg D. The future pattern of psychiatric provision in England. Eur Arch Psychiatry Clin Neurosci. 1999;249(3):123–7.

49. Rivett G. From cradle to grave: fifty years of the NHS. repr. London: King's Fund; 1998.

50. Glover G. Mental illness needs index. In: Thornicroft G, Strathdee G, editors. Commissioning mental health services. London: HMSO; 1996. p. 53–8.

51. Johnson S, Zinkler M, Priebe S. Mental health service provision in England. Acta Psychiatr Scand Suppl. 2001;410:47–55.
52. Joseph R, Birchwood M. The national policy reforms for mental health services and the story of early intervention services in the United Kingdom. J Psychiatry Neurosci. 2005;30(5):362–5.
53. Department of Health. A National Service Framework for Mental Health. London: National Health Service; 1999. https://assets.publishing.service.gov.uk/government/uploads/system/uploads/attachment_data/file/198051/National_Service_Framework_for_Mental_Health.pdf
54. Iliffe S, Davies SL, Gordon AL, Schneider J, Dening T, Bowman C, et al. Provision of NHS generalist and specialist services to care homes in England: review of surveys. Prim Health Care Res Dev. 2016;17(2):122–37.
55. Burns T. Community-based mental health care in Britain. Consortium psychiatricum. 2020;1(2):14–20. https://pubmed.ncbi.nlm.nih.gov/39006898/
56. Chen S, Cardinal Rudolf N. Accessibility and efficiency of mental health services, United Kingdom of Great Britain and Northern Ireland. Bull World Health Organ. 2021;99(9):674–9.
57. Clark DM. Transparency about the outcomes of mental health services (IAPT approach): an analysis of public data. Lancet. 2018;391(10121):679–86.
58. Johns L, Jolley S, Garety P, Khondoker M, Fornells-Ambrojo M, Onwumere J, et al. Improving access to psychological therapies for people with severe mental illness (IAPT-SMI): lessons from the South London and Maudsley psychosis demonstration site. Behav Res Ther. 2019;116:104–10.
59. Windfuhr K, Kapur N. Suicide and mental illness: a clinical review of 15 years findings from the UK National Confidential Inquiry into suicide. Br Med Bull. 2011;100:101–21.
60. Anderson M, Pitchforth E, Edwards N, Alderwick H, McGuire A, Mossialos E. United Kingdom: health system review 2022. Health Syst Transit. 2022;24(1):1–192. https://euro-healthobservatory.who.int/publications/i/united-kingdom-health-system-review-2022
61. Millard C, Wessely S. Parity of esteem between mental and physical health. BMJ (Clinical research ed.). 2014;349:g6821.
62. Steinberg H. 25 Jahre nach der "Wiedervereinigung": Versuch einer Übersicht über die Psychiatrie in der DDR. Teil 1: Nachkriegszeit, Pawlowisierung, psychopharmakologische Ära und sozialpsychiatrische Bewegung. Fortschr Neurol Psychiatr. 2016;84(4):196–210.
63. Schmidt G. Selektion in der Heilanstalt 1939–1945: Neuausgabe mit ergänzenden Texten. Berlin, Heidelberg: Springer; 2011. (SpringerLink Bücher).
64. Deutscher Bundestag. Bericht über die Lage der Psychiatrie in der Bundesrepublik Deutschland—Zur psychiatrischen und psychotherapeutisch/psychosomatischen Versorgung der Bevölkerung : Drucksache 7/4201. Bonn: Verlag Dr. Hans Heger; 1975.
65. Bauer M, Kunze H, von Cranach M, Fritze J, Becker T. Psychiatric reform in Germany. Acta Psychiatr Scand. 2001;104(S410):27–34. https://doi.org/10.1034/j.1600-0447.2001.1040s2027.x
66. Peter S von, Ignatyev Y, Johne J, Indefrey S, Kankaya OA, Rehr B, et al. Evaluation of flexible and integrative psychiatric treatment models in Germany—a mixed-method patient and staff-oriented exploratory study. Front Psychol. 2018;9:785.
67. Schwarz J, Wolff J, Heinze M, von Peter S, Habicht JL. How to measure staff continuity in intensive psychiatric home treatment: a routine data and single case analysis. Front Psychiatry. 2023;14:1166197.
68. Kellinghaus C, Eikelmann B, Ohrmann P, Reker T. Wohnungslos und psychisch krank. Uberblick über den Forschungsstand und eigene Ergebnisse zu einer doppelt benachteiligten Randgruppe. Fortschr Neurol Psychiatr 1999; 67(3):108–121.
69. Kallert TW, Leisse M, Kulke C, Kluge H. Evidenzbasierung gemeindepsychiatrischer Versorgungsangebote in Deutschland: eine Bestandsaufnahme. Gesundheitswesen. 2005;67(5):342–54.
70. Melchinger H, Rössler W, Machleidt W. Ausgaben in der psychiatrischen Versorgung Ist die Verteilung der Ressourcen am Bedarf orientiert? Nervenarzt. 2006;77(1):73–80.
71. Kilian R. Gesundheitsökonomische Evaluation gemeindepsychiatrischer Interventionen. Nervenarzt. 2012;83(7):832–9.

72. Grimm-Halkevopoulos B, Brieger P. Gemeindepsychiatrie in zwei europäischen Regionen: Vergleich des Bezirks Reutte in Tirol mit dem südlichen Oberallgäu in Bayern. Bundesgesundheitsblatt Gesundheitsforschung Gesundheitsschutz. 2019;62(2):156–62.

73. Steinhart I, Jenderny S, Wassiliwizky M, Heinz A. Personenzentrierte Hilfen, aber geschlossen untergebracht? Zur Situation der geschlossenen Heime in Deutschland. Nervenarzt. 2021;92(9):941–7.

74. Klocke L, Brieger P, Menzel S, Ketisch E, Hamann J. Stationsäquivalente Behandlung: Ein Überblick zum Status quo. Nervenarzt. 2022;93(5):520–8.

75. Rauschenberg C, Hirjak D, Ganslandt T, Schulte-Strathaus JCC, Schick A, Meyer-Lindenberg A, et al. Digitale Versorgungsformen zur Personalisierung der stationsäquivalenten Behandlung. Nervenarzt. 2022;93(3):279–87.

76. Jalilzadeh Masah D, Schouler-Ocak M, Gutwinski S, Gehrenbeck K, Deutscher K, Schindel D, et al. Homelessness and associated factors over a 13-year period among psychiatric inpatients in Berlin, Germany: routine data analysis. BJPsych Open. 2023;9(4):e118.

77. Bechdolf A, Nikolaidis K, Peter S von, Längle G, Brieger P, Timm J, et al. Utilization of psychiatric hospital services following intensive home treatment: a nonrandomized clinical trial. JAMA Netw Open. 2024;7(11):e2445042. https://jamanetwork.com/journals/jamanetworkopen/fullarticle/2826213

78. Priebe S, Frottier P, Gaddini A, Kilian R, Lauber C, Martínez-Leal R, et al. Mental health care institutions in nine European countries, 2002 to 2006. Psychiatr Serv. 2008;59(5):570–3.

79. Chow WS, Priebe S. How has the extent of institutional mental healthcare changed in Western Europe? Analysis of data since 1990. BMJ Open. 2016;6(4):e010188. https://pubmed.ncbi.nlm.nih.gov/27130161/

80. Priebe S, Badesconyi A, Fioritti A, Hansson L, Kilian R, Torres-Gonzales F, et al. Reinstitutionalisation in mental health care: comparison of data on service provision from six European countries. BMJ (Clinical research ed). 2005;330(7483):123–6. https://pubmed.ncbi.nlm.nih.gov/15567803/

81. Chow WS, Ajaz A, Priebe S. What drives changes in institutionalised mental health care? A qualitative study of the perspectives of professional experts. Soc Psychiatry Psychiatr Epidemiol. 2019;54(6):737–44.

82. Coldefy M. The evolution of psychiatric Care Systems in Germany, England, France and Italy: similarities and differences. Questions d'économie de la Santé. 2012;180:1–8.

83. Knapp M, Beecham J, McDaid D, Matosevic T, Smith M. The economic consequences of deinstitutionalisation of mental health services: lessons from a systematic review of European experience. Health Soc Care Community. 2011;19(2):113–25.

84. Ikkos G, Bouras N. Metacommunity: the current status of psychiatry and mental healthcare and implications for the future. BJPsych International. 2024;21(3):70–3.

85. Freiheit—Ungleichheit—Brüderlichkeit? Teil I; 2022 [Cited 2025 Mar 10]. Available from: URL: https://www.statistik-bw.de/Service/Veroeff/Monatshefte/20120601.

86. DGPPN. Psychische Erkrankungen in Deutschland: Schwerpunkt Versorgung. Berlin: DGPPN [cited 2025 Mar 4]; 2018. https://www.dgppn.de/_Resources/Persistent/f80fb3f112b4e-da48f6c5f3c68d23632a03ba599/DGPPN_Dossier%20web.pdf

87. Salize HJ, Dressing H. Epidemiology of involuntary placement of mentally ill people across the European Union. Br J Psychiatry. 2004;184:163–8.

88. Rössler W, Salize HJ, Riecher-Rössler A. Changing patterns of mental health care in Germany. Int J Law Psychiatry. 1996;19(3–4):391–411.

89. Becker T, Hoffmann H, Puschner B, Weinmann S, Krumm S, Steger F. Versorgungsmodelle in Psychiatrie und Psychotherapie. 1. Auflage. Stuttgart: Kohlhammer Verlag; 2008. http://nbn-resolving.org/urn:nbn:de:bsz:24-epflicht-1282492

90. World Health Organization. WHO European health information at your fingertips; 2025 [Cited 2025 Mar 4]. https://gateway.euro.who.int/en/indicators/hfa_488-5070-psychiatric-hospital-beds-per-100-000/#id=19551.

91. Tooth GC, Brooke EM. Trends in the mental hospital population and their effect on future planning. Lancet. 1961;1(7179):710–3.

92. Turner J, Hayward R, Angel K, Fulford B, Hall J, Millard C, et al. The history of mental health Services in Modern England: practitioner memories and the direction of future research. Med Hist. 2015;59(4):599–624.
93. Kendell RE. The National Health Service celebrates its 50th birthday. Br J Psychiatry. 1998;173:1–3.
94. Bruns G. Empirische Materialien zu Zwangsunterbringungen in der Bundesrepublik Deutschland—der Stand der empirischen Forschung. In: Bruns G, editor. Ordnungsmacht Psychiatrie?: Psychiatrische Zwangseinweisung als soziale Kontrolle. Wiesbaden: VS Verlag für Sozialwissenschaften; 1993. p. 52–74.
95. Kulenkampff C. Wie schlecht ist die Krankenhauspsychiatrie in diesem Lande? Bemerkungen zu dem Buch von Frank Fischer: "Irrenhäuser, Kranke klagen an". Nervenarzt. 1970;41(3):150–2.
96. Bryant W. Mental health day Services in the United Kingdom from 1946 to 1995: an 'Untidy Set of Services'. Br J Occup Ther. 2011;74(12):554–61.
97. Eikelmann B, Albers M. Die psychiatrische Tagesklinik: 16 Tabellen. Stuttgart, New York: Thieme; 1999.
98. World Health Organization Mental Health Determinants and Populations Team. Atlas: country profiles of mental health resources 2001. World Health Organization; 2001. https://iris.who.int/handle/10665/67160.

Open Access   This chapter is licensed under the terms of the Creative Commons Attribution 4.0 International License (http://creativecommons.org/licenses/by/4.0/), which permits use, sharing, adaptation, distribution and reproduction in any medium or format, as long as you give appropriate credit to the original author(s) and the source, provide a link to the Creative Commons license and indicate if changes were made.

The images or other third party material in this chapter are included in the chapter's Creative Commons license, unless indicated otherwise in a credit line to the material. If material is not included in the chapter's Creative Commons license and your intended use is not permitted by statutory regulation or exceeds the permitted use, you will need to obtain permission directly from the copyright holder.

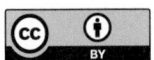

Latin American Psychiatry Reform and the WHO Mental Health Office

22

José Miguel Caldas de Almeida

22.1 Introduction

Latin America is a region with diverse geographical, sociocultural and economic characteristics. It comprises the countries of South America, Central America, the Latin Caribbean and Mexico. Most are low- or middle-income countries, and poverty and wide social inequalities affect a significant proportion of the population. The process of accelerated social change in recent decades, with increasing urbanisation of societies and frequent social conflicts, has had a significant impact on people's mental health.

By the middle of the last century, the countries of the region were faced with the challenges posed by this situation and the difficulties of responding to mental health needs with psychiatric services that, in most countries, were concentrated almost exclusively in large psychiatric hospitals.

The 1960s saw the first attempts to reform psychiatric services in Latin America, influenced by the community mental health movement in the United States and the experience of psychiatric reform in Italy and other European countries.

From the 1960s to the 1980s, the Pan American Health Organization (PAHO), the WHO Regional Office for the Americas, based in Washington DC, but with offices in all countries, provided technical assistance to these early reform projects and sponsored several international conferences to improve mental health care in the countries of the region. These conferences were crucial in defining appropriate reform strategies for Latin America, and drew attention to the need to integrate mental health into primary care and to find alternatives to hospital-based services. Several countries (including Brazil, Honduras and Nicaragua) developed some community mental health services and programmes during this period. In Nicaragua, these initiatives were part of a national mental health policy, but in most cases they

J. M. Caldas de Almeida (✉)
Lisbon Institute of Global Mental Health, Comprehensive Health Research Centre, Nova Medical School, Nova University of Lisbon, Lisbon, Portugal

© The Author(s) 2026
G. Ikkos, T. Becker (eds.), *Psychiatry after Kraepelin*,
https://doi.org/10.1007/978-3-032-09475-9_22

were local projects dependent on circumstantial political support. Despite their local and short-lived nature, these experiences were crucial in disseminating new ideas about community mental health [1, 2].

A regional conference on the restructuring of mental health services in Latin America, organised by the PAHO in Caracas in November 1990, gave new impetus to the process of reform services in the region. The declaration adopted at the end of the conference, known as the Caracas Declaration, has remained the guiding document for the reform movement in this part of the world.

The Caracas Declaration made a clear call for mental health to be integrated into primary care and local health systems, and for psychiatric hospitals to be removed from their central position in the system. It advocated that mental health care should be provided by community-based services, offering accessible, comprehensive, participatory and continuous care, as well as prevention and promotion activities. Another key aspect of the Declaration was its strong commitment to the protection of the human rights of people with mental disorders [3, 4].

The conference came at a critical time. As noted by Itzhak Levav, then Coordinator of the PAHO's Mental Health Unit and principal organiser of the Caracas Conference, 'the opportunity provided by the Conference helped countries to establish a reference framework, outline a programme of action, and effectively mobilise resources from Latin America and from countries outside the Region' [4].

To assist countries in this ambitious project, in 1990 the PAHO promoted a technical cooperation initiative, the Initiative for the Restructuring of Psychiatric Care in Latin America [3, 4], which brought together mental health leaders from their respective countries and many other organisations participating in the Conference. The aim was to initiate a collaborative process involving national, regional and international partners that could contribute to building the capacity of countries to successfully implement mental health reforms based on the principles of the Caracas Declaration.

In the following sections of this chapter, I discuss the roots, conceptual foundations and innovative recommendations of the Caracas Declaration, as well as the main strategic lines developed within the initiative that have contributed most to the reform of mental health services in Latin American countries. I also analyse the impact of the Caracas movement and reflect on the factors that may explain why a process with these characteristics found fertile ground for its development in Latin America, and what contributions it has made to the global mental health movement.

The analyses and discussions presented are based on data on mental health care in the region, collected through the World Health Organization's Atlas of Mental Health, and data on mental health systems in some countries in the region, collected through the Mental Health Systems Assessment Tool (WHO-AIMS). The results of studies and documents on the implementation of mental health reforms in Latin America produced by the World Health Organization and the Pan American Health Organization in recent decades were also considered, as well as other sources of information on these issues.

22.2   The Caracas Declaration

The Caracas Conference, hosted by the PAHO, was attended by representatives of 13 countries in the region, members of parliaments, the Latin American Psychiatric Association and other professional and scientific associations, experts from various disciplines and representatives of users and services that had been involved in mental health reforms in Latin America. Among other institutions and delegations invited, there was an Italian delegation, with representatives from the mental health services of Livorno, Parma, Reggio Emilia and Trieste, and a Spanish delegation from the mental health services of the autonomous communities of Andalusia, Asturias and Valencia. Both delegations brought to the meeting their experiences of how to provide an alternative to psychiatric hospitals and how to develop a community-based model of mental health services.

After 3 days of intense discussion, the participants agreed on the terms of a declaration that would go down in history as the Caracas Declaration. This declaration established a clear 'platform for action' by developing 'a set of principles for the organisation of community-based mental health care, based on various epidemiological, technical and ethical precedents' [4]. The proposed principles emphasise the decentralisation of care by replacing psychiatric hospitals with comprehensive networks of community services that ensure accessibility and continuity of care; the integration of mental health care into primary health care, including prevention and promotion objectives; and the promotion of a legal framework that ensures the protection of the rights of persons with mental disorders [4, 5].

The replacement of long-term psychiatric hospitals, until then the dominant institution in the psychiatric care system in Latin America, by networks of community-based services was based on the recognition of three problems associated with psychiatric hospitals: their inability to meet the care needs of the majority of the population, the frequency with which patients treated in them were victims of poor quality of care and violations of their rights and the fact that these hospitals absorbed almost all the budget available for mental health, leaving almost nothing for the development of other services.

The influence of the Italian experience has been particularly important, which has meant that the concept of deinstitutionalisation adopted in Latin America, far from foreseeing a simple process of de-hospitalisation, has always tended to anticipate deinstitutionalisation as a much more complex process than that. A process that aims not only to reduce the number of beds in psychiatric hospitals and eventually to close them but also to replace them with a network of services in the community, including community mental health centres (or teams), psychiatric units in general hospitals and programmes and facilities specifically designed to support the rehabilitation of users and promote their integration into society. On the other hand, and this point is particularly relevant, according to this conceptualisation, one of the aims of deinstitutionalisation has also been to contribute to a transformation of psychiatric practices in all services, based on the recognition of the centrality of the patient's subjectivity and their right to receive all the support they need to achieve full citizenship status.

The community mental health centres or teams were seen in this model as the core component of the specialised level of care and were expected to be truly 'community-based' mental health services. In other words, they should be 'close to the communities that use them, accessible to all affected people and their families, including but not limited to primary care, developed with the active involvement of affected people, their families and their communities (as well as other stakeholders), and include in vivo services delivered in the places where people live' [6].

The integration of mental health care into primary health care, including prevention and promotion objectives, was part of the primary health care movement then being developed in many Latin American countries, with the support of the PAHO, following the Declaration of Alma-Ata, which had been successfully applied to mental health in the 1980s in several countries (Nicaragua, Brazil, Chile and Cuba, among others).

The inclusion of the promotion of a legal framework to protect the rights of persons with mental disorders is certainly one of the most innovative aspects of the Declaration. In fact, although concerns about violations of the rights of users of mental health services have been present in service reforms since at least the end of the eighteenth century, this point had never been included among the priorities of the reorganisation of mental health services and the need to ensure its implementation through specific legislation had never been recognised.

The process that led to the Caracas Declaration has its deepest roots in the profound social, economic and political changes that took place in Latin America before the 1960s. These made it clear that there was an urgent need to rethink how to respond to the mental health needs of the population.

Latin American psychiatry, as Renato Alarcon shows in his analysis of its evolution, began a process of reflection in the 1960s, in search of a new identity that would reflect the advances in knowledge in the field of social psychiatry and respond to the challenges of building a practice based on the principles of '(a) directing care efforts towards satisfying the needs of the greatest number or, if possible, the entire population; (b) adopting a public health approach to the implementation of effective care and (c) recognising the cultural specificities of the continent's population and the likely genesis of their pathology' [7].

For Itzahk Levav, the Declaration was the culmination of a process influenced by several factors. First, the inadequacy of psychiatric hospitals in most countries to meet the needs of the population, and the realisation that many of the people treated in these hospitals often had their rights violated. Second, the early development of several epidemiological studies which, despite some methodological limitations, had shown that the idea of low-income countries not having significant mental health problems was false, and that the mental health needs of the large majority of people in these countries were not being met. Third, the demonstration that it is possible to create effective alternatives to psychiatric hospitals through well-implemented reforms. Finally, the democratisation processes that were beginning in several countries in the region at the time, which had forced governments to take note of the need to develop services that could better respond to people's mental health problems and defend the rights of those who suffer from them [8].

Another factor that contributed to the emergence of the Caracas Declaration was the technical collaboration of psychiatrists and other professionals from Italy and Spain, who had personal experience of leading mental health reforms in their countries. Franco Basaglia's visits to Brazil played a key role in establishing this collaboration. After a visit to Latin America in the 1960s, Basaglia made several visits in the 1970s, giving lectures in different cities [9]. The text of the transcripts of the Brasilia conferences and the dialogue with the audiences show that the mental health professionals present were very interested in the Italian psychiatric reform and were eager to receive the support of the Trieste team in transforming the services in Brazil, which at that time were almost entirely confined to many poor and overcrowded psychiatric hospitals. This support did not materialise directly from Basaglia, who died shortly afterwards, but his collaborators, led by Franco Rotelli, began a very close collaboration with Brazil, which later extended to other countries [10]. Another process of collaboration was led by Benedetto Saraceno, then at the Mario Negri Institute in Milan, who supported the reforms that were emerging in Nicaragua and other Central American countries [11], work that became a major inspiration for the restructuring of psychiatric services in Latin America that the PAHO led from the 1990s onwards.

22.3 The Initiative for the Restructuring of Psychiatric Services in Latin America

The Caracas Declaration was a platform for action, and at the end of the Conference it was decided to launch an initiative, coordinated by the PAHO, to deepen and extend to all the countries of the region the cooperation already developed in the restructuring of mental health services [4]. The Initiative for the Restructuring of Psychiatric Services in Latin America has facilitated the development of actions aimed at obtaining the political commitment of the governments of the region to transform mental health services in accordance with the principles of the Caracas Declaration. It has mobilised a range of local and international resources, promoted the training of leaders and professionals, supported the improvement of policies and legislation, ensured technical cooperation with countries implementing service reforms, created mental health information systems and contributed to the development of collaborative research projects. Formal agreements were signed between the PAHO and regions in Italy and Spain (e.g. Friuli Venezia, Emilia Romagna, Andalusia and Asturias). These facilitated the organisation of visits by Latin American professionals to innovative services in Europe. They, also, led to the establishment of programmes that guaranteed the provision of regular technical assistance to countries interested in restructuring their services, by psychiatrists with experience in mental health service reform in Europe, who were sent on two or three missions a year to the places they supported. Coordination was carried out by the PAHO, an organisation that, thanks to its long presence in the Region of the Americas (prior to becoming the WHO Regional Office for the Americas, the PAHO had existed since 1902 as the organisation responsible for coordinating all international health cooperation in the Americas), had far greater resources than the other regional offices and a strong influence in all Latin America.

The 1990s saw a further wave of reform as countries adopted new measures to improve their mental health services. National policies were developed and legislation passed in line with the principles set out in the Caracas Declaration. Chile, Cuba, El Salvador, Guatemala and Panama made significant progress, particularly in integrating mental health into primary care. Argentina, Brazil and Belize were particularly successful in developing integrated community mental health services. Of particular note are the reforms in the province of Río Negro, Argentina [12] and the city of Santos, Brazil [13]. These reforms have created a community-based system with a strong psychosocial rehabilitation component and active user participation. Several countries in the region have adopted mental health legislation and improved the protection of the human rights of persons with mental disorders [14, 15].

In 1997, the PAHO Directing Council, which brings together the ministers of health of all the countries in the region, adopted a resolution on mental health reform. This resolution was a political endorsement of the Caracas Declaration and called attention to the urgent need to redouble efforts to provide community services and to enact legislation to protect the rights of persons with mental illness. It also recognised the urgent need to simultaneously implement strategies to respond to the new challenges that had emerged, such as the inclusion of mental health problems in health insurance plans and the development of mental health promotion programmes [16].

22.4   The Impact of WHO 2001 Initiatives

In 2001, the WHO devoted several of its major global initiatives (World Health Day, World Health Report [WHR], special sessions of the World Health Assembly) to mental health. For the first time in history, mental health was recognised as a global health priority. The World Health Report 2001, titled 'Mental health: New understanding, new hope', provided a set of guidelines for action at the country level [17].

The conceptual basis of the reforms advocated in the report and the strategic guidelines it proposed were largely in line with the principles of the Caracas Declaration, and some of the examples of reform presented came from Latin American countries, which naturally provided a great stimulus for the work of the PAHO and the countries of the region.

However, the 2001 WHR was not only a reaffirmation of the Caracas Principles. Its publication was also an opportunity to integrate the process developed in Latin America into the broader global mental health process promoted by the WHO after 2001, under the leadership of Benedetto Saraceno, and made it possible to use many of the initiatives promoted by the WHO since then (the Atlas, MH-Gap and Policy and Services projects, among others) to support the reforms undertaken by various countries in the region.

As early as 2001, analysis of the results of the first regional survey conducted as part of the Atlas project [18] made it possible to assess the progress made in the 1990s and to identify the main difficulties. The Atlas data showed that in 2001, 40% of countries had adopted a national mental health policy since 1990 and 47.7% had adopted a national action plan during the same period. In addition, 20% of the countries had adopted a specific mental health law.

However, in most countries psychiatric hospitals remained the basic structure of the mental health system, with more than 70% of countries having less than 20% of psychiatric beds in general hospitals. Although 70% of countries had community services, in most cases these covered only a small proportion of the population in need. Finally, mental health budgets remained modest in most countries in the region: 30.7% of countries allocated less than 2% of the health budget to mental health, 46.2% allocated between 2% and 5% and only 23.1% allocated more than 5% [18].

All the information available at the time indicated the need to overcome the barriers identified in the establishment of psychiatric units in general hospitals, psychosocial rehabilitation services and programmes, user participation, the development of intersectoral cooperation and the development of specific services and programmes to meet the specific needs of women, children, the elderly, refugees, disaster victims and indigenous peoples [15].

The beginning of the new millennium was therefore a time to reflect on the successes and difficulties of the 1990s and rethink future priorities and strategies in the light of the prospects for global mental health opened by the new approaches introduced by the WHO since 2001.

The strategic lines of action defined at that time were little different from those that had guided PAHO's activities in the 1990s and have remained essentially the same to the present day [19]. However, the activities carried out and the methods and instruments used have changed in line with the evolution of the priorities established, the information and resources available and the political context.

Under the first line of action, 'Building leadership, governance and multisectoral partnerships', several major conferences were organised to broaden partnerships, mobilise resources and build consensus at political and technical levels.

To strengthen country leadership and governance, several training programmes for country directors and members of mental health units in ministries of health were promoted, and countries continued to receive support in the areas of information systems, advocacy and evaluation of services.

In the area of human rights, new projects facilitated the promotion of training activities and supported the development of mental health legislation in many countries.

The transition from hospital-based to community-based mental health care has been at the heart of the collaborative process that has been underway in Latin America for more than three decades. In response to the growing needs in this area, the PAHO Mental Health Unit has increased its staff and created the positions of the PAHO subregional mental health coordinators for Central America, South America and the Caribbean, which have greatly improved the coordination of collaborative activities. The provision of technical assistance to countries for the development of policies and services has also evolved considerably. While in the early days this assistance was dominated by advisers from Europe, from 2001 onwards it has been increasingly provided by advisers from Latin American countries where reforms had begun to take root. New funding mechanisms were also created for collaborative projects between countries, and new programmes were initiated to strengthen the capacity of service managers and to train professionals in the use of MH-GAP tools [14, 15].

The third strand focused on advancing promotion and prevention strategies and activities across the life course, with the expansion of programmes in schools and workplaces, as well as suicide prevention. At the same time, innovative depression prevention projects were launched in Central America.

Within the strategic line of response to the needs of special populations, several initiatives were taken to improve responses to the mental health needs of children and adolescents and the elderly, and to strengthen the integration of mental health and psychosocial support in emergency contexts.

In the area of research, the PAHO supported the participation of several Latin American countries (Argentina, Brazil, Colombia, Mexico, Peru) in the World Mental Health Surveys Initiative and a capacity-building initiative focused on mental health services research for early-career researchers from Latin American countries was promoted in collaboration with the US National Institute of Mental Health, involving Latin American, United States and Canadian universities. Grants and projects have also been awarded in the area of services research [14, 15].

Since the 1990s, a growing number of countries have implemented mental health policies, plans and legislation based on the Caracas Principles. Many have modernised these governance instruments to incorporate new contributions from advances in scientific knowledge and human rights approaches.

Between 2001 and 2011, the proportion of countries that had officially adopted a national mental health policy, a mental health plan and mental health legislation increased from 40.0% to 66.7%, from 47.7% to 72.2% and from 20.0% to 35.3% respectively. Over the same period, the proportion spending more than 1.4% of their total health budget on mental health increased from 25.0% to 40.0% [6]. This trend has continued in recent years: in 2020, the proportion of countries with a national mental health policy was 90% in Central America and 80% in South America [20]. This trend suggests that the strategies developed to support countries in improving their governance instruments have met this goal with considerable success.

However, progress in restructuring services has been more gradual and has varied considerably between countries. Some countries have implemented comprehensive national mental health policies that have involved a profound transformation of mental health services; others have promoted profound reforms, but only in part of the country; and still others have developed reforms that, while important, do not include all the components of reform advocated by the Caracas Declaration.

Six countries—Brazil, Chile, Belize, Panama, Peru and the Dominican Republic—have made significant progress in implementing a comprehensive national reform of their mental health systems, involving a profound transformation of mental health services. The following sections summarise the reforms undertaken in these countries.

22.4.1 Brazil

The implementation of an integrated national policy began in 1980, as part of the democratisation process that took place in the country in that decade. Initially, the reform focused on improving living conditions in psychiatric hospitals and promoting deinstitutionalisation by gradually replacing psychiatric hospitals with a network of community mental health centres, known as CAPS (Centers for Psychosocial Care in Portuguese), residential facilities, mental health care in primary care and psychosocial rehabilitation programmes [21].

Between 2001 and 2014, through a planned and progressive process of deinstitutionalisation, the number of psychiatric hospital beds was drastically reduced from 53,962 to 25,988 [22].

Meanwhile, community-based services were created to replace hospital-based services. At the heart of these services were CAPS, which were designed to meet the key care needs of people with severe and persistent mental disorders. From 2002, new types of CAPS were created to serve populations with special needs: 'CAPS-I' for children and adolescents and 'CAPS-AD' for patients with problems related to alcohol and other forms of substance abuse [21, 22].

Overall, the number of CAPS increased from 148 in 1998 to 2657 in 2020, distributed throughout the country [23].

Residential services have also become an important resource for the deinstitutionalisation of inpatients. In 2004, there were 265 residential services with 1363 residents; by 2017, the total number of residential services had increased to 489 [24].

A particularly innovative deinstitutionalisation strategy was the 'Volta para Casa' (Return Home) programme, which established a financial allowance for deinstitutionalised patients. In 2003, 206 patients were enrolled in the programme, and by 2014 the number had increased to 4349 patients [21, 22].

The progress made by this policy is undeniable. However, the available data show that, despite this progress, there were several weaknesses in the implementation of the policy. Such weaknesses were found in the area of funding. Although funds were correctly allocated to community-based services, many experts felt that the funds were insufficient to fully implement the various components of the reform. Human resource development was also identified as an important issue. Weaknesses were also identified in the quality of information produced by services, the integration of mental health into primary care and the sustainability of patient associations [22, 25].

Changes in the health policy of the Jair Bolsonaro government between 2019 and 2022 have led to various attempts to reduce the role of CAPS, strengthen hospital care and question the continuity of care and coordination between different levels of care. However, these attempts have failed to put into practice an alternative policy to the one that has guided the Brazilian reform, which is still being developed by the current government.

22.4.2 Chile

The transformation of mental health services began in the 1970s, driven by the work of authors such as Marconi [26]. However, it was only with the democratisation of Chile that the implementation of a national policy firmly based on the principles of the Caracas Declaration became a reality. The Chilean reform is undoubtedly one of the most successful and interesting mental health reforms in the world. It is characterised by the rigorous and efficient way in which the country has implemented three successive national mental health plans since the early 1990s.

These plans have led to the implementation of a comprehensive model that articulates mental health promotion, prevention and treatment of mental disorders, ensuring care in each geographic sector through a network of integrated services (including mental health care in primary care, specialised community mental health centres, psychiatric units in general hospitals, intersectoral collaboration and user participation) [6, 27].

Between 1999 and 2006, the proportion of the health budget allocated to mental health almost doubled, from 1.2% to 2.1%. Over the same period, the proportion of the mental health budget allocated to psychiatric hospitals fell from 57% to 33% [6, 15].

Between 1990 and 2014, the number of short-stay beds in psychiatric hospitals (up to 60 days) decreased from 5.9 to 2.9 per 100,000 inhabitants, while the number of medium- and long-term beds decreased from 25.9 to 4.0. During the same period, short-stay beds in general hospitals increased from 2.5 to 5.3 and beds in group homes increased from 0 to 12.0 per 100,000 inhabitants. Data on the numbers of people with mental disorders treated in different services per 100,000 beneficiaries of the public system in Chile (2004 and 2014) show that there was an increase from 2217 to 4559 in primary care services and from 535 to 1014 in specialised outpatient services. In the same period, the number of people admitted to general hospitals per 100,000 inhabitants increased from 55 to 86, while in psychiatric hospitals it decreased from 48 to 32 [27].

22.4.3 Belize

Although part of Central America, Belize is an English-speaking country with its own cultural and political characteristics. In the early 1990s, its mental health system was reduced almost entirely to one psychiatric hospital with poor physical conditions and very few human resources. Despite these challenges, Belize implemented a mental health reform that resulted in the closure of the psychiatric hospital and the establishment of an integrated system of services that includes an inpatient unit in the general hospital, day hospitals, supported housing, an integrated assertive community service for the severely mentally ill and community teams composed of nurses specially trained to provide basic mental health care throughout the country under the supervision of psychiatrists. Innovative rehabilitation programmes have been developed in Belize City, a users' association has been established and a mental health law has been passed.

To achieve these goals, Belize has relied on strong political support, the excellent and creative leadership of Dr. Claudina Cayetano (for some years the only psychiatrist in the country), the involvement of users and families, the ability to develop a good mental health plan and very good use of international cooperation provided by the WHO, the PAHO and various donors [28].

22.4.4 Panama

Panama is a prime example of how a health system centred on a large psychiatric hospital, with all the problems found in this type of institution in Latin America in the 1960s, can be transformed into a community-based system through a sustained policy of training professionals and reallocating resources.

A first mental health plan in the 1960s led to the integration of mental health care into the health centres that were then being built in the different provinces of the country, the creation of psychiatric units in general hospitals and the sectorisation of psychiatric care provided by mental health teams in the community.

In the 1990s, with the support of the PAHO, the government decided to develop a project to reorganise mental health services. This project led to the start of a process of deinstitutionalisation of patients from the psychiatric hospital, the strengthening of mental health teams integrated into primary care and the creation of psychosocial rehabilitation centres. The hospital was transformed into the National Institute of Mental Health.

In 2007, the budget for mental health was 3% of the health budget, of which 40% went to the National Institute of Mental Health. The country had 103 community mental health teams, 3 day centres and 8 psychiatric units in community general hospitals with 284 beds (8.95 per 100,000 inhabitants), 3 of which were for children and adolescents. The National Institute had 200 beds, 65% fewer than 5 years earlier. The existing intersectoral mental health network at the first level of care developed activities aiming at mental health promotion and prevention of mental disorders, working closely with several organisations in the community. At the second level of care, beds for the treatment of psychiatric cases were available in the internal medicine wards of district hospitals and in the psychiatric units and day clinics of general hospitals [29].

22.4.5 Peru

Peru is one of the countries that has recently begun to implement a national mental health policy. In 2013, in the context of an improved economic situation and several health reforms, the government decided to launch a thorough reform of mental health care.

New legislation was passed to include mental health care in the national health insurance system and to secure the rights of people with mental health problems. A network of mental health centres was established as the basis of the new care system. Community mental health centres (CMHC), staffed by a psychiatrist and a team of other mental health professionals, became responsible for the care of a sector of about 100,000 inhabitants. Their role is to provide specialised outpatient services for children, adolescents, adults and the elderly with mental disorders, psychosocial problems and addictions. A core activity of the CHMCs is also to provide technical assistance to primary care centres, to support community integration and to liaise with other existing services.

To ensure support for recovery and reintegration into society, sheltered or halfway houses have also been established for patients discharged from psychiatric hospitals without family support.

Inpatient treatment has begun to be provided through short-term inpatient units, which have been established in 32 general hospitals across the country to provide 24-h medical care and supervision for patients with acute mental disorders. By 2021, the Ministry of Health aimed to have mental health units in 62 hospitals.

Deinstitutionalisation is a key objective of the reform. For this reason, in parallel with the development of the new community-based services, a process of reform and, in some cases, closure of specialised psychiatric hospitals has begun in different regions of the country, in line with the deinstitutionalisation process [30].

This process has led to significant advancements in resources for the country's mental health system. Between 2014 and 2020, the number of community mental health centres and sheltered homes in the country increased, respectively, from 23 to 208 and from six to 55. During this period, the number of mental health professionals increased from 12.4 to 28 per 100,000 inhabitants, while the proportion of the health budget allocated to mental health rose from 0.3% to 2.3% [23].

One of the key aspects of the reform in Peru is the innovative health financing model created to ensure the sustainability of the process. On the one hand, mental health services have been included in the benefits package of the Peruvian Integrated Health Insurance Scheme (SIS). This has been complemented by the development of a revised reimbursement schedule to cover the cost of services provided in community mental health facilities and specialised psychiatric hospitals, which has helped to reduce patients' out-of-pocket payments for mental health services from 94% of the total of payments in 2013 to 32% in 2016. Meanwhile, a 10-year results-based budget programme approved by the Ministry of Economy and Finance in 2014 exclusively for mental health reform supports its implementation and scalability [30, 31].

22.4.6 Dominican Republic

The Dominican Republic began implementing a mental health plan in 2014 that focuses on closing the country's only psychiatric hospital while building a network of community-based services. These include clinical services in general health facilities, day centres and supported housing services to facilitate psychosocial rehabilitation.

Mental health units in general hospitals play a crucial role in ensuring care for all people with mental health problems who cannot be easily managed in primary care, providing crisis services, including short stay beds where needed, outpatient psychiatric and psychological care for people discharged from hospital and liaison psychiatry with other hospital services.

Since 2008, the number of mental health units in district hospitals has increased from 9 to 15, and the number of available short-stay beds has increased from 76 to 113. Overall, these units account for more than half (53%) of all public mental health beds available in the country, up from 33% in 2008 [23].

22.5   General Comparisons

Other countries have promoted in-depth reforms, but only at the level of one or more of the country's provinces; still others developed reforms that were important but did not include all the components of reform advocated by the Caracas Declaration.

Many countries, including Brazil, Chile, Cuba, El Salvador, Guatemala and Panama, have made significant progress in integrating mental health into primary health care [15].

The development of comprehensive, community-based mental health services that could guarantee mental health care for a given population and replace psychiatric hospitals has been the main objective of several national and regional projects throughout Latin America and the Caribbean. The reform in the Argentine province of Río Negro was one of the first to successfully implement an integrated mental health system without psychiatric hospitals in a large territory, with an important psychosocial rehabilitation component and extensive patient participation. In a short period of time, it has managed to organise a system with 19 community mental health teams, 6 halfway houses, 6 income-generating projects, several consumer and family organisations, 3 homes for care and rehabilitation, 1 community mental health association, 150 mental health workers (distributed in 20 out of 28 provincial hospitals), 60 community mental health workers and 90 other professionals (social workers, psychologists, sociologists, doctors and educational psychologists) [12].

Overall, most Latin American countries have made some progress since 1990 in improving and reducing psychiatric hospitals, either nationally or in some localities, and in developing some community mental health initiatives.

However, as shown in the study led by Minoletti [6], which compared the extent of change in the four countries that had implemented national reforms in 2011 (Belize, Brazil, Chile, Panama) with the average changes in the rest of Latin America, at that time only the first four countries had completely transformed the hospital-based model and ensured the creation of a national community-based model.

While psychiatric hospital beds were eliminated in Belize and reduced by 62.2% (for the three countries combined) in Brazil, Chile and Panama in the first decade of the new millennium, the average reduction in the number of psychiatric hospital beds in the other countries of the region over the same period was only 23.9%.

Over this period, the four countries had replaced psychiatric hospitals with beds in general hospitals, community mental health teams and centres and group homes. In 2011, the share of psychiatric beds in general hospitals, outpatient facilities and day facilities (day centres and day hospitals) in Brazil, Chile and Panama was between two and seven times higher than in other Latin American countries. To achieve this change, these countries had significantly increased the share of public mental health expenditure allocated to general hospitals, outpatient facilities and community services—an increase of 67.7% in Brazil, 88.0% in Chile and 56.0% in Panama.

In order to better understand the reasons that might explain the difficulties encountered by countries that have been less successful in transforming their mental health services, Minoletti [6] also carried out a more detailed analysis of the mental health policies and plans of these countries and found that some of the national policies, plans and legislation in this region were 'not explicit enough to support and facilitate the provision of community mental health services' and 'even when they are explicit, their implementation is usually inadequate'. On the other hand, when comparing the percentage of the health budget allocated to mental health in Latin American countries (mostly low- and upper-middle-income countries) with those in other regions of the world in the same income groups, they found that the median percentage in the former (1.90) was lower than in other countries (2.38). These findings seem to indicate that the historical limitations of mental health funding in Latin America and the lack of clarity about the priorities of mental health policies and plans in some countries have been major barriers to their implementation in these countries.

22.6   Implementation Issues

In addition to these barriers, the centralisation of care in traditional psychiatric hospitals, resistance by professionals to change to new models of care, difficulties in integrating mental health care into primary care and a lack of public leadership in mental health have also been important barriers in Latin America [32]. The existence of a national mental health policy, plan and legislation is an important prerequisite for change, but this has not always translated into additional funding for mental health. The reality is that the health budget allocated to mental health in the region has traditionally been very low and, although it has increased in many countries, few have managed to secure significant additional funding during the transition to a new model of care.

One of the lessons learned in the region is that it is very difficult to achieve full success in implementing mental health reform without a unit within the Ministry of Health with adequate leadership, solid technical capacity, access to policy-making centres and the ability to influence all components of the mental health system.

In terms of enabling factors, the transition from political regimes that paid little attention to mental health and systematically violated human rights to democratic governments more committed to respecting human rights provided an excellent window of opportunity for improving mental health services [8]. Natural disasters have also been important windows of opportunity for the development of new services.

The human rights movement in Latin America and the Caribbean proved to be one of the most powerful tools for change in mental health systems, and some of the most successful reforms have been closely linked to human rights initiatives [33].

The early development of research capacity in Latin American countries, in areas such as psychiatric epidemiology and mental health services research, greatly facilitated the implementation of mental health service reform for several reasons. It contributed to a better assessment of the needs of the population. It helped to understand which services were more appropriate for different specific contexts. And it supported the creation of a critical mass that was important to develop the scientific debate on mental health issues.

Finally, the Initiative for the Restructuring of Psychiatric Care in Latin America demonstrated that international cooperation can be an important facilitator in the implementation of mental health reforms in low- and middle-income countries, especially when, as in Latin America, it is possible to establish a systematic and comprehensive programme at the regional level with the support of the World Health Organization [32].

22.7 Conclusions

Thirty years after the launch of the initiative to reorganise mental health services in Latin America, based on the recommendations of the Caracas Declaration, some conclusions can be drawn about the validity of the principles that guide the framework for action, the results of the reforms carried out in the countries of the region and the impact of this initiative worldwide.

The evolution of societies over the last three decades has created new challenges for the organisation of mental health services. The experience gained in the implementation of the three main principles of the reform proposed by the Caracas Declaration—the shift from hospital to community-based care, the integration of mental health care into primary care and the defence of the rights of users of mental health services—has helped to recognise that their implementation is a more complex process than initially anticipated, and that further critical reflection on the conceptual and operational aspects related to these issues is fundamental [6, 10, 34]. Nevertheless, these principles are not only supported by the available evidence, but remain the pillars of mental health service reform recommended by the World Health Organisation [17, 23] and have been endorsed by both the most recent major international documents on mental health policy and services [35] and the landmark UN Convention on the Rights of Persons with Disabilities adopted in 2008 [36].

The current situation of mental health systems in Latin American countries is very different from that of 30 years ago. Governance tools and organisation of services have improved considerably. Almost all countries now have up-to-date policies, plans and legislation and many have made significant progress in their information systems and financing models. Almost all countries have developed some community services and made some progress in integrating mental health into primary care, although in many of them these new services cover only a modest proportion of the population. Several other countries have managed to implement more in-depth reforms covering the population of one or more provinces. Finally, almost a third of countries have made significant progress in implementing a comprehensive national reform of their mental health system, involving a major transformation of mental health services.

It is difficult to determine the extent to which these results can be attributed to the regional process initiated in Caracas. A significant part of the progress achieved must be attributed to the efforts of the countries themselves and all those who have worked to improve their mental health services. Nevertheless, all the technical, political and, in some cases, financial cooperation activities carried out within the framework of the regional initiative developed since 1990 have undoubtedly contributed to improving the capacity of most countries to implement service reforms. It is therefore reasonable to conclude that the Latin American experience has confirmed the importance of international cooperation in the modernisation of mental health services at country level, especially when it is systematic and includes technical and scientific support from the WHO and other international organisations.

The reforms carried out in Latin America over the past 30 years have resulted in significant progress in the reforms already under way and increasing technical sophistication in the most recent ones. Moreover, the contributions of this experience have extended far beyond the region. Indeed, the process developed in Latin America since the Caracas Declaration is now an essential reference in the discussion of fundamental issues related to deinstitutionalisation, the development of truly community-based services, the organisation of human rights-based mental health services and the future of global mental health.

Key Points
- The restructuring of psychiatric care in Latin America, promoted on the basis of the Caracas Declaration since 1990, demonstrates that collaboration between countries in a region, with the support of the WHO and other international organisations, can make a significant contribution to achieving this goal.
- Throughout this process, six countries have successfully implemented in-depth reforms of their mental health services, and many others have taken significant steps in this direction.
- The primary obstacles encountered pertained to the absence of sustained political endorsement, the absence of a comprehensive consensus among the relevant stakeholders and the dearth of additional financial resources allocated to mental health services.
- Conversely, the key facilitators of these reforms include democratisation processes that occurred in various countries, the public health capacity of mental health leaders and the influence of human rights movements.
- International cooperation proved to be of particular significance in the realms of capacity building, enhancement of governance and research and policy development.

References

1. González Uzcátegui R. Salud mental en la comunidad en América Latina. Ejemplo de Programas. In: Levav I, editor. Temas de salud mental en la comunidad. Washington, D.C.: Pan American Health Organization; 1992. p. 291–312. [In Spanish].
2. Alarcon R, Aguilar-Gaxiola S. Mental health policy developments in Latin America. Bull World Health Organ. 2000;78(4):483–90.
3. González Uzcategui R, Levav I. Reestructuración de la atención psiquiátrica: bases conceptuales y guías para su implementación: memorias de la Conferencia Regional de Reestructuración de la Atención Psiquiatrica. Washington, D.C.: Pan American Health Organization; 1991. [In Spanish]
4. Levav I, Restrepo H, Guerra De Macedo C. The restructuring of psychiatric care in Latin America. A new policy for mental health services. J Public Health Policy. 1994;15(1):71–85.
5. Aparicio V. La Declaración de Caracas desde la perspectiva Europea. Salud Mental y Comunidad. 2020;9:136–42. [In Spanish]
6. Minoletti A, Galea S, Susser E. Community mental health services in Latin America for people with severe mental disorders. Public Health Rev. 2012;34(2):1–23.
7. Alarcon R. Hacia una identidad de la psiquiatria latinoamericana. Boletin de la Oficina Sanitaria Panamericana. 1976;81(2):109–21. [In Spanish]
8. Levav I, González Uzcátegui R. The roots of the Caracas declaration. In: Rodriguez J, editor. Mental health care reform: 15 years after Caracas. Washington DC: Pan American Health Organization; 2007. [In Spanish].
9. Basaglia F. Conferenze Brasiliane. Milan: Raffaello Cortina; 2000.
10. Caldas De Almeida JM. The impact in Latin America of Basaglia and Italian psychiatric reform. In: Burns T, Foot J, editors. Basaglia's international legacy: from asylum to community. Oxford: Oxford University Press; 2020.
11. Saraceno B, Aguilar Briceno R, Asioli F, Liberati A, Tognoni G. Cooperation in mental health: an Italian project in Nicaragua. Soc Sci Med. 1990;31:1067–71.
12. Collins P. Argentina: waving the mental health revolution banner: psychiatric reform and community mental health in the province of Rio Negro. In: Caldas de Almeida JM, Cohen A, editors. Innovative mental health programs in Latin America and the Caribbean. Washington DC: Pan American Health Organization; 2008.
13. Alves D, Valentini W. Mental health policy in Brazil. In: Morral PM, Hazelton M, editors. Mental health policy: international perspectives. London: Whurr; 2002.
14. Caldas de Almeida JM. Estrategias de cooperación técnica de la Organización Panamericana de la Salud en la nueva fase de la reforma de los servicios de salud mental en América Latina y el Caribe. Pan Am J Public Health. 2005;18:314–26. [In Spanish]
15. Caldas De Almeida JM, Horvitz-Lennon M. An overview of mental health care reforms in Latin America and the Caribbean. Psychiatr Serv. 2010;61:218–21.
16. Pan American Health Organization. Resolution CD40.R19 of Directing Council. Washington D.C.: Pan American Health Organization; 1997.
17. World Health Organization. World health report 2001: mental health—new understanding, new hope. Geneva: World Health Organization; 2001a.
18. World Health Organization. Mental health atlas 2001. Geneva: WHO Department of Mental Health and Substance Abuse; 2001b.
19. Pan American Health Organization. Policy for improving mental health. Washington DC: Pan American Health Organization; 2023.
20. Pan American Health Organization. Mental health atlas in the Americas. Washington DC: Pan American Health Organization; 2020.
21. Caldas De Almeida JM. Mental health policy in Brazil: what's at stake in the changes currently under way. Cad Saude Publica. 2019;35(11) Available at https://www.scielo.br/j/csp/a/KMwv8DrW37NzpmvL4WkHcdC/?lang=en

22. Fundação Oswaldo Cruz, Fundação Calouste Gulbenkian. Inovações e desafios em desinsti-
    tucionalização e atenção comunitária no Brasil. Seminário Internacional de Saúde Mental:
    documento técnico final. Rio de Janeiro: Fundação Oswaldo Cruz/Fundação Calouste
    Gulbenkian; 2015. [In Portuguese]. Available at https://www.nuppsam.org/wp-content/
    uploads/2021/05/DESINSTITUCIONALIZACAO-E-ATENCAO-COMUNITARIA-
    FIOCRUZ-GULBENKIAN.pdf
23. World Health Organization. World mental health report: transforming mental health for all.
    Geneva: World Health Organization; 2022.
24. Ministerio da Saude Brasil. Panorama e diagnóstico da Política Nacional de Saúde Mental.
    Brasília: Ministério da Saúde; 2017. [In Portuguese]. Avaliable at https://www.gov.br/saude/
    pt-br/acesso-a-informacao/gestao-do-sus/articulacao-interfederativa/cit/pautas-de-reunioes-e-
    resumos/2017/agosto/2a-apresentacao-cit-final.pdf/view
25. Mateus M, Mari j, Delgado P, Almeida-Filho N, Barrett T, Gerolin J, Goihman S, Razzouk D,
    Rodriguez J, Weber R, Andreoli SB, Saxena S. The mental health system in Brazil: policies
    and future challenges. Int J Ment Health Syst. 2008;2(1):12. https://doi.org/10.1186/1752-
    4458-2-12.
26. Marconi J. Policy of mental health in Latin America. Acta Psiquiatr Psicol Am Lat.
    1976;22(2):112–20. [In Spanish]
27. Minoletti A, Sepúlveda R, Gómez M, Toro O, Irarrázabal M, Díaz R, et al. Análisis de la
    gobernanza en la implementación del modelo comunitario de salud mental en Chile. Rev
    Panam Salud Publica. 2018;42:e131. [In Spanish]. Available at https://iris.paho.org/bitstream/
    handle/10665.2/49515/v42e1312018.pdf?sequence=1&isAllowed=y.
28. Ministry of Health of Belize & Pan American Health Organization/World Health Organization.
    WHO-AIMS report on mental health system in Belize. Washington D.C.: Pan American
    Health Organization; 2009. Available at https://iris.paho.org/bitstream/handle/10665.2/7686/
    AIMS_report_2009.pdf?sequence=1&isAllowed=y
29. Pan American Health Organization. Desarrollo de la Salud mental en Panamá. Organización
    Panamericana de la Salud; 2007. [In Spanish]. Available at https://bdigital.binal.ac.pa/bdp/
    Salud-Mental-en-Panama.pdf
30. Toyama M, Castillo H, Galea JT, Brandt LR, Mendoza M, Herrera V, Mitrani M, Cutipé Y,
    Cavero V, Diez-Canseco F, Miranda F. Peruvian mental health reform: a framework for scal-
    ing-up mental health services. Int J Health Policy Manag. 2017;6(9):501–8.
31. Marquez P, Garcia J. Paradigm shift: Peru leading the way in reforming mental health
    services. World Bank Blogs; 2019. Available at https://blogs.worldbank.org/en/health/
    paradigm-shift-peru-leading-way-reforming-mental-health-services
32. Caldas De Almeida JM. Mental health services development in Latin America and the
    Caribbean: achievements, barriers and facilitating factors. Int Health. 2013;5:15–8.
33. Vásquez J, Caldas de Almeida JM. Salud mental y derechos humanos. Atopos. 2004;2:45–56.
    [In Spanish]
34. Bouras N, Ikkos G, Craig T. From community to meta-community mental health care. Int J
    Environ Res Public Health. 2018;15(4):806.
35. Patel V, Saxena S, Lund C, Thornicroft G, Baingaina F, Bolton P, et al. The Lancet Commission
    on global mental health and sustainable development. Lancet. 2018;392:1553–98.
36. United Nations. Convention on the rights of persons with disabilities. New York: United
    Nations; 2006.

Open Access This chapter is licensed under the terms of the Creative Commons Attribution 4.0 International License (http://creativecommons.org/licenses/by/4.0/), which permits use, sharing, adaptation, distribution and reproduction in any medium or format, as long as you give appropriate credit to the original author(s) and the source, provide a link to the Creative Commons license and indicate if changes were made.

The images or other third party material in this chapter are included in the chapter's Creative Commons license, unless indicated otherwise in a credit line to the material. If material is not included in the chapter's Creative Commons license and your intended use is not permitted by statutory regulation or exceeds the permitted use, you will need to obtain permission directly from the copyright holder.

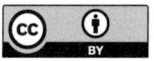

Part VI

Psychiatry and Mental Health Services Today and Tomorrow

This part looks at psychiatry's future from the perspectives of psychiatric research, peer support, clinical treatment and services and justice and vocation.

Chapter 23 shares information on the research programme at the institute that Kraepelin established, now called the Max Planck Institute of Psychiatry, in Munich. Chapter 24 summarises empirical research findings on the engagement and impact of peer support in mental health services. Chapter 25 advocates a future away from the label of schizophrenia and outlines treatment approaches guided by the various aetiological contributions to psychosis. Chapter 26 details the ambitions for major stepwise upgrade and extensions to mental health services in Denmark where, in a country with strong social democratic traditions and policies, professional, service user and political consensus have secured major increases in funding for mental healthcare. Chapter 27 takes a bird's eye view and offers a contemporary montage on the values of the Enlightenment, the evolution of capitalist political economy and the demands for empathy and justice and their importance for the conditions and practice of the psychiatric vocation today and beyond.

Emil Kraepelin and Biological Research in Psychiatry Today

23

Peter Falkai, Lukas Roell, Sergi Papiol, Moritz Rossner, and Andrea Schmitt

23.1 Introduction

As outlined in the foreword to this volume by Allen Frances, Emil Kraepelin's legacy is the classification of mental, especially psychotic disorders based on the clinical symptoms summarised into specific syndromes and their long-term outcome. He believed that in this way he could help define distinct pathophysiologies linked to these subgroups and thus find better treatments. In pursuing the ambition of 'Precision Psychiatry', our field is still looking for clinical, blood-based, neuroimaging and electrophysiological **(bio)-markers** to delimit distinct biological subgroups, leading to mechanistically informed treatments. So far, however, this approach has had limited success. Focusing on schizophrenia, the question arises why it has been so difficult to accomplish these objectives. In this chapter, we will outline conceptual and methodological issues crucial for success in identifying biomarkers. A better understanding of patient subgroups with distinct pathophysiology and treatment responses could lead to mechanistically informed innovative treatment strategies. In summary, in patients with schizophrenia we detected a loss of specific glia cells, the **oligodendrocytes** (Fig. 23.1), in a subregion of the **hippocampus**. This brain structure is responsible for learning and memory. In schizophrenia, it shows a reduced volume, which can be reversed by regular physical exercise training. The underlying mechanisms, for example, improvement in synaptic contacts or energy supply by oligodendrocytes, are currently under investigation.

P. Falkai (✉) · L. Roell · M. Rossner · A. Schmitt
Department of Psychiatry and Psychotherapy, LMU University Hospital, Ludwig-Maximilians-University Munich, Munich, Germany
e-mail: Peter.Falkai@med.uni-muenchen.de; Lukas.Roell@med.uni-muenchen.de; Moritz.Rossner@med.uni-muenchen.de; Andrea.Schmitt@med.uni-muenchen.de

S. Papiol
Max Planck Institute of Psychiatry, Munich, Germany
e-mail: Sergi.Papiol@med.uni-muenchen.de

© The Author(s) 2026
G. Ikkos, T. Becker (eds.), *Psychiatry after Kraepelin*,
https://doi.org/10.1007/978-3-032-09475-9_23

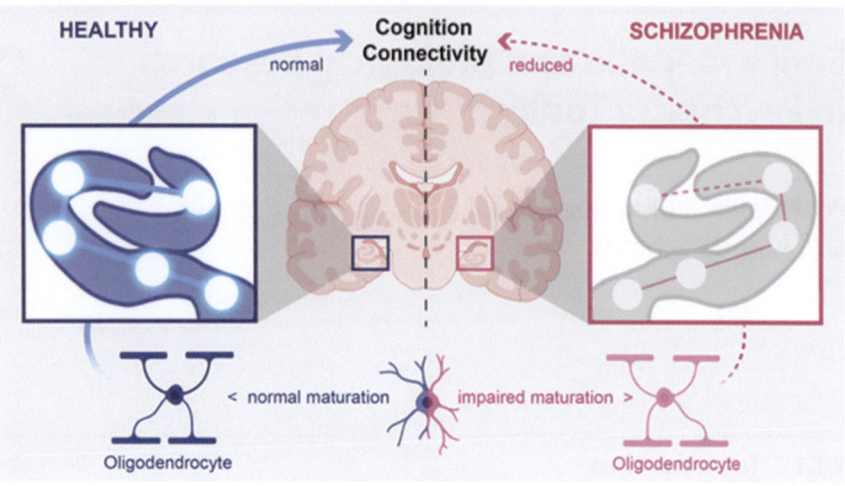

Fig. 23.1 Reduction in oligodendrocytes in the hippocampus

Box 23.1 presents a glossary of the main terms. The terms included in the glossary are printed in bold when first appearing in the text.

23.2 Conceptual Framework: From Degeneration to Disturbed Regeneration

Alois Alzheimer described a thinning of the frontal and parietal cortex in Dementia Praecox (later termed Schizophrenia) [1], which was accompanied by 'deceased cells showing lipoid inclusions'. He interpreted these findings as 'destruction of the nervous cortical elements'. These findings can be compensated by some patients, but in most patients, it leads to 'a peculiar persistent impairment of the psyche' [1, 2]. The conclusion of both scientists, Alzheimer and Kraepelin, was that dementia praecox is a consequence of a 'manifest destruction of the cortex' [1, 3]. Today, we would call this the consequence of a neurodegenerative process, as can be seen in brain disorders such as Parkinson's or Alzheimer's disease. The conclusion that dementia praecox, later called schizophrenia, is a mental illness with an unfavourable outcome and a neurodegenerative basis has continued to influence our way of thinking about this illness ever since. The question remains, however, whether this formulation is correct, or whether schizophrenia should rather be regarded as 'a failure of the regenerative capacities of the human brain' [4, 5].

There are several lines of evidence suggesting a process of disturbed synaptic and myelin plasticity: that is, regenerative rather than degenerative processes.

1. *No progression of cognitive deficits over time.* Cognitive deficits frequently appear years before the manifestation of the first episode of schizophrenia. In about two-thirds of patients, they improve to some extent with the reduction in

the positive symptoms but remain despite antipsychotic treatment with relatively stable residual symptoms. After any initial reduction in cognitive abilities, there is no evidence for further progression over time. This is well documented in several well-controlled studies and summarised in meta-analyses [6–10].

2. *Lack of neuronal loss.* One of the hallmarks of a degenerative process of the brain is loss of neuronal elements over time. Using brain imaging [11, 12] and looking at the pattern of volume changes in brain structures in patients with schizophrenia, the hippocampus, with a Cohen's *d* of 0.5, shows the biggest and most consistent volume reduction, ranging between 5% and 10% [13]. Using state-of-the-art design-based stereological methodology, our own and other studies have demonstrated a lack of neuronal loss in the hippocampus [14, 15], which clearly speaks against a degenerative process affecting neurons.

3. *Lack of astrocytosis or* **microgliosis** *indicative of inflammation.* In a degenerative process with neuronal cell loss, activation and rise of **astrocyte** or **microglia** numbers should occur and be traceable. In our own post-mortem studies [14, 15] and a large meta-analysis [16], no increased number or density of astrocytes has been found in schizophrenia. Moreover, a recent meta-analysis has shown that microglia density was unaltered in schizophrenia and that changes in microglial morphology were also absent. In line with recent **transcriptome** studies however, the expression of microglia-specific genes was decreased in the temporal cortex in schizophrenia [17]. These findings are not indicative of a degenerative process as astrocytosis and microglia activation is lacking. However, we anticipate subgroups of patients may be identified in the future, in which low-grade microgliosis may be found to occur. Microgliosis may play a role in tissue repair, homeostasis, neuroplasticity, synaptic pruning or other neurodevelopmental processes.

4. *Synapse number reduction, but no neurodegenerative changes* per se. Volume reduction in the absence of neuronal loss suggests a reduction in the **neuropil** encompassing synapses, dendrites and axons. Supporting this notion, a meta-analysis has shown a significant reduction in post-synaptic elements in brain regions which are key in schizophrenia pathophysiology [18].

5. *Loss of oligodendrocytes as a sign of impaired myelin homeostasis and plasticity.* Counting all cellular elements of the hippocampal sub-regions using design-based stereological methods, we have found a significant reduction in oligodendrocytes in the CA4 region in schizophrenia and have replicated this finding in an independent sample [14, 15]. These results, together with findings of impaired structural and functional connectivity in neuroimaging studies, have led to the hypothesis of impaired myelin plasticity as the basis of cognitive dysfunction in schizophrenia [5].

6. *Reversibility of structural and functional changes in schizophrenia.* In three subsequent studies which implemented aerobic exercise in patients with schizophrenia, we have demonstrated that hippocampal volume loss especially in the CA4/ Dentate region was reversible [19–21]. We have also found that neuronal circuits of the Default Mode Network could be restored. Such restoration has been associated with improved functioning as measured by the Global Assessment of

Functioning (GAF) [22]. Both findings speak for a regenerative neuroplastic process which occurs during aerobic exercise.

All these findings are compatible with the extensive evidence supporting both the neurodevelopmental hypothesis of schizophrenia and the developmental risk factor model of psychosis [23, 22, 24, 25]. Thus, the genetic and environmental risk of schizophrenia could contribute to neurodevelopmental abnormalities eventually leading to vulnerable synaptic networks and impaired myelination in the adult brain [26]. In this regard, it is noteworthy that Kraepelin was well aware of changes in behaviour long before the onset of psychotic illness and the presence of abnormal developmental trajectories in many of these patients [27, 28].

23.3   Defining a Strong Phenotype: Cognition and Disturbed Myelin Plasticity

One of the major obstacles to understand the pathophysiology of mental disorders is the lack of a strong **phenotype**, contrary to oncological disorders, for example, where the biological underpinnings, for example, the molecular aberrations of a given tumour, are clearly linked to a specific clinical manifestation.

We similarly propose a link of functional outcome, overall psychopathology and cognition in schizophrenia, with the dysfunction of the Default Mode Network [eds: see Fig. 23.2, Chap. 13], the Salience Network and a cognition related network as measured by the Digital Cell Imager (DCI) normalisation [22]. Using transcriptomic imaging the DCI difference was significantly linked to the expression of oligodendrocytes and no other cell types. Interestingly, in our Exercise II study, the volume increase in the hippocampus was linked to the cell-type specific polygenic risk score (**PRS**) of immature oligodendrocyte precursor cells (OPCs) [29]. So far, this finding has been replicated in our Exercise III study in the largest RCT on aerobic exercise [30]. A reduction in oligodendrocytes has been found post-mortem not only in CA4 of the hippocampus [14, 15] but also in the prefrontal cortex and the white matter of the cingulum [31]. Oligodendrocytes provide energetic support to neuron–axonal metabolism through the delivery of lactate for neuronal **mitochondria** to generate adenosine triphosphate (ATP) [32]. The discovery of the metabolic coupling of myelin and axons is an important conceptual advance in neuroscience [33], since it is another example which highlights the intricate interaction of cells within the brain. Using Mendelian randomisation, a relationship between mitochondria-associated proteins and schizophrenia risk has recently been reported [34]. We have proposed a dysfunction of the mitochondria of maturing oligodendrocytes, leading to impaired re-myelination and trophic support of the neurons, as underlying the cognitive dysfunction in schizophrenia (Fig. 23.2) [5].

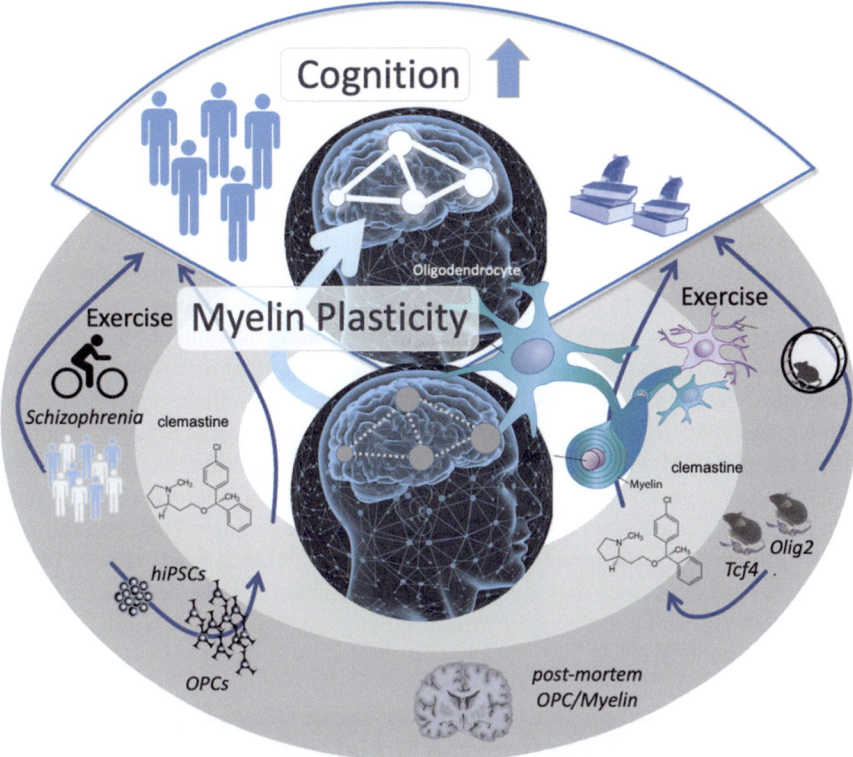

Fig. 23.2 Mechanism through which exercise affects and clemastine may affect cognition. HiPSCs human-induced pluripotent stem cells, OPCs oligodendrocyte progenitor cells, **Tcf4** transcription factor 4, **Olig2** oligodendrocyte transcription factor 2

In the light of the above, we hypothesise that 'disturbed myelin plasticity' (e.g. [5]) is one of the components of a generalised distortion of plastic processes underlying schizophrenia. This would also involve and is likely secondary to 'dysfunctional synaptic plasticity'. As we believe that disturbed myelin plasticity is a prominent pathway that participates in the pathophysiology of schizophrenia, we have initiated a drug repurposing randomised controlled study (RCT) adding the antihistaminergic drug clemastine to aerobic exercise, comparing the combination to placebo. The study aims at clarifying whether this pro-myelinic agent is able to improve cognition in addition to aerobic exercise [5]. Also, presently, a double knock-out mouse (Tcf4/Olig2) under early maternal separation is under investigation to develop a model showing cognitive deficits associated with moderate oligodendrocyte deficits [35].

23.4 Combining Methods and Specialists: Clinical, Neuropsychological, Imaging, Genetic and Animal Model Findings

Emil Kraepelin's big achievement has been to bring scientific methodology into psychiatry and thus move psychiatry into medicine. By inviting top scientists such as Alois Alzheimer to Munich, he eventually took a decisive step by founding a separate research institute, the Max Planck Institute of Psychiatry (Max Planck Institut für Psychiatrie). He, thus, fostered top research in mental disorders, which has led and still leads to important findings. Today, we have a toolbox of advanced technologies (e.g. in genetics/genomics and in neuroimaging) and our institute also has access to large and phenotype-rich clinical data sets. Joint forces are required to understand the functions of risk factors in the brain and thus, their expression at the behavioural level. Specialists in their field need to form networks in order to understand the pathophysiology of mental disorders. At the institute, we have brought together such a group, where clinical (A.S., P.F.), genetics/genomics (S.P.), neuroimaging (L.R.) and animal model (M.R.) expertise is combined. This research network group is complemented by expertise from other fields like data science [4, 5]. With this kind of state-of-the-art assemblies, experiments can be designed, and the data generated can be examined from different perspectives representing specific scientific knowledge.

23.5 Back-Translation from the Model to the Patient: Clinical Studies

If we want to be ambitious in bringing new research findings into clinical reality, as we must, we need to pursue more clinical studies, starting from single patient studies, followed by uni-centric two-arm RCTs leading to large-scale multi-centre RCTs. Clinical studies allow us to discover the end-points of pathophysiological cascades in humans at least. This should then be back-translated to non-human model systems, for example, **transgenic** mice or human stem cell derived models. Only this cycle will allow unravelling the pathophysiology of subgroups of patients with mental disorders, which will eventually lead to **mechanistically** informed specific treatments (Fig. 23.3).

23.6 Conclusion

Cognitive deficits, which entail impairments in learning and memory, are present in most of the patients with schizophrenia and often remain stable even when other symptoms improve. We consider they are responsible for social disintegration, such as a reduced ability to work or to maintain lesser social contacts. Therefore, to develop new treatment strategies, the underlying mechanisms in neuronal brain networks have to be elucidated. In specific brain regions related to learning and

Fig. 23.3 Translation and back-translation: From risk factors to models to clinical studies and back. POP Proof of Principle

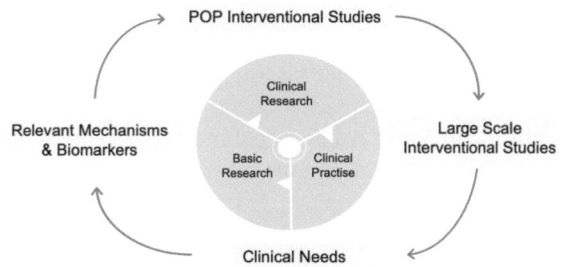

memory such as the hippocampus, we did not detect a loss of neurons in schizophrenia, but a reduction in oligodendrocytes. These build the myelin sheath around neurons; they play an important role in energy supply to neurons and are also responsible for the fast connections to other brain regions. Additionally, reduced synaptic transmission or a mild inflammatory process in the brain may contribute to cognitive deficits. Interestingly, regular physical endurance training improved memory and counteracted the volume loss of the hippocampus in patients with schizophrenia, thereby promoting a regenerative process. In ongoing basic and clinical studies, we want to elucidate these mechanisms in more detail and develop new treatment strategies based on these insights.

Key Points
Nearly, 100 years after Kraepelin, by using state-of-the-art methodology, psychiatry has advanced significantly the understanding of aspects of the pathophysiology of mental disorders. For even more significant progress, we require:

- A better understanding of the pathophysiology: To gain further significant insight into the pathophysiological mechanisms and thus, implement personalised psychiatry.
- The discovery of informative biomarkers: To define pathophysiologically distinct subgroups, (bio)-markers are needed which are pathophysiologically informed and serve as the basis of personalised psychiatry
- The development of mechanistically informed treatments: To prevent mental illness and to treat resistant forms of mental illness, the understanding of risk trajectories and pathophysiological insight is necessary.
- Luck/chance: Serendipity drives innovation. The likelihood of this happening will be increased by publication of negative as well as positive studies.
- Funding: Considering the high societal and economic burden attributable to mental disorders (13% of all medical costs, in Germany, are due to mental ill health), the proportion of less than 1% of the overall research budget going into mental health research is clearly inadequate.

Box 23.1: Glossary

Astrocyte: Any of the star-shaped cells in the tissue supporting the brain and spinal cord.

(Bio)-Markers: A biological molecule found in blood, other body fluids or tissues that is a sign of a normal or abnormal process, or of a condition or disease.

Hippocampus: Small part of the brain responsible for learning and memory.

Mechanistic: A method of understanding or studying how something works by focusing on the underlying mechanisms or processes that drive its behaviour or outcomes.

Mendelian randomisation: Method using measured variation in genes to examine the causal effect of an exposure on an outcome.

Microglia: Cells of the brain that regulate brain development, maintenance of neuronal networks and injury repair.

Microgliosis: An accumulation of microglial cells in nervous tissue as a result of injury.

Mitochondria: Often referred to as the powerhouses of the cell; their main function is to generate the energy necessary to power cells.

Myelin: Insulating layer that forms around nerves, including those in the brain and spinal cord, made up of protein and fatty substances.

Neuropil: Dense network of interwoven nerve fibres and their branches and synapses.

Oligodendrocytes: Essential central nervous system (CNS) cells that form myelin, ensuring fast neural signals, vital for the nervous system.

Olig2: Transcription factor that plays a crucial role in the development of oligodendrocytes.

Phenotype: An individual's observable traits, such as height, eye colour or blood type.

PRS: An estimate of an individual's genetic liability to a trait or disease.

TCF4: Protein that in humans is encoded by the TCF4 gene, involved in neurological development.

Transcriptome: Collection of all the gene readouts present in a cell.

Transgenic: One or more DNA sequences from another species have been introduced by artificial means.

References

1. Alzheimer A. Neuere Arbeiten über die Dementia senilis [recent works on senile dementia]. Monatsschr Psychiatr Neurol. 1893;3:101–15.
2. Kraepelin E. Psychiatrie: ein Lehrbuch für Studirende und Aertze [Psychiatry: A Textbook for Students and Doctors]. 6th ed. Lepizig, Germany: JA Barth; 1899.
3. Kraepelin E. Lehrbuch der Psychiatrie [Textbook of psychiatry]. 8th ed. Leipzig, Germany: JA Barth; 1913.

4. Falkai P, Rossner MJ, Schulze TG, Hasan A, Brzózka MM, Malchow B, Honer WG, Schmitt A. Kraepelin revisited: schizophrenia from degeneration to failed regeneration. Mol Psychiatry. 2015;20(6):671–6.
5. Falkai P, Rossner MJ, Raabe FJ, Wagner E, Keeser D, Maurus I, Roell L, Chang E, Seitz-Holland J, Schulze TG, Schmitt A. Disturbed oligodendroglial maturation causes cognitive dysfunction in schizophrenia: a new hypothesis. Schizophr Bull. 2023;49(6):1614–24.
6. Hoff AL, Sakuma M, Wieneke M, Horon R, Kushner M, DeLisi LE. Longitudinal neuropsychological follow-up study of patients with first-episode schizophrenia. Am J Psychiatry. 1999;156(9):1336–41.
7. Hoff AL, Svetina C, Shields G, Stewart J, DeLisi LE. Ten year longitudinal study of neuropsychological functioning subsequent to a first episode of schizophrenia. Schizophr Res. 2005;78(1):27–34.
8. Falkai P, Maurus I, Schmitt A, Malchow B, Schneider-Axmann T, Röll L, Papiol S, Wobrock T, Hasan A, Keeser D. Improvement in daily functioning after aerobic exercise training in schizophrenia is sustained after exercise cessation. Eur Arch Psychiatry Clin Neurosci. 2021;271(7):1201–3.
9. Heilbronner U, Samara M, Leucht S, Falkai P, Schulze TG. The longitudinal course of schizophrenia across the lifespan: clinical, cognitive, and neurobiological aspects. Harv Rev Psychiatry. 2016;24(2):118–28.
10. Feber L, Peter NL, Chiocchia V, Schneider-Thoma J, Siafis S, Bighelli I, Hansen WP, Lin X, Prates-Baldez D, Salanti G, Keefe RSE, Engel RR, Leucht S. Antipsychotic drugs and cognitive function: a systematic review and network meta-analysis. JAMA Psychiatr. 2025;82(1):47–56.
11. Goodkind M, Eickhoff SB, Oathes DJ, Jiang Y, Chang A, Jones-Hagata LB, Ortega BN, Zaiko YV, Roach EL, Korgaonkar MS, Grieve SM, Galatzer-Levy I, Fox PT, Etkin A. Identification of a common neurobiological substrate for mental illness. JAMA Psychiatry. 2015;72(4):305–15.
12. Sha Z, Wager TD, Mechelli A, He Y. Common dysfunction of large-scale neurocognitive networks across psychiatric disorders. Biol Psychiatry. 2019;85(5):379–88.
13. van Erp TG, Hibar DP, Rasmussen JM, Glahn DC, Pearlson GD, Andreassen OA, Agartz I, Westlye LT, Haukvik UK, Dale AM, Melle I, Hartberg CB, Gruber O, Kraemer B, Zilles D, Donohoe G, Kelly S, McDonald C, Morris DW, Cannon DM, Corvin A, Machielsen MW, Koenders L, de Haan L, Veltman DJ, Satterthwaite TD, Wolf DH, Gur RC, Gur RE, Potkin SG, Mathalon DH, Mueller BA, Preda A, Macciardi F, Ehrlich S, Walton E, Hass J, Calhoun VD, Bockholt HJ, Sponheim SR, Shoemaker JM, van Haren NE, Hulshoff Pol HE, Ophoff RA, Kahn RS, Roiz-Santiañez R, Crespo-Facorro B, Wang L, Alpert KI, Jönsson EG, Dimitrova R, Bois C, Whalley HC, McIntosh AM, Lawrie SM, Hashimoto R, Thompson PM, Turner JA. Subcortical brain volume abnormalities in 2028 individuals with schizophrenia and 2540 healthy controls via the ENIGMA consortium. Mol Psychiatry. 2016;21(4):547–53.
14. Schmitt A, Steyskal C, Bernstein HG, Schneider-Axmann T, Parlapani E, Schaeffer EL, Gattaz WF, Bogerts B, Schmitz C, Falkai P. Stereologic investigation of the posterior part of the hippocampus in schizophrenia. Acta Neuropathol. 2009;117(4):395–407.
15. Schmitt A, Tatsch L, Vollhardt A, Schneider-Axmann T, Raabe FJ, Roell L, Heinsen H, Hof PR, Falkai P, Schmitz C. Decreased oligodendrocyte number in hippocampal subfield CA4 in schizophrenia: a replication study. Cells. 2022;11(20):3242.
16. van Kesteren CF, Gremmels H, de Witte LD, Hol EM, Van Gool AR, Falkai PG, Kahn RS, Sommer IE. Immune involvement in the pathogenesis of schizophrenia: a meta-analysis on postmortem brain studies. Transl Psychiatry. 2017;7(3):e1075.
17. Snijders GJLJ, van Zuiden W, Sneeboer MAM, Berdenis van Berlekom A, van der Geest AT, Schnieder T, MacIntyre DJ, Hol EM, Kahn RS, de Witte LD. A loss of mature microglial markers without immune activation in schizophrenia. Glia. 2021;69(5):1251–67.
18. Berdenis van Berlekom A, Muflihah CH, Snijders GJLJ, MacGillavry HD, Middeldorp J, Hol EM, Kahn RS, de Witte LD. Synapse pathology in schizophrenia: a meta-analysis of postsynaptic elements in postmortem brain studies. Schizophr Bull. 2020;46(2):374–86.

19. Pajonk FG, Wobrock T, Gruber O, Scherk H, Berner D, Kaizl I, Kierer A, Müller S, Oest M, Meyer T, Backens M, Schneider-Axmann T, Thornton AE, Honer WG, Falkai P. Hippocampal plasticity in response to exercise in schizophrenia. Arch Gen Psychiatry. 2010;67(2):133–43.
20. Malchow B, Keeser D, Keller K, Hasan A, Rauchmann BS, Kimura H, Schneider-Axmann T, Dechent P, Gruber O, Ertl-Wagner B, Honer WG, Hillmer-Vogel U, Schmitt A, Wobrock T, Niklas A, Falkai P. Effects of endurance training on brain structures in chronic schizophrenia patients and healthy controls. Schizophr Res. 2016;173(3):182–91.
21. Maurus I, Roell L, Lembeck M, Papazova I, Greska D, Muenz S, Wagner E, Campana M, Schwaiger R, Schneider-Axmann T, Rosenberger K, Hellmich M, Sykorova E, Thieme CE, Vogel BO, Harder C, Mohnke S, Huppertz C, Roeh A, Keller-Varady K, Malchow B, Walter H, Wolfarth B, Wölwer W, Henkel K, Hirjak D, Schmitt A, Hasan A, Meyer-Lindenberg A, Falkai P. Exercise as an add-on treatment in individuals with schizophrenia: results from a large multicenter randomized controlled trial. Psychiatry Res. 2023;328:115480.
22. Wunderlich S, Keeser D, Spaeth J, Maurus I, Alici C, Schmitt A, Falkai P, Stoecklein S, Roell L. Reducing functional dysconnectivity in schizophrenia spectrum disorders. medRxiv 2024.09.26.24314430; https://doi.org/10.1101/2024.09.26.24314430; preprint.
23. Murray RM, Bhavsar V, Tripoli G, Howes O. 30 years on: how the neurodevelopmental hypothesis of schizophrenia morphed into the developmental risk factor model of psychosis. Schizophr Bull. 2017;43(6):1190–6.
24. Weinberger DR. Implications of normal brain development for the pathogenesis of schizophrenia. Arch Gen Psychiatry. 1987;44:660–9.
25. Murray RM, Lewis SW. Is schizophrenia a neurodevelopmental disorder? BMJ (Clin Res Ed). 1988;296:63.
26. Schmitt A, Falkai P, Papiol S. Neurodevelopmental disturbances in schizophrenia: evidence from genetic and environmental factors. J Neural Transm (Vienna). 2023;130(3):195–205.
27. Owen MJ, O'Donovan MC. Schizophrenia and the neurodevelopmental continuum: evidence from genomics. World Psychiatry. 2017;16(3):227–35.
28. Adityanjee AYA, Theodoridis D, Vieweg VR. Dementia praecox to schizophrenia: the first 100 years. Psychiatry Clin Neurosci. 1999;53(4):437–48.
29. Papiol S, Keeser D, Hasan A, Schneider-Axmann T, Raabe F, Degenhardt F, Rossner MJ, Bickeböller H, Cantuti-Castelvetri L, Simons M, Wobrock T, Schmitt A, Malchow B, Falkai P. Polygenic burden associated to oligodendrocyte precursor cells and radial glia influences the hippocampal volume changes induced by aerobic exercise in schizophrenia patients. Transl Psychiatry. 2019;9(1):284.
30. Papiol S, Roell L, Maurus I, Hirjak D, Keeser D, Schmitt A, Meyer-Lindenberg A, Falkai P. Cell type-specific polygenic burden modulates exercise effects in schizophrenia patients: further evidence on volumes of hippocampal subfields. Eur Arch Psychiatry Clin Neurosci. 2024;274(6):1241–4.
31. Schmitt A, Ammann K, Vollhardt A, Schneider-Axmann T, Raabe FJ, Yakimov V, Heinsen H, Hof PR, Falkai P, Schmitz C. Reduced number of oligodendrocytes in the cingulum in schizophrenia: a design-based stereology study. J Biomed Res Environ Sci. 2024;5(9):1089–103.
32. Fünfschilling U, Supplie LM, Mahad D, Boretius S, Saab AS, Edgar J, Brinkmann BG, Kassmann CM, Tzvetanova ID, Möbius W, Diaz F, Meijer D, Suter U, Hamprecht B, Sereda MW, Moraes CT, Frahm J, Goebbels S, Nave KA. Glycolytic oligodendrocytes maintain myelin and long-term axonal integrity. Nature. 2012;485(7399):517–21.
33. Nave KA. Myelination and support of axonal integrity by glia. Nature. 2010;468(7321):244–52.
34. Sun W, Sun P, Li J, Yang Q, Tian Q, Yuan S, Zhang X, Chen P, Li C, Zhang X. Exploring genetic associations and drug targets for mitochondrial proteins and schizophrenia risk. Schizophrenia (Heidelb). 2025;11(1):10.
35. Rossner M, et al. 2025; personal communication, study in progress.

Open Access   This chapter is licensed under the terms of the Creative Commons Attribution 4.0 International License (http://creativecommons.org/licenses/by/4.0/), which permits use, sharing, adaptation, distribution and reproduction in any medium or format, as long as you give appropriate credit to the original author(s) and the source, provide a link to the Creative Commons license and indicate if changes were made.

The images or other third party material in this chapter are included in the chapter's Creative Commons license, unless indicated otherwise in a credit line to the material. If material is not included in the chapter's Creative Commons license and your intended use is not permitted by statutory regulation or exceeds the permitted use, you will need to obtain permission directly from the copyright holder.

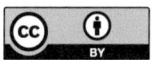

What Does Research Tell Us About Peer Support, Its Strengths and Potential Risks?

24

Chalotte Heinsvig Poulsen and Lene Falgaard Eplov

24.1 Introduction

In the evolving landscape of psychiatry, the recovery model has emerged as a transformative paradigm, challenging traditional approaches to mental illness treatment and support [1–5]. The recovery model in mental health care is predicated on the belief that individuals with mental health conditions can lead fulfilling, hopeful and self-determined lives. This approach shifts focus from symptom management to holistic well-being, emphasising personal strengths and empowering individuals to take an active role in their treatment and recovery journey [6–8]. Central to this model is the recognition of lived experience as a valuable form of expertise because it provides diverse unique insights into the recovery journey that cannot be gained through clinical training alone [9, 10].

Peer support, which may be practiced both within and beyond the formal health care sector, is regarded a central element in recovery-oriented practice and has been defined by the founder of the trauma-informed 'Intentional Peer Support' (IPS) Organisation [11] Shery Mead as '*a system of giving and receiving help founded on key principles of respect, shared responsibility, and mutual agreement of what is helpful*' [12–14]. Thus, peer support is a compassionate and empowering practice, where peers equally and reciprocally share their lived experiences of being in recovery of mental illness with each other in a safe, trustful and valid space, which allows for personal growth [6, 15]. This trauma-informed approach has gained increased recognition for its potential to foster hope, promote recovery and complement traditional mental health services. Thus, research evidence has shown that peer support interventions improve subjective outcomes of personal recovery among individuals with mental illness [16–19], defined by the individuals themselves as: '*A way of*

C. H. Poulsen (✉) · L. F. Eplov
Mental Health Center Amager, Copenhagen University Hospital-Amager and Hvidovre, Research in Recovery and Mental Health Promotion (FORMS), Copenhagen S, Denmark
e-mail: chalotte.heinsvig.poulsen.01@regionh.dk

© The Author(s) 2026
G. Ikkos, T. Becker (eds.), *Psychiatry after Kraepelin*,
https://doi.org/10.1007/978-3-032-09475-9_24

living satisfying, hopeful, and reciprocal lives, together with others even though we may still experience distress' [20].

Admittedly, the peer support effect on indicators of objective outcomes of clinical recovery such as psychiatric symptoms, functional capacity and hospitalisations remains suggestive or in-conclusive [16, 17, 19]. Nevertheless, the peer support approach extends beyond symptom resolution, focusing instead on building resilience and developing social skills that enable individuals to lead meaningful lives within their communities. This approach advocates for person-centred care, viewing individuals holistically rather than through the limited lens of a diagnosis or symptom checklist that may be found in mental health services. Rooted in civil rights advocacy, peer support challenges the reductionist view of defining individuals by their diagnoses [7]. By modelling recovery and championing person-centred care, peer support specialists play a crucial role in transforming the lives of those experiencing mental health challenges [6, 21].

The above notwithstanding, it is crucial to acknowledge that peer support is not without challenges. Potential downsides may include role confusion, variability in training and implementation of peer support programmes, potential exacerbation of symptoms, as well as challenges in maintaining boundaries and managing dual relationships [22–25]. This chapter, therefore, explores the current state of knowledge regarding peer support. As peer support continues to evolve and integrate into mental health systems, understanding its strengths and potential limitations and adverse effects becomes increasingly important for effective implementation and optimisation of mental health care.

24.1.1 Theory and Concepts

Across the world, national organisations are working to disseminate and train peer support workers (PSWs) in the concepts, principles and core values of peer support, providing a structured approach to implementation. For example, Implementing Recovery through Organizational Change (IMROC) is a non-profit UK initiative focused on transforming mental health services to support recovery-oriented practices such as peer support [26]; and The IPS organisation in the United States is focused on transforming mental health through training in trauma-informed transformative peer support relationships [11]. Additionally, national lived experience peer workforce practice guidelines have been developed by The National Mental Health Commission (NMHC) in Australia [27], the non-profit for example national workforce development centre in New Zealand [28], the mental health commission of Canada [29] and in the United States the non-profit National Association of Peer Supporters (N.A.P.S.) [30]. These different frameworks and guidelines aim to standardise peer support practices, define values, roles and responsibilities and ensure ethical conduct in peer support work across various mental health and substance use support settings. Key common elements, theories and concepts across these frameworks and guidelines will be elaborated below.

24.1.1.1 Recovery-Focused Approach

Peer support is grounded in a recovery-focused approach, which posits that individuals with mental health challenges can lead to fulfilling lives despite ongoing symptoms [1–4]. Central to peer support theory is the concept of mutual empowerment, described as a process where both individuals in a peer relationship can connect and grow and develop new beliefs, thoughts and behaviours beyond previously held self-concepts based on disability, stigma and diagnosis [12, 14, 15]. Thus, peer support emphasises personal growth and the development of a positive self-identity beyond the confines of a diagnosis. It focuses on strengths, resilience and the potential for recovery, rather than solely on symptom management and remission. Moreover, the recovery-focused approach embeds a trauma-informed approach to peer support that recognises the high prevalence of trauma among individuals accessing mental health services and seeks to create a safe, supportive and empowering environment that minimises the risk of re-traumatisation [6]. It acknowledges the impact of trauma on individuals' mental, emotional and physical well-being, and integrates this understanding into all aspects of peer support practice.

24.1.1.2 Lived Experience as Expertise

Peer support recognises the value of experiential knowledge in building trusting relationships [21]. This approach acknowledges that individuals who have navigated their own mental health journeys possess invaluable diverse insights, hope and skills that can benefit others facing similar challenges [9, 10, 31]. PSWs draw on their personal experiences of mental distress, service use and recovery to inform their practice. This firsthand knowledge allows them to offer authentic empathy and understanding that may be difficult for traditional mental health professionals to provide [6, 32]. Lived experience provides a distinct viewpoint on mental health challenges, often highlighting aspects of recovery that may be overlooked in traditional clinical approaches. By sharing their own stories of recovery, PSWs demonstrate that improvement and meaningful life are possible, inspiring hope in those currently struggling. The shared experiences between PSWs and service users create a foundation for trust and rapport, often leading to feelings of connectedness, relationship building and more open and honest communication [21, 33].

24.1.1.3 Reciprocity and Mutuality

Unlike traditional mental health provider–patient relationships, peer support is built on reciprocity and mutuality [13, 26]. Thus, both parties contribute equally and receive mutual learning from the relationship engaging in a shared process of exploring and navigating each other's understanding of the world, fostering growth [15]. Reciprocity describes the balanced exchange of understanding, learning, and insight within the peer relationship, where both individuals engage in giving and receiving support. Closely related, mutuality highlights the fundamental equality of the relationship, ensuring both parties are seen as equally capable contributors who engage in a shared process of exploring and navigating different perspectives [15]. The benefits of reciprocity and mutuality in peer support include the possibilities of creating a safe, confidential and supportive environment for open expression fostering empathy and deeper understanding, promoting personal growth and empowerment. "Potentially strengthening the connection to mental health professionals, peer networks, and engagement within the wider community" [21].

24.1.1.4 Transformative Potential and Inclusion

Peer support has the potential to transform mental health care by challenging traditional power dynamics and promoting a culture of health and ability, rather than illness and disability [7, 11, 26]. It complements clinical knowledge with lived experience expertise, offering a more holistic approach to care [9]. Peer support recognises the importance of understanding mental health experiences within broader social and cultural contexts, creating inclusive environments that validate individual experiences and challenge societal stigma. It encourages diversity, recognises individual strengths and supports community re-integration and social inclusion. Lived experience experts are well-positioned to advocate for systemic changes and empower others in their recovery journeys.

The theory and concepts of peer support in mental health represent a paradigm shift in how we approach recovery and well-being. By valuing lived experience, promoting mutuality and focusing on strengths and possibilities, peer support offers a powerful complement to traditional mental health services. As research in this field continues to evolve, the integration of peer support into mental health systems holds promise for more holistic, empowering and effective approaches to mental health care.

24.1.2 Key Findings

24.1.2.1 Effectiveness of Peer Support

Recent research has demonstrated the efficacy of peer support interventions in mental health contexts, with several key findings emerging from large-scale reviews and meta-analyses. A comprehensive umbrella review published in February 2024, analysing 35 existing reviews encompassing 426 primary studies, revealed evidence that peer support can positively improve self-efficacy and personal recovery, as well as improve particularly perinatal depression [22].

However, peer support interventions vary widely in their approach, delivery method and organisational structure making it challenging to compare their effectiveness across different forms of implementation [34, 35]. These variations include one-on-one peer mentoring, group-based peer support and online peer communities. Moreover, peer support can be delivered as face-to-face interactions, telephone support, digital platforms (e.g. video calls, messaging apps etc.) [36] and be organised as programmes within health care systems, community-based initiatives or within grassroots peer-led organisations. This diversity in peer support models reflects adaptations to different contexts, needs and resources across various mental health settings.

24.1.2.2 Overall Personal Recovery Outcomes

The effectiveness of peer support interventions on self-reported overall personal recovery among individuals with mental health diagnoses, including severe mental illness (SMI), has been examined in several meta-analyses [22]. Most of these reported positive outcomes, with six out of seven meta-analyses demonstrating improvements in personal recovery outcomes [19, 34, 37–40]. Longitudinal data from three meta-analyses indicated sustained improvements in personal recovery outcomes for adults with mental health diagnoses. These improvements were observed at follow-up periods of 6 months [34], 3–6 months [39] and 12–18 months [40]. The interventions examined encompassed both individual and group-based peer support formats. Additionally, it has been reported that peer support delivered online had a small but nonsignificant positive effect on personal recovery [19, 36]. However, it is important to note that most of these meta-analyses were rated as critically low or low quality, with one exception receiving a high-quality rating [16]. This high-quality review, based on evidence from three studies, found no effect of peer support on personal recovery in the medium term for adults with schizophrenia or similar SMI diagnoses.

Taken together, these findings underscore the potential efficacy of peer support interventions in promoting personal recovery among individuals with mental health conditions, while also highlighting the need for more high-quality research to establish the long-term effectiveness and optimal implementation strategies for these interventions.

24.1.2.3 Specific Personal Recovery and Psychosocial Outcomes

The effectiveness of peer support on various types of outcomes related to personal recovery in mental health contexts has yielded mixed evidence. Several meta-analyses have reported improvements in hope and hopefulness for adults with SMI [19, 34, 35, 37, 38], while others found no effect in populations with SMI and other mental health diagnoses [16, 39, 41]. The long-term effects on hope remain inconsistent across studies.

Regarding empowerment, some meta-analyses demonstrated improvements for adults with various mental health diagnoses [38, 42], while others reported no effects [19, 34, 37, 39, 41]. Follow-up data on empowerment showed mixed results. One review found that peer support delivered in peer-designed or cocreated interventions such as 'Wellness Recovery Action Planning' (WRAP) and 'Building Recovery and Individual Dreams and Goals Through Education and Support' (BRIDGES) provided in community settings had a modest positive effect on self-advocacy [19].

Self-efficacy consistently improved across various mental health conditions in all meta-analyses reporting on this outcome [19, 37, 41, 42]. A meta-analysis examining the impact of peer support integrated into hospital mental health services revealed a small-to-medium positive effect on self-efficacy [19]. This finding suggests that incorporating peer support within inpatient mental health settings may enhance patients' confidence in self-managing their mental health challenges.

Decreases in self-stigma and stigma-related stress in adults and adolescents with any mental health problem were found by one review with meta-analysis of group-based peer support [41]. However, no significant improvements were found for satisfaction with care or relational outcomes such as social network and relationship building [19, 37, 40, 43]. Quality of life improvements were reported in some meta-analyses for adults with SMI [35, 37], but others found no evidence of improvement, and follow-up data showed no sustained effects.

These findings underscore the need for more rigorous research to establish the effectiveness of peer support across various outcomes and populations. Future studies should focus on improving methodological quality to provide more definitive evidence on the impact of peer support interventions in mental health contexts.

24.1.2.4 Clinical Recovery Outcomes

Meta-analytic evidence suggests that peer support interventions are particularly effective in ameliorating perinatal depression [44, 45]. The reviews suggest that peer support during the perinatal period using Internet or telephone approaches, and combining group and individual sessions at least weekly, may have the potential to effectively prevent perinatal depression or reduce the harm of perinatal depression. However, the efficacy for other depressive disorders is less clear [34, 39]. While some reviews reported no immediate post-intervention effects on depression for adults and adolescents with mental health problems, including those with SMI [19, 37, 41, 43], one study noted improvements at six-month follow-up, despite reporting no effects at immediately post-intervention [34]. This suggests potential delayed benefits of peer support interventions.

One review examining overall clinical recovery in adults with diverse mental health diagnoses reported small improvements in effect sizes at post-intervention and at six to nine months follow-up [17]. However, these benefits were not sustained at 12–18 months, indicating a potential time-limited effect of peer support on clinical recovery.

Most of the evidence suggests no significant effect of peer support on mental health symptom severity among adults and adolescents with mental health diagnoses or those utilising mental health services, with the notable exception of perinatal depression [34, 37, 39, 41, 43]. However, some nuanced findings have emerged: Individual and group-based peer support for adults primarily with SMI diagnoses showed improvements in mental health symptom severity [19, 38]. Additionally, family-led peer support for adults with SMI demonstrated symptom improvements, while individual-led peer support did not show significant effects [37].

Peer support interventions showed mixed results regarding service use. While associated with a reduced risk of hospitalisation [37, 40], no significant effect was found on length of stay [43]. This suggests that peer support may influence the frequency but not the duration of hospitalisations. Lastly, a high-quality review found no effect of peer support on patient activation when this was defined as a person's perceived ability to manage their illness and approach to health care at one to six months follow-up in adults with schizophrenia or similar SMI diagnoses [16].

In conclusion, while peer support shows promise in certain areas, particularly perinatal depression, as well as self-efficacy and overall personal recovery, evidence of its efficacy across other mental health domains remains inconsistent. Future research should focus on improving methodological rigor, for example, through the Medical Research Council (MRC) framework of development and evaluation of complex interventions [46], and given the gradual nature of personal recovery [5], longitudinal measurement is crucial to better understand the role of peer support in comprehensive mental health care.

A co-creation approach is recommended involving peers and researchers to develop and evaluate interventions, leveraging lived experiences to inform pro-gramme theory and design [32, 47, 48]. For example, it has been noted that it is essential to clarify whether peers are employed or volunteers, as this distinction could impact the effective mechanisms of the peer support provided [19]. This approach should include a clear theory of change and hypotheses about intervention mechanisms of change and effects, guiding high-quality randomised controlled tri-als (RCTs), fidelity measures and process evaluations. Additionally, identifying fac-tors that hinder or facilitate implementation and conducting cost-effectiveness studies are key priorities.

24.1.3 Mechanisms of Change in Peer Support

Understanding the mechanisms by which peer support fosters positive change is crucial for optimising its implementation and maximising benefits in mental health services [32, 49]. While the value of peer support is increasingly recognised, the specific processes that drive its effectiveness remain an area of ongoing investigation.

In literature reviews examining the mechanisms that underpin peer support some key mechanisms that contribute to the success and challenges associated with peer support have been identified [21, 32, 33, 50–52]. Thus, the mutual sharing of experi-ences of mental health challenges between peer support workers (PSWs) and ser-vice users is fundamental. This shared understanding fosters trust, empathy and a sense of connection that can induce change and be transformative [32, 33, 53]. Furthermore, the emotional connection that PSWs invest in their relationships with service users encompasses empathy, compassion and a genuine mutual desire to support and empower others in their recovery journey [33]. PSWs provide support that focuses on the strengths and abilities of service users, rather than solely on their deficits or challenges, emphasising a whole-person approach. This approach pro-motes self-efficacy and fosters a sense of hope and agency. PSWs also offer practi-cal assistance in navigating mental health services and accessing community resources [21, 33, 52]. supporting others can be therapeutic for PSWs, contributing to their own recovery and well-being [33]. This mutuality and shared power in the relationship is a core principle of peer support, where both the helper and the recipi-ent experience positive benefits and growth [15]. PSWs often occupy a unique posi-tion between traditional mental health professionals and service users. This 'in-between' status can allow them to bridge gaps in understanding and communication; however, it can also create challenges related to role clarity and acceptance within the mental health professional team [32, 33].

While existing research has illuminated key change mechanisms within one-to-one peer support, particularly from the perspective of PSWs employed in formal mental health settings, a significant gap remains in our understanding of the broader landscape of peer support. Thus, the evidence reviewed potentially overlooks valuable insights from other forms of peer support and the experiences of the recipients of peer support. Future systematic reviews must clarify the contributing mechanisms of peer support in diverse contexts, specifically focusing on independent and online settings. Furthermore, these reviews need to explore a broader range of available literature.

24.1.4 Implementation Factors

The successful implementation of peer support interventions in mental health settings is contingent upon a multitude of factors reviewed in a comprehensive umbrella review [22]. The findings highlight several critical elements that contribute to the effective integration of PSWs within mental health services. Key facilitators for successful implementation include:

- Comprehensive training and supervision for PSWs.
- Recovery-oriented organisational structure.
- Strong leadership commitment.
- Supportive and trusting workplace culture.
- Effective collaboration between PSWs and non-peer staff.

Conversely, significant barriers to implementation were identified: Insufficient time and resources, inadequate funding mechanisms and lack of standardised PSW certification [22].

24.1.4.1 Stakeholder Perspectives in Implementation

The integration of peer support in mental health services reveals a complex array of experiences from PSWs, service users and non-peer staff. Peer support offers numerous benefits, including facilitating PSWs' personal recovery, providing employment pathways and enhancing functioning [24, 54, 55]. One qualitative meta synthesis [24] found that service users benefit from recovery role models. However, some service users expressed reservations about PSWs as role models and found it challenging to view them as professionals. These concerns stemmed from perceptions of inadequate training and concerns about their mental illness histories, challenging the trust and credibility of PSWs in their professional capacity. From working with PSWs, non-peer staff gained enriched perspectives, increased empathy towards service users and a belief in recovery [24]. A central theme is the ambiguity surrounding the PSW role, including unclear job descriptions and boundary issues [22, 23, 54, 55]. This ambiguity allows for flexibility but can lead to perceptions of tokenism and confusion among PSWs, impacting their own recovery.

Organisational issues include inadequate support, training and supervision for PSWs, as well as low compensation, leading to feelings of undervaluation [22]. Non-peer staff attitudes vary; some PSWs feel accepted, while others face negative attitudes. Organisations must prepare structurally and culturally to ensure PSW well-being and reduce sickness-related absences [25, 56, 57].

In conclusion, while peer support offers benefits, its successful implementation requires addressing role ambiguity, organisational challenges and attitudinal barriers. Future research should focus on optimising PSW integration strategies, emphasising role clarity, professional development and cultural change.

24.1.5 Debates and Controversies

In the rapidly evolving field of peer support in mental health, several key debates and controversies have emerged, reflecting the complex nature of integrating lived experience into formal mental health care systems. One central issue is the lack of consensus on the definition and standardisation of peer support. While some argue for clear, standardised roles to ensure quality and consistency, others contend that flexibility and diversity are crucial to maintain the unique value of peer support [31, 32, 58]. This debate extends to the professionalisation of peer roles and adequate lived experience workforce training [59], with concerns about maintaining authenticity and avoiding co-optation by traditional mental health systems.

The effectiveness of peer support interventions remains a contentious topic. As outlined in the key findings above, research studies have yielded mixed results, leading to debates about appropriate outcome measures and the need for more rigorous evaluation methodologies [22, 58]. This controversy is closely tied to discussions about the integration of peer workers into traditional mental health services, where power dynamics and role clarity present significant challenges.

Training and certification for peer supporters are another area of debate. While formal qualifications may enhance credibility and ensure a baseline of knowledge [59], there are concerns that over-emphasising training may diminish the value of lived experience. This relates to broader discussions about boundaries and disclosure, as peer supporters navigate the delicate balance between sharing personal experiences and maintaining professional relationships.

The tension between recovery-oriented approaches championed by many peer support programmes and the medical model prevalent in traditional mental health care is a significant point of contention [6, 8]. This debate often centres on the role of medication and diagnosis in peer support interventions. Ethical considerations, including protecting but not over-protecting individuals in peer support relationships and addressing potential conflicts of interest, remain at the forefront of many debates in the field. These controversies highlight the dynamic nature of peer support in mental health and underscore the need for continued research, dialogue and innovation to address these complex issues.

24.2   Discussion

Our exploration of peer support in mental health services has revealed a complex landscape with both significant strengths and potential risks. This chapter has highlighted several key findings that contribute to our understanding of peer support interventions.

24.2.1 Strengths and Potential Adverse Effects of Peer Support

One of the most consistent findings across studies is the unique value that lived experience brings to mental health services. PSWs offer a perspective that traditional clinical staff cannot, fostering hope and providing relatable role models for recovery [32, 33, 51]. This aspect of peer support appears to be particularly effective in preventing perinatal depression among mothers using internet or telephone-based approaches, as well as in promoting outcomes of personal recovery and self-efficacy [22] among service users receiving peer support within traditional mental health services [19].

Despite these strengths, this chapter has also uncovered potential adverse outcomes that warrant careful consideration. Role ambiguity remains a significant challenge, often leading to confusion among PSWs, service users and non-peer staff. This ambiguity can result in unrealistic expectations, boundary issues and in some cases, may compromise the well-being of PSWs [22–24]. The integration of PSWs into traditional mental health teams has not been without difficulties. Issues of stigma, power imbalances and lack of role clarity can lead to tension within teams and potentially undermine the effectiveness of peer support interventions. In some cases, this has resulted in PSWs feeling marginalised or undervalued within their organisations [23].

Another concern is the potential for peer support to inadvertently reinforce a focus on illness rather than recovery if not implemented thoughtfully [26]. There is a delicate balance between utilising lived experience of mental health challenges and avoiding an over-emphasis on past difficulties.

The issue of professionalisation presents a double-edged sword. While it can enhance the credibility and sustainability of peer support roles, there are concerns that excessive formalisation may dilute the unique qualities that make peer support effective. Nevertheless, given the relatively nascent and inconsistent implementation of peer support within mental health services, many existing trials may have evaluated its effectiveness in environments lacking full organisational and cultural integration [22, 58]. This limited embedding could obscure potential benefits that are not easily captured through conventional quantitative measures. Indeed, peer support may exert positive influences on the broader functioning of mental health services, such as fostering a stronger culture of person-centred care, which are not typically assessed as quantitative outcomes in current research. As peer support becomes more deeply and systematically integrated into mental health care systems, more consistent quantitative evidence demonstrating its benefits may emerge, reflecting its full potential within a supportive and receptive environment.

24.2.2 Successful Implementation of Peer Support

The outlined significant facilitators and barriers to implementation of peer support derived from stakeholders within the mental health services align with recommendations from policy, research and advocacy groups. For instance, as mentioned earlier the ImROC initiative [26], which supports global peer support implementation, emphasises the importance of a recovery-focused approach. Similarly, international competence frameworks, such as those developed in New Zealand [28] and Australia [29] underscore recovery orientation as a core principle of peer support and emphasise the necessity of ongoing professional development. Peer support practice guidelines delineate the importance of supervision and provide specific recommendations for its implementation [30, 60, 61]. These guidelines reflect a growing recognition of the need for structured support systems for PSWs. Additionally, the IPS organisation advocates for a powerful framework of creating mutual transformative peer support relationships where people learn and grow together and offer online opportunities of IPS training and co-reflection [11]. To address some of the identified barriers, the development of formalised career pathways for PSWs has been proposed [62]. While still in early stages, such pathways could potentially mitigate challenges related to role definition, professional recognition and career progression for PSWs [57].

The congruence between our findings and existing implementation frameworks underscores the importance of a systematic approach to integrating peer support within mental health services. Future research should focus on evaluating the effectiveness of these implementation strategies across diverse health care settings and cultural contexts, with particular attention to the long-term sustainability of peer support programmes.

24.2.2.1 Gaps in Knowledge and Future Directions

This chapter has identified several areas where further research is needed. The long-term impacts of peer support interventions remain understudied, particularly in terms of sustained recovery outcomes. Additionally, more rigorous research is required to understand the specific mechanisms through which peer support affects various outcomes—especially from the peer support recipient's perspective. The optimal methods for training, supervising and supporting PSWs are still being debated. Future studies should focus on identifying best practices in these areas to maximise the benefits of peer support while minimising potential adverse effects. Cultural competence in peer support is an area requiring further exploration, particularly in diverse and multicultural settings. Understanding how peer support can be adapted to different cultural contexts without losing its core principles is crucial for its broader application.

24.3 Conclusion

Peer support in mental health services offers unique and valuable contributions to recovery-oriented care. Its strengths lie in the authenticity of shared experience, the promotion of hope and self-efficacy and its potential to complement traditional services. However, the field must address challenges such as role ambiguity, integration issues and the balance between professionalisation and maintaining the essence of peer support. As we move forward, it is crucial to continue refining our understanding of peer support through rigorous research and thoughtful implementation. By addressing the potential downsides and building on the strengths identified, peer support can evolve into an even more effective and integral component of comprehensive mental health care.

Key Points
- Unique value of lived experience as an expertise: Peer support's core strength is the distinct expertise gained from personal recovery journeys. This lived experience provides unique empathy and understanding that traditional training lacks, fostering crucial trust and hope.
- Complementary to traditional services: Peer support effectively enhances, rather than replaces, traditional mental health care. It offers a unique, experience-focused approach that promotes hope and empowerment, leading to more holistic and person-centred recovery.
- Role ambiguity challenges: The role of peer support workers often lacks clear definition within traditional settings. This ambiguity can hinder team collaboration, supervision and the optimal use of their valuable skills.
- Integration and implementation difficulties: Successfully incorporating peer support into existing systems faces challenges. These include organisational culture, insufficient role-specific training and supervision and inadequate funding for sustainable initiatives.
- Need for further research: More rigorous research is crucial to fully understand and optimise peer support's impact. Future studies should clarify its mechanisms of change, long-term effects across diverse contexts and best practices for training and integration.

References

1. Anthony WA. Recovery from mental illness: the guiding vision of the mental health service system in the 1990s. Psychosoc Rehabil J. 1993;16:11–23.
2. Le Boutillier C, Leamy M, Bird VJ, Davidson L, Williams J, Slade M. What does recovery mean in practice? A qualitative analysis of international recovery-oriented practice guidance. Psychiatr Serv. 2011;62:1470–6.
3. Slade M, Amering M, Farkas M, Hamilton B, O'Hagan M, Panther G, et al. Uses and abuses of recovery: implementing recovery-oriented practices in mental health systems. World Psychiatry. 2014;13:12–20.

4. Winsper C, Crawford-Docherty A, Weich S, Fenton SJ, Singh SP. How do recovery-oriented interventions contribute to personal mental health recovery? A systematic review and logic model. Clin Psychol Rev. 2020;76:101815.
5. Leamy M, Bird V, Le BC, Williams J, Slade M. Conceptual framework for personal recovery in mental health: systematic review and narrative synthesis. Br J Psychiatry. 2011;199:445–52.
6. Sweeney A, Filson B, Kennedy A, Collinson L, Gillard S. A paradigm shift: relationships in trauma-informed mental health services. BJPsych Adv. 2018;24:319–33. https://doi.org/10.1192/bja.2018.29.
7. World Health Organization. World mental health report: transforming mental health for all. Geneva; 2022.
8. Leonhardt BL, Huling K, Hamm JA, Roe D, Hasson-Ohayon I, McLeod HJ, et al. Recovery and serious mental illness: a review of current clinical and research paradigms and future directions. Expert Rev Neurother. 2017;17:1117–30.
9. Moitra M, Owens S, Hailemariam M, Wilson KS, Mensa-Kwao A, Gonese G, et al. Global mental health: where we are and where we are going. Curr Psychiatry Rep. 2023;25:301.
10. Davis S, Pinfold V, Catchpole J, Lovelock C, Senthi B, Kenny A. Reporting lived experience work. Lancet Psychiatry. 2024;11:8–9.
11. Intentional Peer Support (IPS) organization. n.d. https://intentionalpeersupport.org/. Accessed 18 Feb 2025.
12. Mead S, Hilton D, Curtis L. Peer support: a theoretical perspective. Psychiatr Rehabil J. 2001;25
13. Repper J, Carter T. A review of the literature on peer support in mental health services. J Ment Health. 2011;20:392–411.
14. Mead S. Defining peer support. 2003.
15. Mead S, Filson B. Mutuality and shared power as an alternative to coercion and force. Ment Health Soc Incl. 2017;21:144–52. https://doi.org/10.1108/MHSI-03-2017-0011.
16. Chien WT, Clifton AV, Zhao S, Lui S. Peer support for people with schizophrenia or other serious mental illness. Cochrane Database Syst Rev. 2019; https://doi.org/10.1002/14651858.CD010880.pub2.
17. Smit D, Miguel C, Vrijsen JN, Groeneweg B, Spijker J, Cuijpers P. The effectiveness of peer support for individuals with mental illness: systematic review and meta-analysis. Psychol Med. 2022:1–10.
18. Jambawo SM, Owolewa R, Jambawo TT. The effectiveness of peer support on the recovery and empowerment of people with schizophrenia: a systematic review and meta-analysis. Schizophr Res. 2024;274:270–9.
19. Høgh Egmose C, Heinsvig Poulsen C, Hjorthøj C, Skriver Mundy S, Hellström L, Nørgaard Nielsen M, et al. The effectiveness of peer support in personal and clinical recovery: systematic review and meta-analysis. Psychiatr Serv. 2023;74:847.
20. Topor A, Borg M, Di Girolamo S, Davidson L. Not just an individual journey: social aspects of recovery. Int J Soc Psychiatry. 2011;57:90–9.
21. Gillard S, Gibson SL, Holley J, Lucock M. Developing a change model for peer worker interventions in mental health services: a qualitative research study. Epidemiol Psychiatr Sci. 2015;24:435–45.
22. Cooper RE, Saunders KRK, Greenburgh A, Shah P, Appleton R, Machin K, et al. The effectiveness, implementation, and experiences of peer support approaches for mental health: a systematic umbrella review. BMC Med. 2024;22:1–45.
23. Vandewalle J, Debyser B, Beeckman D, Vandecasteele T, Van Hecke A, Verhaeghe S. Peer workers' perceptions and experiences of barriers to implementation of peer worker roles in mental health services: a literature review. Int J Nurs Stud. 2016;60:234–50.
24. Walker G, Bryant W. Peer support in adult mental health services: a metasynthesis of qualitative findings. Psychiatr Rehabil J. 2013;36:28–34.
25. Reeves V, McIntyre H, Loughhead M, Halpin MA, Procter N. Actions targeting the integration of peer workforces in mental health organisations: a mixed-methods systematic review. BMC Psychiatry. 2024;24:211.

26. Imroc. n.d. https://www.imroc.org/. Accessed 18 Feb 2025.
27. Mental Health Commission N. National Mental Health Commission // National Lived Experience (Peer) Workforce Development Guidelines. 2021.
28. Competencies for the consumer, peer support and lived… | Te Pou. n.d. https://www.tepou.co.nz/resources/competencies-for-the-mental-health-and-addiction-consumer-peer-support-and-lived-experience-workforce-1. Accessed 26 Feb 2025.
29. Sunderland KMWPLG. Guidelines for the practice and training of peer support. Mental Health Commission of Canada. 2013;
30. N.A.P.S. National Association of Peer Supporters. National Practice Guidelines for peer specialists and supervisors. Washington, DC; 2019.
31. Speyer H, Ustrup M. Embracing dissensus in lived experience research: the power of conflicting experiential knowledge. Lancet Psychiatry. 2025.
32. Gillard S, Foster R, Gibson S, Goldsmith L, Marks J, White S. Describing a principles-based approach to developing and evaluating peer worker roles as peer support moves into mainstream mental health services. Ment Health Soc Incl. 2017;21:133–43.
33. Watson E. The mechanisms underpinning peer support: a literature review. J Ment Health. 2019;28:677–88. https://doi.org/10.1080/09638237.2017.1417559.
34. Lloyd-Evans B, Mayo-Wilson E, Harrison B, Istead H, Brown E, Pilling S, et al. A systematic review and meta-analysis of randomised controlled trials of peer support for people with severe mental illness. BMC Psychiatry. 2014;14:39.
35. Fuhr DC, Salisbury TT, De Silva MJ, Atif N, van Ginneken N, Rahman A, et al. Effectiveness of peer-delivered interventions for severe mental illness and depression on clinical and psychosocial outcomes: a systematic review and meta-analysis. Soc Psychiatry Psychiatr Epidemiol. 2014;49:1691–702.
36. Fortuna KL, Naslund JA, LaCroix JM, Bianco CL, Brooks JM, Zisman-Ilani Y, et al. Digital peer support mental health interventions for people with a lived experience of a serious mental illness: systematic review. JMIR Ment Health. 2020;7:e16460. https://doi.org/10.2196/16460.
37. Wang Y, Chen Y, Deng H. Effectiveness of family- and individual-led peer support for people with serious mental illness: a meta-analysis. J Psychosoc Nurs Ment Health Serv. 2022;60:20–6.
38. Peck CKH, Thangavelu DP, Li Z, Goh YS. Effects of peer-delivered self-management, recovery education interventions for individuals with severe and enduring mental health challenges: a meta-analysis. J Psychiatr Ment Health Nurs. 2023;30:54–73.
39. Lyons N, Cooper C, Lloyd-Evans B. A systematic review and meta-analysis of group peer support interventions for people experiencing mental health conditions. BMC Psychiatry. 2021;21:315.
40. White S, Foster R, Marks J, Morshead R, Goldsmith L, Barlow S, et al. The effectiveness of one-to-one peer support in mental health services: a systematic review and meta-analysis. BMC Psychiatry. 2020;20 https://doi.org/10.1186/s12888-020-02923-3.
41. Sun J, Yin X, Li C, Liu W, Sun H. Stigma and peer-led interventions: a systematic review and meta-analysis. Front Psychiatry. 2022;13:915617.
42. Burke E, Pyle M, Machin K, Varese F, Morrison AP. The effects of peer support on empowerment, self-efficacy, and internalized stigma: a narrative synthesis and meta-analysis. Stigma Health. 2019:337–56.
43. Pitt V, Lowe D, Hill S, Prictor M, Hetrick SE, Ryan R, et al. Consumer-providers of care for adult clients of statutory mental health services. Cochrane Database Syst Rev. 2013;2013:CD004807.
44. Fang Q, Lin L, Chen Q, Yuan Y, Wang S, Zhang Y, et al. Effect of peer support intervention on perinatal depression: a meta-analysis. Gen Hosp Psychiatry. 2022;74:78–87.
45. Huang R, Yan C, Tian Y, Lei B, Yang D, Liu D, et al. Effectiveness of peer support intervention on perinatal depression: a systematic review and meta-analysis. J Affect Disord. 2020;276:788–96.
46. Skivington K, Matthews L, Simpson SA, Craig P, Baird J, Blazeby JM, et al. A new framework for developing and evaluating complex interventions: update of Medical Research Council guidance. BMJ. 2021;374:n2061. https://doi.org/10.1136/bmj.n2061.

47. Poulsen CH, Egmose CH, Ebersbach BK, Hjorthøj C, Eplov LF. A community-based PEER-support group intervention "Paths to EvERyday life" (PEER) added to service as usual for adults with vulnerability to mental health difficulties—a study protocol for a randomized controlled trial. Trials. 2022;23:727.
48. Osborne SP, Radnor Z, Strokosch K. Co-production and the co-creation of value in public services: a suitable case for treatment? Public Manag Rev. 2016;18:639–53. https://doi.org/10.1080/14719037.2015.1111927.
49. Moore GF, Audrey S, Barker M, Bond L, Bonell C, Hardeman W, et al. Process evaluation of complex interventions: Medical Research Council guidance. BMJ. 2015;350.
50. Gillard S, Banach N, Barlow E, Byrne J, Foster R, Goldsmith L, et al. Developing and testing a principle-based fidelity index for peer support in mental health services. Soc Psychiatry Psychiatr Epidemiol. 2021;56:1903–11.
51. Chinman M, McCarthy S, Mitchell-Miland C, Daniels K, Youk A, Edelen M. Early stages of development of a peer specialist fidelity measure. Psychiatr Rehabil J. 2016;39:256.
52. Jacobson N, Trojanowski L, Dewa CS. What do peer support workers do? A job description. BMC Health Serv Res. 2012;12:1–11.
53. Egmose CH, Poulsen CH, Bjørkedal S-TB, Eplov LF. The 'Paths to everyday life' (PEER) trial—a qualitative study of mechanisms of change from the perspectives of individuals with mental health difficulties participating in peer support groups led by volunteer peers. BMC Psychiatry. 2024;24:1–12.
54. Bailie HA, Tickle A. Effects of employment as a peer support worker on personal recovery: a review of qualitative evidence. Ment Health Rev J. 2015;20:48–64.
55. du Plessis C, Whitaker L, Hurley J. Peer support workers in substance abuse treatment services: a systematic review of the literature. J Subst Use. 2020;25:225–30.
56. Poremski D, Kuek JHL, Yuan Q, Li Z, Yow KL, Eu PW, et al. The impact of peer support work on the mental health of peer support specialists. Int J Ment Health Syst. 2022;16:1–8.
57. Repper J Gilfoyle S Gillard S Perkins R Rennison J. Peer Support Workers: a practical guide to implementation. 2013.
58. Gillard S. Peer support in mental health services: where is the research taking us, and do we want to go there? J Ment Health. 2019;28:341–4.
59. Opie JE, McLean SA, Vuong AT, Pickard H, McIntosh JE. Training of lived experience workforces: a rapid review of content and outcomes. Admin Pol Ment Health. 2023;50:177–211.
60. Watson S. The consumer perspective supervision. An annotated summary of resources. 2019.
61. Watson E, Bowyer D, Cooper S, Dodd Z, Manning E, Morgan G, et al. Supervision for Peer workers. IMROC; n.d.
62. Ball M; Skinner S. Raising the glass ceiling: considering a career pathway for peer support workers. 2021.

Open Access   This chapter is licensed under the terms of the Creative Commons Attribution 4.0 International License (http://creativecommons.org/licenses/by/4.0/), which permits use, sharing, adaptation, distribution and reproduction in any medium or format, as long as you give appropriate credit to the original author(s) and the source, provide a link to the Creative Commons license and indicate if changes were made.

The images or other third party material in this chapter are included in the chapter's Creative Commons license, unless indicated otherwise in a credit line to the material. If material is not included in the chapter's Creative Commons license and your intended use is not permitted by statutory regulation or exceeds the permitted use, you will need to obtain permission directly from the copyright holder.

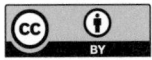

Beyond Kraepelin: An Aetiological Approach to the Typology and Treatment of Psychosis

25

Robin M. Murray, Luis Alameda, Aikaterini Dima, and Dominic Oliver

25.1   Introduction

One of the main purposes of diagnosis in medicine is to predict response to treatment and outcome [1]. Unfortunately, current ways of classifying the psychoses in the Diagnostic and Statistical Manual of Mental Disorders, Fifth Edition (DSM-5) and International Classification of Diseases, Eleventh Revision (ICD-11) do not achieve these aims, nor do they relate to aetiology. Consequently, the current classification of psychosis has been increasingly regarded as unsatisfactory (e.g. [2, 3]). Perhaps the most heartfelt description of its inadequacies is to be found in the paper by Goloksuz and Van Os [4] entitled 'The slow death of the concept of schizophrenia'.

As a result, some authorities have advocated abandoning the traditional Kraepelinian classification system and moving to other schemes. Leucht et al. [5] reviewed the better-known schemes including the Research Domain Criteria (RDoC), the Hierarchical Taxonomy of Psychopathology (HiTOP), Network

R. M. Murray (✉)
Institute of Psychiatry, Psychology and Neuroscience (IoPPN), King's College London, London, UK
e-mail: robin.murray@kcl.ac.uk

L. Alameda
Department of Psychosis Studies at the IoPPN at King's College London, London, UK
Service of General Psychiatry, Treatment and Early Intervention in Psychosis Program, Lausanne University Hospital (CHUV), Lausanne, Switzerland
Centro Investigacion Biomedica en Red de Salud Mental (CIBERSAM); Instituto de Biomedicina de Sevilla (IBIS), Hospital Universitario Virgen del Rocio, Departamento de Psiquiatria, Universidad de Sevilla, Sevilla, Spain

A. Dima
South London and Maudsley Psychiatric (SLaM) Training Programme, Maudsley Hospital, London, UK

D. Oliver
Department of Psychiatry, University of Oxford, Oxford, UK

© The Author(s) 2026
G. Ikkos, T. Becker (eds.), *Psychiatry after Kraepelin*,
https://doi.org/10.1007/978-3-032-09475-9_25

Approaches and clinical staging. They concluded that all these approaches have merits but also deficiencies, and therefore have themselves gone on to advocate [6] a 'Problem, resources and goals oriented multidimensional framework (PRoGO)' which considers not only symptoms but also a wider range of factors such as adverse life-style or social conditions.

Other investigators tried to subdivide psychosis and/or its subcategories into discrete entities. The 1980s saw several such approaches. Andreasen et al. [7] built on Crow's concept of positive and negative syndromes to reify these into discrete subtypes of schizophrenia; Murray et al. [8] distinguished between familial and non-familial cases of schizophrenia; while Carpenter and his colleagues [9] subdivided patients with schizophrenia into those with and without the 'deficit syndrome'. None of these proved satisfactory.

More recently, biological markers have been used to try to distinguish meaningful subgroups [10]. It has been common to subdivide patients on the basis of MRI (magnetic resonance imaging) scan findings. For example, Chand et al. [11] used machine learning to subdivide schizophrenia into two distinct neuroanatomical subtypes, while Clementz and his colleagues [12] in the Bipolar–Schizophrenia Network on Intermediate Phenotypes (B-SNIP) consortium, combined imaging with neuropsychology to subdivide psychosis into three main types. Howes et al. [13] subdivided schizophrenia into those with and without mesostriatal hyperdopaminergia. Peripheral blood markers such as cytokines have also been used to identify those psychotic patients with and without evidence of possible inflammation [14, 15].

Unfortunately, while such subdivisions have helped to advance the careers of those academic psychiatrists who developed them, they have not been found to have clinical utility, neither delineating clearcut subgroups with defined aetiology nor accurately predicting treatment response or outcome.

25.2   Precedents from General Medicine

When we compare psychiatry with general medicine, we see that in the latter, classification moved long ago from clinical syndromes to diseases. While psychiatric disorders continue to be diagnosed on the basis of signs and symptoms, many medical diseases have come to be diagnosed following investigations, for example, the varieties of renal or chest disease distinguished by radiography. Other diseases were delineated by cause. For example, Vitamin C deficiency and scurvy. The futility of relying purely on symptomology became apparent when conditions such as tuberculosis or syphilis were shown to produce a wide range of manifestations which are unified by having a single identifiable cause.

Many disorders are multifactorial in cause. If we take coronary artery disease (CAD) as an example, the initial presentation with chest pain is confirmed by electrocardiogram (ECG) or angiography. Immediate treatment may address the thrombosis in the coronary artery, the final common pathway which mediates the cardiac muscle damage. However, this does not mean that cardiologists are disinterested in the causes of the thrombosis. On the contrary, once they have made a diagnosis of CAD, they seek out the risk factors which have led to this endpoint and attempt to address these too: hyperlipidaemia, hypertension, diabetes, cigarette smoking, obesity, lack of exercise [16].

Thus, once CAD is diagnosed, an attempt is made to establish and then address the external and internal causal factors that are likely to exacerbate it. Physicians take a similar approach for many medical disorders.

25.3   The Final Common Pathway to Psychosis

Is there an equivalent common pathway for psychosis to the coronary artery thrombosis? Evidence points to striatal dopaminergic abnormalities as representing this final common pathway in the vast majority of psychotic patients; a possible exception is a subset of patients with treatment-resistant schizophrenia. Initially it was thought that the locus of abnormality in most patients might be in the D2 dopamine receptor since positron emission tomography (PET) studies showed an upregulation of these receptors. However, subsequently it was realised that this was the case only for those patients who had already received antipsychotics and therefore this was best considered a consequence of the D2 dopamine blockade [17]. Subsequent attention switched to presynaptic mechanisms and it has been consistently found that most patients with acute psychosis (both schizophrenia and manic) show an excess synthesis of dopamine in the dorsal striatum [18].

The striatal dopamine abnormalities are likely caused by disrupted GABAergic and glutamatergic signalling in the hippocampus [19]. This imbalance between inhibitory and excitatory signalling causes increased activity in midbrain dopaminergic neurons that project to the striatum, leading to positive symptoms [20, 21]. Hyperactivity of the ventral subiculum may further disrupt basolateral amygdala and prefrontal cortex function, impairing emotional reactivity control and cognition, respectively [20, 21]. However, the evidence is more secure for positive symptoms than for negative symptoms or impaired cognition (Fig. 25.1) [22–25].

But how does abnormal striatal dopamine give rise to psychotic symptoms? We learn and update our beliefs through prediction error. We constantly predict what we expect to happen in our environment—but if our predictions do not match up to reality, this results in surprise! Dopamine neurons fire to unexpected (surprise), but not to expected, events. Unmedicated patients, with early psychosis show increased striatal dopamine and prediction error abnormalities [26, 27]. The increased dopamine signalling leads to aberrant assignment of importance (salience) to unimportant stimuli. In this way Increased dopamine signalling leads to an aberrant assignment of salience to otherwise insignificant stimuli, resulting in the formation of spurious meaningful connections between coincident external impressions, perceptions, thoughts, and recollections that happen to occur simultaneously in consciousness [28].

So we now have an understanding that abnormal reward learning consequent upon increase in dopamine synthesis in the associative striatum is commonly the final common pathway to the positive symptoms of psychosis, the equivalent of the

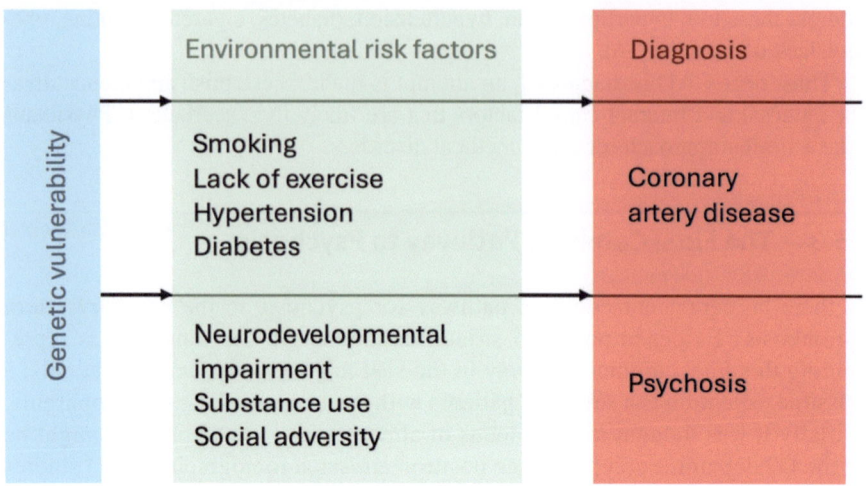

Fig. 25.1 Pathways to illness: a comparison of coronary artery disease and psychosis

coronary artery thrombosis. And as with the risk factors for CAD, we now have relatively good knowledge of the aetiological factors which drive the psychosis. We will now briefly review the main risk factors.

25.4   Genetic Risk

Psychosis is in the most part polygenic as discussed by Owen and colleagues [30] (Eds: see also Chap. 6). For example, the most recent large collaborative genome-wide association studies (GWAS) identified common variants associated with schizophrenia at 287 genomic loci [29]. We can now measure the extent of genetic load using polygenic risk scores (PRSs) for schizophrenia, bipolar disorder and depressive psychosis. Analyses have shown a significant overlap of polygenic risk across schizophrenia and bipolar disorder (approximately two-thirds of genes overlap), and to a lesser extent with depression [31, 32]. Thus, polygenic predisposition forms a background of susceptibility on which the effects of environmental risk factors act.

GWAS show that the associations with schizophrenia are enriched in neuronal genes, those involved in neurodevelopment and those with high expression in excitatory glutamatergic neurons from cerebral cortex and hippocampus, but also in cortical inhibitory interneurons Gamma-Aminobutyric Acid (GABA) as well as calcium channel genes [29, 30]. Gamma-Aminobutyric Acid (GABA) and gluta-matergic systems have important effects on dopaminergic function, suggesting that the genetic variants in these systems may alter the regulation of dopamine in psychosis. One analysis of the GWAS data pointed to 11 genes more directly related to dopamine synthesis, metabolism and neurotransmission [33]. Recently, Sportelli et al. identified a set of genes predominantly expressed in the caudate nucleus and associated with both clinical state and genetic risk for schizophrenia that shows dopaminergic selectivity [34]. A higher polygenic risk score for schizophrenia parsed by this set of genes predicts greater dopamine synthesis in the striatum and greater striatal activation during reward anticipation.

About 2% of schizophrenic patients show a copy number variant (CNV) which has a much greater effect on the phenotype. Evidence from over 11,000 patients has shown an enrichment of CNVs involving glutamatergic and GABAergic systems [30, 35]. Interestingly, the most common CNV is 22q11.2 deletion where up to 25% of carriers develop psychosis; in contrast individuals with 22q11.2 duplication are protected from risk of schizophrenia [36]. Rogdaki et al. [37] have shown that non-psychotic individuals who carry the deletion show an excess of striatal dopamine while those with the duplication have lower striatal dopamine than normals.

25.5   Environmental Risk

It has become increasingly obvious that environmental factors play an important role in the aetiology of psychosis. Numerous risk factors have been reported. Arango et al. [38] carried out an umbrella review of meta-analyses concerning these risk factors and classified them by extent of supportive evidence. Many were discarded as having insufficient evidence. For the purposes of this review, we have compressed these factors which they considered to have consistent, or highly suggestive, evidence into three overall types (Fig. 25.1):

A. *Those adversely affecting neurodevelopment*: obstetric complications (OCs), minor physical abnormalities, low premorbid intelligence quotient (IQ).
B. *Drug Use, especially Cannabis use.*
C. *Social adversity* including adversities in childhood, being a migrant or from an ethnic minority, stressful life events.

We will now describe the main risks and possible mechanistic pathways whereby these can disrupt dopamine dysregulation.

25.5.1 Neurodevelopmental Risk Pathway

Prenatal and perinatal complications, often collectively termed obstetric complications (OCs), are among the best replicated environmental risk factors for psychosis. Two detailed meta-analyses have been carried out. The earlier one [39] reported that three groups of complications were significantly associated with later schizophrenia: a) *complications of pregnancy* (bleeding, diabetes, Rh incompatibility, preeclampsia); b) *abnormal foetal growth and development* (low birthweight, congenital malformations, reduced head circumference); and c) *complications of delivery* (uterine atony, asphyxia, emergency caesarean section). Estimates of effect sizes were generally less than 2. The more recent meta-analysis by Davies et al. [40]

included a greater number of studies ($n = 152$), and largely replicated Cannon's findings. Both meta-analyses concluded that foetal hypoxia and anoxia-related factors, where the developing brain is deprived of oxygen, were those most consistently implicated.

Minor physical abnormalities have long been reported as in excess in psychosis [41–43], one of the first reports being from Thomas Clouston in 1891 [44]. These may arise from genetic factors such as CNVs or from adverse environmental factors operating in utero [45]. They are not infrequently associated with minor neurological signs [46]. Structural abnormalities in the olfactory bulb and related areas are commonly seen in patients with schizophrenia [47, 48]. These regions are rich in dopaminergic neurons, and disruptions in dopaminergic signalling relate to impairments in olfactory identification [49].

Premorbid IQ tends to be lower in individuals who later develop schizophrenia, compared to the general population. Many people diagnosed with schizophrenia exhibit cognitive impairments before the onset of full-blown psychosis [50]. This lower premorbid IQ is not necessarily caused by genetic predisposition to schizophrenia itself but may be a reflection of polygenic inheritance of IQ [51], or may be consequent upon obstetric events [52].

Of course, the physical and cognitive abnormalities noted above may be reflective of the underlying neurobiological changes preceding psychosis, rather than specifically increase risk themselves.

It is now well established that early hazards can cause subtle brain damage, and resultant neurodevelopmental impairment [53]. For example, asphyxia-related obstetric complications result in smaller brain volumes and lower cognitive abilities [54]. Moreover, exposure to obstetric complications is associated with adult enlarged striatal volumes [55, 56] as well as altered striatal dopaminergic activity, potentially related to salience processing [19, 57, 58].

As long ago as 1971, Mednick et al. suggested that pre- and perinatal complications might damage the hippocampus thus increasing risk of psychosis [59]. Subsequently, Stefanis and colleagues [60] reported that schizophrenic patients who had been exposed to obstetric difficulties had smaller hippocampi than both normal subjects and those patients without OCs. In the early 2000s, there was a flurry of animal research assessing whether early hippocampal lesions were associated with dopaminergic abnormalities and psychosis-like behaviour when the animals matured. Evidence came from perinatal administration of methylazoxymethanol acetate (MAM) in pregnant rats, or lesioning the hippocampus in neonatal rats, both of which led to psychosis-like behaviour and dopaminergic abnormalities in adult rats [61–63]. Interestingly, Froudist-Walsh et al. [64] who studied adults who had been born preterm, showed that neonatal hippocampal injury was associated with adult dopamine dysfunction, thus providing a potential mechanism linking early life risk factors to adult psychotic illness.

Prenatal maternal infection could have a distinct mechanism through altering foetal brain development [65]. Two prominent preclinical models of psychosis rely on infection during gestation in rodents: maternal gestational exposure to the human influenza virus and administration of the viral mimic polyriboinosinic-polyribocytidilic acid (Poly[I:C]) [63]. Both models result in GABAergic abnormalities, particularly a reduced number of GABAergic hippocampal neurons. The resulting inhibition results in dopaminergic and glutamatergic dysfunction downstream, as seen in patients with psychosis [66–68]. These models also result in behavioural abnormalities, including impaired prepulse inhibition, reduced exploration and reduced social interaction [69, 70], as seen in patients with psychosis [71–76]. The severity of these alterations appears to be dependent on the intensity of a cytokine-mediated immune response [77], suggesting a role of inflammation in psychosis aetiopathology. Peripheral blood cytokines and markers of chronic low-grade inflammation (i.e. C-reactive protein) are similarly elevated in medication-naïve First-Episode Psychosis (FEP) patients [78, 79].

25.5.2 Substance Use Pathway

There is good evidence that psycho-stimulants (such as amphetamines and cocaine) can induce psychosis; methamphetamine psychosis is a major problem in the Far East, Australia, South Africa and parts of North America [80–82].

Prospective and case-control epidemiological studies have consistently shown a relationship between cannabis use and the development of psychosis with increased risks ranging from 1.5 to 19 depending on the frequency of use and the potency of the cannabis used [83, 84]. Meta-analyses have demonstrated a clear dose–response relationship between the level of use and the risk for psychosis [85].

Transient psychotic-like experiences can be induced in healthy individuals by the administration of Δ9-tetrahydrocannabinol (THC), the main psychoactive ingredient of cannabis [86]. Furthermore, continued cannabis use by those with psychosis is associated with increased risk of medication non-response, medication non-adherence, as well as higher rates of recurrence of psychosis symptoms, and rehospitalisations [87].

The prevalence of cannabis use has been shown to impact on the incidence of psychosis. Thus the European Network of National Schizophrenia Networks Studying Gene–Environment Interactions (EU-GEI) study found that if high-potency cannabis were no longer available, around 12% of first-episode psychosis cases across 11 Europe-wide sites could be prevented, rising to 30% in London and 50% in Amsterdam [83]. A registry-linked national cohort study from Denmark examined the population-attributable risk fraction (PARF) of cannabis use disorder on schizophrenia in Denmark. The PARF increased over time as the use and potency of cannabis increased [88]. The potency and availability of cannabis continues to increase [89] particularly in legalised markets, increasing the incidence of psychosis.

25.5.2.1 How Does Drug Abuse Increase Risk of Psychosis?

It is easy to understand the mechanistic link between abuse of amphetamines and psychosis. After being taken up into dopamine varicosities, amphetamine displaces dopamine from the intracellular vesicles; it also reverses the direction of the dopamine transporter (DAT) on the cell surface, so that rather than being recycled, dopamine is instead pumped out of the varicosity onto recipient neurons. The knowledge of the effects of amphetamines on dopamine has long been one of the planks of the dopamine hypothesis of schizophrenia.

The neurochemical basis of cannabis-related psychosis is more complex but animal studies show that the endogenous cannabinoid system interacts with the dopamine system in the basal ganglia. THC stimulates CB_1 receptors which are targets for the endogenous cannabinoids. These receptors are widely distributed throughout the brain, and upon stimulation by cannabinoids, they decrease presynaptic glutamate or Gamma-Aminobutyric Acid (GABA) release. The glutamate and Gamma-Aminobutyric Acid (GABA) inputs to the dopamine neurons in the ventral midbrain express CB_1 receptors, and therefore THC alters the balance of excitation and inhibition reaching dopamine cells with an increase in firing and resultant elevations of dopamine release. Because both endocannabinoid and dopamine systems actively participate in maturation, it is likely that any interference with this signalling during adolescence will result in psychopathological phenotypes later in life. Thus in juvenile rodents, exposure to THC disinhibits prefrontal cortex network function with consequent hyperactivity of subcortical dopaminergic activity accompanying a range of cognitive and affective phenotypes resembling those observed in schizophrenia [90].

THC administration to humans is associated with medial temporal and striatal activation which is specifically correlated with transient psychotic symptoms [91]. Some [92, 93] but not other [94] studies in healthy volunteers have reported that acute administration of THC leads to increased striatal dopamine release. Most recently, the group of Palaniyappan has used neuromelanin-sensitive MRI, which reflects dopamine synthesis and release, to scan cannabis users [94]. The users showed higher neuromelanin signal in the substantia nigra/ventral tegmental area (VTA), as did people with early schizophrenia. Heavy chronic cannabis users appear to show compensatory mechanisms, with reduced striatal dopamine synthesis capacity and release [95], and reduced glutamate-derived metabolites in cortical and subcortical brain areas [96]. This may seem the opposite of what is usually associated with psychosis risk but animal studies suggest that the explanation may be that chronic use leads to dopamine receptor supersensitivity [97].

25.5.3 Social Adversity Pathway

25.5.3.1 Childhood Adversity

This concept includes exposure to a broad range of potentially traumatic events in childhood and adolescence (Eds: see also Chap. 13). In the field of psychosis, it usually refers to moderate or severe degrees of exposure to sexual abuse, physical abuse, emotional/psychological abuse, physical and emotional neglect etc. [98], although more recently bullying and household discord have been incorporated into the construct [99]. In a seminal meta-analysis, Varese et al. [100] reported strong evidence that childhood adversity (abuse, neglect and bullying) was associated with increased risk for psychosis in adulthood (overall odds ratio [OR] = 2.78). Dragioti et al. [101] claimed that 38% of schizophrenia cases could be prevented if childhood trauma were eradicated.

These findings have been replicated in a recent updated meta-analysis [102] which confirmed the link between childhood trauma and psychosis (OR = 2.8). The relationship between childhood trauma and psychosis appears to be dose-dependent, with evidence supporting the presence of a dose–response relationship. Moreover, this study showed differential effects of trauma subtypes. For example, emotional abuse was associated with the largest increase in risk (OR = 3.5) and parental antipathy with the lowest (OR = 1.58). Additionally, there is evidence suggesting that above a certain threshold of cumulative exposure, the risk of developing psychosis increases more sharply, indicating a non-linear relationship.

25.5.3.2 Adverse Recent Life Events

While childhood adversity often refers to exposure prior the age of 18, life events are more proximal to the onset of illness and include exposures in adulthood. A meta-analysis by Beards et al. showed a threefold increased odds of life events in the period prior to psychosis onset [103]. First-episode psychosis patients are also more likely to live alone, be single or unemployed, live in a rented accommodation, live in overcrowded conditions and receive an income below official poverty level, not only at first contact with psychiatric services but up to 5 years prior to the onset of psychosis [104]. There is some evidence that recent life events may in some cases mediate or interact with childhood adversity in psychosis risk [105, 106]. Although evidence exploring the interplay between childhood trauma and adverse life events in psychosis risk is surprisingly limited, it is reasonable to hypothesise that some individuals may need both insults to trigger psychosis.

25.5.3.3 Migration and Ethnicity

Selten et al. [107] conducted a meta-analysis of psychosis incidence studies and migration, across multiple countries. They found an increased risk of developing psychosis among first- and second-generation migrants, with an overall relative risk (RR) of 2.9 for migration to Europe from non-European countries. The RR was higher where migrants originated from developing versus developed countries. The risk was highest among those with black skin colour (RR 4.19). This effect was attenuated but remained after the authors adjusted for socioeconomic status (RR 1.8).

In Western countries, individuals from ethnic minority backgrounds are at greater risk of developing psychosis compared to White individuals [108, 109]. This risk is more pronounced when living in an area alongside relatively few other ethnic minority individuals relative to the White majority (low ethnic density), but psychosis risk remains substantial even in high ethnic density areas [110, 111].

25.5.3.4 How Does Social Adversity Increase Psychosis Risk?

The psychological mechanisms proposed to explain the association between childhood adversity (mainly focused on abuse) and psychotic disorders have been

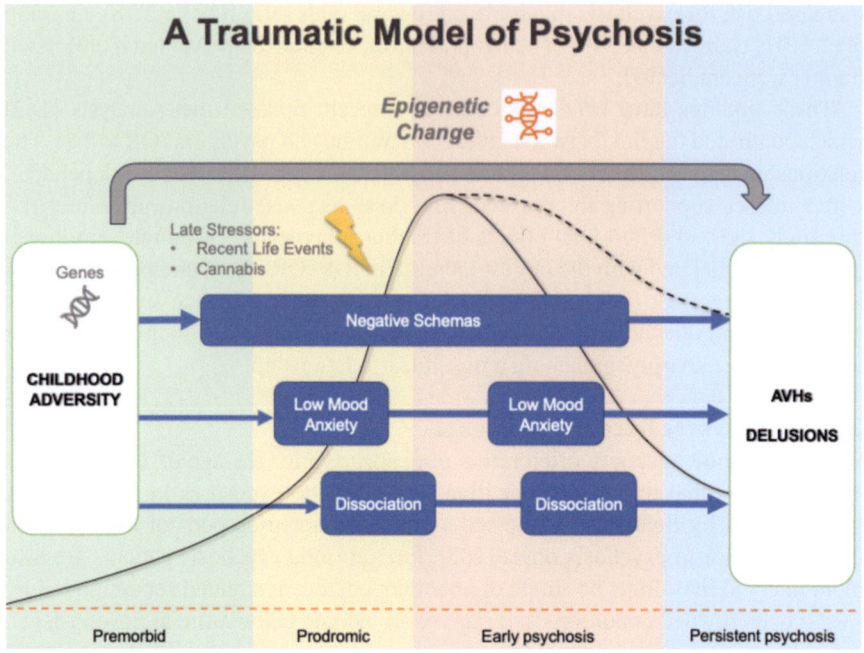

Fig. 25.2 A traumatic model of psychosis. This figure illustrates how childhood trauma leads to epigenetic changes, mood changes, dissociation and dysfunctional cognitive processes that make individuals vulnerable to psychosis, particularly auditory verbal hallucinations (AVHs) and delusions. Later stressors in those with a genetic vulnerability will accentuate mood problems and/or increase dissociation, leading to the first episode of psychosis. While for many patients, the outcome will be good (dotted line), for others this will not be the case (poor outcome, straight line), marking the beginning of a poor trajectory and even treatment resistance

reviewed in three systematic reviews [112–114] and one meta-analysis [115]. Evidence converges on the importance of negative cognitive schemas about the self, the world and others—post-traumatic stress symptoms with dissociation being the strongest and most replicated mediator. There is also evidence suggesting that low mood and anxiety mediate the abuse–psychosis association, which supports an affective pathway linking abuse and psychosis. Obviously, there may be more than one pathway operating in an individual, and some pathways may overlap—for example, the affective and schema-based pathways. Along similar lines, individuals with post-traumatic stress symptoms often hold negative schemas about the self, the world and others. So these mechanism should be considered in an integrated way (see therapeutic implications below and Fig. 25.2).

From a biological perspective, it is hypothesised that trauma causes a dysregulation of the hypothalamic–pituitary–adrenal (HPA) axis [116] through its action on stress responsive brain structures such as hippocampus and amygdala; childhood trauma has been associated with decreased volume of the former [117]. People with childhood adversity tend to have smaller hippocampi and amygdalae, areas of the brain that regulate emotions, memory and stress. Psychotic patients who had been subject to severe physical or sexual abuse in childhood show elevated dopamine function in the associative striatum in adulthood [118, 119]. Because these regions are enriched with glucocorticoid receptors, which mediate the HPA axis, it is hypothesised that dysregulation of this axis may lead to hypersensitivity, resulting in downregulation of glucocorticoid receptors and, in turn, an excess of glucocorticoids in these stress-sensitive regions.

Chronic activation of the HPA axis following repeated exposure to psychosocial stressors is characterised by high basal/unstimulated cortisol levels [120]. Individuals with psychosis have higher concentrations of blood and salivary cortisol in comparison to healthy controls [121–123]. Conversely, cortisol responses to awakening and in response to psychosocial stressor tasks are attenuated among individuals with psychosis relative to controls [124–127]. These high cortisol levels reduce the ability of the HPA axis to mount an appropriate response when faced with acute stressors. Such stressors may result in less effective behavioural and psychological responses [128, 129].

The timing of chronic exposure to stress hormones can have differential effects on brain areas, particularly when they are undergoing development. For example, the hippocampus is particularly vulnerable to stressors occurring in the first 2 years of life when it undergoes significant development [130]. Exposure to the same stressors during late childhood and adolescence might lead to changes in amygdala volume and the frontal cortex, respectively, during their key stages of development.

With regard to Involvement of dopamine, Selten et al. [131] suggested that the long-term experience of being excluded from the majority group (causing social defeat) increases risk via effects on the dopamine system. In accord with this, Egerton et al. [132] showed that immigrants showed elevated striatal stress-induced dopamine release and dopamine synthesis capacity compared to non-immigrants, independent of clinical status. Discrimination is correlated with higher amygdala activity and increased functional connectivity between the amygdala and other brain regions, particularly the thalamus [133], similar to findings in psychosis patients experiencing paranoid symptoms [134]. Stress and trauma combined with low socioeconomic status throughout adolescence is linked to earlier completion of brain development and lower brain volume [135], indicating a neurodevelopmental link, either due to earlier curbing of synaptic density increases or greater synaptic pruning throughout adolescence. Morgan et al. [136] proposed a socio-developmental pathway in which exposure to adversity and trauma interacts with underlying genetic risk and impacts on neurobiological development (in particular the stress response and dopamine systems) to create an enduring liability to psychosis. Psychosocial stress, partly generated through discrimination [137], which is directly associated with psychosis [138–140], may be a key driver of psychosis risk in individuals from ethnic minority backgrounds.

Epigenetic changes, especially DNA methylation (DNAm), may help clarify how trauma contributes to the development of psychosis. DNAm plays a key role in mediating the interaction between genetic vulnerability and environmental influences in the risk for psychosis and schizophrenia. Exposure to childhood trauma can trigger lasting epigenetic modifications that persist into adulthood, potentially

Aetiological Pathways to Psychosis

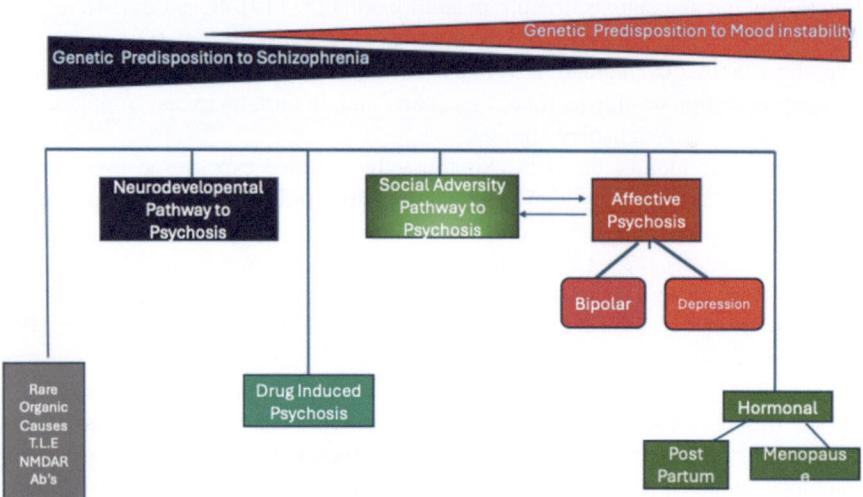

Fig. 25.3 Aetiological pathways to psychosis

increasing vulnerability to further stress or cannabis use (Fig. 25.3) [141]. These factors may then contribute to psychosis by disrupting biological pathways, such as those involving dopamine regulation.

These epigenetic changes can increase the impact of later exposures on increasing psychosis risk. For example, there is an emerging pathway of interest linking trauma and psychosis via cannabis use. In a study of 881 individuals with first-episode psychosis and 1231 healthy controls, Trotta et al. [142] suggest that childhood trauma, particularly experiences such as abuse and household discord, is strongly associated with psychosis, both directly and via increased cannabis use.

Figure 25.2 illustrates how genetic and social adversity may interplay along with other risk factors in contributing to psychosis and poor outcome, with psychological and biological pathways operating simultaneously.

25.6   Advantages of an Approach to Psychosis Based on Aetiology

It is clear from the above that much evidence implicates dopamine dysregulation as the final common pathway in most cases of psychosis, and that there is increasing evidence that both susceptibility genes and environmental risk factors contribute to this [143]. Treatment for psychosis generally focusses on blocking the dopamine receptor but rarely addresses the environmental factors which increase risk and often predispose to poorer outcome.

An approach based on risk factors offers obvious benefits for research. The usual approach of studying patients by diagnosis results in substantial heterogeneity with the inclusion of patients whose psychosis has resulted from quite different risk factors. Most studies of schizophrenia or of psychosis consider the syndrome as a whole, and therefore it is likely that, for example, neuropsychological or imaging characteristics of the individual risk groups are obscured by being merged with patients with which they have little in common aetiologically. A more appropriate research strategy would be to identify patients whose psychosis appears to have resulted predominantly from one particular risk factor and then study the psychological and biological characteristics in patients associated with this risk factor.

An aetiological approach to treating psychosis enables the psychiatrist to consider more targeted treatment rather than the one-size-fits all model. Obviously, all people with psychosis should be offered antipsychotics. But in addition, it is important that those underlying risk factors which are driving the psychosis should also be addressed. This could involve putting in place strategies to avoid exposure to the risk factor (e.g. public health measures concerning the risks of heavy cannabis use) but also to target the mechanisms (if these are well studied) that are operating as mediators between the risk factor and psychosis and its related clinical manifestations (e.g. low mood or dissociation mediate the association between childhood abuse and psychosis).

Figure 25.3 shows a possible method of subdividing people experiencing psychosis into aetiological prototypes. Of course, we know that frequently an individual with psychosis has been exposed to a number of risk factors. However, this is also the case for the model medical disorder, coronary artery disease (CAD) which we discussed earlier; this has not prevented it being highly productive to consider the different risk factors for CAD and their mechanistic pathways separately.

25.6.1 Neurodevelopmental Prototypical Patients: Characteristics and Care

Psychotic patients who have experienced neurodevelopmental delay or deviance tend to show particular characteristics (Fig. 25.4). Such patients show poorer premorbid social function and IQ [144], minor physical and neurological abnormalities, and present with earlier age at illness onset [145], and more neurocognitive [52] and MRI abnormalities [53, 54, 146].

A meta-analysis by Forte et al. [147] compared psychotic individuals with and without exposure to obstetric complications. Obstetric complications were associated with more severe psychopathology as compared with non-exposed people with psychosis. The better-quality studies showed an association with negative symptoms. Patients with a copy number variant (CNV) gene also tend to have a poor response to antipsychotics and to be more likely to be classified as having treatment-resistant schizophrenia. Patients with poorer premorbid function, and those with cognitive deficits are associated with poor response to antipsychotics [148–150]; so also are brain structural abnormalities [151, 152]. The above factors have led us to

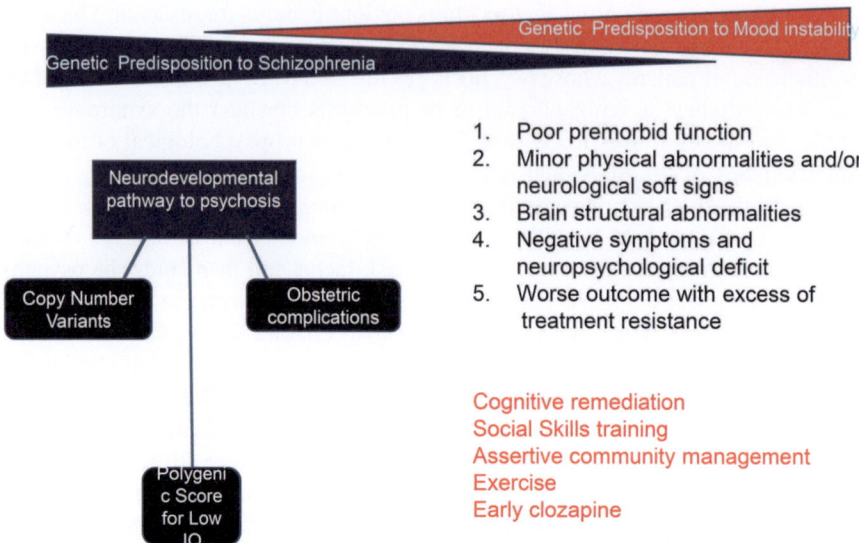

Fig. 25.4 Characteristics and treatment of neurodevelopmental psychosis

point out that many of those with treatment-resistant psychosis may be neurodevelopmentally impaired [149, 150].

Useful treatment approaches to patients with neurodevelopmental damage are cognitive remediation [153, 154] to maximise their intellectual function, and assertive community outreach to help them negotiate the complexities of society [155]. Social skills training can be effective in improving social and communication functioning [156].

Introducing physical exercise is a simple and cost-effective intervention that can be implemented in both inpatient and outpatient settings. Three systematic reviews have supported its role in improving cognition [157–159]. A recent review of 22 randomised controlled trials (RCTs) confirmed these findings—physical exercise significantly improved cognition, with aerobic exercise having the greatest effect [160]. Physical activity has also been shown to be effective on improving executive function among individuals with a wide range of neurodevelopmental disorders [161, 162].

Clozapine should be considered early in the course of the care of patients with neurodevelopmental impairment and indeed should be more often implemented by early intervention services [163]. However, in recent years, multiple pharmacological agents have been studied to tackle cognitive deficits in psychosis although none has of yet shown conclusive evidence of efficacy [164].

25.6.2 Drug Abuse Prototypical Patients: Characteristics and Care

Patients who have developed psychosis following drug abuse show a very different profile from those with neurodevelopmental impairment (Fig. 25.5). They are more likely to have had good premorbid social and academic function, and normal

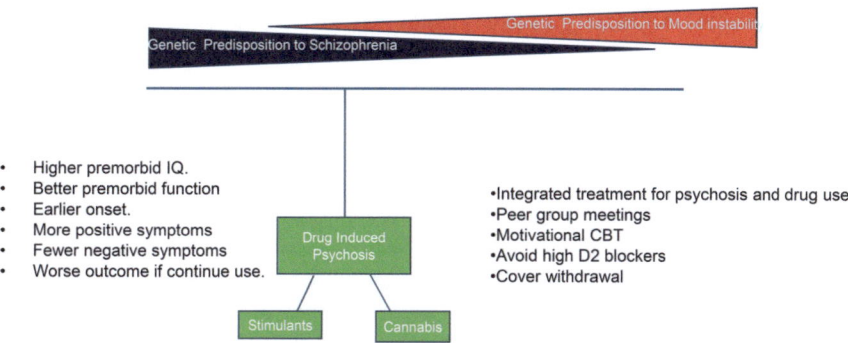

Fig. 25.5 Characteristics and treatment of drug-induced psychosis

premorbid IQ [165, 166]; the former ensures that they have friends who can introduce them to drug taking while the latter enables them to conceal their drug taking for a prolonged period. Cannabis-using psychotic patients present earlier than their non-using counterparts [167], their cognition is better [168–173] and at least at onset MRI is normal [174, 175]. Their outcome depends greatly on whether they continue or stop their drug use [176].

There is evidence that the choice of antipsychotics has a bearing on likelihood of relapse into drug taking. Heavy drug users show low dopamine in the ventral striatum, which results in continued craving to use drugs [95, 177, 178]. This can be exacerbated by antipsychotics, especially those which cause high D2 [179]. Consequently, there is some evidence that partial agonists such as aripiprazole [180] or clozapine [181] are associated with a better outcome. Pharmacological help with a drug such as Sativex (containing low dose THC and cannabidiol [CBD]) to cover drug withdrawal, can also be helpful [182].

Patients with psychosis associated with cannabis use frequently fall between general adult psychiatry and drug addiction services, the former treating the psychosis but doing nothing to help the patients overcome their dependence while the latter often declining to treat the dependence because the patients are psychotic. To overcome such difficulties, Di Forti et al. [183] established a specialised clinic for such dual diagnosis patients. This offers weekly one-to-one therapy with motivational interviewing and cognitive behavioural therapy (CBT) as well as attendance at a weekly peer group. A reduction in dependence was observed with 74% of participants achieving abstinence and 26% reducing the frequency and potency of their use. Significant improvements in psychosis and with functional outcomes were observed, with 91% returning to work or education. Thus, such an integrated setting provides the necessary support for those with heavy use or dependence to gradually reduce their consumption and avoid cannabis withdrawal and its associated problems.

25.6.3 Social Adversity Prototypical Patients: Characteristics and Care

Meta-analysis has shown that childhood abuse is associated with more severe positive and depressive symptoms [184]; abuse and, more strongly, neglect are associated with poorer neurocognition [185], neglect is associated with more severe negative symptoms [184, 186] and both abuse and neglect are associated with poor social functioning at onset and during follow-up in prospective studies [187, 188].

Research on treatment focused on those patients with psychosis who suffered childhood adversity is at an early stage. Following findings suggesting a mediating role from negative schemas, post-traumatic stress disorder (PTSD) symptoms and dissociation, two trials using trauma-focused cognitive behavioural therapy and Eye Movement Desensitization and Reprocessing (EMDR), respectively, are being conducted [189, 190]. These trials postulate that treating PTSD symptoms including dissociation may improve not only these, but also the related symptoms of psychosis. Dissociation puts reality testing under pressure and may alter the ability of a traumatised individual to distinguish traumatic experience from post-traumatic intrusions as such, externalising them in the form of a perceptual abnormality. Preliminary findings support the value of these therapies [191, 192] in those psychotic patients with child abuse and PTSD symptoms.

Much research in recent years has focussed on an affective pathway to psychosis (Fig. 25.6). This postulates that people with trauma will often develop low mood and anxiety, which makes them vulnerable to developing and maintaining delusions and hallucinations [191, 193]. It is well accepted that when a patient with bipolar disorder or psychotic depression has mood-congruent delusions or perceptual abnormalities, not only positive symptoms but also the underlying mood component need to be addressed. However, it is often overlooked that people with trauma and psychosis can have subdiagnostic levels of depression and anxiety, that may have

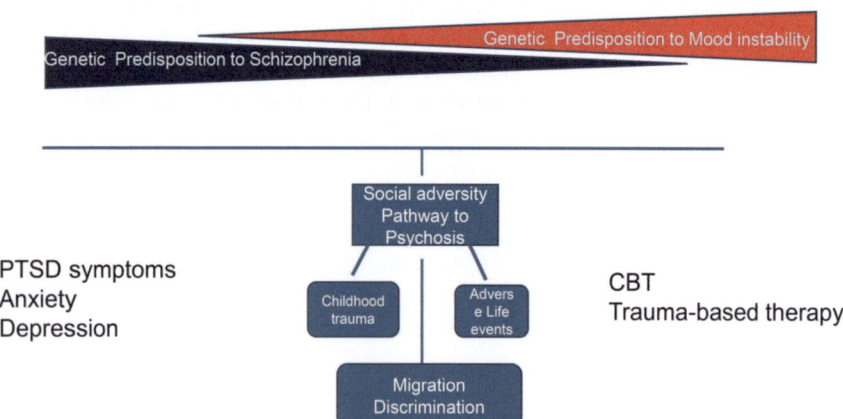

Fig. 25.6 Characteristics and treatment of social adversity psychosis

not reached the severity of a formal moderate or major depressive episode, or an anxiety disorder, but that may be enough to affect reality testing and precipitate onset or relapse, or the maintenance, of positive symptoms of psychosis as well as poor functioning [194, 195]. Therefore, people with trauma and psychosis, mood and anxiety phenomena, even at subdiagnostic levels, should be carefully assessed and treated not only with CBT (including mindfulness) but also with antidepressants where appropriate, of course along with antipsychotics. See Fig. 25.2 for an illustration of how these different pathways may operate as mediators between trauma and psychosis and outcome.

25.7   Affective Psychosis

In their meta-analysis of risk factors for psychosis, Arango et al. [38] did not consider other psychiatric disorders or hormonal factors. However, to have a complete picture of risk factors for psychosis, we should remind ourselves that people who are diagnosed as having a primary affective disorder may develop a secondary psychosis. This is commonly the case for bipolar disorder and less commonly for major depression. In such patients, clearly the mood disorder should be treated along with the psychosis. However, as these facts are well known, we will not discuss them further here.

25.8   Psychoses Affecting Women Specifically

Women are, of course, subject to additional types of psychosis (Fig. 25.3).

25.8.1 Postpartum Psychosis

The period following childbirth is when a woman is at maximal risk of psychosis in her life. Hormonal factors are key. During pregnancy, levels of oestrogen and progesterone rise significantly. After childbirth, the rapid drop in these hormone levels especially oestrogen can trigger psychotic symptoms. These disorders most frequently have an affective basis [196], so a mood stabiliser such as lithium or/and an antidepressant is generally required to treat the mood component [197] with due attention to patient information, breastfeeding and plasma levels.

25.8.2 Psychosis in Perimenopausal Period

Epidemiological studies have shown that during the perimenopausal period, typically occurring around the age of 50, there is a period of increased risk of psychosis in women. At this time, there are decreases in oestrogen and progesterone. Oestrogen has been shown to have neuroprotective properties [198], influencing neurotransmitter systems, and may affect dopamine receptor activity [199], so its lack may facilitate the development of psychosis. Recent trials have investigated the role of oestrogen therapy [200] and raloxifene, a selective oestrogen receptor modulator [201, 202], as adjunctive treatment for schizophrenia. Results have been promising for female patients across most studies. Most recently, Hormone Replacement Therapy (HRT) was associated with a 16% lower risk of psychotic relapse in menopausal women [203].

25.8.3 Menstrual-Related Psychosis

Many women experience exacerbations of psychosis in synchrony with the menstrual cycle.

25.9 Organic Causes

As noted in Fig. 25.3, there are also rare organic causes of functional psychosis. These include temporal lobe epilepsy [204] and N-Methyl-D-Aspartate (NMDA) auto-antibodies [205]. Although rare, these need to be identified as appropriate treatment can transform them (Eds: see Chap. 8).

25.10 Exposure to Multiple Genetic and Environmental Risk Factors

When considering environmental risk, it is important to remember that many patients with psychosis have inherited some genetic vulnerability to illness. As we noted earlier, susceptibility genes for schizophrenia and affective psychosis overlap [32] (Fig. 25.3). Furthermore, an increasing number of studies have been examining the relationship between genetic and environmental risk. For example, the polygenic risk for schizophrenia and heavy cannabis use appear to act as independent risk factors for psychosis. Many people with a high polygenic risk score for schizophrenia develop psychosis without ever using cannabis while others with a low polygenic risk score only develop psychosis following very heavy cannabis use; in the majority of cases, the two combine to push the individual over the threshold for expressing psychosis [206]. In carrying out such studies, we need to take care that genetic predisposition does not predispose the individual to exposure to environmental factors. Gene–environmental correlation was not of importance in this last study by Austin-Zimmerman, Spinazzola et al., that is, polygenic risk for schizophrenia did not predispose to cannabis use.

As yet, we measure polygenic predisposition in a very crude global manner. However, it is possible that different environmental risk factors may interact with different genetic pathways; for example, one might speculate that cannabis use might interact with the geneset for the endocannabinoid system, or childhood adversity with genes influencing the HPA axis.

Experienced clinicians will recognise the typological subgroups that we have just described where exposure to a particular risk factor has shaped the clinical picture of a patient with psychosis. In such cases, the treatment should follow along the lines we have outlined above. However, clinicians may point out that many patients with psychosis have a history of exposure to several environmental risk factors. These may be of similar type, for example, those who had premature birth may have also suffered asphyxia and postnatal complications. Alternatively, those who were abused as a child may have then encountered bullying and adverse life events in adulthood. But in addition, individuals may have been exposed to different types of risk factors. For example, young people exposed to childhood adversity at home may gravitate in their adolescence to gang membership and consequent exposure to drug use and violence. Thus, they will then share some of the specificities of those from the childhood adversity group and those from the drug abuse pathway, that is, more than one pathway to dopamine dysregulation may be operating in the same patient.

Researchers have examined the cumulative effect of multiple environmental factors on risk of psychosis as aggregate index of total number of risk factors or weighted sum. For example, Cougnard et al. [207] reported an additive effect of exposure to three risk factors—childhood trauma, urbanicity, and cannabis use—in predicting persistent psychotic symptoms in the general population. Stepniak et al. found that individuals who had been exposed to four or more environmental risk factors had a significantly lower age of onset than those exposed to three factors. Several different measures that sum environmental risk have been developed including the Maudsley Environmental Risk Score [208], the Exposome [209], and the Psychosis Polyrisk Score [210].

Those patients who have been exposed to a number of risk factors deserve to have attention directed to each of these in the same way that cardiologists will address several risk factors for coronary artery disease (CAD), for example, hyperlipidaemia, cigarette smoking and lack of exercise in the same individual (Fig. 25.1). This situation requires a flexible and integrative approach where the treatment priorities can be set hierarchically based on the predominant feature. For example, an initial focus on drug abuse could be followed by psychological therapy addressing the consequences of childhood adversity once drug abuse ceases or at least decreases substantially.

Finally, it is worth reflecting on the fact that the importance of individual risk factors for psychosis varies both geographically and temporally (e.g. methamphetamine psychosis). This means that the clinical and biological characteristics of psychosis will not be constant across countries and time but will reflect the relative prevalence of the different risk factors in that place or time. It also reminds us of the importance of primary prevention, that is, of attempting to decrease the likelihood of exposure to risk factors. Perhaps, the most clear-cut opportunity is public health education aimed at informing the population about the risks of heavy cannabis use.

Sadly, current trends in cannabis use and consequent rates of psychosis are going in exactly the wrong direction [211].

25.11 Conclusion

Current treatment of psychosis is hindered by the fact that it rarely addresses the risk factors that underlie the onset and persistence of the patient's psychosis. We consider that the best way to improve the care of patients is not only to prescribe antipsychotics but also to attend to the causal factors. The major types of environmental risk factors (or component causes) comprise neurodevelopmental hazards, drug abuse and social adversity. We advocate identifying patients whose psychosis has resulted predominantly from exposure to one particular risk factor. For example, those patients who are neurodevelopmentally impaired typically show premorbid social abnormalities, prominent negative symptoms, cognitive and brain structural abnormalities and poorer long-term outcome. Secondly, at the start of their illness, those patients whose psychosis results from drug abuse (amphetamines and cannabis especially) show largely normal premorbid social function and cognition, but prominent positive symptoms. Thirdly, patients who have been exposed to social adversity often present with PTSD symptoms or anxiety and depression as part of their psychosis. Appropriate interventions should be offered, in addition to antipsychotics, to patients in accord with their exposure to the different risk factors. For example, the patient who had been abused in childhood should be offered trauma-based therapy, and antidepressants as appropriate, while the patient who continues to abuse cannabis should be offered CBT/motivational therapy to decrease his/her drug consumption. Those patients who have been exposed to several risk factors deserve to have attention directed to each of these in turn.

Key Points
- Treatment of psychosis generally neglects the factors which cause its onset and persistence.
- Patients should be offered interventions addressing the following causal risk factors; neurodevelopmental impairment, drug abuse and social adversity.
- For example, those who were exposed to social adversity may benefit from trauma-based therapy, and antidepressants as appropriate.
- Those who developed psychosis following cannabis abuse should be offered CBT/motivational interviews to help them reduce/stop their drug use.
- Patients with neurodevelopmental impairment may benefit from cognitive remediation, intensive social support and early clozapine.

References

1. Kendell R, Jablensky A. Distinguishing between the validity and utility of psychiatric diagnoses. Am J Psychiatry. 2003;160(1):4–12.
2. Brockington I. Schizophrenia: yesterday's concept. Eur Psychiatry. 1992;7(5):203–7.
3. Murray RM, Quattrone D. The Kraepelian concept of schizophrenia: dying but not yet dead. Schizophr Res. 2022;242:102–5.
4. Goloksuz S, Van Os J. The slow death of the concept of schizophrenia and the painful birth of the psychosis spectrum. Psychol Med. 2018;48(2):229–44. https://doi.org/10.1017/S0033291717001775. Epub 2017 Jul 10
5. Leucht S, van Os J, Jäger M, Davis JM. Prioritization of psychopathological symptoms and clinical characterization in psychiatric diagnoses: a narrative review. JAMA Psychiatr. 2024;81(11):1149–58. https://doi.org/10.1001/jamapsychiatry.2024.2652.
6. Leicht S, Konig B, Francesco A, Rodolioco A, Priller J, Boge K, et al. Enhancing mental health care: a problem, resources and goals oriented multidimensional framework (PRoGO). Eur Arch Psychiatry Clin Neurosci. 2025; https://doi.org/10.1007/s00406-025-02045-5. Online ahead of print
7. Andreasen NC. Positive vs. negative schizophrenia: a critical evaluation. Schizophr Bull. 1985;11(3):380–9. https://doi.org/10.1093/schbul/11.3.380.
8. Murray RM, Lewis SW, Reveley AM. Towards an aetiological classification of schizopohrenia. Lancet. 1985;325(8436):1023–6. https://doi.org/10.1016/S0140-6736(85)91623-X.
9. Carpenter WT, Heinrichs DW, Wagman AM. Deficit and nondeficit forms of schizophrenia. Am J Psychiatry. 1988;145(5):578–83. https://doi.org/10.1176/ajp.145.5.578.
10. Abi-Dargham A, Moeller SJ, Ali F, DeLorenzo C, Domschke K, Horga G, et al. Candidate biomarkers in psychiatric disorders: state of the field. World Psychiatry. 2023;22(2):236–62.
11. Chand GB, Dwyer DB, Erus G, Sotiras A, Varol E, Srinivasan D, et al. Two distinct neuroanatomical subtypes of schizophrenia revealed using machine learning. Brain. 2020;143(3):1027–38.
12. Clementz BA, Parker DA, Trotti RL, JE MD, Keedy SK, Keshavan MS, et al. Psychosis biotypes: replication and validation from the B-SNIP consortium. Schizophr Bull. 2021;48(1):56–68.
13. Howes OD, Bukala BR, Jauhar S, McCutcheon RA. The hypothesis of biologically based subtypes of schizophrenia: a 10-year update. World Psychiatry. 2025;24(1):46–7.
14. Zhang L, Lizano P, Guo B, Xu Y, Rubin LH, Hill SK, et al. Inflammation subtypes in psychosis and their relationships with genetic risk for psychiatric and cardiometabolic disorders. Brain Behav Immun Health. 2022;22:100459.
15. Nasrallah HA. Psychosis, inflammatory biomarkers, and subtypes of childhood trauma. J Clin Psychiatry. 2024;85(2):24com15310.
16. O'Gara PT. The COURAGE (Clinical Outcomes Utilizing Revascularization and Aggressive Drug Evaluation) trial: can we deliver on its promise? J Am Coll Cardiol. 2010;55(13):1359–61.
17. Howes OD, Kambeitz J, Kim E, Stahl D, Slifstein M, Abi-Dargham A, et al. The nature of dopamine dysfunction in schizophrenia and what this means for treatment. Arch Gen Psychiatry. 2012;69(8):776–86.
18. Jauhar S, Nour MM, Veronese M, Rogdaki M, Bonoldi I, Azis M, et al. A test of the transdiagnostic dopamine hypothesis of psychosis using positron emission tomographic imaging in bipolar affective disorder and schizophrenia. JAMA Psychiatr. 2017;74(12):1206–13.
19. Howes OD, Shatalina E. Integrating the neurodevelopmental and dopamine hypotheses of schizophrenia and the role of cortical excitation-inhibition balance. Biol Psychiatry. 2022;92(6):501–13.

20. Grace AA. Dysregulation of the dopamine system in the pathophysiology of schizophrenia and depression. Nat Rev Neurosci. 2016;17(8):524–32.
21. Grace AA, Gomes FV. The circuitry of dopamine system regulation and its disruption in schizophrenia: insights into treatment and prevention. Schizophr Bull. 2019;45(1):148–57.
22. Javitt DC. Glutamatergic theories of schizophrenia. Isr J Psychiatry Relat Sci. 2010;47(1):4–16.
23. RA MC, Keefe RSE, McGuire PK. Cognitive impairment in schizophrenia: aetiology, pathophysiology, and treatment. Mol Psychiatry. 2023;28(5):1902–18.
24. Merritt K, McGuire PK, Egerton A, Aleman A, Block W, Bloemen OJN, et al. Association of age, antipsychotic medication, and symptom severity in schizophrenia with proton magnetic resonance spectroscopy brain glutamate level: a mega-analysis of individual participant-level data. JAMA Psychiatr. 2021;78(6):667–81.
25. Moghaddam B, Krystal JH. Capturing the angel in "angel dust": twenty years of translational neuroscience studies of NMDA receptor antagonists in animals and humans. Schizophr Bull. 2012;38(5):942–9.
26. Murray GK, Corlett PR, Clark L, Pessiglione M, Blackwell AD, Honey G, et al. Substantia nigra/ventral tegmental reward prediction error disruption in psychosis. Mol Psychiatry. 2008;13(3):239. 267–76
27. Haarsma J, Fletcher PC, Griffin JD, Taverne HJ, Ziauddeen H, Spencer TJ, et al. Precision weighting of cortical unsigned prediction error signals benefits learning, is mediated by dopamine, and is impaired in psychosis. Mol Psychiatry. 2021;26(9):5320–33.
28. Gray JA, Feldon J, Rawlins JN, Hemsley DR, Smith AD. The neuropsychology of schizophrenia. Behav Brain Sci. 1991;14(1):1–84.
29. Trubetskoy V, Pardiñas AF, Qi T, Panagiotaropoulou G, Awasthi S, Bigdeli TB, et al. Mapping genomic loci implicates genes and synaptic biology in schizophrenia. Nature. 2022;604(7906):502–8.
30. Owen MJ, Bray NJ, JTR W, O'Donovan MC. Genomics of schizophrenia, bipolar disorder and major depressive disorder. Nat Rev Genet. 2025; https://doi.org/10.1038/s41576-025-00843-0.
31. Scott J, Crouse JJ, Medland S, Byrne E, Iorfino F, Mitchell B, et al. Polygenic risk scores and the prediction of onset of mood and psychotic disorders in adolescents and young adults. Early Interv Psychiatry. 2024;18(6):397–405.
32. Rodriguez V, Alameda L, Quattrone D, Tripoli G, Gayer-Anderson C, Spinazzola E, et al. Use of multiple polygenic risk scores for distinguishing schizophrenia-spectrum disorder and affective psychosis categories in a first-episode sample; the EU-GEI study. Psychol Med. 2023;53(8):3396–405.
33. Edwards AC, Bacanu SA, Bigdeli TB, Moscati A, Kendler KS. Evaluating the dopamine hypothesis of schizophrenia in a large-scale genome-wide association study. Schizophr Res. 2016;176(2–3):136–40.
34. Sportelli L, Eisenberg DP, Passiatore R, D'Ambrosio E, Antonucci LA, Bettina JS, et al. Dopamine signaling enriched striatal gene set predicts striatal dopamine synthesis and physiological activity in vivo. Nat Commun. 2024;15(1):3342.
35. Pocklington AJ, Rees E, Walters JT, Han J, Kavanagh DH, Chambert KD, et al. Novel findings from CNVs implicate inhibitory and excitatory signaling complexes in schizophrenia. Neuron. 2015;86(5):1203–14.
36. Rees E, Kirov G, Sanders A, Walters JTR, Chambert KD, Shi J, et al. Evidence that duplications of 22q11.2 protect against schizophrenia. Mol Psychiatry. 2014;19(1):37–40.
37. Rogdaki M, Devroye C, Ciampoli M, Veronese M, Ashok AH, McCutcheon RA, et al. Striatal dopaminergic alterations in individuals with copy number variants at the 22q11.2 genetic locus and their implications for psychosis risk: a [18F]-DOPA PET study. Mol Psychiatry. 2023;28(5):1995–2006.
38. Arango C, Dragioti E, Solmi M, Cortese S, Domschke K, Murray RM, et al. Risk and protective factors for mental disorders beyond genetics: an evidence-based atlas. World Psychiatry. 2021;20(3):417–36.

39. Cannon M, Jones PB, Murray RM. Obstetric complications and schizophrenia: historical and meta-analytic review. Am J Psychiatry. 2002;159(7):1080–92.
40. Davies C, Segre G, Estradé A, Radua J, De Micheli A, Provenzani U, et al. Prenatal and perinatal risk and protective factors for psychosis: a systematic review and meta-analysis. Lancet Psychiatry. 2020;7(5):399–410.
41. Weinberg SM, Jenkins EA, Marazita ML, Maher BS. Minor physical anomalies in schizophrenia: a meta-analysis. Schizophr Res. 2007;89(1–3):72–85.
42. Xu T, Chan RC, Compton MT. Minor physical anomalies in patients with schizophrenia, unaffected first-degree relatives, and healthy controls: a meta-analysis. PLoS One. 2011;6(9):e24129.
43. Sut E, Akgül Ö, Bora E. Minor physical anomalies in schizophrenia and first-degree relatives in comparison to healthy controls: a systematic review and meta-analysis. Eur Neuropsychopharmacol. 2024;86:55–64.
44. O'Connell P, Woodruff PW, Wright I, Jones P, Murray RM. Developmental insanity or dementia praecox: was the wrong concept adopted? Schizophr Res. 1997;23(2):97–106.
45. Compton MT, Walker EF. Physical manifestations of neurodevelopmental disruption: are minor physical anomalies part of the syndrome of schizophrenia? Schizophr Bull. 2009;35(2):425–36.
46. Dazzan P, Murray RM. Neurological soft signs in first-episode psychosis: a systematic review. Br J Psychiatry Suppl. 2002;43:s50–7.
47. Nguyen AD, Pelavin PE, Shenton ME, Chilakamarri P, McCarley RW, Nestor PG, et al. Olfactory sulcal depth and olfactory bulb volume in patients with schizophrenia: an MRI study. Brain Imaging Behav. 2011;5(4):252–61.
48. Turetsky BI, Crutchley P, Walker J, Gur RE, Moberg PJ. Depth of the olfactory sulcus: a marker of early embryonic disruption in schizophrenia? Schizophr Res. 2009;115(1):8–11.
49. Kamath V, Moberg PJ, Gur RE, Doty RL, Turetsky BI. Effects of the val(158)met catechol-O-methyltransferase gene polymorphism on olfactory processing in schizophrenia. Behav Neurosci. 2012;126(1):209–15.
50. Jones P, Rodgers B, Murray R, Marmot M. Child development risk factors for adult schizophrenia in the British 1946 birth cohort. Lancet. 1994;344(8934):1398–402.
51. Legge SE, Cardno AG, Allardyce J, Dennison C, Hubbard L, Pardiñas AF, et al. Associations between schizophrenia polygenic liability, symptom dimensions, and cognitive ability in schizophrenia. JAMA Psychiatry. 2021;78(10):1143–51.
52. Amoretti S, Rabelo-da-Ponte FD, Garriga M, Forte MF, Penadés R, Vieta E, et al. Obstetric complications and cognition in schizophrenia: a systematic review and meta-analysis. Psychol Med. 2022;52(14):2874–84.
53. Vanes LD, Murray RM, Nosarti C. Adult outcome of preterm birth: Implications for neurodevelopmental theories of psychosis. Schizophr Res. 2022;247:41–54.
54. Costas-Carrera A, Garcia-Rizo C, Bitanihirwe B, Penadés R. Obstetric complications and brain imaging in schizophrenia: a systematic review. Biol Psychiatry Cogn Neurosci Neuroimaging. 2020;5(12):1077–84.
55. Holz NE, Zabihi M, Kia SM, Monninger M, Aggensteiner PM, Siehl S, et al. A stable and replicable neural signature of lifespan adversity in the adult brain. Nat Neurosci. 2023;26(9):1603–12.
56. Merritt K, Luque Laguna P, Sethi A, Drakesmith M, Ashley SA, Bloomfield M, et al. The impact of cumulative obstetric complications and childhood trauma on brain volume in young people with psychotic experiences. Mol Psychiatry. 2023;28(9):3688–97.
57. Davis KL, Kahn RS, Ko G, Davidson M. Dopamine in schizophrenia: a review and reconceptualization. Am J Psychiatry. 1991;148(11):1474–86.
58. Kapur S. Psychosis as a state of aberrant salience: a framework linking biology, phenomenology, and pharmacology in schizophrenia. Am J Psychiatry. 2003;160(1):13–23.
59. Mednick SA. Breakdown in individuals at high risk for schizophrenia: Possible predispositional perinatal factors. Ment Hyg. 1970;54(1):50–63.

60. Stefanis N, Frangou S, Yakeley J, Sharma T, O'Connell P, Morgan K, et al. Hippocampal volume reduction in schizophrenia: effects of genetic risk and pregnancy and birth complications. Biol Psychiatry. 1999;46(5):697–702.
61. Lipska BK, Weinberger DR. A neurodevelopmental model of schizophrenia: neonatal disconnection of the hippocampus. Neurotox Res. 2002;4(5–6):469–75.
62. Lodge DJ, Grace AA. Hippocampal dysfunction and disruption of dopamine system regulation in an animal model of schizophrenia. Neurotox Res. 2008;14(2–3):97–104.
63. Oliver D, Modinos G, McGuire P. Chapter 12 - Neurochemical models of psychosis risk and onset. In: Risk factors for psychosis. Academic Press; 2020. p. 229–47.
64. Froudist-Walsh S, Bloomfield MA, Veronese M, Kroll J, Karolis VR, Jauhar S, et al. The effect of perinatal brain injury on dopaminergic function and hippocampal volume in adult life. Elife. 2017;6
65. Meyer U, Yee BK, Feldon J. The neurodevelopmental impact of prenatal infections at different times of pregnancy: the earlier the worse? Neuroscientist. 2007;13(3):241–56.
66. Lieberman JA, Girgis RR, Brucato G, Moore H, Provenzano F, Kegeles L, et al. Hippocampal dysfunction in the pathophysiology of schizophrenia: a selective review and hypothesis for early detection and intervention. Mol Psychiatry. 2018;23(8):1764–72.
67. Manoach DS. Prefrontal cortex dysfunction during working memory performance in schizophrenia: reconciling discrepant findings. Schizophr Res. 2003;60(2–3):285–98.
68. Schobel SA, Chaudhury NH, Khan UA, Paniagua B, Styner MA, Asllani I, et al. Imaging patients with psychosis and a mouse model establishes a spreading pattern of hippocampal dysfunction and implicates glutamate as a driver. Neuron. 2013;78(1):81–93.
69. Meyer U, Feldon J, Fatemi SH. In-vivo rodent models for the experimental investigation of prenatal immune activation effects in neurodevelopmental brain disorders. Neurosci Biobehav Rev. 2009;33(7):1061–79.
70. Shi L, Fatemi SH, Sidwell RW, Patterson PH. Maternal influenza infection causes marked behavioral and pharmacological changes in the offspring. J Neurosci. 2003;23(1):297–302.
71. Bolino F, Di Michele V, Di Cicco L, Manna V, Daneluzzo E, Casacchia M. Sensorimotor gating and habituation evoked by electro-cutaneous stimulation in schizophrenia. Biol Psychiatry. 1994;36(10):670–9.
72. Braff DL, Stone C, Callaway E, Geyer M, Glick I, Bali L. Prestimulus effects on human startle reflex in normals and schizophrenics. Psychophysiology. 1978;15(4):339–43.
73. Braff DL, Grillon C, Geyer MA. Gating and habituation of the startle reflex in schizophrenic patients. Arch Gen Psychiatry. 1992;49(3):206–15.
74. Catalan A, Salazar de Pablo G, Aymerich C, Damiani S, Sordi V, Radua J, et al. Neurocognitive functioning in individuals at clinical high risk for psychosis: a systematic review and meta-analysis. JAMA Psychiatry. 2021;78(8):859–67.
75. Cornblatt BA, Carrión RE, Addington J, Seidman L, Walker EF, Cannon TD, et al. Risk factors for psychosis: impaired social and role functioning. Schizophr Bull. 2012;38(6):1247–57.
76. Perry W, Braff DL. Information-processing deficits and thought disorder in schizophrenia. Am J Psychiatry. 1994;151(3):363–7.
77. Meyer U, Feldon J, Schedlowski M, Yee BK. Towards an immuno-precipitated neurodevelopmental animal model of schizophrenia. Neurosci Biobehav Rev. 2005;29(6):913–47.
78. Mondelli V. From stress to psychosis: whom, how, when and why? Epidemiol Psychiatr Sci. 2014;23(3):215–8.
79. Pillinger T, Osimo EF, Brugger S, Mondelli V, McCutcheon RA, Howes OD. A meta-analysis of immune parameters, variability, and assessment of modal distribution in psychosis and test of the immune subgroup hypothesis. Schizophr Bull. 2019;45(5):1120–33.
80. Chen CK, Lin SK, Sham PC, Ball D, Loh EW, Hsiao CC, et al. Pre-morbid characteristics and co-morbidity of methamphetamine users with and without psychosis. Psychol Med. 2003;33(8):1407–14.
81. McKetin R, McLaren J, Lubman DI, Hides L. The prevalence of psychotic symptoms among methamphetamine users. Addiction. 2006;101(10):1473–8.

82. Tardelli VS, Johnstone S, Xu B, Kim S, Kim H, Gratzer D, George TP, Le Foll B, Castle DJ. Marked increase in amphetamine-related emergency department visits and inpatient admissions in Toronto, Canada, 2014–2021. Can J Psychiatry. 2023;68(4):249–56.

83. Di Forti M, Quattrone D, Freeman TP, Tripoli G, Gayer-Anderson C, Quigley H, et al. The contribution of cannabis use to variation in the incidence of psychotic disorder across Europe (EU-GEI): a multicentre case-control study. Lancet Psychiatry. 2019;6(5):427–36.

84. Robinson N, Ploner A, Leone M, Lichtenstein P, Kendler KS, Bergen SE. Environmental risk factors for schizophrenia and bipolar disorder from childhood to diagnosis: a Swedish nested case-control study. Psychol Med. 2024;54(9):2162–71.

85. Marconi A, Di Forti M, Lewis CM, Murray RM, Vassos E. Meta-analysis of the association between the level of cannabis use and risk of psychosis. Schizophr Bull. 2016;42(5):1262–9.

86. Morrison PD, Zois V, McKeown DA, Lee TD, Holt DW, Powell JF, et al. The acute effects of synthetic intravenous Delta9-tetrahydrocannabinol on psychosis, mood and cognitive functioning. Psychol Med. 2009;39(10):1607–16.

87. Schoeler T, Petros N, Di Forti M, Klamerus E, Foglia E, Ajnakina O, et al. Effects of continuation, frequency, and type of cannabis use on relapse in the first 2 years after onset of psychosis: an observational study. Lancet Psychiatry. 2016;3(10):947–53.

88. Hjorthøj C, Posselt CM, Nordentoft M. Development over time of the population-attributable risk fraction for cannabis use disorder in schizophrenia in Denmark. JAMA Psychiatr. 2021;78(9):1013–9.

89. Freeman TP, Craft S, Wilson J, Stylianou S, ElSohly M, Di Forti M, et al. Changes in delta-9-tetrahydrocannabinol (THC) and cannabidiol (CBD) concentrations in cannabis over time: systematic review and meta-analysis. Addiction. 2021;116(5):1000–10.

90. Solinas M, Melis M. Developmental exposure to cannabis compromises dopamine system function and behavior. Curr Opin Behav Sci. 2024;59:101442.

91. Bhattacharyya S, Fusar-Poli P, Borgwardt S, Martin-Santos R, Nosarti C, O'Carroll C, et al. Modulation of mediotemporal and ventrostriatal function in humans by Delta9-tetrahydrocannabinol: a neural basis for the effects of Cannabis sativa on learning and psychosis. Arch Gen Psychiatry. 2009;66(4):442–51.

92. Bossong MG, Mehta MA, van Berckel BN, Howes OD, Kahn RS, Stokes PR. Further human evidence for striatal dopamine release induced by administration of Δ9-tetrahydrocannabinol (THC): selectivity to limbic striatum. Psychopharmacology (Berl). 2015;232(15):2723–9.

93. Stokes PR, Mehta MA, Curran HV, Breen G, Grasby PM. Can recreational doses of THC produce significant dopamine release in the human striatum? Neuroimage. 2009;48(1):186–90.

94. Ahrens J, Ford SD, Schaefer B, Reese D, Khan AR, Tibbo P, et al. Convergence of cannabis and psychosis on the dopamine system. JAMA Psychiatry. 2025;82(6):609–17. https://doi.org/10.1001/jamapsychiatry.2025.0432.

95. Bloomfield MA, Morgan CJ, Egerton A, Kapur S, Curran HV, Howes OD. Dopaminergic function in cannabis users and its relationship to cannabis-induced psychotic symptoms. Biol Psychiatry. 2014;75(6):470–8.

96. Colizzi M, McGuire P, Pertwee RG, Bhattacharyya S. Effect of cannabis on glutamate signalling in the brain: a systematic review of human and animal evidence. Neurosci Biobehav Rev. 2016;64:359–81.

97. Ginovart N, Kapur S. Role of dopamine D(2) receptors for antipsychotic activity. In: Handb Exp Pharmacol, vol. 212; 2012. p. 27–52.

98. Sætren SS, Bjørnestad JR, Ottesen AA, Fisher HL, DAS O, Hølland K, et al. Unraveling the concept of childhood adversity in Psychosis pesearch: a systematic review. Schizophr Bull. 2024;50(5):1055–66.

99. Morgan C, Gayer-Anderson C, Beards S, Hubbard K, Mondelli V, Di Forti M, et al. Threat, hostility and violence in childhood and later psychotic disorder: population-based case-control study. Br J Psychiatry. 2020;217(4):575–82.

100. Varese F, Smeets F, Drukker M, Lieverse R, Lataster T, Viechtbauer W, et al. Childhood adversities increase the risk of psychosis: a meta-analysis of patient-control, prospective- and cross-sectional cohort studies. Schizophr Bull. 2012;38(4):661–71.

101. Dragioti E, Radua J, Solmi M, Arango C, Oliver D, Cortese S, et al. Global population attributable fraction of potentially modifiable risk factors for mental disorders: a meta-umbrella systematic review. Mol Psychiatry. 2022;27(8):3510–9.
102. Zhou L, IEC S, Yang P, Sikirin LV, Van Os J, Bentall R, et al. What do four decades of research tell us about the association between childhood adversity and psychosis? An updated and extended multi-level meta-analysis. Am J Psychiatry. 2025;182(4):360–72. https://doi.org/10.1176/appi.ajp.20240456.
103. Beards S, Gayer-Anderson C, Borges S, Dewey ME, Fisher HL, Morgan C. Life events and psychosis: a review and meta-analysis. Schizophr Bull. 2013;39(4):740–7.
104. Stilo SA, Murray RM. Non-genetic factors in schizophrenia. Curr Psychiatry Rep. 2019;21(10):100.
105. Ayesa-Arriola R, Setién-Suero E, Marques-Feixa L, Neergaard K, Butjosa A, Vázquez-Bourgon J, et al. The synergetic effect of childhood trauma and recent stressful events in psychosis: associated neurocognitive dysfunction. Acta Psychiatr Scand. 2020;141(1):43–51.
106. Bhavsar V, Boydell J, McGuire P, Harris V, Hotopf M, Hatch SL, et al. Childhood abuse and psychotic experiences - evidence for mediation by adulthood adverse life events. Epidemiol Psychiatr Sci. 2019;28(3):300–9.
107. Selten JP, van der Ven E, Termorshuizen F. Migration and psychosis: a meta-analysis of incidence studies. Psychol Med. 2020;50(2):303–13.
108. Kirkbride JB, Errazuriz A, Croudace TJ, Morgan C, Jackson D, Boydell J, et al. Incidence of schizophrenia and other psychoses in England, 1950–2009: a systematic review and meta-analyses. PLoS One. 2012;7(3):e31660.
109. Radua J, Ramella-Cravaro V, Ioannidis JPA, Reichenberg A, Phiphopthatsanee N, Amir T, et al. What causes psychosis? An umbrella review of risk and protective factors. World Psychiatry. 2018;17(1):49–66.
110. Tortelli A, Errazuriz A, Croudace T, Morgan C, Murray RM, Jones PB, et al. Schizophrenia and other psychotic disorders in Caribbean-born migrants and their descendants in England: systematic review and meta-analysis of incidence rates, 1950–2013. Soc Psychiatry Psychiatr Epidemiol. 2015;50(7):1039–55.
111. Bosqui TJ, Hoy K, Shannon C. A systematic review and meta-analysis of the ethnic density effect in psychotic disorders. Soc Psychiatry Psychiatr Epidemiol. 2014;49(4):519–29.
112. Alameda L, Rodriguez V, Carr E, Aas M, Trotta G, Marino P, et al. A systematic review on mediators between adversity and psychosis: potential targets for treatment. Psychol Med. 2020;50(12):1966–76.
113. Sideli L, Murray RM, Schimmenti A, Corso M, La Barbera D, Trotta A, et al. Childhood adversity and psychosis: a systematic review of bio-psycho-social mediators and moderators. Psychol Med. 2020;50(11):1761–82.
114. Williams J, Bucci S, Berry K, Varese F. Psychological mediators of the association between childhood adversities and psychosis: a systematic review. Clin Psychol Rev. 2018;65:175–96.
115. Bloomfield MA, Chang T, Woodl MJ, Lyons LM, Cheng Z, Bauer-Staeb C, et al. Psychological processes mediating the association between developmental trauma and specific psychotic symptoms in adults: a systematic review and meta-analysis. World Psychiatry. 2021;20(1):107–23.
116. Murphy F, Nasa A, Cullinane D, Raajakesary K, Gazzaz A, Sooknarine V, et al. Childhood trauma, the HPA axis and psychiatric illnesses: a targeted literature synthesis. Front Psychiatry. 2022;13:748372.
117. Aas M, Navari S, Gibbs A, Mondelli V, Fisher HL, Morgan C, et al. Is there a link between childhood trauma, cognition, and amygdala and hippocampus volume in first-episode psychosis? Schizophr Res. 2012;137(1–3):73–9.
118. Dahoun T, Nour MM, RA MC, Adams RA, MAP B, Howes OD. The relationship between childhood trauma, dopamine release and dexamphetamine-induced positive psychotic symptoms: a [(11)C]-(+)-PHNO PET study. Transl Psychiatry. 2019;9(1):287.

119. Egerton A, Valmaggia LR, Howes OD, Day F, Chaddock CA, Allen P, et al. Adversity in childhood linked to elevated striatal dopamine function in adulthood. Schizophr Res. 2016;176(2–3):171–6.
120. Shah JL, Malla AK. Much ado about much: stress, dynamic biomarkers and HPA axis dysregulation along the trajectory to psychosis. Schizophr Res. 2015;162(1–3):253–60.
121. Girshkin L, Matheson SL, Shepherd AM, Green MJ. Morning cortisol levels in schizophrenia and bipolar disorder: a meta-analysis. Psychoneuroendocrinology. 2014;49:187–206.
122. Hubbard DB, Miller BJ. Meta-analysis of blood cortisol levels in individuals with first-episode psychosis. Psychoneuroendocrinology. 2019;104:269–75.
123. Misiak B, Pruessner M, Samochowiec J, Wiśniewski M, Reginia A, Stańczykiewicz B. A meta-analysis of blood and salivary cortisol levels in first-episode psychosis and high-risk individuals. Front Neuroendocrinol. 2021;62:100930.
124. Berger M, Kraeuter AK, Romanik D, Malouf P, Amminger GP, Sarnyai Z. Cortisol awakening response in patients with psychosis: systematic review and meta-analysis. Neurosci Biobehav Rev. 2016;68:157–66.
125. Ciufolini S, Dazzan P, Kempton MJ, Pariante C, Mondelli V. HPA axis response to social stress is attenuated in schizophrenia but normal in depression: evidence from a meta-analysis of existing studies. Neurosci Biobehav Rev. 2014;47:359–68.
126. Dauvermann MR, Donohoe G. Cortisol stress response in psychosis from the high-risk to the chronic stage: a systematic review. Ir J Psychol Med. 2019;36(4):305–15.
127. Zorn JV, Schür RR, Boks MP, Kahn RS, Joëls M, Vinkers CH. Cortisol stress reactivity across psychiatric disorders: a systematic review and meta-analysis. Psychoneuroendocrinology. 2017;77:25–36.
128. Pruessner M, Béchard-Evans L, Boekestyn L, Iyer SN, Pruessner JC, Malla AK. Attenuated cortisol response to acute psychosocial stress in individuals at ultra-high risk for psychosis. Schizophr Res. 2013;146(1–3):79–86.
129. Pruessner M, Cullen AE, Aas M, Walker EF. The neural diathesis-stress model of schizophrenia revisited: an update on recent findings considering illness stage and neurobiological and methodological complexities. Neurosci Biobehav Rev. 2017;73:191–218.
130. Lupien SJ, Juster RP, Raymond C, Marin MF. The effects of chronic stress on the human brain: from neurotoxicity, to vulnerability, to opportunity. Front Neuroendocrinol. 2018;49:91–105.
131. Selten JP, van Os J, Cantor-Graae E. The social defeat hypothesis of schizophrenia: issues of measurement and reverse causality. World Psychiatry. 2016;15(3):294–5.
132. Egerton A, Howes OD, Houle S, McKenzie K, Valmaggia LR, Bagby MR, et al. Elevated striatal dopamine function in immigrants and their children: a risk mechanism for psychosis. Schizophr Bull. 2017;43(2):293–301.
133. Clark US, Miller ER, Hegde RR. Experiences of discrimination are associated with greater resting amygdala activity and functional connectivity. Biol Psychiatry Cogn Neurosci Neuroimaging. 2018;3(4):367–78.
134. Walther S, Lefebvre S, Conring F, Gangl N, Nadesalingam N, Alexaki D, et al. Limbic links to paranoia: increased resting-state functional connectivity between amygdala, hippocampus and orbitofrontal cortex in schizophrenia patients with paranoia. Eur Arch Psychiatry Clin Neurosci. 2022;272(6):1021–32.
135. Gur RE, Moore TM, Rosen AFG, Barzilay R, Roalf DR, Calkins ME, et al. Burden of environmental adversity associated with psychopathology, maturation, and brain behavior parameters in youths. JAMA Psychiatr. 2019;76(9):966–75.
136. Morgan C, Charalambides M, Hutchinson G, Murray RM. Migration, ethnicity, and psychosis: toward a sociodevelopmental model. Schizophr Bull. 2010;36(4):655–64.
137. Anglin DM, Ereshefsky S, Klaunig MJ, Bridgwater MA, Niendam TA, Ellman LM, et al. From womb to neighborhood: a racial analysis of social determinants of psychosis in the United States. Am J Psychiatry. 2021;178(7):599–610.
138. Anglin DM, Lighty Q, Greenspoon M, Ellman LM. Racial discrimination is associated with distressing subthreshold positive psychotic symptoms among US urban ethnic minority young adults. Soc Psychiatry Psychiatr Epidemiol. 2014;49(10):1545–55.

139. Oh H, Yang LH, Anglin DM, DeVylder JE. Perceived discrimination and psychotic experiences across multiple ethnic groups in the United States. Schizophr Res. 2014;157(1–3):259–65.
140. Stowkowy J, Liu L, Cadenhead KS, Cannon TD, Cornblatt BA, McGlashan TH, et al. Early traumatic experiences, perceived discrimination and conversion to psychosis in those at clinical high risk for psychosis. Soc Psychiatry Psychiatr Epidemiol. 2016;51(4):497–503.
141. Alameda L, Liu Z, Sham PC, Aas M, Trotta G, Rodriguez V, et al. Exploring the mediation of DNA methylation across the epigenome between childhood adversity and First Episode of Psychosis-findings from the EU-GEI study. Mol Psychiatry. 2023;28(5):2095–106.
142. Trotta G, Rodriguez V, Quattrone D, Spinazzolla E, Tripoli G, Gayer-Anderson CG, et al. Cannabis use as a potential mediator between childhood adversity and first-episode psychosis: results from the EU-GEI case-control study. Psychol Med. 2023;53(15):7375–84. https://doi.org/10.1017/S0033291723000995. Epub 2023 May 4
143. Heinz A, Murray GK, Schlagenhauf F, Sterzer P, Grace AA, Waltz JA. Towards a unifying cognitive, neurophysiological, and computational neuroscience account of schizophrenia. Schizophr Bull. 2019;45(5):1092–100.
144. Wortinger LA, Engen K, Barth C, Lonning V, Jørgensen KN, Andreassen OA, et al. Obstetric complications and intelligence in patients on the schizophrenia-bipolar spectrum and healthy participants. Psychol Med. 2020;50(11):1914–22.
145. Baeza I, de la Serna E, Amoretti S, Cuesta MJ, Díaz-Caneja CM, Mezquida G, et al. Premorbid characteristics as predictors of early onset versus adult onset in patients with a first episode of psychosis. J Clin Psychiatry. 2021;82(6)
146. Costas-Carrera A, Verdolini N, Garcia-Rizo C, Mezquida G, Janssen J, Valli I, et al. Difficulties during delivery, brain ventricle enlargement and cognitive impairment in first episode psychosis. Psychol Med. 2024;54(7):1339–49.
147. Forte MF, Oliva V, De Prisco M, Garriga M, Bitanihirwe B, Alameda L, et al. Obstetric complications and psychopathology in schizophrenia: a systematic review and meta-analysis. Neurosci Biobehav Rev. 2024;167:105913.
148. Millgate E, Smart SE, Pardiñas AF, Kravariti E, Ajnakina O, Kępińska AP, et al. Cognitive performance at first episode of psychosis and the relationship with future treatment resistance: evidence from an international prospective cohort study. Schizophr Res. 2023;255:173–81.
149. Demjaha A, Lappin JM, Stahl D, Patel MX, MacCabe JH, Howes OD, et al. Antipsychotic treatment resistance in first-episode psychosis: prevalence, subtypes and predictors. Psychol Med. 2017;47(11):1981–9.
150. Lally J, Ajnakina O, Di Forti M, Trotta A, Demjaha A, Kolliakou A, et al. Two distinct patterns of treatment resistance: clinical predictors of treatment resistance in first-episode schizophrenia spectrum psychoses. Psychol Med. 2016;46(15):3231–40.
151. Mouchlianitis E, Bloomfield MA, Law V, Beck K, Selvaraj S, Rasquinha N, et al. Treatment-resistant schizophrenia patients show elevated anterior cingulate cortex glutamate compared to treatment-responsive. Schizophr Bull. 2016;42(3):744–52.
152. Vita A, Minelli A, Barlati S, Deste G, Giacopuzzi E, Valsecchi P, et al. Treatment-resistant schizophrenia: genetic and neuroimaging correlates. Front Pharmacol. 2019;10:402.
153. Cella M, Preti A, Edwards C, Dow T, Wykes T. Cognitive remediation for negative symptoms of schizophrenia: a network meta-analysis. Clin Psychol Rev. 2017;52:43–51.
154. Lejeune JA, Northrop A, Kurtz MM. A meta-analysis of cognitive remediation for schizophrenia: efficacy and the role of participant and treatment factors. Schizophr Bull. 2021;47(4):997–1006.
155. Hassiotis A, Ukoumunne OC, Byford S, Tyrer P, Harvey K, Piachaud J, et al. Intellectual functioning and outcome of patients with severe psychotic illness randomised to intensive case management. Report from the UK700 trial. Br J Psychiatry. 2001;178:166–71.
156. Turner DT, McGlanaghy E, Cuijpers P, van der Gaag M, Karyotaki E, MacBeth A. A meta-analysis of social skills training and related interventions for psychosis. Schizophr Bull. 2018;44(3):475–91.

157. Dauwan M, Begemann MJ, Heringa SM, Sommer IE. Exercise improves clinical symptoms, quality of life, global functioning, and depression in schizophrenia: a systematic review and meta-analysis. Schizophr Bull. 2016;42(3):588–99.

158. Firth J, Stubbs B, Rosenbaum S, Vancampfort D, Malchow B, Schuch F, et al. Aerobic exercise improves cognitive functioning in people with schizophrenia: a systematic review and meta-analysis. Schizophr Bull. 2017;43(3):546–56.

159. Fernández-Abascal B, Suárez-Pinilla P, Cobo-Corrales C, Crespo-Facorro B, Suárez-Pinilla M. In- and outpatient lifestyle interventions on diet and exercise and their effect on physical and psychological health: a systematic review and meta-analysis of randomised controlled trials in patients with schizophrenia spectrum disorders and first episode of psychosis. Neurosci Biobehav Rev. 2021;125:535–68.

160. Lak M, Jafarpour A, Shahrbaf MA, Lak M, Dolatshahi B. The effect of physical exercise on cognitive function in schizophrenia patients: a GRADE assessed systematic review and meta-analysis of controlled clinical trials. Schizophr Res. 2024;271:81–90.

161. Sung MC, Ku B, Leung W, MacDonald M. The effect of physical activity interventions on executive function among people with neurodevelopmental disorders: a meta-analysis. J Autism Dev Disord. 2022;52(3):1030–50.

162. Su WC, Amonkar N, Cleffi C, Srinivasan S, Bhat A. Neural effects of physical activity and movement interventions in individuals with developmental disabilities-a systematic review. Front Psychiatry. 2022;13:794652.

163. Casetta C, Santosh P, Bayley R, Bisson J, Byford S, Dixon C, et al. CLEAR - clozapine in early psychosis: study protocol for a multi-centre, randomised controlled trial of clozapine vs other antipsychotics for young people with treatment resistant schizophrenia in real world settings. BMC Psychiatry. 2024;24(1):122.

164. Vita A, Nibbio G, Barlati S. Pharmacological treatment of cognitive impairment associated with schizophrenia: state of the art and future perspectives. Schizophr Bull Open. 2024;5(1):sgae013.

165. Ferraro L, Russo M, O'Connor J, Wiffen BD, Falcone MA, Sideli L, et al. Cannabis users have higher premorbid IQ than other patients with first onset psychosis. Schizophr Res. 2013;150(1):129–35.

166. Ferraro L, Di Forti M, La Barbera D, La Cascia C, Morgan C, Tripoli G, et al. Cognitive presentation at psychosis onset through premorbid deterioration and exposure to environmental risk factors. Psychol Med. 2025;55:e12.

167. Di Forti M, Sallis H, Allegri F, Trotta A, Ferraro L, Stilo SA, et al. Daily use, especially of high-potency cannabis, drives the earlier onset of psychosis in cannabis users. Schizophr Bull. 2014;40(6):1509–17.

168. Ferraro L, Murray RM, Di Forti M, Quattrone D, Tripoli G, Sideli L, et al. IQ differences between patients with first episode psychosis in London and Palermo reflect differences in patterns of cannabis use. Schizophr Res. 2019;210:81–8.

169. Menendez-Miranda I, Garcia-Alvarez L, Garcia-Portilla MP, Gonzalez-Blanco L, Saiz PA, Bobes J. History of lifetime cannabis use is associated with better cognition and worse real-world functioning in schizophrenia spectrum disorders. Eur Addict Res. 2019;25(3):111–8.

170. Yücel M, Bora E, Lubman DI, Solowij N, Brewer WJ, Cotton SM, et al. The impact of cannabis use on cognitive functioning in patients with schizophrenia: a meta-analysis of existing findings and new data in a first-episode sample. Schizophr Bull. 2012;38(2):316–30.

171. Schnakenberg MAM, Bonfils KA, Davis BJ, Smith EA, Schuder K, Lysaker PH. Compared to high and low cannabis use, moderate use is associated with fewer cognitive deficits in psychosis. Schizophr Res Cogn. 2016;6:15–21.

172. Rabin RA, Zakzanis KK, George TP. The effects of cannabis use on neurocognition in schizophrenia: a meta-analysis. Schizophr Res. 2011;128(1–3):111–6.

173. Schnell T, Koethe D, Daumann J, Gouzoulis-Mayfrank E. The role of cannabis in cognitive functioning of patients with schizophrenia. Psychopharmacology (Berl). 2009;205(1):45–52.

174. Cunha PJ, Rosa PG, Ayres Ade M, Duran FL, Santos LC, Scazufca M, et al. Cannabis use, cognition and brain structure in first-episode psychosis. Schizophr Res. 2013;147(2–3):209–15.

175. Malchow B, Hasan A, Fusar-Poli P, Schmitt A, Falkai P, Wobrock T. Cannabis abuse and brain morphology in schizophrenia: a review of the available evidence. Eur Arch Psychiatry Clin Neurosci. 2013;263(1):3–13.

176. Schoeler T, Monk A, Sami MB, Klamerus E, Foglia E, Brown R, et al. Continued versus discontinued cannabis use in patients with psychosis: a systematic review and meta-analysis. Lancet Psychiatry. 2016;3(3):215–25.

177. Volkow ND, Wang GJ, Fowler JS, Tomasi D, Telang F. Addiction: beyond dopamine reward circuitry. Proc Natl Acad Sci U S A. 2011;108(37):15037–42.

178. Proebstl L, Kamp F, Manz K, Krause D, Adorjan K, Pogarell O, et al. Effects of stimulant drug use on the dopaminergic system: a systematic review and meta-analysis of in vivo neuroimaging studies. Eur Psychiatry. 2019;59:15–24.

179. Voruganti LN, Heslegrave RJ, Awad AG. Neuroleptic dysphoria may be the missing link between schizophrenia and substance abuse. J Nerv Ment Dis. 1997;185(7):463–5.

180. Moreira FA, Dalley JW. Dopamine receptor partial agonists and addiction. Eur J Pharmacol. 2015;752:112–5.

181. Rafizadeh R, Danilewitz M, Bousman CA, Mathew N, White RF, Bahji A, et al. Effects of clozapine treatment on the improvement of substance use disorders other than nicotine in individuals with schizophrenia spectrum disorders: a systematic review and meta-analysis. J Psychopharmacol. 2023;37(2):135–43.

182. Trigo JM, Lagzdins D, Rehm J, Selby P, Gamaleddin I, Fischer B, et al. Effects of fixed or self-titrated dosages of Sativex on cannabis withdrawal and cravings. Drug Alcohol Depend. 2016;161:298–306.

183. Di Forti M, Bond BW, Spinazzola E, Trotta G, Lynn J, Malkin R, et al. A proof-of-concept analysis of data from the first NHS clinic for young adults with comorbid cannabis use and psychotic disorders. BJPsych Open. 2024;11(1):e1.

184. Alameda L, Christy A, Rodriguez V, Salazar de Pablo G, Thrush M, Shen Y, et al. Association between specific childhood adversities and symptom dimensions in people with psychosis: systematic review and meta-analysis. Schizophr Bull. 2021;47(4):975–85.

185. Vargas T, Lam PH, Azis M, Osborne KJ, Lieberman A, Mittal VA. Childhood trauma and neurocognition in adults with psychotic disorders: a systematic review and meta-analysis. Schizophr Bull. 2019;45(6):1195–208.

186. Bailey T, Alvarez-Jimenez M, Garcia-Sanchez AM, Hulbert C, Barlow E, Bendall S. Childhood trauma is associated with severity of hallucinations and delusions in psychotic disorders: a systematic review and meta-aAnalysis. Schizophr Bull. 2018;44(5):1111–22.

187. Christy A, Cavero D, Navajeeva S, Murray-O'Shea R, Rodriguez V, Aas M, et al. Association between childhood adversity and functional outcomes in people with psychosis: a meta-analysis. Schizophr Bull. 2023;49(2):285–96.

188. Fares-Otero NE, Alameda L, Pfaltz MC, Martinez-Aran A, Schäfer I, Vieta E. Examining associations, moderators and mediators between childhood maltreatment, social functioning, and social cognition in psychotic disorders: a systematic review and meta-analysis. Psychol Med. 2023;53(13):5909–32.

189. Peters E, Hardy A, Dudley R, Varese F, Greenwood K, Steel C, et al. Multisite randomised controlled trial of trauma-focused cognitive behaviour therapy for psychosis to reduce post-traumatic stress symptoms in people with co-morbid post-traumatic stress disorder and psychosis, compared to treatment as usual: study protocol for the STAR (Study of Trauma And Recovery) trial. Trials. 2022;23(1):429.

190. Varese F, Sellwood W, Aseem S, Awenat Y, Bird L, Bhutani G, et al. Eye movement desensitization and reprocessing therapy for psychosis (EMDRp): protocol of a feasibility randomized controlled trial with early intervention service users. Early Interv Psychiatry. 2021;15(5):1224–33.

191. Peters E. Findings from STAR TRIAL presented at Institute of Psychiatry, Psychology and Nueoroscience; 2025.

192. Varese F, Sellwood W, Pulford D, Awenat Y, Bird L, Bhutani G, et al. Trauma-focused therapy in early psychosis: results of a feasibility randomized controlled trial of EMDR for psychosis (EMDRp) in early intervention settings. Psychol Med. 2024;54(5):874–85.

193. van Os J, Pries LK, Ten Have M, de Graaf R, van Dorsselaer S, Delespaul P, et al. Evidence, and replication thereof, that molecular-genetic and environmental risks for psychosis impact through an affective pathway. Psychol Med. 2020:1–13.
194. Alameda L, Conus P, Ramain J, Solida A, Golay P. Evidence of mediation of severity of anxiety and depressive symptoms between abuse and positive symptoms of psychosis. J Psychiatr Res. 2022;150:353–9.
195. Alameda L, Golay P, Baumann PS, Progin P, Mebdouhi N, Elowe J, et al. Mild depressive symptoms mediate the impact of childhood trauma on long-term functional outcome in early psychosis patients. Schizophr Bull. 2017;43(5):1027–35.
196. Bergink V, Rasgon N, Wisner KL. Postpartum psychosis: madness, mania, and melancholia in motherhood. Am J Psychiatry. 2016;173(12):1179–88.
197. Jairaj C, Seneviratne G, Bergink V, Sommer IE, Dazzan P. Postpartum psychosis: a proposed treatment algorithm. J Psychopharmacol. 2023;37(10):960–70.
198. Wise PM, Dubal DB, Rau SW, Brown CM, Suzuki S. Are estrogens protective or risk factors in brain injury and neurodegeneration? Reevaluation after the Women's health initiative. Endocr Rev. 2005;26(3):308–12.
199. Bendis PC, Zimmerman S, Onisiforou A, Zanos P, Georgiou P. The impact of estradiol on serotonin, glutamate, and dopamine systems. Front Neurosci. 2024;18:1348551.
200. Brand BA, EJM W, IMH H, Sommer IE. Evidence-based recommendations for the pharmacological treatment of women with shizophrenia spectrum disorders. Curr Psychiatry Rep. 2023;25(11):723–33.
201. de Boer J, Prikken M, Lei WU, Begemann M, Sommer I. The effect of raloxifene augmentation in men and women with a schizophrenia spectrum disorder: a systematic review and meta-analysis. NPJ Schizophr. 2018;4(1):1.
202. Brand BA, de Boer JN, Marcelis MC, Grootens KP, Luykx JJ, Sommer IE. The direct and long-term effects of raloxifene as adjunctive treatment for schizophrenia-spectrum disorders: a double-blind, randomized clinical trial. Schizophr Bull. 2023;49(6):1579–90.
203. Brand BA, Sommer IE, Gangadin SS, Tanskanen A, Tiihonen J, Taipale H. Real-world effectiveness of menopausal hormone therapy in preventing relapse in women with schizophrenia or schizoaffective disorder. Am J Psychiatry. 2024;181(10):893–900.
204. Clancy MJ, Clarke MC, Connor DJ, Cannon M, Cotter DR. The prevalence of psychosis in epilepsy; a systematic review and meta-analysis. BMC Psychiatry. 2014;14:75.
205. Lennox BR, Palmer-Cooper EC, Pollak T, Hainsworth J, Marks J, Jacobson L, et al. Prevalence and clinical characteristics of serum neuronal cell surface antibodies in first-episode psychosis: a case-control study. Lancet Psychiatry. 2017;4(1):42–8.
206. Austin-Zimmerman I, Spinazzola E, Quattrone D, Wu-Choi B, Trotta G, Li Z, et al. The impact of schizophrenia genetic load and heavy cannabis use on the risk of psychotic disorder in the EU-GEI case-control and UK Biobank studies. Psychol Med. 2024;54(15):1–13. https://doi.org/10.1017/S0033291724002058.
207. Cougnard A, Marcelis M, Myin-Germeys I, De Graaf R, Vollebergh W, Krabbendam L, et al. Does normal developmental expression of psychosis combine with environmental risk to cause persistence of psychosis? A psychosis proneness-persistence model. Psychol Med. 2007;37(4):513–27.
208. Vassos E, Sham P, Kempton M, Trotta A, Stilo SA, Gayer-Anderson C, et al. The Maudsley environmental risk score for psychosis. Psychol Med. 2020;50(13):2213–20.
209. Pries LK, Erzin G, Rutten BPF, van Os J, Guloksuz S. Estimating aggregate environmental risk score in psychiatry: the exposome score for schizophrenia. Front Psychiatry. 2021;12:671334.
210. Oliver D, Radua J, Reichenberg A, Uher R, Fusar-Poli P. Psychosis Polyrisk Score (PPS) for the detection of individuals at-risk and the prediction of their outcomes. Front Psychiatry. 2019;10 https://doi.org/10.3389/fpsyt.2019.00174.
211. Murray RM, Paparelli A, Di Forti M, Morrison PD. The rising tide of drug-induced psychosis. Neuropsychiatrie. 2025; In Press

Open Access This chapter is licensed under the terms of the Creative Commons Attribution 4.0 International License (http://creativecommons.org/licenses/by/4.0/), which permits use, sharing, adaptation, distribution and reproduction in any medium or format, as long as you give appropriate credit to the original author(s) and the source, provide a link to the Creative Commons license and indicate if changes were made.

The images or other third party material in this chapter are included in the chapter's Creative Commons license, unless indicated otherwise in a credit line to the material. If material is not included in the chapter's Creative Commons license and your intended use is not permitted by statutory regulation or exceeds the permitted use, you will need to obtain permission directly from the copyright holder.

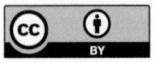

The Best Psychiatry in the World: Ambition and Achievement in Denmark

26

Merete Nordentoft

26.1 The Best Psychiatry in the World: Nirvana or Denmark?

When the editors invited me to write this chapter, my initial thought was that they were envisioning some Nirvana-like utopian ideal in the distant future. However, I soon realised they were referring to Denmark. Upon reflection, I began to consider that, despite the many ongoing challenges and complaints voiced by both patients and professionals, Danish psychiatry might indeed be among the best in the world. Sadly, these considerations reflect that even though Denmark is not a perfect place, it could be much worse.

Denmark, with a population of six million, has approximately 14,000 supported accommodation facilities and 3000 psychiatric beds. The psychiatric secondary healthcare sector employs around 11,000 clinical staff members, including nurses, psychiatrists, psychologists, nurse aides, occupational therapists, social workers and others. However, outpatient services are often perceived as understaffed, while the number of inpatient facilities is frequently considered insufficient to meet the population's needs.

I realise how much worse conditions can be elsewhere. In some countries, deinstitutionalisation has nearly eliminated all hospital beds and outpatient services are severely understaffed, underfunded and unable to adequately care for the most severely ill patients. In many countries, the public sector often struggles to employ enough psychiatrists, with many instead working in private practice, and the reliance on temporary locum doctors undermines organisational continuity, professionalism and long-term improvements. Furthermore, social services in many places are insufficient, lacking supported accommodation or well-managed programmes for

M. Nordentoft (✉)
Copenhagen Research Center for Mental Health, Mental Health Center Copenhagen, Bispebjerg and Frederiksberg Hospital, Copenhagen, Denmark
e-mail: merete.nordentoft@dadlnet.dk

© The Author(s) 2026
G. Ikkos, T. Becker (eds.), *Psychiatry after Kraepelin*,
https://doi.org/10.1007/978-3-032-09475-9_26

homeless individuals, which further exacerbates the challenges faced by vulnerable populations.

Denmark is a welfare state characterised by one of the world's lowest levels of inequality (Gini coefficient = 0.25) and a low level of corruption. The country also boasts high levels of safety, minimal crime, low murder rates and a small prison population. Additionally, Denmark has a high literacy rate and, for several years, has consistently ranked as one of the happiest nations in the world according to the World Happiness Report [1].

We have a well-developed general practice system, free maternity care, free health visitor services for small children with a very high acceptance rate, school nurses and well-trained staff in childcare institutions. We also have a rather well-developed system with psychologists employed by municipalities to address mental health issues in schools. We have good access to a highly skilled workforce. Additionally, we have unique research opportunities thanks to Danish registries and biobanks, a large pool of talented researchers, world-class research environments, PhD programmes and other networks at universities. All of this has given us a strong foundation to build world-class psychiatry.

With this background, I chose to approach this chapter as both a reflection on the current state of Danish psychiatry and an exploration of the potential improvements outlined in the 10-year plan for Psychiatry [2]. This plan includes a significant commitment to increasing the state budget for psychiatry by 35% annually, a measure aimed at addressing existing challenges and ensuring substantial, sustained improvements. By examining how this increased funding will enhance services and infrastructure, I also consider how Danish psychiatry could ideally evolve in the future.

In this chapter, I will mainly focus on the services for people aged 18 years and older.

26.1.1 Equal Rights to Healthcare

At the heart of any great mental health system lies the principle of equal access to care.

In an ideal world, mental health services would be universally accessible and equitably distributed, ensuring that every citizen has access to the support they need regardless of socioeconomic status.

In many parts of the world, access to high-quality mental health services is often reserved for the wealthy or those with comprehensive health insurance—whether privately obtained or linked to employment. In some cases, insurance is only available to those without pre-existing conditions and coverage often comes with strict limitations on the duration or cost of treatment. In the most unequal systems, as much as 80% of psychiatrists serve the wealthiest 20% of the population, leaving just 20% of professionals to address the needs of the remaining 80% [3].

In Denmark, as in other Nordic countries, the healthcare system is funded through taxes and is primarily owned and managed by the state, regions, or municipalities. This structure ensures that services are generally universally accessible without direct out-of-pocket payments. Philosophically, the Danish model reflects a social contract approach: all citizens contribute through taxes to a shared healthcare system, not knowing who will ultimately require its services [4]. In this way, healthcare and care for the elderly, is treated as a collective responsibility.

Suffering from a mental illness can be profoundly challenging, reflecting a sad and difficult aspect of the human condition. However, it is reassuring to know that the healthcare system is doing everything in its power to provide support and care. The combination of a comprehensive social security system and the right to free treatment for psychiatric and somatic disorders establishes a solid foundation for primary, secondary and tertiary prevention. In an ideal world, mental health services should be equally and easily available for all citizens.

A tax-financed system can be very cost-effective. Administrative overhead is minimised, and service providers are incentivised to deliver the most cost-effective treatments. One could add that this occurs with an understanding that resources are managed optimally and that the trust between citizens and the healthcare system leads to a reduced tendency to practice defensive medicine. There is trust that the healthcare system manages resources efficiently, and the extent of defensive medical practices has decreased. As a result, Denmark's healthcare expenditure per capita is roughly half that of the United States. Discussions of costs often overlook the broader implications—such as the emotional and financial toll on individuals and families, or the expenses borne by other societal institutions like foster care, homeless shelters and prisons, which frequently absorb the unmet needs of those with severe mental illness. However, in more recent years, in Denmark as elsewhere private health insurance and private practitioner has increased inequality in mental health by making mental health services more available for privileged citizens. This has especially been relevant for children being referred to child and adolescent psychiatry, as waiting lists in public services have increased.

26.1.2 Diversity, Equity and Inclusion

The Danish government works with equity and inclusion in various areas, for example, through equality policies, anti-discrimination legislation and initiatives to promote diversity in the labour market.

For people with mental illness and neurodivergence, legislation provides access to financial support and coaching within the educational system and labour market. One example of this is the nationwide rollout of the Individual Placement and Support (IPS) programme [5].

However, even in Denmark, which boasts universal healthcare funded by taxes, disparities in access to care exist. Key structural barriers include availability, accessibility and affordability [6]. Accessibility issues, such as access to transportation or challenges stemming from physical or mental disabilities, affect various groups. These groups include individuals living in supported accommodations and shelters, experiencing homelessness, or those serving a court sentence [7–9]. Some structural changes have been implemented for selected groups of patients to ensure better access to healthcare services in Denmark. One example of such interventions is included in the collective agreement with Danish General Practitioners (GPs) on a more extensive physical examination of people with mental illness in general practice. Another example is implementation of housing first policy [10] to improve living conditions of homeless people with mental disorders.

26.1.3 A Healthcare System Taking Care of All Phases of Mental Illness

The Danish healthcare system is designed to address all phases of mental illness, ensuring comprehensive care tailored to each stage of a person's condition. Even before the onset of illness, interventions aimed at primary prevention can be implemented. These might include school-based programmes and visiting nurses focusing on the mental health of children and young people. For individuals in the early phases, characterised by subtle symptoms, the primary point of entry is often through primary care or school health services. From there, referrals can be made to private psychiatrists or secondary healthcare services for further assessment and treatment.

A variety of specialised services are in place to support severely ill individuals at every stage of their illness. These include early intervention programmes, such as OPUS for first-episode psychosis and similar initiatives for the first episode of bipolar disorder. Continuous treatment is available for individuals with long-term mental illness and significant challenges in daily functioning. Additionally, the system provides access to inpatient facilities, including specialised units, supported accommodation and outreach teams for homeless individuals. Programmes such as Housing First and acute psychiatric emergency outreach further enhance the ability to deliver timely and effective care to those in need.

In the following, some of the most important elements in Danish mental healthcare system will be mentioned.

26.1.4 Right to Evidence-Based Treatment

Equal right to treatment is only meaningful if it is linked to high quality of care. In Denmark, psychiatric disorders have since 2013 been covered by a guarantee of individual evaluation and treatment within 30 days in the secondary health sector. If the local regional facility cannot meet this timeframe, patients can receive evaluation and treatment at another hospital or a private hospital free of charge. Overall, in secondary healthcare, more than 90% of adult patients begin treatment within the 30-day timeframe. Between 2007 and 2022, the number of patients receiving treatment increased by 33%, primarily due to improved access to outpatient services and increased public and professional awareness of ADHD, autism spectrum disorders and Post Tramumatic Stress Disorder (PTSD). Patients benefit from guaranteed quick access to evaluation and evidence-based treatment without individual payment or concerns about insurance coverage.

Evidence-based medicine serves as the cornerstone of service delivery. The Danish Health Authority has established national guidelines covering a wide range of psychiatric conditions, including schizophrenia, bipolar disorder, major depression, ADHD, autism, anxiety disorders, eating disorders, borderline personality disorder, Obsessive Compulsive Disorder (OCD), and dual diagnosis. These guidelines are grounded in systematic reviews and meta-analyses, ensuring a rigorous and scientifically supported foundation for care [11]. Building on these national guidelines, more detailed recommendations for treatment are outlined in national programmes addressing various psychiatric and child and adolescent psychiatric conditions. Currently, 15 programmes are in place, covering conditions such as first-episode schizophrenia, bipolar disorder, anxiety, depression, eating disorders, PTSD, OCD, ADHD and emotionally unstable personality disorder. Each programme provides a concise description of the recommended treatment elements and their duration. Evidence-based treatments, such as cognitive behavioural therapy (CBT) and dialectical behaviour therapy (DBT), are recommended for conditions where their effectiveness has been scientifically demonstrated.

Across the national regions, these programmes are implemented through structured 'treatment packages', which vary in length depending on the condition. For example, the programme for first-episode schizophrenia is designed to last up to 2 years and includes the same elements as OPUS, Denmark's early intervention service for psychosis [12].

Treatment packages for moderate and severe anxiety and depression are typically shorter, lasting around 14 weeks and involving weekly sessions. Regional health authorities determine the organisation of these treatments, which may be delivered in group settings, individualised formats, or a combination of both. Currently, it is obvious that not all patients included in these treatment packages will gain a satisfactory treatment outcome after treatment has ended. In future planning, the packages will be revised so that they become more flexible and include principles of continuity of care to a higher degree.

Mild depression is generally managed within the primary healthcare sector, either by general practitioners (GPs), private psychologists, or private psychiatric practitioners. Both GPs and private psychiatrists operate under agreements with the regional healthcare system, ensuring that treatment remains free of charge.

Mental health services are provided by regional health authorities. In 2022, the secondary mental health sector treated 145,000 patients as inpatients or outpatients, with 25,000 requiring inpatient care.

26.1.5 Acute Psychiatric Outreach

Since 1997, the Capital Region has implemented Acute Psychiatric Outreach, targeting individuals with severe mental illness or those in crisis who cannot resolve their problems through a GP on call or by visiting a psychiatric emergency room. This service is uniquely staffed by a psychiatrist and an ambulance driver, allowing for emergency visits, even in challenging and potentially dangerous situations.

The target group includes individuals in acute need of psychiatric intervention due to mental illness, severe crises, or posing a danger to themselves or others. The service allows patients, relatives, general practitioners, the police and social security services to contact Acute Psychiatric Outreach directly. In cases involving violence or threats, the police collaborate with the psychiatric outreach team to address the situation. This joint approach enables the service to address some of the challenges faced by severely mentally ill individuals in the community, including facilitating referrals, voluntary care, or compulsory admissions when necessary. Acute Psychiatric Outreach can solve some of the problems of the severely mentally ill in the community by organizing referrals to services, voluntary or compulsory admissions. Most calls to the service are highly relevant, involving people who fall within the target group for immediate psychiatric intervention [13].

In addition to Acute Psychiatric Outreach, most psychiatric clinics also have acute teams that can support patients shortly after discharge or provide a short-term alternative to admission.

26.1.6 OPUS: Specialised Assertive Early Intervention

The early phase of psychosis is the most vulnerable phase with high risk of suicidal acts and social marginalisation. The evidence for the effectiveness of specialised assertive early intervention services is supported by the results of the OPUS trial [14] and from findings in other trials such as LEO [15] and RAISE [16]. There are positive effects on psychotic and negative symptoms, on substance abuse and user satisfaction. This is summarised in a comprehensive meta-analysis [17]. Disappointingly, the clinical effects on psychotic and negative symptoms were not sustainable when patients were transferred to standard treatment [18]. However, the positive effects on service use and ability to live independently seem to be durable [19]. Health economic analyses indicate that specialised assertive treatment is better and cheaper than treatment as usual [20]. Implementation of specialised assertive early intervention services is recommended; several trials comparing 2 years of intervention with extended treatment periods indicate that longer treatment is associated with more beneficial outcomes [21–23].

In Denmark, the OPUS programme is the most comprehensive of the treatment packages. It is implemented all over Denmark, and the 10-year plan for Psychiatry is expected to strengthen the implementation even further [24].

26.1.7 Outreach Teams

For patients suffering from severe mental illness, Assertive Community Treeatment (ACT) teams were developed. The originally described ACT method entails that each primary caseworker is responsible for approximately ten patients. However, between 2010 and 2020, ACT in Denmark was gradually replaced by F-ACT (Flexible Assertive Community Treatment). This approach aimed to maintain the same outreach principles, but staff became responsible for a broader patient group, with each caseworker overseeing 30–40 patients. With the 10-year plan for Psychiatry, hopefully more staff can be employed to ensure sufficient level of care for the most disabled patients [2].

Specific and more well-resourced teams are operating for people with dual diagnosis, homeless mentally ill, and people with a court sentence to mandatory psychiatric treatment.

Recently, a political decision was made to integrate the treatment of substance use and mental illness within regional health facilities for individuals with dual diagnoses. This initiative is in its early stages and is expected to enhance the quality of care for this vulnerable group.

In larger Danish cities, there are specialised initiatives for the homeless. These include social interventions from the municipality based on 'housing first' principles [25], as well as regional health teams offering assistance with the treatment of psychiatric health problems [26].

26.1.8 Supported Accommodation Facilities

Supported accommodation is a vital resource for individuals with severe mental illnesses, who often have complex physical and mental health needs. In Denmark, 14,000 people live in such facilities, and the complexity of their situation is reflected in shorter life expectancy than others with similar level of psychiatric hospital contacts. The increased mortality rates are explained by increased rates of suicides, accidents and death by somatic disorders [27]. This population faces higher rates of untreated or undertreated somatic health issues and limited access to preventive care [8, 9, 28, 29]. Many have severe schizophrenia or similar illnesses, often on high-dose antipsychotics or polypharmacy, which are insufficiently monitored [30]. Substance abuse is also common, further increasing mortality [31].

Despite these significant needs, supported accommodation is typically staffed by non-medical personnel, with psychiatric and medical care provided externally. To address this, regional psychiatric outreach teams are being introduced nationwide as part of the 10-year plan for Psychiatry. These teams will offer on-site psychiatric evaluation, treatment and staff supervision. Moreover, when possible, admissions will be at specific wards to ensure continuity of care. Additionally, a new reform will affiliate general practitioners with these facilities to improve access to medical care.

26.1.9 Individual Placement and Support

Compared to prevocational training, there is clear evidence of the positive effects on labour market affiliation of the programme Individual Placement and Support. Most of the literature stems from the United States but a large Danish trial indicates that the same benefits can be achieved in high-welfare countries [5]. The key principle is to offer employment in a competitive labour market or an educational institution with individual adjustments, such as fewer hours per week, or a more protected function/work environment. As part of the 10-year plan for Psychiatry, this approach will gradually be implemented all over Denmark.

26.1.10 Monitoring of Quality

The implementation and quality of treatment are monitored through national quality databases for conditions such as schizophrenia, depression, bipolar disorder, Attention Deficit Hyperactive Disorder (ADHD) and forensic psychiatry. These databases utilise data from sources like the Danish Patient Registry, the National Prescription Registry and the Clinical Laboratory Information System Research Database, which includes laboratory-based biomarkers.

Quality indicators for schizophrenia, for example, include the proportion of first episode patients being interviewed with a diagnostic interview, proportion with family involvement in treatment, assessment of cognitive functioning, appropriate management of hypertension, high cholesterol and diabetes, as well as the rate of suicide attempts or deaths within 30 days of discharge [32, 33]. Each year, the performance of regions and hospitals is assessed against these standards. Overall, quality has been improving—for instance, there has been a significant rise in the proportion of schizophrenia patients receiving adequate monitoring of HbA1c and blood lipids. Systematic data collection supports feedback loops to clinicians, helping to enhance treatment quality.

The universal system includes an obligation to ensure consistent high quality of treatment by providing coordinated training and supervision of healthcare staff, such as nurses and doctors.

26.1.11 Civil Society

Denmark is fortunate to have many volunteer-driven organisations that do invaluable work for individuals with mental illnesses. In some cases, these organisations act as a 'first line of defence', while in others, they play a key role in enhancing the daily lives and well-being of those affected.

A few of the strongest organisations are listed below.

Headspace involves volunteers and offers conversation-based services. Most of Headspace's advisors are volunteers who wish to help and listen. Some are students some are adults interested in youth well-being, and seniors with professional experience working with young people.

Livslinien is a volunteer-driven help line focusing on helping people with suicidal ideation. It has phone and chat options, and work is based on a shared set of values and a common vision of preventing suicide.

The Psychiatric Foundation works broadly to combat mental illness and ensure better conditions for those affected. This is done through counselling, awareness-raising, political advocacy and collaboration with municipalities and other non-governmental organisations (NGOs).

Hope in Psychiatry is a charitable, nationwide association dedicated to improving the conditions for people with mental illness who are undergoing psychiatric treatment. The association's goal is to strengthen the individuals' courage, hope and agency through equal interaction and community-building activities.

OMBOLD is an organisation that organises football training, games, and tournaments for homeless and marginalised individuals. It promotes social inclusion, well-being and community building while fostering confidence, teamwork and a sense of belonging among participants.

Moreover, in addition to advocacy, several NGOs (e.g. SIND and Better Psychiatry) offer activities and support for people with mental illnesses and their relatives.

26.2   Factors Involved in Building the Momentum of the 10-Year Plan for Psychiatry

In 2022, the Danish government made the landmark decision to permanently increase the mental healthcare budget by in the first place approximately 20%, later presented as 35% increase [34]. Several factors contributed to creating the political momentum necessary for this achievement. Efforts to combat stigma, the presentation of compelling evidence on the burden of mental illness, a united front among stakeholders, and active lobbying all played crucial roles in securing this success. The work in these different areas is described in the following sections.

26.2.1 Fighting Stigma: The Cornerstone of Better Mental Healthcare

Stigmatisation of mental illness is an important reason to why treatment of mental illness is often underprioritised. In every classroom, there are almost four children who, before age 18, develop a psychiatric disorder requiring treatment. This is equivalent with 15% of all children being in contact with mental health services sometime during childhood [35]. If the class reunites 50 years later, this figure would be twice as high, as more than 30% will have been in contact with the psychiatric treatment system [36].

Mental illnesses are widespread public health issues—hidden, stigmatised and often kept secret. For example, when I have appeared on television to be interviewed about auditory hallucinations, the makeup artists or the programme hosts discreetly pull me aside to share stories of a son or nephew who hears voices. After every lecture—even at medical societies—someone takes me aside to consult me informally about a niece or stepdaughter experiencing voices, anxiety, or eating disorder.

My husband has a slipped disc. There is nothing secretive about it. It is also hard to hide, but there is no reason to hide it. At times, I almost get the impression he is proud of it. At one point, it was so severe that he could not sit or stand. In this extraordinary situation, his workplace responded by purchasing an expensive, advanced elevation bed for intermittent bed rest in his office, which he used for almost a year, creating a win–win situation for everyone. He returned to work and almost became a mascot for his workplace. The organisation received 100% of his productivity—and then some—while also gaining a sense of pride in being a workplace that accommodated employees with extensive and creative measures.

Why is it shameful to have depression but perfectly acceptable to have a herniated disc? Both conditions represent a vulnerability in human constitution—one affecting the spinal discs, the other involving the complex brain mechanisms that enable us to face life with energy and resilience. Both are influenced by external stressors and can affect relationships, work capacity and personal potential. Yet, mental illness is perceived as striking much closer to the core of what defines a person.

Depression is often viewed by those who suffer from it as a personal failure, a sign of weakness that most try to keep secret from their social circles and workplaces. Episodes of illness are often explained away or disguised, leaving gaps in resumes. Fortunately, some companies are open to hiring individuals with mental health challenges, even engaging with psychiatric professionals to understand how to create supportive work environments. Both small and large organisations take pride in fostering an inclusive society and a job market that accommodates individuals with physical or mental challenges.

Nonetheless, secrecy and fear dominate the conversation. Why must mental health issues remain such a closely guarded secret?

Part of the explanation lies in an implicit devaluation of individuals with mental illnesses. Offhand remarks like 'That must be one of your clients' to a person with colourful clothes or an atypical way of walking or 'I spent a year in a psychiatric ward once—as a doctor, of course', reveal this underlying and often unconscious bias. Such comments suggest a wish to assert, 'We—the normal ones—do not have mental issues'. You would never hear a similar joke about an orthopaedic ward: 'Haha, that must be someone with a broken leg'.

It is worth noting that societal acceptance of cancer is a relatively recent development. Cancer was once a stigmatised and secretive illness, but through extensive public information campaigns, increased funding and improved treatments, public perceptions of cancer have shifted [37].

Prejudice can be challenged through increased awareness of what mental illness truly entails. One of the most effective tools against stigma is education, especially through personal stories. A shining example is the 'OPUS panel', formed by young people treated for psychosis in the OPUS programme. Comprising 40 individuals and some of their relatives, the panel aims to share what it is like to live with an invisible yet severe illness—and to demonstrate that recovery and a good life are possible. They offer training at hospitals and outpatient clinics for staff, patients and relatives, and they engage with the media. Hearing personal accounts from real people significantly impacts societal perceptions of severe mental illnesses.

Fortunately, several renowned Danish artists have openly shared their experiences with anxiety, depression and ADHD. Recently, a prominent Danish author published a book detailing their treatment with electroconvulsive therapy for severe depression accompanied by psychotic delusions [38]. Together, these candid accounts have played a vital role in fostering public recognition of mental illnesses as significant health conditions that deserve appropriate treatment. The fact that one out of every three persons in Denmark will receive treatment from the mental health services, and that one out of every three are currently close to someone struggling with mental illness, tells a clear story: this concerns all of us.

26.2.2 Important Data Highlighted the Need for Investment

Denmark, like other Nordic countries, benefits from exceptional access to register-based data, enabling valuable insights across various areas. Research has shown that mental illnesses account for 25% of the total burden of disease, surpassing cancer (15%) and cardiovascular disease (17%) [2]. Part of the reason for this high figure is that mental illnesses are often long-lasting and tend to manifest early in life. For instance, 50% of all people with mental disorders have their first contact with the secondary health sector before the age of 18 [35]. Additionally, data have revealed a 10–15-year reduction in life expectancy among individuals with mental disorders [39, 40], increased somatic comorbidities [28], and dramatically elevated suicide rates shortly after discharge from psychiatric departments—200–400 times higher than the general population [41]. Also, the increase in the number of forensic patients has raised concerns. These findings have significantly shaped public discourse.

Epidemiological studies have repeatedly underscored that mental illness is a major public health concern. One in six children in Denmark has contact with mental health services before the age of 18 [35], and one-third of the population will receive treatment from mental health services during their lifetime [36]. Furthermore, Danish data indicating a 15–20-year reduction in workforce participation for individuals with mental illnesses have further highlighted the societal impact [42]. Together with WHO (World Health Organization) reports on treatment gaps [43], these findings provided compelling evidence of the urgent need for better mental health services.

This information was also disseminated through a popular Danish book titled *How to Create the Psychiatry of the Future* [44]. The book, part of a series addressing significant societal challenges, outlined the inequalities between somatic and psychiatric healthcare, particularly in terms of access to treatment, quality of care, excess mortality and stigma. It also proposed principles for future solutions.

Additionally, a marked increase in individuals seeking help from psychiatric services and a growing number of young people reporting difficulties thriving [45] raised concerns among healthcare providers, policymakers and the public. An alarming trend was also noted in the rising rates of readmissions within 30 days after discharge from psychiatric departments, which increased from 21% in 2014 to 24% in 2022.

Collectively, these findings underscore the critical need for substantial investment and improvement in psychiatric services.

26.2.3 Uniting All Forces in the Psychiatry Alliance

A key factor in this positive development has been the collaboration among NGOs and various professional groups, culminating in the formation of a unified organisation called the 'Psychiatry Alliance'. This alliance brings together user organisations, including both overarching user and family groups and disease-specific associations, as well as trade unions representing doctors, nurses, social workers, occupational therapists, physiotherapists, pedagogues and nursing aides. It also includes scientific societies for psychiatrists and psychologists.

Achieving this unification has been a long and challenging process. Initially, only a small number of organisations agreed on a limited set of common recommendations. However, in September 2021, 45 organisations came together to endorse a document called *Psykiatriløftet*—a title with a dual meaning in Danish, signifying both 'Promise to Psychiatry' and 'Lifting Psychiatry'. This document outlined eight key recommendations addressing critical priorities for both user groups and professionals.

The united effort played a significant role in garnering broad support for the 10-year plan for Psychiatry, developed by national health and social authorities. This collective action has truly transformed the landscape of mental health advocacy in Denmark. We are immensely proud and grateful to be part of this united movement.

26.2.4 Journalists Were Our Best Friends

Many organisations within the Psychiatry Alliance had established strong relationships with journalists from national television, radio and major newspapers. We frequently participated in interviews and appeared across various media platforms. All the largest organisations employed full-time or part-time journalists who assisted in writing opinion pieces and debate articles, ensuring their publication. Often, multiple organisations in the Psychiatry Alliance collaborated on joint viewpoints. Social media was also leveraged to disseminate key messages and to highlight the unity and mutual support among the organisations.

Many journalists showed a genuine interest in the cause, proactively posing relevant questions to politicians. This engagement made the media a valuable ally in bringing psychiatry to the forefront of public debate and the lead-up to the October 2022 election. Media outlets often reported on scientific findings, facilitated by a constructive collaboration where researchers explained their work, and journalists translated it into compelling news stories.

The central messages we emphasised were that psychiatric illnesses affect everyone, the current health and social care systems are inadequate and meaningful improvements for both patients and society are achievable with the right interventions.

During the general election, psychiatry emerged as the fourth most important issue for voters, ranking just behind climate change, the economy and general healthcare.

26.2.5 Presenting a Calculated Budget

In November 2021, the Danish Psychiatric Society, the Danish Child and Adolescent Psychiatric Society, and a professor in health economics collaborated to present a detailed and realistic budget for addressing the needs of psychiatric care in Denmark. This budget proposed an annual running cost of 4.5 billion Danish Kroner (0.6 billion Euros) and an additional 3.5 billion for capital expenditures. A large part of this tentative budget was set aside to increase capacity in both in- and out-patient treatment. By being the first to present concrete figures, this initiative set a benchmark for public debate and framed the expectations for the announced ten-year plan. The widely cited figures proved pivotal, ensuring the final budget aligned more closely with the identified needs.

26.2.6 An Assertive Approach Towards Politicians

Organisations within the Psychiatry Alliance maintained persistent and structured engagement with politicians across government, supporting parties and opposition. Psychiatry was recognised as a key issue across the political spectrum, and the Alliance effectively emphasised its broad voter base. Regular meetings, as well as continuous communication via phone, e-mail and text, helped maintain focus on the issue throughout the negotiations. This united and assertive strategy ensured psychiatry's prominence in the political agenda and significantly influenced the outcome of the ten-year plan.

26.3   Initiatives in the 10-Year Plan for Psychiatry

The 10-year plan for Psychiatry has several main priorities, which will improve capacity and quality in already existing services and improve research. Together with a strong focus on improvement of treatment for children and adolescents with mental health problems, the most important high priority was to strengthen treatment and care for people with severe mental disorder. This will be ensured by implementing well-described quality standards and requirements for the patient pathway and for the collaboration between professionals and sectors involved during the entire pathway.

26.3.1 Acute Psychiatric Helpline and Acute Outreach

As part of Denmark's 10-year plan for Psychiatry, a national acute psychiatric telephone helpline will be established, along with strengthened acute outreach services. The World Health Organization recommends such helplines as a key element of national suicide prevention strategies [46]. A professional helpline can facilitate timely interventions, including outreach, follow-ups and referrals to other services. It can also manage frequent callers effectively, addressing a common challenge for helplines. The overarching goal is to create more integrated services by coordinating existing resources, such as crisis teams, assertive outreach teams, psychiatric emergency services, suicide prevention clinics and NGO-run helplines. An ambition with a professionally managed psychiatric crisis hotline is to ensure that help and treatment are organised following an acute mental health crisis, and that no one falls through the cracks.

There is a pressing need to strengthen acute psychiatric outreach services, particularly for individuals in severe crises or experiencing acute mental illness. The Danish 10-year plan for Psychiatry has allocated state funding to implement and expand acute psychiatric outreach services across the country. The inclusion of psychiatrists and ambulance drivers in outreach teams ensures that emergency visits are both feasible and effective, even in complex and high-risk situations. For instance, nearly 20% of cases result in involuntary admissions—decisions that require the expertise of a psychiatrist familiar with the legal criteria for such actions. Similarly, expert evaluations are crucial for identifying suicidal cases and providing appropriate interventions. The Capital Region's model demonstrates how a well-structured acute outreach service can fulfil its purpose, offering timely and expert care to those most in need. The model established in the Capital Region of Denmark can serve as a gold standard for such initiatives. In 2025, this service covers only 40% of the Danish population, but with dedicated funding from the ten-year plan, it is being considered how similar principles can be implemented for acute psychiatric services in the rest of the country.

26.3.2 Increased Capacity for Assertive Outreach and Inpatient Facilities

The above-described teams will receive more funding to meet the needs of the most severely ill people. This will increase the capacity in OPUS, F-ACT and outreach teams for homeless people. There will also be investments in specialised inpatient units. Already, specialised units for people with non-suicidal self-harm have been established.

26.3.3 Suicide Prevention

A national plan for suicide prevention was endorsed by the parliament [47] priori- tizing funding of suicide preventive clinics and services for those at highest risk of suicide, immediately after discharge and after having contacted psychiatric emer- gency department [48]. The time change in suicide rates and rates of post-discharge suicide will be monitored yearly by a council for suicide prevention.

Targeted interventions for individuals engaging in non-suicidal self-harm, such as cutting, are being introduced across several Danish regions.

26.3.4 Danish Multidisciplinary Psychiatric Groups Guidelines

Danish Multidisciplinary Psychiatric Groups was established as an umbrella organ- isation. The primary task of the organisation is to develop clinical guidelines, pro- viding clinicians across the country with an updated, evidence-based foundation for maintaining high standards of care. Follow-ups are conducted through clinical data- bases, allowing for professional reflection and ongoing improvement. In the future, the organisation aims to focus on knowledge dissemination and research across the field of psychiatry.

26.3.5 Virtual Reality and Artificial Intelligence

Virtual reality has been explored as a tool to alleviate symptoms in various psychi- atric conditions. While its use has primarily been limited to research settings, grow- ing evidence supports the effectiveness of immersive exposure therapy [49, 50]. As this evidence continues to grow, it is likely that virtual reality will be implemented in clinics across the country for selected conditions.

Artificial intelligence (AI) is increasingly being used in psychotherapy, offering tools to enhance mental healthcare. AI-powered applications, such as chatbots and virtual assistants, deliver evidence-based techniques like cognitive behavioural ther- apy (CBT), providing immediate support and making therapy more accessible. AI can also aid therapists by analysing patient data—such as speech, behaviour and emotions—to tailor treatments and monitor progress. AI should complement, not replace, human therapists, as the therapeutic relationship is central to care.

26.3.6 Research

As part of the 10-year plan for Psychiatry, research in the field has been prioritised. A permanent allocation of 26 million euros per year has been secured in the state budget. This initiative aims to establish a stronger framework for research into the prevention and treatment of mental disorders. It seeks to ensure that individuals with mental illnesses benefit from high-quality professional care while enhancing research into the prevention of poor mental health and the treatment of mental illness. Additionally, the initiative will contribute to strengthening academic and scientific environments, as well as improving the recruitment and retention of employees across the entire field of psychiatry. Moreover, significant contributions from large Danish private funds such as Lundbeck Foundation, Novo Nordisk Foundation and Tryg Foundation further enhance the financial foundation of Danish psychiatric research, making it better funded than in most other countries. This enables Danish researchers to lead global epidemiological research and conduct some of the world's largest clinical trials, despite Denmark's small population of six million.

26.4 The Future Best Psychiatry in the World

26.4.1 Explore All Possibilities for Prevention: More Research Is Needed

Our societal ability to address mental illnesses rationally, constructively and without prejudice will improve if we collectively learn more about their causes, symptoms, treatment options and outcomes. Achieving this requires expanding research and ensuring wider dissemination of existing knowledge. The greatest challenge in psychiatry is that the causes and mechanisms of many mental disorders remain unclear. We have yet to 'crack the code' and understand why some people develop mental illnesses while others do not. If this mystery is solved, it could lead to more rational treatment and prevention, higher prioritisation and a positive influence on societal perceptions of mental health.

Extensive research into genetic and environmental factors is contributing to this understanding, with Danish researchers playing a significant role globally. Breakthroughs are emerging, such as identifying rare genetic variants that increase the risk of schizophrenia and discovering the significant role of genes regulating brain development and immune function. A promising future breakthrough may lie in understanding the role of inflammatory processes and the immune system in mental illnesses.

A solid grasp of the causes can, at best, be applied preventively. However, there is no direct path from identifying causes to understanding disease mechanisms or determining effective prevention and treatment strategies.

26.4.2 Universal Preventive Intervention

Internationally, different indicators point to a mental health crisis in teenagers and young adults. Far too little is known about the roots of this. Possible aetiological factors have been suggested such as too much screentime, to little physical activity, poor sleep and lack of social training through unsupervised play. It could also be too much time spent on social media in an early age, toxins and pesticides in the environment, high pace in society, more 'being watched over' by adults, less freedom to explore and high demands on adolescents in terms of how they look and behave and how to be successful in every dimension of life before age 18, which is stressful for many. At the current stage, we do not know and more research is needed, including randomised clinical trials where different approaches are being tried out.

In Denmark, there is a well-developed system that includes maternity care, public health nurses for babies, school health services, educational psychological support in schools and home care for individuals with reduced functional capacity. Monitoring of emerging mental illness can be integrated into these services to ensure early detection, easy access to healthcare and smooth transitions between systems.

26.4.3 Selective Prevention

Several high-risk groups can be identified already in childhood, including children placed outside of the parental or family home, those with parents who have a mental illness and children who already show signs of mental health issues. It is essential to develop and implement improved interventions for these vulnerable groups.

26.4.4 Children at Familial High Risk of Developing Mental Illness: VIA-Family

There should also be available services tailored to specific high-risk groups, such as children of parents with severe mental illness or substance abuse, children in foster care and children growing up in challenging circumstances, for example, due to trauma, including refugee children.

Children born to parents with mental illnesses is a large and overlooked group in the health system as well as in society. In Denmark, it is estimated that 25,000 children currently have a parent who is being treated in mental health services. At the same time, they represent an unused potential for prevention due to their significantly increased risk of being diagnosed with a mental illness themselves [51–53]. Further, children in families with parental mental illness are more likely to struggle with a range of problems including cognitive problems [54, 55], trauma, periods with impaired parenting [56] and stigmatisation. Despite growing awareness, there is still a lack of evidence on how best to support these children and their families to prevent negative life outcomes, including intergenerational transmission of mental health problems. In Denmark, several randomised clinical trials are underway to evaluate interventions aimed at mitigating disease progression and improving outcomes. The largest of these studies, VIA Family 2.0, plans to include 600 families. This trial seeks to provide evidence on how to ensure effective, holistic and preventive support to families affected by parental mental illness, enable early detection of declining mental health and prevent reduced functioning in at-risk offspring. The ultimate goal is to develop a framework for preventive interventions that can be applied to other high-risk groups.

26.4.5 Indicated Prevention

The psychiatry of the future must ensure easy and straightforward access to help, even for individuals who do not meet the diagnostic criteria for a specific psychiatric disorder. If we aim to intervene early, it must be possible to seek qualified help while symptoms may still be in their early stages.

Early detection of mental illness is crucial for improving long-term outcomes, and Denmark has implemented several programmes to identify emerging conditions at an early stage.

The research programmes TIPS (Early Intervention in Psychosis) and TOP (Early Detection of Psychosis) focus on recognising the first signs of psychosis, providing timely intervention to reduce the impact of the illness. Additionally, UHR (Ultra High Risk) clinics can be designed to identify individuals at high risk of developing psychosis before full-blown symptoms emerge. These services can offer specialised care to prevent or delay the onset of serious mental health conditions, promoting better recovery prospects. This is not implemented in Denmark yet.

26.4.6 Take Good Care of Staff Members

Staff members in mental health services are an undervalued treasure. Most are deeply motivated by a desire to improve the lives of individuals with mental illness, striving daily to make a meaningful difference for those facing challenging life circumstances. Yet, they often feel that their efforts go unrecognised.

There is a risk that policies driven by New Public Management can undermine the joy and fulfilment of their work by emphasising performance metrics that are often seen as less relevant than more meaningful quality indicators, such as patient satisfaction and sustained programme attendance [57].

Staff in the public health sector deserve to be valued and supported. There is no justification for their wages being lower than in the private sector. They should be provided with ample opportunities for education and supervision and have a significant voice in the planning and organisation of their work. This principle should cover doctors, psychologists, nurses, social workers and other health professionals.

26.4.7 Continuity of Care as a General Principle: Do They Have an Elisabeth in School?

When I spoke with my, at that time, six-year-old son about starting school soon, he surprised me with an insightful question that revealed his concerns: 'Do they have an Elisabeth in school?' I immediately understood that he was referring to Elisabeth, the kind and attentive preschool teacher from his kindergarten. Translated into adult terms, he was asking whether there would be a compassionate, reliable and approachable professional at school—someone who would look out for him and be there to help with any problem. Though he could not articulate it fully, what he was longing for were principles like continuity, sensitivity, responsibility and a 'no wrong door' approach in his new environment.

These are the kinds of principles we aim to implement in psychiatric care—a dedicated person available to both patients and carers. This person will often be a part of a multidisciplinary team, ensuring access to different professional expertise and supervision. While challenges like night shifts, sick leave and training obligations make this difficult in practice, we can strive to incorporate these principles as much as possible into mental healthcare.

26.4.8 'By the Way You Saved My Life'

Participants in the original OPUS trial were invited to a follow-up interview 20 years after their inclusion in the study. These interviews were conducted by blinded assessors. As one participant was leaving after completing the interview, he remarked, 'By the way, you saved my life'. Similar statements are frequently reported by patients who have undergone OPUS treatment, highlighting the profound impact that tailored, comprehensive, assertive care can have. When implemented as standard treatment, OPUS has been associated with a reduction in mortality rates [58].

26.4.9 Conclusion

Creating world-class psychiatry means recognising that mental health is a critical public health issue that demands universal care. Provided sufficient funding, a tax-financed system can guarantee equal access, upholding the fundamental right to evaluation and evidence-based treatment. By centring care on service users' perspectives and grounding innovations in rigorous research, we can build a comprehensive, effective and equitable mental healthcare system.

Key Points
- Mental health is a critical public health issue.
- A tax-financed system ensures equal access to treatment and care for all.
- The right to evaluation and evidence-based treatment is fundamental.
- Comprehensive care should be grounded in the perspective of service users.
- Research is the foundation for progress in mental healthcare.

References

1. Helliwell JF, Layard R, Sachs JD, De Neve J-E, Aknin LB, Wang S. World happiness report. United Nations; 2021.
2. Danish_Health_Authority. Strengthening mental health care. Recommendations for a 10-year action plan in Denmark. Copenhagen: Danish_Health_Authority; 2022.
3. Janse van Rensburg B, Kotze C, Moxley K, Subramaney U, Zingela Z, Seedat S. Profile of the current psychiatrist workforce in South Africa: establishing a baseline for human resource planning and strategy. Health Policy Plan. 2022;37(4):492–504.
4. Rawls J. A theory of justice: revised edition. Harvard University Press; 1999.
5. Christensen TN, Wallstrom IG, Stenager E, Bojesen AB, Gluud C, Nordentoft M, Eplov LF. Effects of individual placement and support supplemented with cognitive remediation and work-focused social skills training for people with severe mental illness: a randomized clinical trial. JAMA Psychiatr. 2019;76:1232.
6. Mainz J, Johnsen SP. Befolkningens sundhed og sygdom (Population health and disease). In: Kvalitet og patientsikkerhed. Copenhagen: Munksgaard; 2023.
7. Feodor Nilsson S, Laursen TM, Hjorthoj C, Nordentoft M. Homelessness as a predictor of mortality: an 11-year register-based cohort study. Soc Psychiatry Psychiatr Epidemiol. 2018;53(1):63–75.
8. Nilsson SF, Laursen TM, Osler M, Hjorthoj C, Benros ME, Ethelberg S, et al. Adverse SARS-CoV-2-associated outcomes among people experiencing social marginalisation and psychiatric vulnerability: a population-based cohort study among 4,4 million people. Lancet Reg Health Eur. 2022;20:100421.
9. Nilsson SF, Laursen TM, Osler M, Hjorthoj C, Benros ME, Ethelberg S, et al. Vaccination against SARS-CoV-2 infection among vulnerable and marginalised population groups in Denmark: a nationwide population-based study. Lancet Reg Health Eur. 2022;16:100355.
10. Tsemberis S, Gulcur L, Nakae M. Housing first, consumer choice, and harm reduction for homeless individuals with a dual diagnosis. Am J Public Health. 2004;94(4):651–6.
11. Baandrup L, Ostrup RJ, Klokker L, Austin S, Bjornshave T, Fuglsang BV, et al. Treatment of adult patients with schizophrenia and complex mental health needs – a national clinical guideline. Nord J Psychiatry. 2016;70(3):231–40.
12. Nordentoft M, Melau M, Iversen T, Petersen L, Jeppesen P, Thorup A, et al. From research to practice: how OPUS treatment was accepted and implemented throughout Denmark. Early Interv Psychiatry. 2015;9(2):156–62.
13. Nordentoft M, Bjarking L, Hemmingsen R. Psychiatric emergency outreach: a report on the first 2 years of functioning in Copenhagen. Nord J Psychiatry. 2002;56(6):399–405.
14. Petersen L, Jeppesen P, Thorup A, Abel MB, Ohlenschlaeger J, Christensen TO, et al. A randomised multicentre trial of integrated versus standard treatment for patients with a first episode of psychotic illness. BMJ. 2005;331(7517):602.
15. Craig TK, Garety P, Power P, Rahaman N, Colbert S, Fornells-Ambrojo M, Dunn G. The Lambeth early onset (LEO) team: randomised controlled trial of the effectiveness of specialised care for early psychosis. Br Med J. 2004;329(7474):1067.
16. Kane JM, Robinson DG, Schooler NR, Mueser KT, Penn DL, Rosenheck RA, et al. Comprehensive versus usual community care for first-episode psychosis: 2-year outcomes from the NIMH RAISE early treatment program. Am J Psychiatry. 2016;173(4):362–72.
17. Correll CU, Galling B, Pawar A, Krivko A, Bonetto C, Ruggeri M, et al. Comparison of early intervention services vs treatment as usual for early-phase psychosis: a systematic review, meta-analysis, and meta-regression. JAMA Psychiatry. 2018;75(6):555–65.
18. Puntis S, Minichino A, De Crescenzo F, Cipriani A, Lennox B, Harrison R. Specialised early intervention teams for recent-onset psychosis. Cochrane Database Syst Rev. 2020;11:CD013288.

19. Secher RG, Hjorthoj CR, Austin SF, Thorup A, Jeppesen P, Mors O, Nordentoft M. Ten-year follow-up of the OPUS specialized early intervention trial for patients with a first episode of psychosis. Schizophr Bull. 2015;41(3):617–26.
20. Hastrup LH, Kronborg C, Bertelsen M, Jeppesen P, Jorgensen P, Petersen L, et al. Cost-effectiveness of early intervention in first-episode psychosis: economic evaluation of a randomised controlled trial (the OPUS study). Br J Psychiatry. 2013;202:35–41.
21. Malla A, Joober R, Iyer S, Norman R, Schmitz N, Brown T, et al. Comparing three-year extension of early intervention service to regular care following two years of early intervention service in first-episode psychosis: a randomized single blind clinical trial. World Psychiatry. 2017;16(3):278–86.
22. Chang WC, Chan GH, Jim OT, Lau ES, Hui CL, Chan SK, et al. Optimal duration of an early intervention programme for first-episode psychosis: randomised controlled trial. Br J Psychiatry. 2015;206(6):492–500.
23. Albert N, Melau M, Jensen H, Emborg C, Jepsen JR, Fagerlund B, et al. Five years of specialised early intervention versus two years of specialised early intervention followed by three years of standard treatment for patients with a first episode psychosis: randomised, superiority, parallel group trial in Denmark (OPUS II). BMJ. 2017;356:i6681.
24. Sundhedsstyrelsen, Boligstyrelsen So. Beskrivelse af forløb for voksne med psykoselidelser. Anbefalinger til tilrettelæggelse af tværsektorielle indsatser [WEB]. Sundhedsstyrelsen; 2024.
25. Socialstyrelsen. Styrket implementering af housing first – erfaringer fra danske kommuner. Copenhagen: Socialstyrelsen; 2021.
26. Sundhedsstyrelsen DHA. Afdækning af tværfaglige udgående teams i den regionale psykiatri 2024.
27. Nordentoft M, Pedersen MG, Pedersen CB, Blinkenberg S, Mortensen PB. The new asylums in the community: severely ill psychiatric patients living in psychiatric supported housing facilities. A Danish register-based study of prognostic factors, use of psychiatric services, and mortality. Soc Psychiatry Psychiatr Epidemiol. 2012;47(8):1251–61.
28. Momen NC, Plana-Ripoll O, Agerbo E, Benros ME, Borglum AD, Christensen MK, et al. Association between mental disorders and subsequent medical conditions. N Engl J Med. 2020;382(18):1721–31.
29. Mackenhauer J, Frischknecht Christensen E, Andersen G, Mainz J, Johnsen SP. Disparities in reperfusion therapy and time delays among patients with ischemic stroke and a history of mental illness. Stroke. 2022;53(11):3375–85.
30. Austin SF, Mors O, Budtz-Jorgensen E, Secher RG, Hjorthoj CR, Bertelsen M, et al. Long-term trajectories of positive and negative symptoms in first episode psychosis: a 10 year follow-up study in the OPUS cohort. Schizophr Res. 2015;168(1–2):84–91.
31. Hjorthoj C, Sturup AE, McGrath JJ, Nordentoft M. Years of potential life lost and life expectancy in schizophrenia: a systematic review and meta-analysis. Lancet Psychiatry. 2017;4:295.
32. Kvalitetsinstitut   S.   https://www.sundk.dk/kliniske-kvalitetsdatabaser/den-nationale-skizofrenidatabase/om-databasen/?utm_source 2024. Available from: https://www.sundk.dk/kliniske-kvalitetsdatabaser/den-nationale-skizofrenidatabase/om-databasen/?utm_source.
33. Baandrup L, Cerqueira C, Haller L, Korshoj L, Voldsgaard I, Nordentoft M. The Danish Schizophrenia Registry. Clin Epidemiol. 2016;8:691–5.
34. Nordentoft M, Rasmussen M, Hogh L, Legind C, Kjellberg J. How come Denmark is planning to increase the annual budget for psychiatry with almost 20 percent? Eur Psychiatry. 2023:1–10.
35. Dalsgaard S, Thorsteinsson E, Trabjerg BB, Schullehner J, Plana-Ripoll O, Brikell I, et al. Incidence rates and cumulative incidences of the full spectrum of diagnosed mental disorders in childhood and adolescence. JAMA Psychiatry. 2020;77(2):155–64.
36. Beck C, Pedersen CB, Plana-Ripoll O, Dalsgaard S, Debost JP, Laursen TM, et al. A comprehensive analysis of age of onset and cumulative incidence of mental disorders: a Danish register study. Acta Psychiatr Scand. 2024;149(6):467–78.

37. Mukherjee S. The emperor of all maladies: a biography of cancer. New York: Scribner; 2010. 2010.
38. Øvig P. Jeg er hvad jeg husker. Efter elektrochokket - mellem mirakler og mareridt (I am what I remember. After electroconvulsive treatment – bestween miracles and nightmare). Copenhagen: Gyldendal; 2022.
39. Nordentoft M, Wahlbeck K, Hallgren J, Westman J, Osby U, Alinaghizadeh H, et al. Excess mortality, causes of death and life expectancy in 270,770 patients with recent onset of mental disorders in Denmark, Finland and Sweden. PLoS One. 2013;8(1):e55176.
40. Plana-Ripoll O, Pedersen CB, Agerbo E, Holtz Y, Erlangsen A, Canudas-Romo V, et al. A comprehensive analysis of mortality-related health metrics associated with mental disorders: a nationwide, register-based cohort study. Lancet. 2019;394(10211):1827–35.
41. Madsen T, Erlangsen A, Hjorthoj C, Nordentoft M. High suicide rates during psychiatric inpatient stay and shortly after discharge. Acta Psychiatr Scand. 2020;142(5):355–65.
42. Plana-Ripoll O, Weye N, Knudsen AK, Hakulinen C, Madsen KB, Christensen MK, et al. The association between mental disorders and subsequent years of working life: a Danish population-based cohort study. Lancet Psychiatry. 2023;10(1):30–9.
43. Patel V, Saxena S, Lund C, Thornicroft G, Baingana F, Bolton P, et al. The lancet commission on global mental health and sustainable development. Lancet. 2018;392(10157):1553–98.
44. Nordentoft M. Fremtidens psykiatri (Future of psychiatry). Copenhagen: Informations forlag; 2018.
45. Sundhedsstyrelsen; SDU SIfF. Danskernes sundhed. Den nationale sundhedsprofil 2021. København: Sundhedsstyrelsen; SDU SIfF; 2022.
46. World Health Organization. National suicide prevention strategies: progress, examples and indicators. World Health Organization; 2018.
47. Sundhedsstyrelsen. Prevention of suicide and suicide attempt. Copenhagen: Sundhedsstyrelsen; 2024.
48. Nordentoft M, Erlangsen A, Madsen T. More coherent treatment needed for people at high risk of suicide. Lancet Psychiatry. 2022;9(4):263–4.
49. Craig TK, Rus-Calafell M, Ward T, Leff JP, Huckvale M, Howarth E, et al. AVATAR therapy for auditory verbal hallucinations in people with psychosis: a single-blind, randomised controlled trial. Lancet Psychiatry. 2018;5(1):31–40.
50. Garety PA, Edwards CJ, Jafari H, Emsley R, Huckvale M, Rus-Calafell M, et al. Digital AVATAR therapy for distressing voices in psychosis: the phase 2/3 AVATAR2 trial. Nat Med. 2024;30(12):3658–68.
51. Thorup AAE, Laursen TM, Munk-Olsen T, Ranning A, Mortensen PB, Plessen KJ, Nordentoft M. Incidence of child and adolescent mental disorders in children aged 0-17 with familial high risk for severe mental illness – a Danish register study. Schizophr Res. 2018;197:298–304.
52. Paananen R, Tuulio-Henriksson A, Merikukka M, Gissler M. Intergenerational transmission of psychiatric disorders: the 1987 Finnish birth cohort study. Eur Child Adolesc Psychiatry. 2021;30:381–9.
53. Ellersgaard D, Jessica Plessen K, Richardt Jepsen J, Soeborg Spang K, Hemager N, Klee Burton B, et al. Psychopathology in 7-year-old children with familial high risk of developing schizophrenia spectrum psychosis or bipolar disorder – the Danish high risk and resilience study – VIA 7, a population-based cohort study. World Psychiatry. 2018;17(2):210–9.
54. Hemager N, Christiani CJ, Thorup AAE, Spang KS, Ellersgaard D, Burton BK, et al. Neurocognitive heterogeneity in 7-year-old children at familial high risk of schizophrenia or bipolar disorder: the Danish high risk and resilience study – VIA 7. J Affect Disord. 2022;302:214–23.
55. Knudsen CB, Greve AN, Jepsen JRM, Lambek R, Andreassen AK, Veddum L, et al. Neurocognitive subgroups in children at familial high-risk of schizophrenia or bipolar disorder: subgroup membership stability or change from age 7 to 11-the Danish high risk and resilience study. Schizophr Bull. 2022.
56. Sherman MD, Hooker SA. Supporting families managing parental mental illness: challenges and resources. Int J Psychiatry Med. 2018;53(5–6):361–70.

57. Bjørnholt B, Larsen F. The politics of performance measurement: 'evaluation use as mediator for politics'. Evaluation. 2014;20(4):400.
58. Posselt CM, Albert N, Nordentoft M, Hjorthoj C. The Danish OPUS early intervention services for first-episode psychosis: a phase 4 prospective cohort study with comparison of randomized trial and real-world data. Am J Psychiatry. 2021;178(10):941–51.

Open Access   This chapter is licensed under the terms of the Creative Commons Attribution 4.0 International License (http://creativecommons.org/licenses/by/4.0/), which permits use, sharing, adaptation, distribution and reproduction in any medium or format, as long as you give appropriate credit to the original author(s) and the source, provide a link to the Creative Commons license and indicate if changes were made.

The images or other third party material in this chapter are included in the chapter's Creative Commons license, unless indicated otherwise in a credit line to the material. If material is not included in the chapter's Creative Commons license and your intended use is not permitted by statutory regulation or exceeds the permitted use, you will need to obtain permission directly from the copyright holder.

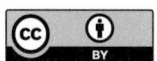

Doing Justice: Psychiatry as a Vocation

27

George Ikkos, Thomas Becker, Francesca Brencio,
Paul Hoff, Alastair Morgan, and Giovanni Stanghellini

Truth is the significance of fact. (Mies van der Rohe [1])

[…] truth is not an unveiling that destroys the mystery but a revelation that does it justice. (Walter Benjamin [2])

The authors are the European members of the international collaboration group "The Precision of Images: Emil Kraepelin, Walter Benjamin and the History of Psychiatry 1926–2026" which has been meeting since 2022. GI suggested the chapter theme, led the scoping review and produced the first draft outline. All members of the group have contributed equally to the text.

G. Ikkos
Department of Liaison Psychiatry, Royal National Orthopaedic Hospital, Stanmore, UK
e-mail: ikkos@doctors.org.uk

T. Becker
Department of Psychiatry and Psychotherapy, Univesity of Leipzig Medical Center,
Leipzig, Germany
e-mail: Thomas.Becker@medizin.uni-leipzig.de

F. Brencio (✉)
Institute for Mental Health, School of Psychology, University of Birmingham,
Birmingham, UK
e-mail: f.brencio@bham.ac.uk

P. Hoff
University Hospital of Psychiatry Zurich, Zurich, Switzerland
e-mail: paul.hoff.zollikon@gmail.com

A. Morgan
School of Health Sciences, Division of Nursing, Midwifery and Social Work, University of
Manchester, Manchester, UK
e-mail: alastair.morgan@manchester.ac.uk

G. Stanghellini
Department of Health Sciences, University of Florence, Florence, Italy
e-mail: giostan@libero.it

© The Author(s) 2026
G. Ikkos, T. Becker (eds.), *Psychiatry after Kraepelin*,
https://doi.org/10.1007/978-3-032-09475-9_27

27.1   Introduction

How may we think of psychiatry as a vocation and its relation to justice in the twenty-first century? In seeking answers to our question, we make no apologies for a wide-ranging discourse. This includes: the broad sweep of the legacy of the Enlightenment; the emergence of modernity; the political economy of late capitalism; their relation to mental (ill) health and services; patient autonomy; empathy and more. As the field is necessarily broad, the different sections of this long chapter are best read as pieces of a montage. That is, the full picture should emerge from their juxtaposition, like that of stones in a mosaic. We do hope, however, that the narrative threads we have tried to draw between them will add depth and conviction. Box 27.1 offers an outline of our approach, and we recommend the reader turns attentively to it as a start.

Box 27.1: Chapter Outline

27.1. Introduction
27.2. Emil Kraepelin, Max Weber and Walter Benjamin: modern era pioneers in the scholarly and scientific investigation of psychiatry, society and experience respectively
    27.2.1. Emil Kraepelin
    27.2.2. Max Weber
    27.2.3. Walter Benjamin
27.3. Beyond Walter Benjamin: Justice and Empathy as Philosophical Foundations of Psychiatric Vocation
    27.3.1. Justice
    27.3.2. Vocation and Empathy
27.4. Social Justice: Political Economy, Mental Health and Psychiatry
    27.4.1. Political Economy
    27.4.2. Political Economy and Progress
    27.4.3. Social Determinants of Mental Health
27.5. What is to be done?
    27.5.1. Personal Autonomy and Psychiatric Care
    27.5.2. Disenchantment and Utopia
    27.5.3. Marginalisation
27.6. Summary and Discussion: Dialectical Pessimism
27.7. Conclusion
Key Points
Disclosures
Author Contributions
References

We first take our cue from Emil Kraepelin and two of his German contemporaries—Max Weber and Walter Benjamin—who were all born during the nineteenth century and each set a direction for their respective disciplines of psychiatry, sociology and cultural theory in the twentieth century. There are some large themes that pervade their works that remain contemporary, including their relationship to the philosophical tradition of the Enlightenment, and the intellectual and cultural movement that emerged in Europe during the late seventeenth and early eighteenth centuries whose key tenets include the valorisation of reason, science, humanism, individual rights and the critique of tradition. However, it is not our intention to dwell on these authors but to employ them as points of departure at the beginning of the 100 years this book surveys to help trace and measure the distance both psychiatry and society have travelled since.

In the second section we briefly present the three towering innovators and their relevance to the perspective adopted in this chapter. Then, we comment on philosophical and conceptual aspects of justice, vocation and empathy. Next, we discuss factors relating to social justice: political economy and the social determinants of mental health. In the following section, which addresses 'what is to be done', we urge that psychiatry embraces the personhood of the autonomous subject, whether lacking mental capacity or not, as the central pillar of its clinical identity combined with radical or *critical disenchantment* with established social forces of domination and a *vocational passion for (micro) utopia*. Ultimately clinical care is about resonant encounters and healing.

Mistrustful of recurrent macro-utopias in the history of psychiatry, we conclude the chapter by suggesting that doing justice to psychiatry as a vocation in the foreseeable future mandates an outlook of *dialectical pessimism*, which requires sustaining professionally the powerful tension between the need for radical or *critical disenchantment* with today's societies on the one hand, and a *vocational passion for (micro) utopias*, on the other.

27.2 Emil Kraepelin, Max Weber and Walter Benjamin: Modern Era Pioneers in the Scholarly and Scientific Investigation of Psychiatry, Society and Experience, Respectively

Emil Kraepelin (1856–1926) and Max Weber (1864–1924) were practically exact contemporaries, Walter Benjamin (1892–1940) significantly younger. Whereas Kraepelin was a psychiatrist, both Weber and Benjamin suffered from severe mood disorders [3, 4]. Elsewhere, we have sought affinities in and differences between the work of Kraepelin and Benjamin [5].

27.2.1 Emil Kraepelin

The immediate relevance of Emil Kraepelin to this chapter includes his agenda for psychiatric professionalism, that is, his determination to establish psychiatry firmly as a legitimate medical specialty, twinned with his interest in improving public mental health, which, for him, was 'national mental health', with the 'image' of the German nation as a body. Though he engaged briefly when he was 20 years old with

philosophy [6], and his revered mentor Wilhelm Wundt (1832–1920) did extensively so, within the tradition of the Enlightenment Kraepelin had more narrowly
scientific interests. Nonetheless—and this is a central point to understanding
Kraepelin's work appropriately—decisive, but often unexplained, epistemological
presuppositions became the cornerstones of his thinking [7]. At least four of these
are important:

- Realism: For Kraepelin, there was a *real world* existing in full independence
  from persons perceiving it, describing it, or doing research on it. This world
  included other people and their healthy or disturbed mental processes. In his
  view, the psychiatric researcher must describe objectively what 'really' exists.
  Consequently, he favoured a descriptive approach in psychopathology and psychiatric diagnosis.
- Parallelism: Kraepelin advocated the concept of psychophysical parallelism: for
  him, mental and physical (neurobiological) events are *separate, but closely
  linked* and act as 'parallel' phenomena. However, his position regarding the
  mind–body relationship might be called ambivalent, if not blurry. There is an
  implicit tendency towards monism in Kraepelin's writings, particularly when it
  understands psychology as a natural science. However, his monistic tendency
  was not metaphysical but only methodological [8].
- 'Experimentalism': Kraepelin strongly supported the development and implementation of psychological and psychophysiological experiments in psychiatric
  research. He saw this approach as the via *regia* to any profound understanding of
  disturbed but also of healthy mental processes. Both Wundt and he, as the paral-
  lelists they were, did realise the epistemological difference between a physical
  and a psychological experiment but did not consider the respective experimental
  designs as significantly different.
- Naturalism: The question of how far the explanatory power of physical, chemical
  and, especially, biological findings might reach was a major issue at the end of
  the nineteenth century. The answers of leading authors not only in biology and
  medicine, but also in philosophy, often favoured a strong version of naturalism,
  as Kraepelin did. For him, man is nothing but a part of nature, and anything man
  can do is a product of this natural existence. Later in his life, he became more
  cautious in this respect, but did not substantially change his position.

Despite a frequently encountered misconception, Kraepelin's central motivation
during his nearly five decades of psychiatric work was *not* to create new disease
entities. Rather, he wanted to establish a self-confident scientific identity for psychiatry that would be widely recognised in medical faculties and in the field of
practical medical care. To do this, he believed that psychiatry should be methodologically aligned as closely as possible with other medical subjects and, particularly, be open to empirical–quantitative work.

Kraepelin arrived early on at the striking thesis of the existence and scientific
recognisability of *objectively existing—in his diction: 'natural'—disease entities* to
explain insanity, and this shaped his later life's academic work, and it was thus only

logical for him to postulate that psychiatric research would necessarily arrive at the same nosological entities, regardless of whether it used the perspectives of pathological anatomy of the central nervous system, or other aetiology, or the monitoring of the course of illness—precisely because these entities existed independently of any conceptualisation and empirical research.

In his late programmatic works, published between 1918 and 1920, because of various objections Kraepelin began to question his nosological concept and accommodated his critics on individual points. However, he *did not abandon* the basic postulate of the existence of 'naturally' given disease entities [9, 10].

27.2.2 Max Weber

The title of Max Weber's seminal *Economy and Society* [11] speaks for itself, and his work stands at the European foundations of Sociology as a science, on a par with Karl Marx's *Capital* [12, 13] and Emile Durkheim's wide range of contributions [14]. Durkheim is best known in psychiatry for his study of suicide and his related concept of *anomie* (normlessness) [15], a concept of continuing key contemporary significance for psychiatry, as we shall see. Working firmly within the tradition of Enlightenment, Weber researched the dynamics of science, technology, economy and society. Though disputed, his ideas on *The Protestant Ethic and the 'Spirit' of Capitalism* [16] have been hugely influential.

Weber was interested not only in what may have been gained through the Enlightenment but also in what might have been lost, including particularly through the processes of secularisation of society. He captured this loss with his striking reference to the 'disenchantment of the world', something of great relevance to psychiatry and indeed to this chapter. Weber's immediate relevance to our chapter also stems from the titles of two of his seminal lectures, later published as essays, namely *Science as a Vocation* [17] and *Politics as a Vocation* [18]. Interestingly, he begins the first by stating: 'You wish me to speak about "Science as a Vocation". Now, we political economists have a pedantic custom, which I should like to follow, of always beginning with the external conditions. In this case, we begin with the question: What are the conditions of science as a vocation in the material sense of the term?' [17]. Though none of us is a social scientist and we do not start from the exact same point, we will also refer extensively to the conditions for psychiatry as a vocation today 'in the material sense of the term'. This is essential to both understanding the history and addressing the challenges of psychiatry today.

27.2.3 Walter Benjamin

Benjamin, a Jewish Marxist with an enduring interest in Biblical Messianic Mysticism, cuts a complex intellectual figure. Notwithstanding his enormous respect for the towering Enlightenment philosopher Immanuel Kant (1724–1804), his work may be understood as an attempt to overcome the limitations of the latter's thought and that of his own Neo-Kantian teachers. Elsewhere, in a series of papers we introduce his work for psychiatry [19–21] and psychotherapy [22].

Though consistently secular in his orientation, Benjamin's avid intellectual interest in the Absolute, spirituality and theology, together with his critique of the erosion of tradition and accelerating pace of change and industrialisation under capitalism and what he diagnosed as the impoverishment of daily experience [*Erfahrung*], makes it tempting to think of him as someone in search of re-enchantment of the world and there is truth in this. However, in his terms, it would be equally accurate to say that he attempted disenchantment from what he summarised as the 'phantasmagorias' of capitalism. Following Marx, he explored how capitalism fostered certain religious attitudes and practices towards property and commodities [e.g. 23]. This, he believed, enchants us with the promises of the ever new and veils our disappointment with failed promises. The phantasmagorias of capitalism, he argued, have prevented protest or revolt against the injustices of the class or, we would now add, the imperial oppressions of his times and ecological catastrophes of ours. He was, therefore, profoundly interested in social justice, a key theme of this chapter.

Benjamin was not hostile to technology; indeed, he wrote pioneering cultural criticism on its social potential as well as risks [24–26]. In an important sense what he was most consistently interested in was human fulfilment [27, 28] and what he lamented as the repeated social unfulfillment of the potential of technology. Because of the circumstances of both his life and death, Benjamin's intellectual legacy had been at great risk of being lost. It was salvaged by three friends and collaborators, Gershom Scholem (1897–1982), Theodor Adorno (1903–1969) and Hannah Arendt (1906–1975). Arendt, a philosopher and political theorist of equal stature in her field to that of the three male pioneers in theirs, is referred to immediately below in her own right.

In general terms then, though we will also address the significant new concerns that have arisen since their times, the broad themes of the Enlightenment that concerned Kraepelin, Weber and Benjamin, including those of science and professionalism, technology and society, disenchantment and phantasmagoria, injustice and fulfilment, remain of contemporary relevance and will be explored here. In the next section we discuss concepts of justice, vocation and empathy.

27.3 Beyond Walter Benjamin: Justice and Empathy as Philosophical Foundations of Psychiatric Vocation

27.3.1 Justice

In philosophy, the concept of justice is complex and multifaceted, with various interpretations and theories developed over centuries. However, justice is not primarily a concept but lived experience. For example, in the postscript to her *Walter Benjamin's Other History: Of Stones, Animals, Human Beings and Angels* [29], Beatrice Hansen refers to French philosopher Emmanuel Levinas' abject experience in a Nazi camp for Jewish prisoners during WWII, as recounted in his essay 'The Name of a Dog, or Natural Rights'. Here, Levinas contrasted the utterly dehumanizing treatment of the prisoners by the civilian staff in the camp with the way a stray dog treated the captives. Unlike the humans who ignored, humiliated or otherwise abused them when they returned from their day's forced labour, 'Bobby' greeted those interned joyfully, jumping around and wagging his tail. Arguably, Bobby, a dog, specifically recognised their humanity and did justice to it in a way that other humans failed to do.

Addressing the major question 'what is justice?' necessitates also a second question, immediately related to the first one: 'what is injustice?' As two sides of the same coin, definitions of justice and injustice cannot be separated, rather they are alive with reciprocal implications that characterise mutually the definition of each pole. Moreover, the characterisation of what is justice requires the recognition of a plural dimension, without which any possible definition risks being isolated and reduced only to one of several moral virtues. This is, for example, what happens if we consider Aristotle's meditation on justice. He developed a nuanced theory of justice (in classical Greek δικαιοσύνη; dikaiosune) not merely confined to a legal or political concept, but a fundamental *moral virtue*. He considered it to be the most complete virtue, insofar as it is exercised in relation to *others*. Recognising that strict adherence to law can sometimes lead to injustice, Aristotle introduced the concept of equity (επιείκεια; epieikeia), which allows for the correction of law where it falls short due to its generality in adapting justice to circumstances.

A substantial contribution to discourse on the relationship between a notion of justice as moral virtue and as social outcome is offered by Hannah Arendt. Central to her understanding of justice is the conception of the public realm. For Arendt, justice is not merely a matter of individual morality or legal procedures but is fundamentally tied to the existence of a shared, political world. In *The Human Condition* she argues that justice emerges from the *plurality* of human perspectives coming together in the public sphere. It is through public debate, discussion and collective action that we can arrive at a sense of what is just. Genuine power emerges when people act together in concert, and this collective power is the basis for establishing and maintaining institutions: 'human power corresponds to the condition of plurality to begin with' [30].

One of Arendt's most significant contributions to thinking about justice is her concept of 'the right to have rights'. Developed in response to the plight of stateless people after World War II, this idea suggests that the most fundamental form of justice is the *recognition* of an individual's right to belong to a political community. Arendt argued that without membership in a political community, individuals lose not only their legal rights but also their ability to act in the world in a meaningful way. It is especially in her coverage of the trial of Adolf Eichmann that she developed her concept of 'the banality of evil' [31]. She argued that great evils are not necessarily committed by monsters, but often by ordinary people who fail to think critically about their actions. As she writes in *The Life of the Mind*, 'The manifestation of the wind of thought is not knowledge; it is the ability to tell right from wrong, beautiful from ugly. And this, at the rare moments when the stakes are on the table, may indeed prevent catastrophes, at least for the self' [32].

This insight has significant implications for how we think about justice. It suggests that justice requires not only adherence to laws, but also active *engagement in moral thinking and judgement*. It also raises questions about the nature of responsibility and culpability in systems of injustice. By situating justice firmly within the realm of human affairs and political action, Arendt reminds us that it is not an abstract ideal, but something that must be *constantly negotiated and enacted* in the public sphere. Precisely because of these remarks, we cannot discuss a general and metaphysical conception of justice disentangled from the notions of *plurality, recognition and public space*, central themes also in the field of healthcare. Justice in healthcare is a critical yet complex concept that underpins many ethical decisions and policy choices. As resources are currently limited when measured against healthcare needs, questions of fair distribution, equal access and equitable treatment become paramount.

Perhaps we can unpack the issue of justice in healthcare through three often referred to perspectives, such as distributive justice, procedural justice, and social justice. Distributive justice concerns the fair allocation of healthcare resources, while procedural justice in medical decision-making relies on fair processes related to informed consent, patient autonomy, transparency in resource allocation decisions and fair hearing in medical disputes. Social justice is strictly linked to health equity, the cardinal elements of which are access to healthcare, understanding of social and economic factors affecting health outcomes and overcoming discrimination and bias in healthcare. If the implications of all these aspects are delicate and complex in healthcare in general, they are more problematic in the field of mental health. Perhaps we could ask: How can we do justice to psychiatry: to patients, services and practitioners? Possible answers to this question depend on the perspective we embrace, as mental health users, as mental health clinicians, as social community, as political decision makers.

In recent years, Miranda Fricker has introduced the notion of *epistemic injustice* in mental health, which refers to unfair treatment of individuals with mental health conditions in their capacity as knowers or sources of knowledge [33]. Very briefly we may say that this concept has two main forms when it comes to mental health: on the one hand, it assumes the guise of *testimonial injustice*, when a person's testimony or account of their experiences is given less credibility due to prejudice against their mental health status. For example, a patient's description of their symptoms might be dismissed or downplayed by healthcare professionals because of their psychiatric diagnosis. On the other hand, it may assume the form of *hermeneutical injustice* when there is a gap in collective understanding that puts someone with a mental health condition at an unfair disadvantage. For instance, a person might struggle to articulate their experiences due to a lack of appropriate concepts or language in society to describe mental health issues. More specifically, in the context of mental health, epistemic injustice can manifest in several ways: disbelieving or minimising patients' reported symptoms or experiences; attributing physical symptoms to mental health conditions without proper investigation (diagnostic overshadowing); excluding individuals with mental health conditions from participating in research or policy-making about mental health; stigmatising certain diagnoses, leading to self-doubt and internalised stigma in patients; prioritising clinical knowledge over lived experience in treatment decisions. In essence, Sect. 5 of this chapter on 'What Is to Be Done' offers ways to avoid and overcome these.

27.3.2 Vocation and Empathy

The concept of vocation (from Latin, *vocatio*, literally 'a calling, a being called') in medicine goes far beyond the notion of a mere career or job. It is also different to profession. To draw a fundamental distinction, we may say that it relates to fulfilment, whereas professionalism refers to fulfilment of contract [34, 35].

Vocation embodies a profound sense of calling, purpose and dedication that has been integral to the medical profession for centuries. The idea of medicine as a vocation has roots in ancient traditions, where healers were often seen as having a divine calling. Hippocrates emphasised the sacred nature of the medical profession, setting forth ethical principles that still guide the field today. If we adopt Durkheim's secular definition of the 'sacred' whereby it refers to things that are set apart, revered, and treated with a sense of awe, respect, or fear, as opposed to things that are 'profane', that is, the ordinary, mundane, or everyday aspects of life, then vocation continues to relate to something sacred today [36, 37]. In medicine it involves a sense of moral obligation and personal fulfilment derived from putting one's own clinical knowledge in the service of others. This profound meaning of vocation contributes to the impact of patient care: it implies great empathy and compassion, a strong resilience in the face of challenges and setbacks, the imperative to maintain a patient-centred focus in one's own practice.

The notion of vocation in medicine (generally speaking) and in psychiatry is rooted in the dialogue that these disciplines have with the humanities (generally speaking) and with philosophy, a dialogue often overlooked due to the nature of modern healthcare systems, with their focus on efficiency and productivity, that can sometimes conflict with the vocational nature of medicine. One of us recalls when he was a Team leader of an Assertive Outreach team, one of the first teams set up in the UK, who was berated at a management meeting for not reducing the number of 'bed days' for acute admissions. He pointed out that the team had not reduced the number but had managed to shift the balance from formal to informal admissions for many of the patients. 'That's nothing at all' was the reply—of no consequence to us.

It is in this context that the link between vocation and empathy must be considered: The preliminary act of every medical action is an act of empathy [38]. Whoever wants to commit to the care of men, women and children must acknowledge the other. The key word in the description of the act of empathy is to become aware (*Gewahren*). Empathy (*Einfühlung*) means to feel the presence of the other, let it stand out against the background as a proper figure, drag it out of insignificance, or, better, out of non-existence. Empathy is a form of mimetic practice; even if it is not synonymous with warmth or welcoming, empathy is, rather, a special kind of intentional experience in which my perception of the other leads me to grasp (or to feel that I grasp) his personal experience and to feel how the other is an embodied person like me, animated by his own feelings and sensations and capable of voluntary movements and of expressing his experience. The intentional movement entailed in the experience of empathy is twofold: either I may (temporarily) feel that I incorporate the other's way of experiencing, or I may feel that I am transposed to the place or into the body of the other. In both cases, empathy implies a special kind of immediate resonance between my self (and especially my embodied self) and that of the other person and, through this, I feel that I understand him (or her) [39].

Usually, empathy does not require any voluntary and explicit effort. We may call this type of empathy, which is at play since the first seconds of our life, 'non-conative' or 'first-order' empathy—a kind of spontaneous and pre-reflexive attunement between embodied selves through which we implicitly make sense of the other's behaviour. But in some cases, the other's behaviour becomes elusive. In these situations, while we deliberately make every effort to thematically understand the other (which may be called 'conative' empathy), we also experience the limitations of this mode of understanding, In some cases—maybe the most relevant in clinical practice—we do not feel immediately in touch with the other, we do not immediately grasp the reasons and meaning of their actions, and thus purposively and knowingly attempt to put ourselves in their place. As an example, understanding psychotic experiences requires a kind of training that goes beyond non-conative, spontaneous and '*naïf*' empathic skills, and at the same time avoids the pitfalls of conative empathy based on the clinician's personal experiences and common-sense categories [40, 41].

The clinician's empathic capacities need some kind of education. In the clinical setting we cannot simply rely on standard empathic capacities. To achieve this 'second order' empathic capacity is a complex process. First, I need to acknowledge that the 'life-world' inhabited by the other person is not like my own. The supposition that the other lives in a world like my own—that is, that he lives time, space, his own body, others, the materiality of objects etc. just like I do—is often the source of serious misunderstanding. To empathise with others, I must acknowledge an 'existential difference' that separates me from the way of being in the world that characterises each of them. Any forgetting of this ontological difference, for instance between my own world and that of an anxious or psychotic patient (but, also between my own and an adolescent's or an old man's world), will be an obstacle to empathic understanding, since these people live in a life-world whose structure is (at least in part) different from my own. Achieving second-order empathy thus requires me to bracket my own pre-reflexive, natural attitude (in which my first-order empathic capacities are rooted), and to approach the other's world as I would do while exploring an unknown and alien country [42].

Through empathy I become aware that the other and his pain constitute an event in front of me, that while taking place and happening breaks the continuity of my experience. 'Empathy, thus, is a fracture in the continuity of the single through which the other enters predominantly in sight, where looking becomes seeing, among all senses the most specially connected to the activities of the mind' [43]. Regarded as a *fracture* in the continuity of our professions/practices/life, empathy may contribute to nourishing the sense of vocation at the core of the medical enterprise. As vocation, the practice of medicine unveils its nature in terms of a moral enterprise grounded on an intersubjective dimension, a paradigm often not considered in medicine in general and in mental health in particular. In some ways, and rightly so, psychiatry as a science must live up to the demands of natural scientific progress and be measured against the successes of other fields of medicine. But how can we measure the healing encounter in terms that progress understands, and should we want to?

The psychiatrist Jean Oury provided one answer when he spoke about clinical encounters as opening 'spaces of the saying' [44]. He recounted a story of working with a patient: '(Oury presents a photograph)—during the war, this man had been an engineer, working with solar energy, a very intelligent man, completely mad. He could not be anywhere, not in his bedroom, not at the table, not in his bed … to see him in my office was not possible, so much so that I had to write to him asking him if we could meet under a tree. So, he arrived and we kept at a distance. If I approached him too closely he would walk away; we had to maintain a distance … We worked with him for one year … Anyway, one night, after a year of working with him, I was told that he had arrived at the chateau [where the clinic was based], that he had sat down in a chair, and that he had opened a newspaper to read. The same night, another patient—not schizophrenic, but slightly melancholic—told me she had sat down in her usual chair and begun to knit when she saw a man she had never seen before sitting beside her who looked extremely comfortable within the chair, contented, reading the paper. This is the space of the saying, he sat in the chair, he unfolded the paper, there was a desire here, but it didn't last. To work for a year to see five minutes like this is worth every effort'.

Many of the best moments in our clinical work have all been like this, small, ephemeral and impossible to quantify. Moments of professional encounter always occur in the context of wider social fields and such deeply fulfilling professional moments do not always have to be intersubjective dialogues either, as there is also the possibility of redeeming collective moments [45]. Furthermore, whether in dialogue or collective happening, such moments often arise through dissension, through conflict. Lyotard writes that 'invention is always born of dissension' [46].

27.4 Social Justice: Political Economy, Mental Health and Psychiatry

We have referred already to the tension between justice and vocation and current health service realities. In this section we pull back from both abstract concepts and concrete clinical encounters to focus on mental (ill) health in the light of political economy and the social determinants of mental (ill) health. Because of their importance, we will attend to the evolution of current dominant forces in the political economy first and then to the implications of political economy and social determinants for mental health and services today. In Sect. 5, on 'What Is to Be Done', we will return to issues of justice in the clinical relationship in their social context.

27.4.1 Political Economy

Contemporary medicine is the fruit of the interplay of the Enlightenment (as both science and culture) with capital and society. The Enlightenment's relation to technology, capitalism and society is complex but Bernstein summarises succinctly some of Max Weber's views: 'Weber argued that the hope and expectation of the Enlightenment thinkers was a bitter and ironic illusion. They maintained a strong necessary linkage between the growth of science, rationality, and universal human freedom. But when unmasked and understood, the legacy of the Enlightenment was the triumph of … purposive- instrumental rationality. This form of rationality affects and infects the entire range of social and cultural life encompassing economic structures, law, bureaucratic administration, and even the arts. The growth of [purposive-instrumental rationality] does not lead to the concrete realisation of universal freedom but to the creation of an 'iron cage' of bureaucratic rationality from which there is no escape' [47]. In other words, to the extent that this formulation holds true and whatever the upsides to this transformation may have been, human worth has now come to be assessed through citizens' performance within one or more instrumentally designed but imperfect systems. Over recent decades, whether as efficiency, efficacy or effectiveness, performance has continued to advance increasingly as the organising principle of business, politics and even art [48].

Within the above framework, the dynamism unleashed by the interaction of science, technology and capital has made it more difficult to discern the meaning that helps us shape our identity and be confident about the shared values that should guide people's lives. In Henri Lefebvre's words: 'Around 1910 a certain space was shattered. It was the space of common sense, of knowledge, of social practice, of political power, a space hitherto enshrined in everyday discourse, just as in abstract thought, as the environment of and channel for communication… Euclidian and perspectivist space have disappeared as systems of reference, along with other former 'common places' such as town, history, paternity, the tonal system in music, traditional morality, and so forth. This was a truly crucial moment' [49]. Such fundamental changes in daily environment and experience emphasise the necessity to continue interrogating critically the assumptions and practices of Kraepelin, which were formed in the nineteenth century but were carried forward in psychiatry's twentieth, even twenty-first.

Writing in 1983 about the onset of WWI, S. Kern noted 'the men in power lost their bearing in the hectic rush paced by flurries of telegrams, telephone conversations, memos, and press releases; hard boiled politicians broke down and seasoned negotiators cracked under the pressure of tense confrontations and sleepless nights, agonising over the probable disastrous consequences of their snap judgements and hasty actions' [50]. Harvey adds 'Newspapers fed popular anger, swift military mobilisations were set in motion, thus contributing to the frenzy of diplomatic activity that broke down simply because enough decisions could not be made fast enough in enough locations to bring the warlike stresses under collective control. Global war was the result. It seemed, to both Gertrude Stein and Picasso, a cubist war, and was fought on so many fronts and in so many spaces that the denotation appears reasonable even on a global scale' [51].

Crucial to success in capitalism is the shrinking of time and space. The profit imperative mandates ever quicker innovation and access to both resources and markets across the globe. The outcome can be greater ease in our daily life with sanitation, transport and domestic appliances being emblematic in this respect until the 1990s or so. However, the 1970s, the very decade when Lefebvre was writing, prepared the ground for further monumental changes in economy, technology and culture, often summarised under the label 'neoliberalism' [52, 53]. Writing in 1990, Harvey commented 'The half-life of a typical Fordist product was, for example, from five to seven years, but flexible accumulation has more than cut that in half in certain sectors (such as textile and clothing industries), while in others—such as the so-called 'thought-ware' industries (e.g. video games and computer software programmes)- the half-life is down to less than eighteen months. Flexible accumulation has been accompanied on the consumption side, therefore, by much greater attention to quick-changing fashions and the mobilisation of all the artifices of need inducement and cultural transformation that this implies. The relatively stable aesthetic of Fordist modernism has given way to all the ferment, instability, and fleeting qualities of a postmodernist aesthetic that celebrates difference, ephemerality, spectacle, fashion, and the commodification of cultural forms' [54]. Fordist accumulation here refers to capital based on gold and machine-plant as opposed to abstract finance. Flexible accumulation refers to financialisation, global chains and just-in-time production processes.

Crucial to changes since 1990 have been big data and digitisation. The first mobile phone call was made in the 1970s. The 1990s saw its general use, the widespread availability of the World Wide Web and the increasing use of e-mail. Kornbluh writes 'The suite of i-tech- including smartphone and social media- began broadly in 2006–7, with the iPhone launch in June 2007 and the opening of Facebook beyond Harvard University's walls in September 2006. In 2010, Instagram kicked off, gaining 10 million users within its first year and selling to Facebook in 2012. Twitter started in 2006, adding photo sharing in 2011, growing to 330 million users at its peak' [55]. OpenAI released ChatGPT in November 2022. All these have generated a culture demanding 'Immediacy' [55].

The acceleration of time, shrinking of space and demand for immediacy are of direct relevance to psychiatry. For example, whatever its bona fide credentials as a mental ill health condition may or may not be, the current social media and other clamour for ADHD (attention deficit/hyperactivity disorder) and the related stimulant overprescription rates [56, 57] make best sense in the light of demands for performance and immediacy. 'Attention must not even waver for a minute' was an attitude presumably unthinkable, even counter-adaptive, in the Environment of Evolutionary Adaptiveness (EAA) [58]. Arguably, this is a key example of how economy and culture both generate and define but also set the parameters for the treatment of 'psychopathology'. For the avoidance of doubt: professional guidelines find evidence that prescription of medication for ADHD is indicated at times. However, major problems arise at the margins. Here the margins are wide [56], especially as the putative neuropathology of the condition remains elusive [59] and, perhaps, will never materialise. In any case, a lot of psychiatry is practiced at the margins. This has always been the case because of the nature of its object and expertise [60–63].

In his admirably detailed account, Reckwitz has described some key societal outcomes of changes in recent decades [64]. He highlights the evolution from materially based 'modern'/'Fordist' industrial societies to what, via processes of increasing 'culturalisation' enabled by digital and communication media, he refers to as our contemporary 'society of singularities'. He describes a transformation from conditions of physical scarcity in the 'modern'/'Fordist' materially driven economy to one of overabundance of cultural products in the new one. The availability of secure corporate careers has declined. Contemporaneously, future success has become more difficult to predict and plan for. Increasingly unpredictable but exceptional singularities (e.g. 'influencers', Amazon, Taylor Swift, specific Universities, Greek holiday islands, new terrorist organisations, Donald Trump, anything) achieve remarkable success while many more citizens, start-ups, even established businesses and other institutions are destined to fail. Failure and disappointment can occur in any stratum of society and any stage of a career, but it is cushioned more in some circumstances and less in others. It is from the pool of demands for ever-improving performance, uncertainty, failure and defeat, combined with the loss of support occasioned by the fragmentation of family and community, that mental ill health often arises [65].

Bhargava and colleagues [66] summarise vividly the increase in mental health problems, addictions, overdoses, suicide and alienation during the neoliberal decades in the USA, undoubtedly the most consequential country since WWII and, perhaps, one destined to remain so in the foreseeable future [67, 68], though some confidently foresee its imminent demise [69]. Bhargava et al. emphasise that the neoliberal social conditions, twinned with the ideologies and politics associated with them, have led to the failure of policy to comfort those most in need. This, even, includes the failure of well-intended policies such as provision of state benefits.

Though they may have cause to be, this does not mean that all Americans are unhappy [70, 71]. Even if they are not, however, the above facts are still of fundamental importance for psychiatry, both today and beyond. A landmark Lancet Commission report has shown that beginning with the election of Ronald Reagan in the early 1980s and the consequent dominance of neoliberalism, there have been accelerating excess mortality rates in the USA compared to the other G7 most developed economies. In 2018 for example, before the Coronavirus Disease-2019 (COVID-19) Pandemic, the excess annual mortality was well over 400,000. Cumulatively during the years 1980–2020, it has been approximately 900,000,000

[72]. Bhargava et al. identify the increasing prevalence of Durkheim's *anomie* as a key explanatory concept and advocate community activism as a remedy.

Bhargava et al.'s call for socially committed activism resonates with the one advocated for mental health professionals by Ikkos and Bouras. In 'Metacommunity: The status of psychiatry today and implications for the future' [73], they have proposed that in developed countries we may broadly think of the history of psychiatry as divided into three eras: the asylum, community, and *metacommunity* eras. In Greek, meta ($\mu\varepsilon\tau\alpha$) means after, in this case after community psychiatry. They argue that, though community psychiatry has met some of its objectives, it has essentially failed in terms of its own ambitions. For those with severely disabling mental health conditions this has meant fragmentation of care, neglect and markedly reduced lifespans compared to the general population. To a significant extent this has been because of the evolution of neoliberalism that has brought about very different circumstances, perhaps entirely unforeseen by the pioneers of community psychiatry.

The first shoots of the metacommunity era of psychiatry became discernible in the 1990s, at the same time as the demise of the USSR, the triumph of neoliberalism and the forward leap of online communication technology, but Ikkos and Bouras suggest it has only been since the COVID-19 pandemic, today's cracks in globalisation, and with the arrival of ChatGPT that we have entered it fully. Metacommunity psychiatry is the condition of the specialty as we find it today. Ikkos and Bouras propose that because of increasing inequality, instability and breakdown of communities, the disappointment of the aspirations for the decade of the brain, and the emergence of big data, social media and the dominant power of big tech [67], the already well-understood imperatives for commitment to clinical ethics, scientific integrity and evidence-based practice are not enough. The metacommunity era demands a more socially critical orientation than hitherto, as well. Others have added that the narrative of metacommunity psychiatry requires appropriate recalibration if it is to be of global relevance [74].

As a profession, psychiatrists (after some deferred gratification) achieve a reasonable material renumeration. But, what about moral comfort? This is another matter altogether. Trainees very rapidly come face to face with the violence of mental healthcare and how this is situated within the everyday violence of modern life. Two related issues arise: one adverse and the other potentially liberating. The first issue is that of moral injury, and the demoralisation and burnout associated with it [75]. Burnout due to overwhelming workloads and administrative burdens distracts clinicians from patient care and contributes to the erosion of physician autonomy and empathy. The second issue is that of critical social thinking and grassroots activism as possible responses to social injustice and moral injury. Social critique and communal activism offer the opportunity to counter injury and prevent burnout. Indeed, even the possibility of bringing about exceptional professional fulfilment. Such fulfilment might not be available the same way in other specialties in medicine and is potentially achievable even in cases where clinical psychiatric outcomes do not amount to what we would all like to see.

27.4.2 Political Economy and Progress

By 2018, decades of social and political change and wealth creation had almost halved the proportion of people living in absolute poverty, enhanced the education and social position of women and ensured 80% of children had at least one vaccination worldwide. Global life expectancy had increased to 70 years [76]. China's economy having grown 25 times during the period 1978–2013 and its share of global GDP having shot up from under 3% in 1978 to almost 15% in 2015, has contributed the lion's share of this advance [77]. Because of their immediate challenge to psychiatry, we have emphasised the failures and casualties of neoliberalism in the preceding section. It is important to acknowledge in parallel, however, its significant successes. In this section, we will comment on neoliberalism's successes and their antinomies in relation to psychiatry.

When thinking about political economy and society, matters are invariably dialectical, that is, internally contradictory rather than straight forward. This is captured well by Benavav when he writes that 'the share of the world's population suffering from the most extreme forms of poverty has declined over time, alongside the urbanisation of the world's population... incomes for the poorest half of the global populations doubled between 1980 and 2016 (although rising by only a tiny amount in absolute terms), but that accounted for only 12 percent of overall income growth; the richest 1 percent captured more than twice that share- 27 percent- over the same period. As inequality has risen, social mobility has fallen. Whether working as home health aides in Minnesota, adjunct university lecturers in Italy, fruit vendors in Tunisia, or construction workers in India, more and more people feel that they are stuck in place' [78]. 'Most people are scraping by, earning additional minutes of life one at a time...The vast majority of the world's underemployed workers therefore end up employed in the heterogeneous service sector, which accounts for between 70 and 80 percent of total employment in high income countries and the majority of workers in Iran, Nigeria, Turkey, the Philippines, Mexico, Brazil, and South Africa' [79]. There are winners and losers in capitalism and the gap is widening with increasingly adverse consequences for the losers. And, paradoxically perhaps, as the paper by Bhargava et al. highlights, this holds even, maybe above all, in the most economically and technologically advanced country in the world. Even in China, its outstanding economic and technological achievements notwithstanding, historian Klaus Mühlhahn describes vividly the anxieties generated internally by its ambitions and progress in recent decades [77].

With respect to increasing inequality, it is important to consider the relative social positions of psychiatrists and their patients. This is because inequality has improved the circumstances of those with higher degrees in education and adversely affected those with less or minimal education [80]. In addition, medicine still offers relatively stable corporate or professional career structures with reasonably predictable pathways to success. Therefore, in any equitably accessible mental health system, psychiatrists may be expected to belong to the more privileged, highest income and career security brackets but their patients disproportionately the opposite. This raises questions about psychiatrists' ability to understand their patients' struggles and form truly empathic relationships and underscores the shortcomings of a purely science, policy and technical skills approach to professional life. Critical social awareness and community engagement are not simply 'good to have' but essential requirements.

With respect to the increase in knowledge and improvements in technology, one area where it has been translated to outstanding improvements is clinical outcomes in medicine. Unfortunately, this is an area where psychiatry has lagged. This is both because of the complexity of the brain [81] that was truly unforeseen even as late as the 1990s, the 'decade of the brain', and the importance of social factors that have worked precisely against that group of citizens who develop mental ill health [62, 73]. This, of course, poses a challenge to those like Kraepelin who wish to see psychiatry 'just like any other medical specialty' and further reinforces the need for broader perspectives.

The descriptive changes outlined previously in relation to the neoliberal and metacommunity eras, especially towards culturalisation and symbolic products, should not obscure the fact that throughout, and still today, capital remains a dominant driving force, now increasingly abstract in the form of finance and digital data rather than as tangible commodities and machinery-plant in the ownership of industrial barons. David Harvey comments: 'If we view culture as that complex of signs and significations (including language) that mesh into codes of transmission of social values and meanings, then we can at least begin upon the task of unravelling its complexities under present-day conditions by recognising that money and commodities are themselves the primary bearers of cultural codes. Since money and commodities are entirely bound up with the circulation of capital, it follows that cultural forms are firmly rooted in the daily circulation process of capital. It is, therefore, with the daily experience of money and the commodity that we should begin, no matter if special commodities or even whole sign systems may be extracted from the common herd and made the basis of 'high' culture or that specialised 'imaging' which we have already commented on' [82].

It is this, together with our technology, ideology and the mass media that are dependent on it, that determines the daily structures within which we live. These structures are not exclusively premised on reason or even performativity, but too often on violence in the service of interests, hegemony and domination [83]. The ever-expanding debt invested in the military of the USA since the Viet Nam war and continuing to grow today is testimony to this. A robustly documented but less well-understood reality is the interdependence of the US national security establishment with private business interests and the flow of funds from state assets that help generate profits for the latter [84]. In turn, those businesses directly underpin and serve the country's status as global hegemon. This is what General Dwight Eisenhower, the Republican former US President, referred to in the 1950s as the 'Military Industrial Complex'. Ominously, Harvey discusses in detail how this deficit-funded public–private defence industry and finance nexus has been crucial to the function of the whole world economy [85].

The determining power of capital accounts decisively for the reality of both domestic and international inequalities. It is also important to emphasise that although symbolic products and communication have become increasingly prevalent there have remained extensive industrial and corporate structures, with the former often transferred to China or the Global South. Most recently, the transfer has even been from China to Viet Nam and other more economically peripheral countries. Furthermore, though society has evolved towards increasingly symbolic products and processes, the related technologies both depend on natural mineral resources and pose a threat to sustainability [86]. Because of its gigantic energy demands, the recent explosion of AI brings threats to sustainability. It also brings threats to democracy. The relative significance of promises and threats remains impossible to compute today [87].

Whether it is deaths of despair in the USA, trauma related conditions due to war or immiseration globally, or hunger, illegal migration and people smuggling because of ecological catastrophe, it is relations of power and domination that have a major role to play in bringing people (and peoples, or populations) to psychiatrists' attention [88]. In the next section we summarise how political economic factors interdigitate with psychiatry through the social determinants of mental (ill) health.

27.4.3 Social Determinants of Mental Health

The evidence base for social determinants of mental health is substantial. These determinants include wider social, economic, environmental, cultural and political factors. These factors contribute to shaping health-related behaviours and (physical and mental) health outcomes [89]. Frameworks have been developed that help to conceptualise the (down-stream) effects of social determinants. Such frameworks reach from generic structural drivers, e.g. socioeconomic, environmental and cultural contexts, via mechanisms of social stratification and a range of determining factors (e.g. ethnic group, gender, social class and sexuality—see the issue of intersectionality immediately below), and they lead towards daily living conditions across the life span that, in their turn, interact with health behaviours and funnel into the differential distributions of health and mental health. Structural drivers include economic instability, and a surge in suicide rates was documented in England, Greece, Spain and the USA following the economic calamities set off by the financial crisis of 2008 [89].

Social strata refer to ethnicity, gender, sexuality, social class, income and educational levels. Common mental disorders are more prevalent among women than men. The level of gender inequality within countries has been found to be associated with gender inequality with respect to mental health outcomes, and wealth inequality associated with male but not female rates of depression [90]. Among high-income countries, those characterised by greater income inequality have higher rates of mental distress and ill health [91]. Low socio-economic status is associated with low education, fewer well-paid jobs, less good-quality work, low-quality housing and dietary problems. Racial discrimination has been identified as a mental health stressor, and racism affects outcomes such as depression, anxiety and stress while emotional support may attenuate such associations. A combination of issues related to different aspects of social position and identity (e.g. ethnicity, social class and gender) is referred to as intersectionality [92].

Daily living conditions are important determinants of mental health in early life and adolescence. Parental love and attention interact with family income, education and housing in shaping resilience and mental (ill) health. Biological mechanisms such as stress responses are affected by adverse living conditions. Childhood adversity is associated with mental disorders at all stages of life, and childhood adversity is related to socioeconomic disadvantages. Family social disadvantages are reflected in mental ill health at adolescence, and in obesity and relationship problems.

Later in life, working conditions characterised by a combination of 'low control and high demand' or by 'high effort and low reward' lead to work stress and impact negatively on employee mental health. Unemployment is associated with a higher prevalence of common mental disorders, and the economic consequences of the COVID-19 pandemic have had negative mental health effects. Financial debt has been shown to be an important lever in the relationship between low income and mental ill health in adulthood.

There is, however, evidence that policy measures targeted at social protection can mitigate such effects [93]. Welfare regimes can mitigate gender (and other) inequalities in mental well-being. Both childhood and adult green living space and the quality of housing and living environments are associated with levels of mental ill health. The general sense of control over one's life or, alternatively, of a lack of control, has an important role in creating health inequalities while close and supportive social relationships can buffer such effects, and protective effects have been identified for stable, loving childhood relationships [89].

In conclusion, mental health professionals operate within the complexity of multiple components of the wider social and cultural context, that is, of risk factors, buffers and mechanisms of the 'social' impinging on individual (and group) mental ill health. They are also faced with a high level of societal (national), regional and local factors shaping mental health service systems in different countries and settings. In the next section, we ask 'what is to be done'?

27.5 What Is to Be Done?

In relation to the question of what is to be done, for example, Johnson and colleagues offer extensive advice with respect to acute psychiatric care [94]. They see it as the responsibility of the profession to develop flexible and accessible local area crisis care systems offering a variety of options to meet service user needs and preferences. Coproduction with the people using services and their communities and with multiprofessional staff in all relevant sectors is considered an important prerequisite. Below, however, we want to answer the question at a different register: not that of policy and service provision themselves but the vocational ethics, clinical relationships and cultural know-how required to get them right. Here Horkheimer and Adorno's telling phrase of 'Dialectic of the Enlightenment' [95] remains relevant to psychiatry today. This should become apparent as we address below issues of personal autonomy, social critique and disenchantment, clinical utopias and the importance of social marginalisation and Mad Studies.

27.5.1 Personal Autonomy and Psychiatric Care

On the positive side of the dialectic, a big step forward has been closely linked with Enlightenment's core topic: a powerful image has emerged of the autonomous, responsible citizen, citoyen/citoyenne who is not simply called upon to accept the decisions of the secular and spiritual authorities, but to question and help shape them. Immanuel Kant, when writing about 'Answering the question: What is enlightenment?', quite deliberately included the injunction, '*Sapere aude!*' ('Dare to know'), which goes back to the Roman poet Horace [96]. In this way, reason has been advanced as the actual core of what makes a person, the centre of the *Conditio Humana* (the condition of the human).

Though this has not been consistently the case, from the above perspective, illnesses may be considered as causing citizens to be temporarily unable to use their reason or to use it only to a limited extent, without fundamentally affecting their status as a person. As a result, some of those who were previously considered as 'possessed', as punished by God, or simply as criminals gradually came to be seen as sick, suffering human beings with a genuine claim to social acceptance, support and, above all, treatment, guaranteed solely by their recognised status as patients. From this perspective, the *insane*, as they were then called, were suffering individuals who were *dependent on* and *entitled to* help. Newly built psychiatric hospitals stimulated the conceptual, that is, scientific and ethical, examination of the young field. Probably the best-known representative of this development is Philippe Pinel (1745–1826), the French psychiatrist who in 1793 ordered the Bicêtre clinic in Paris to stop using coercive measures wherever possible, particularly the chaining of patients, which was common practice at the time.

To avoid misunderstandings: any idealised or hagiographic description of psychiatry's conceptual history during this period must be nipped in the bud since the discipline has truly shown itself not only in its bright, but also in its dark sides [97]. Crucially, and this is a point often missed, ideals of enlightenment have by no means guaranteed that daily practice in dealing with mentally ill people would meet ethical standards. Indeed, there have been some methods of 'therapy' that were based on a supposedly rational attitude but were in fact naïve and bluntly paternalistic and strike us as barbaric today. For example, assuming that manic-depressive illness, bipolar disorder nowadays, was due to a disordered blood flow to the brain, sufferers were placed on a so-called 'rotating chair' and spun in rapid rotation to positively influence blood circulation. And then, of course, beyond such examples, there have been practices that cannot be considered as anything other than abuse or criminality [98, 99].

In the light of this complex dialectic, any proposal linking the Enlightenment positively with psychiatry might be greeted with some scepticism, if not open hostility. However, some recent publications highlight the continuing potential for a positive Enlightenment legacy for science and society in the twenty-first century [100]. From a Kantian philosophical perspective, the basic idea of Enlightenment, that is, the strengthened position of the autonomous citizen with his or her inalienable rights and duties, has not only contributed significantly to the emergence and sustainable establishment of the new discipline of psychiatry, but also has the potential to strengthen its currently fragile scientific identity.

Psychiatry is necessarily a multidimensional science and practice. If we want to counter the 'centrifugal' thinning out or even dissolution of the specialty to the detriment of many citizens in distress, we need a unifying bracket. One such device could be the very concept of the autonomous person. Specifically with respect to psychopathology, this could pave the way for the integration of subjective experiences, objectifiable somatic findings and interpersonal, that is, social, domains. This approach rejects any reductionist attempt to fully replace one of these perspectives with another [63, 101]. Before, during and after any mental ill health condition, next or opposite to the psychiatrist sits or agitates a person. And the clinician is a person herself.

This is not exclusively about epistemology. It is also about the imperatives of psychiatry, as a profession and as a vocation, and about individual and social justice. Moving within this broad field of theoretical tensions in an undogmatic and responsible manner is (and will remain) a core task of psychiatry—an obligatory and a challenging one. But how can we translate such abstract considerations into concrete acts, especially in relation to epistemic justice, second-order empathy and healing in today's shared political worlds? It is here, as part of the negative side of our dialectic, that disenchantment comes in. And so do possible responses to it through demand for (micro) utopias, and attention to issues of marginalisation and Mad Studies.

27.5.2 Disenchantment and Utopia

Late capitalist societies are not *communities* of people cooperating and in dialogue with each other but primarily collections of isolated individuals. In an individualistic society, each individual plays for him- or herself and not for the team. Yet, at the same time this very society has been constructing a cult for itself. More important than individuals, society has become that on which everything is justified. However, in yet another twist, even society itself is a means not an end. Society, demanding efficient performance in the service of capital, is a phantasmagoria [102] that regiments and channels the desire of all to produce and consume goods, activities whose greatest value increasingly accrues to the few.

In this kind of 'society', the very word *individual* has become ambiguous: on the one hand it means personal particularity and autonomy but on the other it encourages the assertion of oneself over others. And it may appear a paradox but, though driven by the ideology of individualism [103], capitalism has constructed and simultaneously been dependent on the increasingly complex and organised liberal states (and empires) of the nineteenth and twentieth centuries [104, 105]. In this process, despite its roots in the Enlightenment critique of tradition, in order to resolve the contradiction between the ideology of ragged individualism and the collectivity of the nation in the service of capital, the liberal state (and its neoliberal successors and their market orientated authoritarian variants) has borrowed formally and brutally from a hybrid of nationalism and religion (for instance, sacrifice for the homeland, for the one true God etc.) [106]. Subsequently, in the name of the ever more efficient functioning of society they have required the ironing of every anomalous crease that, in fact, is individuality. Being 'antisocial' has become the equivalent of a sin in the religious sense of the term. In this sense, 'sinning' consists in being unable or unwilling to submit to and conform to social codes.

From the perspective of psychopathology, we might contrast two instructive groups. On the one hand, there are the *compliant individuals*—sometimes so compliant that they become submissive: they are the officials, the clerks of the system and the skeleton on which it is supported. They unknowingly efface themselves as autonomous individuals. The prototype is Tellenbach's *typus melancholicus*, rigidly conscientious, very respectful of social order and above all heteronomous, that is, unreflectively respectful of what he/she assumes are societal norms [107]. Too subjugated to openly rebel, they may 'sin' as they sink into depression or present as 'neurotic'. They are the majority. Next is the group of openly *rebellious individuals*. Desperate or exalted dissidents, weird or eccentric, angry and sometimes violent, they are the ones that are most scary for the devotees of society and risk, therefore, being categorised as 'psychotic' or on the verge of psychosis—'borderline'.

A word of caution. We must not fall prey to simplistic and romantic idealisation. Symptoms of psychopathology are not just the reaction of a healthy mind to a sick society. They are, rather, signs of the struggle of a human subject to cope with the vulnerability inherent in his (or her) humanity. Looking at it from this perspective, we may find something we might call beautiful, to which we must do justice. One may ask what is beautiful about suffering and what is called mental illness? Little or nothing if the phenomenon is taken in and for itself, that is, suffering, deviance or diversity, or the abnormal thoughts and behaviour of an isolated individual. Much, on the other hand, if another individual comes into play who, standing in front of the sufferer, engages in dialogue with him and questions the personal and human meaning of such suffering. It is this struggle and the opportunity that psychiatrists are afforded to witness and join in with that are beautiful.

Note: we will be better able to engage fully in the way suggested above if disenchanted with society. Otherwise, we will risk falling prey to distraction and prattle. That is, unless disenchanted we will continue to fantasise about the next discovery, product, policy, plan or service development instead, and miss the chance right in front of us. After all, more than two centuries of psychiatry, more than a century of psychoanalysis, more than half a century of antipsychiatry, and decades of cognitive behavioural therapy (CBT), positive thinking and intensive neuroscientific research, have not prevented the increasing prevalence of psychopathology (and utilisation of services of various kinds) nor lessened the yawning mortality gap between those living with severe mental ill health and the general population. It is such outcomes that require psychiatrists to turn to disenchantment, even pessimism. However, the pessimism required is dialectical. That is, radical or *critical disenchantment with society* is only one side, the other, intensely contrary to it, is passion, the *vocational passion for (micro) utopia*.

But beware of utopia, the reader may say, and she will be right! Ideology is an enemy of truth, freedom and beauty. In his scholarly and original history of psychiatry, Warren [108] argues that all major initiatives in psychiatry (asylum, community, biological and antipsychiatry included) began as utopias but turned into dystopias. We have become disenchanted with the macro-utopias of the past. Two personal examples, indicative of the experiences of many:

First dystopia: in the 1980s and 1990s, in Italy but not only, reaching a diagnosis and admitting a patient for treatment was considered by some to be a reactionary gesture and was sanctioned by the 'top' as a shameful act on the part of the psychiatrist who had ordered the hospitalisation. Beds per inhabitant had to be below 1 in 10,000. In order not to hospitalise patients in an acute state, however, in a town in central Italy the patient was carried around in an ambulance throughout the night and administered high doses of neuroleptics. In the same psychiatric service, the medical records avoided any psychopathological annotation. Psychopathology was considered a bourgeois and reactionary science. Clinicians limited themselves to recording that 'the patient is better' or 'the patient is worse'.

Second dystopia: that of community psychiatry intent on integrating individual mental sufferers into a sick and pathogenic society in a top-down operation. One of us had the good fortune, or misfortune, to have witnessed—at his young age when he worked in the psychiatric services of the Italian Mental Health Service— some excesses of *psichiatria territotiale* (community or catchment area psychiatry). It was in the mid-nineties when the head of his psychiatric service proudly showed him a map of the territory of Livorno—a Tuscan seaside known for the famous congress of 1921 in which the Italian Communist Party was founded by a split in the Socialist Party. A city, therefore, with a strong 'progressive' vocation. The boss said, 'Look at this map!'. The younger psychiatrist asked, 'So what?'. 'This is my utopia: four psychiatric wards at the four cardinal points of the city: north, south, east, west. Because the psychiatry of the territory must give the same guarantees as the asylum'. Ideology really is an ugly beast, isn't it? Whatever colour she is dressed in. To supervise the territory, therefore, to guard it, to control it. *Surveiller et punir: Naissance de la prison* ('To Discipline and Punish: The Birth of the Prison') by Michel Foucault [109] was published in 1975! Is this what survives of Foucault's legacy in the folds of 'democratic psychiatry'? Territorial psychiatric services risk becoming a bureaucratic and/or authoritarian institution in their turn. When such risks materialise, they are a utopia that should not be denied but overcome.

Ideology does not make mental health services a place that favours encounters between human beings. Nevertheless, psychiatrists' critical disenchantment must not reach the extreme of the renunciation of politics. We must stand in solidarity with the denunciation of injustice and join in giving voice to the offended and stand for their right to be 'antisocial'. The dream (and hope) of eliminating (or alleviating) mental suffering with the use of diagnosis, psychotherapy, social interventions and psychopharmacological treatments is a utopia that should not be abandoned. But we must also recognise the dystopian nature of this utopia when it has transformed into a device for the 'normalisation' of deviant people according to common sense and the social norms to which psychiatric categories have too often been tailored [110, 111].

Good social functioning has become a must for contemporary psychiatry. But what does 'good social functioning' mean if not adapting to the dominant social norms and customs of society? Psychiatry should also focus beyond these, even against them, as necessary sometimes. Utopia becomes dystopia when psychotropic drugs are only used as devices to eliminate symptoms because they hinder the proper functioning of individuals within the production chain. Crucially, when constraining, restraining or medicating people with the kind of madness we call psychosis, as is necessary at times, we must not forget that inherent in madness there is a complex and powerful dialectic of its own [112]!

As a profession and vocation, psychiatrists should be part of a third group, equidistant between the conforming and rebelling, one that recognises the physiological incompatibility between the dictates and rules of society and some individuals who do not recognise themselves in it and instead require 'the right to get sick'. Therefore, the our proposed critical disenchantment psychiatry with society and the passion for a (clinical) utopia are the two arms of an inseparable pair (both disenchantment and utopia, not disenchantment or utopia). But it is a utopia of a specific psychiatric vocational kind.

Psychopathology is a knowledge ($\lambda \acute{o} \gamma o \varsigma$; logos) that concerns the suffering ($\pi \acute{a} \theta o \varsigma$; pathos) of the human psyche. In Minkowski's words, it should not be a pathology of the psychological (a field of knowledge that seeks the pathological as a distortion of the human), but a psychology of the pathological—that is, a field of knowledge that strives to trace what is considered pathological back to the fundamental questions of human existence [113]. Psychopathology should not aim to establish a clear separation between the normal and the pathological, nor should it deny the presence of a vulnerability intrinsic to the human condition. But it should try to give psychopathological phenomena a more precise foundation, that is, to extend them not so much towards normal as towards life with the structures and organisation upon which human life, in all its complexity, rests. The overall aim of this operation is that psychopathology thus remains in contact in permanent interaction with living reality [114]. Which is to say that the psychopathologists who find themselves in front of someone who suffers should have the task of searching for the 'critically human' in this suffering. In doing so, they will discover that the sufferer embodies a fundamental knot of human existence, a way of facing his suffering, however ineffective it may seem or be. Both involuntary and voluntary to some extent, in Binswanger's words it is a form of *unfortunate existence* [115]. A way of being in the world of someone who is lost while trying to carve out a path through the aporias of existence.

With such an approach to psychopathology, as we have suggested, mental suffering may be said to be 'beautiful'. A terrible beauty, no doubt, but what makes mental suffering 'beautiful' is this gaze—first and foremost, our gaze as psychiatrists—which sees in it the figure of the human. It is to this reevaluating gaze that young psychiatrists must be educated. Patients are not mere carriers of symptoms to be eliminated, like nefarious Christmas trees from which, when Christmas ends, their unfortunate decorations must be removed. Symptoms are not sick additions to a healthy organism, but the expression of a vulnerable organism that reacts to a real or imaginary threat.

Treating symptoms without questioning their causes is clearly a mistake in medicine, and treating symptoms without questioning their meaning is equally so in psychiatry. Psychiatrists, then, will have to educate everyone—the 'citizens'—to look at mental suffering with this gaze. A gaze that is not merely compassionate or generically empathetic. And, of course, not a cynically aestheticising gaze either but an interested gaze, engaged, committed to grasping in the other—in his symptom—his humanity and to care for it. A gaze capable of grasping the aura of humanity inherent in mental suffering. This is the (micro) utopia to which passion in psychiatric vocation must and can lead, and it must be inseparable from the radical disenchantment of dialectical pessimism.

The (micro) utopia that we propose is that psychiatric services should be places designated to build encounters between human beings, Oury's 'spaces of the saying', and spaces of dialogue [44]. Institutions are fortunately made up of people. And even medications are substances prescribed by people to other people. Good enough institutions for practices of care can only be based on the good enough training of the people who work in them. In our opinion, good training begins by enabling medical doctors, psychologists, nurses, social workers etc. to recognise what is human in the condition of those suffering from mental health problems. This is an essential requirement for the fulfilment of psychiatric vocation.

How can we not grasp the humanity of the people some call 'schizophrenic', at loggerheads with questions that if we listened to them could distress us all, such as the one on the 'reality of reality', or on the splitting of our consciousness, or on the boundaries between words, images and things [116]? How can we not recognise the human in the theme of guilt that distresses melancholic people—a major group of 'compliant' individuals? Grappling with the uncertain boundary between responsibility and guilt, between voluntary and involuntary in relation to our actions, and between reversible and definitive relative to their consequences and their outcomes? How can we not recognise the human in the visceral need for recognition by the other, in the constitutive power of the gaze to confer an identity on oneself, which we find in the existence of people in hysterical predicaments [117]? How can we not recognise a human aspiration to become disconnected from one's personal history and operate outside temporal and social constraints and the laws of responsibility and, thus, give rein to uncontrollable passion as happens to the significant group among the 'rebellious' we call 'borderline'? [118]?

We need a psychopathology that, more than establishing boundaries between what is normal and what is pathological, more than finding early alarm bells in the history of an individual in order to prevent illness, is devoted to an anthropology, that is to an in-depth knowledge of the *Conditio Humana* in its vulnerability, as well as its resilience that some of us often admire in our patients. But, if this is so, how can we prepare ourselves to extend our understanding to reach some of the people we have been talking about here, especially those socially disadvantaged, abused, oppressed, marginalised or excluded? In the next section we suggest one potential facilitating perspective, namely attention to issues of social marginalisation.

27.5.3 Marginalisation

In their review, Johnson and colleagues emphasise the lack of evidence-based guidelines and systematic knowledge on crisis care in low- and middle-income countries. Furthermore, a 'Systematic Review with Qualitative Evidence Synthesis' has confirmed that discriminatory practices in mental healthcare lead to specific barriers to care for multiply marginalised service users [119]. Therefore, in dealing with the real social context in which people with mental conditions live, it may be helpful to turn to a construct developed by Antonio Gramsci (1891–1937) in the 1920s and 1930s when he confronted the situation of social groups that were under-privileged and marginal in Italian society at the time.

Gramsci used the term of the 'subaltern' to refer to the problem (and scandal) of exclusion of the urban and rural poor from the socio-economic institutions of Italian society [120]. His practice of avoiding terms such as the 'industrial and rural prole-tariat' was, in part, owed to his being a prisoner in Fascist pre-WWII Italy and having to evade the censors. However, Gramsci's thinking also took note of the historic defeat of the (orthodox) socialist–communist project of overthrowing capitalism in highly industrialised countries. His thinking, therefore, has been understood as the formulation of a non-dogmatic Marxist analysis of modern society that attributes a key role to cultural factors. He offered a differentiated analysis of societal elites in the economic, professional, cultural and spiritual spheres, focusing on conceptual constructs such as political and cultural 'hegemony' and the role of what he called 'classical' and 'organic' intellectuals.

Becker et al. [121] refer to Gramsci's (and Walter Benjamin's) potential contri-butions to the understanding of (international) psychiatric care and mental health reform. They discuss the role of some aspects of Gramsci's thinking during Italy's mental health reform of the 1960s–1980s as embodied in the closure of mental hos-pitals and a new mental health legislation (Law 180 of 1978). This reading of psy-chiatric reform positions the field of mental health and mental healthcare firmly in a wider socio-economic, cultural and political context. In such a reading of mental health issues, we can ask what other fields of societal activism and social–cultural–political movements could be relevant as partners within a wider coalition towards a more inclusive society.

The field of interest of subaltern studies is not far from the study of transregional (social and political) movements [122] that include political alliances and groups such as the anti-apartheid movement, the fair-trade movement, anti-debt campaigns, human rights NGOs (non-governmental organisations) and transregional environmental NGOs. It is a field of research full of lively and heated debate. However, no strong link with critical thought within and about psychiatry, no links with mental health activism and no alliances with mental health peer organisations can readily be found—although there are tenuous links in the literature [123]. Therefore, looking towards subaltern studies may appear far-fetched for the psychiatric profession(s) when facing current challenges. Such reality notwithstanding, or perhaps because of it, the onus should be on local and regional initiatives in psychiatry and the wider field of mental health (and pertinent fields of science and researchers working in them) to pick up on and join in the potential for new forms of joint activism and research around inclusion and the cultural forces hidden in marginal groups, their experience and reservoirs of resilience and survival. Such initiatives, movements and researchers might turn out to be key partners for the profession in its struggle to balance its bodies of positive scientific knowledge and professional practice with the potential for critical scrutiny of society. And, of course, it is here that service user movements and organisations and Mad Studies [124] must play a major role, too.

Any extension of our discourse from the Global North to the South requires much greater focus and detail but also promises new insights and opportunities. For example, against a background of wider socio-cultural-political debates, there is recent literature suggesting that the development of Western societies' modern understanding of mental illness may have been related to internalising the colonialists' concepts of 'race' and 'differentness' thus leading to the exclusion and extermination of those humans considered 'of lesser value' (both in the global North and South). There are also authors who fear that, with a new focus on 'culture', the old stereotypes, prejudices, stigma and danger of 'exclusion' of minority groups may come to the fore again [125, 126]. In other worlds, there are obvious and significant mental health issues to be addressed in understanding the history of Western psychiatry as well as colonialism. And, in a reversal of what has been happening to date, some other authors have suggested that innovative developments in low- and middle-income countries may have the potential to serve as templates for more inclusive collaborative practices of crisis care in high-income countries themselves [127].

27.6   Summary and Discussion: Dialectical Pessimism

In the Introduction and Sect. 2, we posited issues of justice and vocation for psychiatry in the context of the contributions of Emil Kraepelin, Max Weber and Walter Benjamin: modern era pioneers in the scholarly and scientific investigation of psychiatry, society and experience, respectively. Within this context, we reviewed Kraepelin's unexamined philosophical and scientific assumptions and the ambiguous legacy of the Enlightenment. We found any benefits arising out of the valorisation of reason, science, humanism and individual rights and the critique of tradition to have been accompanied by the disenchantment of the world and the spread of the phantasmagorias of commodity capitalism. We highlighted Kraepelin's early striking belief in the existence and scientific recognisability of objectively identifiable—in his diction: 'natural'—disease entities to explain insanity, which shaped his later life's academic work. Though not necessarily always explicitly so, in one way or another the remaining chapter has been a meditation on how the implications of this assumption have worked out in the context of evolving ethics, society and the constraints and opportunities of psychiatric practice. Looking back, we might consider the outcome as an example of the farsightedness of a key pre-occupation of Walter Benjamin, namely the social unfulfillment of science and technology. That is, the unfulfillment of the technologies of psychopharmacology, genetics, neuroscience and social science in psychiatry in the time of advanced and late capitalism.

In Sect. 3, we discussed conceptual and experiential issues in relation to empathy and vocation. We emphasised the essence of justice, not as an abstract moral virtue or character trait, but as lived experience in relation to others in contexts of citizenship and community. Here we highlighted Miranda Fricker's recent contribution of the idea of epistemic injustice, that is, the unfair treatment of individuals with mental health conditions in their capacity as knowers or sources of knowledge. The preliminary act of every medical action is or should be an act of empathy, that is, the fullest possible encounter with the other person's humanity. We emphasised that empathy in psychiatric practice requires highly complex skills and that, assuming they are present, their application is often obstructed by service and social circumstances. Sections 4 and 5 that followed may be considered an investigation into these obstructions and how they may be overcome.

In Sect. 4, we outlined the evolution of political economy and society since Kraepelin's times and their relation to mental (ill) health and services today. We highlighted elements of capitalism, technology, innovation, the shrinking of time and space and the ever-increasing demands for constant high performance. We focused particularly on the developments of neoliberalism, globalisation and digitisation in recent decades and on some key associated phenomena such as increasing inequality, fragmentation of communities, decreasing social mobility and marginalisation of large sections of the population. These have had demonstrably adverse effects on the epidemiology of mental ill health. In addition, patients with severe mental disorders continue to die one or two decades earlier than the general population. We have confirmed the importance of social determinants of mental (ill) health and some potential for remedial action. As a result, we found that, following its community psychiatry era, the profession has moved on to a new one, the metacommunity era. Metacommunity psychiatry is what psychiatry is today, together with the opportunities in sight and the demands that confront it.

In Sect. 5, we asked: what is to be done? Here we returned to the Enlightenment ideal of the autonomous person and emphasised the imperative of its centrality to psychiatry, whether the patient is legally incapacitated by illness or trauma or not. In part due to the legacy of Kraepelin's narrow biomedical assumptions, to date psychiatric training, research and clinical practice have too often fallen short in this, sometimes woefully so. We have argued that to remedy the shortfall and to do justice to psychiatry's vocation require broad understanding of the human condition in our contemporary social circumstances.

In view of our findings, we advocate that psychiatrists must adopt a critical stance to society and adopt an equidistant position between the struggles of patients who are alternatively 'compliant' or 'rebellious' in their societies. We labelled this aspect of psychiatry's stance as one of radical or *critical disenchantment*. Within such a context and with unflinching commitment to professional standards, the psychiatrist must not seek too rigid a boundary between normality and not. Clinicians must attend empathically to what is critical in their patients' humanity. Psychopathology is a knowledge (*λόγος*; logos) that concerns the suffering (*πάθος*; pathos) of the human psyche, a field of knowledge that strives to trace what is considered pathological back to the fundamental questions of human existence. We labelled this the vocational *passion for (micro) utopia*. These two, critical disenchantment and passion for utopia, make up the *dialectical pessimism* that is necessary for doing justice to psychiatry as a vocation. We consider commitment to coproduction, and Mad Studies as key emerging tools to help achieve this.

27.7 Conclusion

In this chapter, in significant part, we have offered a critique of neoliberal economy in relation to psychiatry but not an alternative political vision. That would be beyond the scope of psychiatry. Nevertheless, despite its length, our chapter has limitations. For example, irrespective of any wider social critique, we have not detailed positive research strategies nor tactical opportunities for treatment and development of mental healthcare within the framework of current social structures. Indeed, such research and reform remain essential to justice and vocation today and are discussed elsewhere in this volume (Eds: e.g. Chaps. 23, 24, 25, and 26). However, they have not been proven sufficient to date. Therefore, the limitations of our approach notwithstanding, we trust that the broad thrust of our appeal holds and will help move psychiatry forward.

To conform to and pacify the dominant positivist strain of medicine, psychiatric training of all types has felt compelled to hide (part of) its true heart and beliefs and engage in subterfuge. Socially, entering a career in psychiatry and related fields means that we are entering professions that are burdened and sometimes overwhelmed by trying to soothe the distress caused by an increasingly atomised and uncaring society. Though this is relevant to all of medicine, psychiatry is the place where the arts of attention and empathic reconstruction find shelter within the broader profession. But we must constantly fight for recognition for these central and important aspects of medical care (although the rise of the medical humanities in the last 20 years has improved the situation). In the light of this, whatever else psychiatry may be, and it is many things, it must be an act of resistance.

We remain fully committed to professionalism in psychiatry as commonly understood both within and beyond the profession. However, we also agree with Poole and Robinson that professionalism should not be erected as a citadel [128] in which mental health professionals barricade themselves against a hostile world and set up shops to trade their skills or join corporations to meet targets in the marketplace of healthcare or out of which they venture mainly to negotiate policy with the hegemonic powers that set the rules, whether governments, funding agencies or regulators. It is from this perspective that we advocate dialectical pessimism. This captures creatively the energy at the heart of the tension that pitches critical disenchantment with the forces of social domination in interaction with the (micro) utopian ambitions of vocation. This requires clinicians to engage in public discourse and listen, speak with, give voice, and join in solidarity with those who for whatever reasons and in different ways are unwell, suffer mental illness, or feel sick from and sick with how the social field is set for them.

In her Tanner lectures on ethics, the distinguished American political scientist Wendy Brown has warned against 'cruel optimism' when she commented that it is 'too much for many young spirits' to demand that they 'put one entrepreneurial foot in front of the other as if they were not walking toward catastrophe. Build your resume, cultivate your networks, find your mate… but also, save for an unaffordable home and unlikely retirement, plan for the end of democracy, and an uninhabitable planet. Most young people are in a mode of pre-apocalyptic survivalism, as are we all to some extent' [129]. In truth, the only alternatives to dialectical pessimism in psychiatry today are cruel optimism or a cynicism that accepts twenty-first century social injustices as they are.

Key Points

- We have examined aspects of Emil Kraepelin's legacy in psychiatry within the broad context of the dialectics of the Enlightenment. In the century since his death, psychiatry has benefited from his inspiration in establishing itself as a medical specialty. However, it has also been weighed down by it when it has continued espousing his unexamined and unwarranted assumptions. Together with the evolving nature of healthcare, this has led to the true vocation of the specialty having been veiled or obscured.
- In recent decades, both biological and community psychiatry have fallen short of their aspirations. This, together with the effective triumph of the neoliberal political economy and globalisation, has been associated with increased prevalence of mental health problems and continuing markedly premature mortality of those with severe mental health conditions. Therefore, there is an urgent need to displace the Kraepelin-inspired narrow medical model at the heart of psychiatry. This is consistent with emerging findings in evolutionary biology and neuroscience and does not reject the continued importance of biomedical care. Psychiatry must remain a medical specialty and, indeed, the change we advocate should lead to smarter therapeutic implementation of biomedical advances too.
- It has been argued that, in the context of accelerating changes in society, technology, consumption and unsustainable ecology, psychiatry has moved into its new metacommunity era. In this era, compassionate and relational care demands that psychiatry places engagement with the autonomous person firmly at the centre of its concerns, integrating the diverse factors bearing on each person's

predicament. Citizens presenting as patients require clinicians who do not espouse arbitrarily sharp boundaries of normality but are able to engage empathically with critically human factors, including when working with those living with extreme mental distress.

- In psychiatry's metacommunity era of ever-increasing displacement, digitisation, dizzying speed of change, demands for immediacy, grotesque inequalities and social exclusion, the specialty must find an actively critical social register and give voice to what matters to those who use its services. Inter alia, this requires including Mad Studies in the training and continuing professional development curriculum.
- To do justice to psychiatry as a vocation in the twenty-first century demands an outlook of *dialectical pessimism*: that is, radical or *critical disenchantment* with the determining forces of injustice in society on the one hand, and an insistence on a *vocational passion for (micro) utopia* on the other.

Disclosure All authors are the European members of the international collaboration group 'The Precision of Images: Emil Kraepelin, Walter Benjamin and the History of Psychiatry 1926–2026', which has been meeting since 2022.

Author Contributions GI suggested the chapter theme, led the scoping review and produced the first draft outline. All members of the group have contributed equally to the text.

References

1. quoted in Harvey, D. The condition of postmodernity. Oxford: Blackwell; 1990. p. 32.
2. quoted in Oyarzun, P. Doing justice: three essays on Walter Benjamin. Polity; 2020. p. 107.
3. Radkau J. Max Weber: a biography. Polity; 2011.
4. Eiland H, Jennings MW. Walter Benjamin: a critical life. Harvard University Press; 2016.
5. Becker T, Hoff P. Emil Kraepelin and Walter Benjamin: distant contemporaries, diverse working methods, any resonance? Int Rev Psychiatry. 2024:1–17. https://doi.org/10.1080/09540261.2024.2355994.
6. Kraepelin E. Memoirs. Ed. by Hippius H, Peters G, Ploog D in collaboration with Hoff P, Kreuter A. Translated by Wooding-Deane C. Berlin/Heidelberg: Springer; 1987. pp. 3–4.
7. Hoff P. Emil Kraepelin und die Psychiatrie als klinische Wissenschaft. Ein Beitrag zum Selbstverständnis psychiatrischer Forschung. Monographien aus dem Gesamtgebiete der Psychiatrie, vol. 73. Berlin/Heidelberg/New York: Springer; 1994: pp 47 ff
8. Hoff P, Hippius H. Wilhelm Griesinger (1817–1868)—sein Psychiatrieverständnis aus historischer und aktueller Perspektive. Nervenarzt. 2001;72:885–92.
9. Hoff P. Nosologische Grundpostulate bei Kraepelin—Versuch einer kritischen Würdigung des Kraepelinschen Spätwerkes. Z Klin Psychol Psychopathol Psychother. 1988;36:328–36.
10. Kraepelin E. Die Erscheinungsformen des Irreseins. Zeitschrift für die gesamte Neurologie und Psychiatrie. 1920;62:1–2.
11. Weber M. Tr tribe, K., economy and society. Harvard University Press; 2019.
12. Marx K. Tr Fowkes, M., capital: critique of political economy v.1. Penguin Classics; 1990.
13. Harvey D. A companion to Marx's capital: the complete edition. Verso; 2018.
14. Fournier M. Émile Durkheim: a biography. Polity. 2012;

15. Durkheim E. On suicide. Penguin Classics; 2006.
16. Weber M. The protestant ethic and the 'spirit' of capitalism. Penguin; 2002.
17. Weber M. Science as a vocation tr. Eds. H.H. Gerth and C. Wright Mills (Translated and edited), From Max Weber: Essays in Sociology. Oxford University Press; 1946. p. 212.
18. Weber M. Politics as a vocation tr. Eds. H.H. Gerth and C. Wright Mills (Translated and edited), From Max Weber: Essays in Sociology. Oxford University Press; 1946.
19. Ikkos G, Stanghellini G, Morgan A. History, 'nowtime' (jetztzeit) and dialectical images: introduction to Walter Benjamin for psychiatry (I). Int Rev Psychiatry. 2024:1–15. https://doi.org/10.1080/09540261.2024.2359468.
20. Stanghellini G. The psychiatrist as a ragpicker. Introduction to Walter Benjamin for psychiatrists (II): the dialectics between the fragment and the whole. Int Rev Psychiatry. 2024:1–12. https://doi.org/10.1080/09540261.2024.2354368.
21. Morgan A. '… the most complex and lyrical song of experience': Walter Benjamin and a dialectical image of madness. Introduction to Walter Benjamin for psychiatry (III). Int Rev Psychiatry. 2024:1–14. https://doi.org/10.1080/09540261.2024.2354375.
22. Ikkos G, Stanghellini G. Images of the past: introduction to Walter Benjamin and "Berlin childhood around 1900". Psychoanal Inq. 2024:1–12. https://doi.org/10.1080/07351690.2024.2383512.
23. Benjamin W. Capitalism as religion, tr Livingstone, R. in eds Bullock, M., Jennings, M., W. Selected Writings, volume 1, 1913–1926; 1996. pp. 288–91.
24. Benjamin W. Little history of photography, tr Jephcott, E. and Shorter, K. in in eds Jennings, M, W., Smith, G. Selected Writings, volume 2, Pat 2 1931–1931; 1999. pp. 506–30.
25. Benjamin W. The work of art in the age of its technical reproducibility, tr Zohn, H., Jephcott, in eds Eiland, H., Jennings, M. W., Selected Writings, volume 4, 1938–1940; 2003. pp. 251–83.
26. Buck-Morss. The dialectics of seeing: Walter Benjamin and the arcades project. MIT Press; 1991.
27. Ikkos G. Fulfilling experience: Walter Benjamin—psychiatry in philosophy. Br J Psychiatry. 2021;219(1):367. https://doi.org/10.1192/bjp.2021.35.
28. Ikkos G, Stanghellini G, Ikkos-Serrano A. The drama of fulfilment: reflection on Walter Benjamins "Fate and Character" (1921)- psychiatry in philosophy. Br J Psychiatry. 2026, in press.
29. Hansen B. Walter Benjamin's other history: of stones, animals, human beings, and angels. University of California Press; 2000. p. 163–5.
30. Arendt H. The human condition. London: The University of Chicago Press; 1958. p. 201.
31. Arendt H. Eichmann in Jerusalem: a report on the banality of evil. Penguin Classics; 1984.
32. Arendt H. The life of the mind. London: Harcourt Publication; 1984. p. 193.
33. Fricker M. Epistemic injustice: power and the ethics of knowing. Oxford University Press; 2007.
34. Bhugra D, Malik A, Ikkos G, editors. Psychiatry's contract with society: concepts, controversies and consequences. Oxford University Press; 2010.
35. Ikkos G, McQueen D, St. John-Smith P. Psychiatry's contract with society: what is expected? Acta Psychiatr Scand. 2011;124:1–3. https://doi.org/10.1111/j.1600-0447.2011.01678.x.
36. Durkheim E. tr Fields, K. E. The elementary forms of religious life. Free Press; 1995.
37. Ikkos G, McQueen D. Reflections on the elementary forms of religious life—reflections. Br J Psychiatry. 2019;214(5):304. https://doi.org/10.1192/bjp.2019.71.
38. Englander M, Ferrarello S. Empathy and ethics. Rowman & Littlefield Publishers; 2021.
39. Fuchs T. 'Intercorporeality and interaffectivity', in Ch. 1. In: Meyer C, Streeck J, Scott Jordan J, editors. Intercorporeality: emerging socialities in interaction, foundations of human interaction. New York: Oxford Academic; 2017. https://doi.org/10.1093/acprof:oso/9780190210465.003.0001.
40. Lucas R. The psychotic wavelength. Psychoanal Psychother. 1993;7(1):15–24. https://doi.org/10.1080/02668739300700021.

41. Ikkos G, Wee C. Mental illness, the psychotic wavelength and the mental health act (1983). Psychoanal Psychother. 2003;17(4):342–51. https://doi.org/10.108 0/14749730310001609744.
42. Stanghellini G. Philosophical resources for the psychiatric interview. In: Fulford KWM, Davies M, Gipps RGT, Graham G, Sadler JZ, Stanghellini G, Thornton T, editors. The Oxford handbook of philosophy and psychiatry. Oxford; 2013.
43. Brencio F. Heidegger and Binswanger: just a misunderstanding? Humanist Psychol. 2015;43(3):287–8. https://doi.org/10.1080/08873267.2014.993069.
44. Oury J. 'The hospital is ill', interview with David Reggio and Mauricio Novello. Radic Philos. 2007;143(32–45):44–5.
45. Brencio F. Bildwissenschaft and revolution. The story of Marco Cavallo and its significance in the history of psychiatry. Int Rev Psychiatry. 2024:1–8. https://doi.org/10.1080/0954026 1.2024.2356686.
46. Lyotard J-P. The postmodern condition—a report on knowledge, Trans. Geoffrey Bennington and Brian Massumi, with a foreword by Frederic Jameson. Manchester: Manchester University Press; 1979. p. 46.
47. quoted in Harvey D. The condition of postmodernity. Blackwell; 1990. p. 15.
48. Schechner R, Lucie S. Performance studies: an introduction. Routledge; 2020. p. 249.
49. Lefebvre, 1974 quoted Harvey D. The condition of postmodernity. Blackwell; 1990. p. 266.
50. quoted in Harvey D. The condition of postmodernity. Blackwell; 1990. p. 278.
51. Harvey D. The condition of postmodernity. Blackwell; 1990. p. 278.
52. Harvey D. A brief history of neoliberalism. Oxford University Press; 2005.
53. Slobodian Q. Globalists: the end of empire and the birth of neoliberalism. Harvard University Press; 2018.
54. Harvey D. The condition of postmodernity. Blackwell; 1990. p. 156.
55. Kornbluh A. Immediacy or the style of too late capitalism. Verso; 2023. p. 36.
56. te Meerman S, Batstra L, Grietens H, Frances A. ADHD: a critical update for educational professionals. Int J Qual Stud Health Well Being. 2017;12(sup1) https://doi.org/10.108 0/17482631.2017.1298267.
57. Reuben C, Nazik Elgaddal N. Attention-deficit/hyperactivity disorder in children ages 5–17 years: United States, 2020–2022. NCHS Data Brief, No. 499, 2024 March.
58. Barack DL, Ludwig VW, Parodi F, et al. Attention deficits linked with proclivity to explore while foraging. Proc R Soc B Biol Sci. 2024, published 21 February. https://doi.org/10.1098/rspb.2022.2584.
59. Koirala S, Grimsrud G, Mooney MA, et al. Neurobiology of attention-deficit hyperactivity disorder: historical challenges and emerging frontiers. Nat Rev Neurosci. 2024;25:759–75. https://doi.org/10.1038/s41583-024-00869-z.
60. Iliopoulos J. Is Foucault an anti-psychiatrist? Ch 4. In: The history of reason in the age of madness: Foucault's enlightenment and the radical critique of psychiatry. Bloomsbury; 2019.
61. Ikkos G. Psychiatric expertise. Br J Psychiatry. 2015;207(5):399. https://doi.org/10.1192/bjp.bp.115.169946.
62. Ikkos G. Not doomed: sociology and psychiatry, and ignorance and expertise. BJPsych Bulletin. 2023;47(2):90–4. https://doi.org/10.1192/bjb.2022.60.
63. Hoff P. Arthur Kronfeld und die Identität der Psychiatrie—Denkwege vom 18. bis zum 21. Jahrhundert. Stuttgart: Kohlhammer; 2023.
64. Reckwitz A. The society of singularities. Polity. 2020;
65. Kirkbride JB, Anglin DM, Colman I, Dykxhoorn J, Jones PB, Patalay P, Pitman A, Soneson E, Steare T, Wright T, Griffiths SL. The social determinants of mental health and disorder: evidence, prevention and recommendations. World Psychiatry. 2024;23(1):58–90. https://doi.org/10.1002/wps.21160. PMID: 38214615; PMCID: PMC10786006.
66. Bhargava D Shams S, Hanbury H. The death of "Deliverism". Democracy: A Journal of Ideas. 2023, June 22. https://democracyjournal.org/arguments/the-death-of-deliverism/.

67. Rikap C. The interplays of the United States, China and their intellectual monopolies, Ch 4. In: Capitalism, power and innovation: intellectual monopoly capitalism uncovered. Routledge; 2021.

68. Stevenson T. Someone Else's empire: British illusions and American hegemony. Verso; 2023.

69. Rapley J, Heather P. Why empires fail: Rome, America and the future of the west. Penguin; 2024.

70. Jagger A. Hyperpolitics USA. New Left Rev. 2024;149:5–16.

71. Peltzman S. The socio-political demography of happiness (July 12, 2023). George J. Stigler Center for the Study of the Economy & the State Working Paper No. 331, Available at SSRN: https://ssrn.com/abstract=4508123 or https://doi.org/10.2139/ssrn.4508123.

72. see Fig 2 in Woolhandler S, Himmelstein DU, Ahmed S, et al. Public policy and health in the Trump era. 2021;397(10275):705–53. https://doi.org/10.1016/S0140-6736(20)32545-9.

73. Ikkos G, Bouras N. Metacommunity: the current status of psychiatry and mental health-care and implications for the future. BJPsych Int. Published online 2024:1–4. https://doi.org/10.1192/bji.2024.15.

74. Reba YA, Muttaqin MZ, Prasetya YY. Towards democratised psychiatry: building metacom-munities for inclusive and equitable global mental health. BJPsych Int. Published online 2024:1–3. https://doi.org/10.1192/bji.2024.3075.

75. Broome M, Rodrigues J, Ritunnano R, Humpston C. Psychiatry as a vocation: moral injury, Covid-19 and the phenomenology of clinical practice. Clinical Ethics. 2024;19(2):157–70.

76. Rosling H. Introduction factfulness: ten reasons we're wrong about the world—and why things are better that you think. Sceptre; 2019.

77. Mühlhahn K. Ambitions and anxieties: contemporary China, Ch. 12. In: Making China modern: from the great Qing to xi Jinping. The Belknap Press of Harvard University Press; 2019. p. 607.

78. Benavav A. Automation and the future of work. Verso; 2020. p. 63.

79. Benavav A. Automation and the future of work. Verso; 2020. p. 56.

80. Acemoglu D, Restrepo P. Tasks, automation, and the rise in US wage inequality. NBER Working Paper No. 28920, JEL No. J23, J31, O33. 2021. http://www.nber.org/papers/w28920.

81. Marcus G, Freeman J, editors. The future of brain: essays by the world's leading neuroscien-tists. Princeton University Press; 2015.

82. Harvey D. The condition of postmodernity. Blackwell; 1990. p. 299.

83. Toscano A. A phantom with limbs of steel, Ch 4. In: Late Fascism. Verso; 2023. p. 91.

84. Weiss L. America Inc.? Innovation and enterprise in the national security state. Cornel University Press; 2014.

85. Harvey D. The political economic transformation of late twentieth century capitalism, part II. In: The condition of postmodernity. Blackwell; 1990.

86. Parikka J. A geology of media. University of Minesota Press; 2015.

87. Bostrom N. Is the default outcome doom? Ch 8. In: Superintelligence: paths, dangers, strate-gies. Oxford University Press; 2014.

88. Persaud A, Day G, Gupta S, et al. Geopolitical factors and mental health I. Int J Soc Psychiatry. 2018;64(8):778–85. https://doi.org/10.1177/0020764018808548.

89. Bell R, Marmot M. Social determinants and mental health. In: Bhugra D, Moussaoui D, Craig TJ, editors. Oxford textbook of social psychiatry. Oxford: Oxford University Press; 2022. p. 171–9.

90. Yu S. Uncovering the hidden impacts of inequality on mental health: a global study. Transl Psychiatry. 2018;8:98.

91. Pickett KE, Wilkinson R. Inequality: an underacknowledged source of mental illness and distress. Br J Psychiatry. 2019;197:426–8.

92. Cole ER. Intersectionality and research in psychology. Am Psychol. 2009;64(3):170–80. https://doi.org/10.1037/a0014564.

93. Wahlbeck K, McDaid D. Actions to alleviate the mental health impact of the economic crisis. World Psychiatry. 2012;11(3):139–45.

94. Johnson S, Dalton-Locke C, Baker J, et al. Acute psychiatric care: approaches to increasing the range of services and improving access and quality of care. World Psychiatry. 2022;21(2):220–36.

95. Horkheimer M, Adorno TW. Dialektik der Aufklärung. Philosophische Fragmente. Frankfurt am Main: Fischer Taschenbuch; 1988, ISBN 978-3-596-27404-8.

96. Kant I. Beantwortung der Frage: Was ist Aufklärung? Berlinische Monatsschrift, Heft 12. 1784:481–94.

97. Scull A. Madness in civilization: a cultural history of insanity from the bible to Freud, from the madhouse to modern medicine. Thames and Hudson; 2020.

98. Jones K. Asylums and after: a revised history of the mental health services: from the early 18th century to the 1990's. Athlone Press; 1993.

99. Turda M. Degeneration and eugenics, Ch 3. In: Ikkos G, Becker T, editors. Psychiatry after Kraepelin: ambition images practices 1926–2026. Springer Nature; this volume.

100. Boehm O. (4th ed) Radikaler Universalismus. Berlin: Ullstein; 2022.

101. Hoff P. Psychopathologie: operationalisiertes Werkzeug oder „Denkstil"? Eine Reflexion zum diagnostischen Prozess (auch) in der forensischen Psychiatrie. Forens Psychiatr Psychol Kriminologie. 2024;18:332–40.

102. Buck-Morss S. Mythic history: fetish, Ch. 4. In: The dialectics of seeing: Walter Benjamin and the arcades project. MIT Press; 1991.

103. MacPherson CB. The political theory of possessive individualism: Hobbes to Locke. Hassel Street Press; 2021.

104. Wallerstein I. The second era of great expansion of the capitalist world-econom, 1730's–1840's, volume 3. In: The modern world system. University of California; 2011.

105. Wallerstein I. Centrist liberalism triumphant 1789–1914, volume 4. In: The modern world system. University of California; 2011.

106. Byung-Chul H. The crisis of narration. Polity Press; 2024.

107. Tellenbach H. Melancholy. Pittsburgh: Duquesne University Press; 1961, 1980.

108. Warren S. The white rat, Ch. 1. In: Storming bedlam: madness, utopia and revolt. Common Notions; 2024.

109. Foucault M. Surveiller et punir: Naissance de la prison. Gallimard; 1975.

110. Warren S. Barefoot therapeutics, Ch. 2. In: Storming bedlam: madness, utopia and revolt. Common Notions; 2024; Warren, S. (2024) Another Name for Losing our Shirt, Storming Bedlam: Madness, Utopia and Revolt, Common Notions, p. 175.

111. Ings S. Stalin and the Scientists: a History of Triumph and Tragedy 1905–1953; 2016. pp. 426–429; Dole, R. (2024) I accuse psychiatry of murder, Mad in America, 19 November, accessed online 26/11/24.

112. Morgan A. '… the most complex and lyrical song of experience': Walter Benjamin and a dialectical image of madness. Introduction to Walter Benjamin for psychiatry (III). Int Rev Psychiatry. 2024;36(6):612–25. https://doi.org/10.1080/09540261.2024.2354375.

113. Stanghellini G, Mancini M. The therapeutic interview in mental health: a values-based and person-centered approach. Cambridge University Press; 2017.

114. Minkowski E. Traité de psychopathologie. Paris: Empécheurs de penser rond; 1999.

115. Binswanger L. Drei Formen missglückten Daseins: Verstiegenheit, Verschrobenheit, Manieriertheit. De Gruyter; 1956.

116. Stanghellini G. Disembodied spirits and deanimated bodies: the psychopathology of common sense. Oxford University Press; 2004.

117. Esposito CM, Stanghellini G. The pathogenic and therapeutic potential of the gaze of the other in the clinic of "eating disorders". Psychopathology. 2020;53(5–6):291–7.

118. Stanghellini G. Homo dissipans: excess and expenditure as keys for understanding the borderline condition? Psychopathology. 2023. https://doi.org/10.1159/000529130.

119. Christin Hempeler BA, Lydia Schneider-Reuter MA, Anne-Sophie Windel MD, Jona Carlet BA, et al. Psychiatric services. 2024, published online 28 June. https://doi.org/10.1176/appi.ps.20230252.

120. Forgacs D, editor. The Gramsci reader: selected writings, 1916–1935. New York University Press; 2000.
121. Becker T, Müller T, Ikkos G, Speerforck S. Radical social theorists Antonio Gramsci and Walter Benjamin: can they help understand and power effective mental health reform? Int Rev Psychiatry. 2024. https://doi.org/10.1080/09540261.2024.23648446
122. Flam H. The study of transnational movements. In: Middell M, editor. The Routledge handbook of transregional studies. London: Routledge; 2018. p. 82–90. https://doi.org/10.4324/9780429438233.
123. e.g.,Dube S. Figures of immanence. In: Dube S, Seth S, Skaria A, editors. Dipesh Chakrabarty and the global south. Subaltern studies, postcolonial perspectives, and the Anthropocene. New York: Routledge; 2020. p. 232–47.
124. Beresford P. Mad people and mad studies, Ch 12. In: Ikkos G, Becker T, editors. Psychiatry after Kraepelin: ambition images practices 1926–2026. Springer Nature; this volume.
125. Heinz A. Das kolonialisierte Gehirn und die Wege der Revolte. suhrkamp taschenbuch wissenschaft. Berlin: Suhrkamp Verlag; 2023, ISBN 978-3-518-30003-9
126. Heinz A, Müller DJ, Krach S, Cabanis M, Kluge UP. The uncanny return of the race concept. Front Hum Neurosci. 2014;8:836. https://doi.org/10.3389/fnhum.2014.00836. eCollection 2014. PMID: 25408642
127. Satram V. Decolonising our minds: what UK psychiatry needs to (un)learn. BJPsych Bulletin. 2024;48(4):261–3. https://doi.org/10.1192/bjb.2024.62.
128. Poole R, Robinson CA. Breaking out of the citadel: social theory and psychiatry. BJPsych Bulletin. 2023;47(3):146–9. https://doi.org/10.1192/bjb.2022.17.
129. Brown W. Nihilistic times: thinking with max Weber, Belknap. Cambridge, MA: Harvard University Press; 2023. p. 104.

Open Access This chapter is licensed under the terms of the Creative Commons Attribution 4.0 International License (http://creativecommons.org/licenses/by/4.0/), which permits use, sharing, adaptation, distribution and reproduction in any medium or format, as long as you give appropriate credit to the original author(s) and the source, provide a link to the Creative Commons license and indicate if changes were made.

The images or other third party material in this chapter are included in the chapter's Creative Commons license, unless indicated otherwise in a credit line to the material. If material is not included in the chapter's Creative Commons license and your intended use is not permitted by statutory regulation or exceeds the permitted use, you will need to obtain permission directly from the copyright holder.

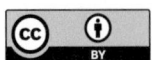

Afterword: Psychiatry's Long Twentieth Century—Kraepelin, Methods and Metaphysics

Matthew R. Broome

It was a great privilege to both be part of the excellent conference *AfterKraepelin: Ambitions, Images, Practices and the History of Psychiatry 1926–2026* at the Royal Society of Medicine in March 2025,[1] and to be asked to write an afterword for this incredible volume, marking the centenary of Kraepelin's death.

Given the geopolitical turmoil currently, a striking impression I had of the event in London was how the global intellectual community can transcend international concerns, and how clinicians, historians, philosophers, social scientists, biological researchers, service users, experts by experience can meet to discuss important academic issues that, although seemingly of primarily historical relevance, are of pressing importance to mental health science and practice now and into the future. To keep this time frame in mind, I was stimulated by the closing chapter of the volume (Chap. 27, Ikkos et al.,) which discusses the long twentieth century in their closing comments (I would extend this from roughly 1870 to the present). This struck me as a useful temporal lens that allows us to go back into the latter part of the nineteenth century, the period when Kraepelin began as a researcher and psychiatrist, and to consider psychiatry as it is practiced today, in the first part of the twenty-first century.

---

[1] An account of this conference can be read at Mason, J. (2026) Kraepelin 2026, HOPSIG Newsletter: Newsletter of the RCPsych's History of Psychiatry Special Interest Group, 20, 28–22 https://www.rcpsych.ac.uk/docs/default-source/members/sigs/hopsig/newsletters/hopsig-newsletter%2D%2D-spring-2025.pdf?sfvrsn=8e6340d3_3

M. R. Broome
Institute for Mental Health, University of Birmingham, Birmingham, UK

Birmingham and Solihull Mental Health NHS Foundation Trust, Birmingham, UK
e-mail: m.r.broome@bham.ac.uk

© The Editor(s) (if applicable) and The Author(s) 2026
G. Ikkos, T. Becker (eds.), *Psychiatry after Kraepelin*,
https://doi.org/10.1007/978-3-032-09475-9

509

The contributions to this book are rich and varied and I commend the authors and editors for doing such an excellent job in bringing the volume together. I believe it will serve internationally as a powerful reminder, spur and warning, for us to work together, across practice, policy, research and advocacy, to improve the lives of those with mental ill health and think how we can also change society to achieve that aim. Although I am unable to do justice to all the chapters, I have picked out several themes which particularly interested me as a researcher, a psychiatrist who works with young people with psychosis and as someone interested in the history and philosophy of psychiatry.

Responses to the First Biological Psychiatry

As Nietzsche repeatedly reminds us, nihilism and the loss of values may be a requirement for a rebirth for a new system of thought and morality. Hoff (Chap. 3) discusses connections between Emil Kraepelin, Karl Jaspers (1883–1969) and Arthur Kronfeld (1886–1941). Work on the history of psychiatry suggests a period of intense research in biological psychiatry in the middle of the nineteenth century [1, 2], but one where progress slows and therapeutic pessimism replaces the previous scientific optimism. A key figure in this 'first biological psychiatry' was Wilhelm Griesinger (1817–1868). In 1845 Griesinger stated that *Psychische Krankheiten sind Erkrankungen des Gehirns* (Mental Illnesses are Diseases of the Brain), setting out a programme of neuropathological research for psychiatry. Alongside his clinical and academic work, Griesinger worked institutionally to reform psychiatry in Germany, moving the speciality from a focus on alienists in asylums to 'cerebral pathologists' working in university clinics. With this professional shift, came an emphasis on the tools of histopathology as the main route to study mental illness and the brain. Engstrom describes psychiatrists in this period, thus:

> Their observations were directed not so much at institutionalized patients, as at histological specimens, and vivisected animals. They drew less upon skills derived from years of asylum experience and more upon practices and techniques learned as students and honed in rudimentary laboratory facilities. Their ideal was not the practicing alienist, but rather the diligent researcher who spent long hours in front of the microscope and at the autopsy table. The psychiatric knowledge that they extracted from their objects of study was the product of disciplined laboratory conduct in handling microscopes and specimens, in opening the cranium, in applying electrodes. For them, psychiatry was a natural science with its own rigorous techniques and modes of observation. [2, pg. 89]

Although many gains were made in an intense period of a few decades, for the young Kraepelin and Jaspers, this approach seemed to be running out of steam, and they turned to alternative or adjunctive approaches to neuropathological psychiatry to reinvigorate their speciality. Jaspers, in his own autobiographical writings, describes his experience of psychiatry:

> The realization that scientific investigation and therapy were in a state of stagnation was widespread in German psychiatric clinics at that time. The large institutions for the

mentally ill were built constantly more hygienic and more magnificent. The lives of the unfortunate inmates, which could not be changed essentially, were controlled […]. In view of the exceedingly small amount of knowledge and technical knowhow, intelligent, yet unproductive psychiatrists, such as Hoche, took recourse to a sceptical attitude and to elegant sounding phrases of gentlemanly superiority. In Nissl's hospital too, therapeutic resignation was dominant. In therapeutics we were basically without hope, but we were humane and kind and prevented, as far as possible, any calamity which might unnecessarily result from the condition of the mentally ill [3, pg. 16]

With Griesinger, Kraepelin would have been concerned with the isolation of the alienists and, as drawn out in multiple chapters of this volume, was concerned with reconnecting psychiatry with medicine, and making psychiatry a key part of the medical profession and research endeavour. Jaspers takes a different route, and one to which, inspired Iby Fulford and colleagues [4, 5], I am sympathetic to—psychiatry is medicine, but not just medicine as narrowly conceived. It has to draw on philosophy and social sciences to address the real complexity of psychiatry's subject matter, and the object of its investigation, namely the person rather than just the brain [6]. Jaspers turns to phenomenology and hermeneutics, and, as helpfully outlined by Steinberg and Schomerus (Chap. 1), Kraepelin was similarly dissatisfied with the approach of Gudden and Flechsig and the brain-anatomical school, and he turned to the experimental psychology of Wundt, psychopharmacology (Ferrier, Chap. 2), and subsequently nosology and longitudinal studies (Frances, Foreword) as methods to advance scientific psychiatry. Hence, as argued by Hoff (Chap. 3), both Jaspers and Kraepelin are united in their disappointment with the first biological psychiatry and the brain-anatomical school and concerns regarding 'brain mythology' and both serve as 'heterological thinkers', in Kronfeld's taxonomy, in their response—drawing on concepts and methods from related scientific disciplines, but with each prioritising different allied areas of research.

Kraepelin's Methods and Metaphysics

Reading Steinberg and Schomerus (Chap. 1), it is interesting how Kraepelin was able to dissect Wundt's work, taking what was useful to psychiatry and stretching the methods and objectives beyond Wundt's intentions. Hence, Kraepelin began using the techniques of experimental psychology not only to study those with mental illnesses but also to adapt experimental techniques accordingly to this participant group, and to go beyond Wundt in studying higher mental functions. As Frances notes (foreword), Kraepelin was an epistemological and naïve realist, or perhaps what I'd refer to as a common-sense realist. He viewed the entities of psychiatry as real objects, like others in the world, where different modes of perception or investigation will reveal the same construct and this construct tends to endure over time. Such constructs are discrete and demarcated from others, and if they have a single defining feature or rigid essence, can be thought of as natural kinds, in the language of contemporary metaphysics and philosophy of science. However, when Steinberg and Schomerus helpfully cite Kraepelin's compendium, he goes further in that he seems to view that this realist structure is replicated, in a meaningful pattern, at different levels of explanation and analysis, and further that mental disorders can be broken down into their constituent symptoms, which in turn can be understood as variations from normal psychological functioning. Kraepelin writes (cited in Chap. 1):

> In order to fully understand mental disorders, it is essential to break down given symptoms into their smallest components and to ascribe these elementary alterations of mental processes to pathological changes of basic mental functions in general. The clinical approach in psychiatry can only prove successful if it is coupled with an exact analysis of basic mental phenomena and a profound knowledge of basic mental functions established by scientifically based psychology. Without this, facing mental disorders […] will be like trying to analyse urine without the help of our chemical and physiological knowledge. It would be totally impossible to identify the real pathological components, let alone to ascribe them to a specific organic illness.

Reading this passage, and perhaps emphasising the contemporary timeliness of Kraepelin's thinking, I felt as if I could be reading a paper from the early part of this century, where cognitive neuropsychiatry [7] became an important research endeavour. This approach, as Kraepelin and Wundt's experimental psychology, connected psychopathology with normal cognitive function. Halligan and David define cognitive neuropsychiatry as 'a systematic and theoretically driven approach to explain clinical psychopathologies in terms of deficits to normal cognitive mechanisms'. They continue: 'A concern with the neural substrates of impaired cognitive mechanisms links cognitive neuropsychiatry to the basic neurosciences' [7 , p. 209]. The authors go on to describe the methodology of such a paradigm, according to which psychiatric disorders need to be understood within the framework of cognitive psychology and by referring to the pathology of brain structures [7, 8]. Hence, as with Kraepelin, cognitive neuropsychiatry sees the symptoms of mental illness as understandable and explainable within our existing psychological frameworks and characterises the symptoms of mental illnesses as being consequent on deficits and biases of normal psychological function, and thus due to similar mechanisms. On this account, psychopathology is not something qualitatively different from the rest of mental life and experience.

This approach of Kraepelin, and cognitive neuropsychiatry, outlines a scientific approach that has been incredibly fertile and broadly fits under the rubric of 'reductionism' that, although not wholly smooth, suggests that constructs at the syndromal level (our diagnoses) can be reduced to symptoms, which in turn can be reduced to changes in psychological processes, and then can relate to neuroscience and brain function. Such an approach methodologically reveals Kraepelin's covert, and possibly unexamined, metaphysics and is not unusual in science, as Dennett writes:

> Scientists sometimes deceive themselves into thinking that philosophical ideas are only, at best, decorations or parasitic commentaries on the hard, objective triumphs of science, and that they themselves are immune to the confusions that philosophers devote their lives to dissolving. But there is no such thing as philosophy-free science; there is only science whose philosophical baggage is taken on board without examination. [9, pg. 21].

The philosophy of psychiatry has however been aware of the complexity of the nature of mental disorder and offers various responses to this [10]. A recent important work by Jefferson [11, 12] goes back to the clarion call of Griesinger and examines whether mental disorders are indeed brain disorders. Jefferson's novelty is that rather than firstly focusing on what a mental disorder may be, she interrogates the concept of brain disorder. In doing this, she examines a 'narrow' view of brain disorder, dominated by the example of neurosyphilis and offers an 'expansive' conception [13]. On this account brain disorders can be seen as brain dysfunction- brain difference, which in turn realises psychological dysfunction, which if harmful would also be understood as mental disorders. And this 'realisation' or instantiation can be multiple (i.e. there may be multiple ways a brain can be different to lead to a similar psychological dysfunction and hence is less tightly linked to a single unitary cause).

This approach has the important conceptual gain of expanding our theoretical scope in that, although it may be the case that some mental disorders can also be brain disorders (where there is difference/dysfunction realising harmful psychological dysfunction), on this analysis, there can also be mental disorders that are not brain disorders, and conversely, as we know from neurology, brain disorders that aren't mental disorders, and are psychologically silent. Hence, this approach moves us beyond the dichotomy of 'are mental disorders brain disorders or psychological disorders?', with the answer, that they can be both, with both physiological and psychological properties and modes of investigation. Despite Jefferson herself endorsing a physicalist conception of mental disorder, she acknowledges that her own conceptual analysis aligns with a subtype of property dualism, where psychological dysfunction could occur theoretically in the absence of brain difference. Further, she endorses the conception of mental disorder as 'autonomous' from the notion of brain disorder: concepts of mental disorders do not rely on the state of the brain for their status, but rather normative claims about psychological function and distress.

This idea of the 'autonomy of the mental' can perhaps couple with a more phenomenological view that mental disorders are disorders of the person, or the being-in-the-world. Psychological dysfunction, given its status being linked to normative claims, could be thought to only be apparent in the context of a person engaged in meaningful tasks that link to a project over time, and which rely on a wider interpersonal and social context. Hence, and picking up on Jefferson's conceptual separation of brain and psychological difference-dysfunction and multiple realisability, this allows a conception of psychological dysfunction and harm that is not linked necessarily to brain difference but rather to changes in the embodied, embedded, enactive and extended mind [14]. Externalism in the philosophy of mind offers a potential expansion of her views on multiple realisability of psychological dysfunction and would offer the view that it is not only the brain that acts as a realiser of such change but the body-world too. This would take seriously the claims of extended mind/vehicle externalism hypotheses whereby the structure of the world, how we navigate it, and the tools we use, instantiate our mental acts, processes and states. On this account, some mental states are, at least in part, *constituted* by factors that are located outside the brain, or the biological boundaries of the individuals who have those mental states.

This recognition of a complex and multiple causality in psychiatry resonates with many contributors to this volume (e.g. Owen, Chap. 6; Lawrie, Chap. 7; Heckers, Chap. 14; Falkai, Chap. 23; and Murray et al., Chap. 25) and is relevant to what is perhaps seen as Kraepelin's greatest contribution to psychiatry, namely the so-called Kraepelinian dichotomy and the demarcation of dementia praecox from manic-depressive insanity, or schizophrenia from bipolar disorders.

The Concept of Schizophrenia

In their chapter, Ramirez-Bermudez and Aftab (Chap. 8) examine how the notion of schizophrenia has changed over time, and whether we should see this as a unitary, continuous concept and construct over time or if there is discontinuity. I came into psychiatry when the Kraepelinian dichotomy was under serious assault from several areas of research—neuroimaging, neuropsychology, outcome studies, genetics and clinical psychopathology—with an important paper by Craddock and Owen summarising many of the key issues [15]. This critique of the clear demarcation of schizophrenia and bipolar led to a reconceptualising of both disorders, recognising features that had been thought to be archetypal in one, being present in the other and vice versa. Schizophrenia, thus, became affective and bipolar, cognitive. Rather than a dichotomy, a variety of continua or, as Owen helpfully characterises it (Chap. 6), a range of orthogonal dimensions, which, in how they are weighted and combine in a given individual, will create a specific syndrome, which may be more or less like the classical descriptions of schizophrenia or bipolar. Thinking back to Kraepelin, here the realism is pushed back from level of syndrome or diagnosis to these orthogonal transdiagnostic dimensions which underpin our diagnoses. With ideas of multiple realisability and complex causality, this opens new avenues of intervention, in addition to antipsychotics, as described by Murray and colleagues (Chap. 25).

As a psychiatry trainee at the close of the last century and the beginning of this one, as well as the pressure on the dichotomy and the boundaries of established psychiatric illnesses, I saw there was also an expansion of the psychosis concept and a blurring between caseness and non-caseness. Here, I am thinking of the expansion of scientific work on the prodromal phase of psychosis [16] and clinical staging [17], but also the recognition of psychotic-like experiences occurring in a non-help seeking proportion of the population [18], leading to ideas around a continuum or continua of psychosis, from health and full function to distress and marked impairment. Despite these pressures on the core schizophrenia concept—both from bipolar disorder, and from prodromal or psychotic experiences in the general population—I still find it a useful notion. As in comments above around Kraepelin, depending on one's philosophical position, a concept can still be useful without committing one to realist or natural kind view of psychiatric disorders. Schizophrenia can be fuzzy construct with blurred boundaries, and one perhaps that changes over time as Ramirez-Bermudez and Aftab suggest (Chap. 8). In their closing contribution, Ikkos et al. (Chap. 27) discuss the work of the social scientist Max Weber, and it is Weber and his concept of ideal types that I find particularly useful here [10]. For Weber, ideal types do not exist in reality ('In its conceptual purity, this mental construct [*Gedankenbild*] cannot be found anywhere in reality. It is a utopia'). Burger offers a useful definition of Weber's notoriously hard to pin down idea:

> Ideal types are statements of general form asserting the existence of certain constellations of elements which are empirically only approximated by the instances of the class of phenomena to which each type refers. [19, pg. 134].

Hence, an ideal type is an intellectual construct which we may not expect to find replicated in reality as such but can still guide our research. And this is where I think schizophrenia can still be a helpful concept in research and practice, albeit with the caveat that there may be multiple, differing, partially unexamined, concepts in existence at once in our field, and certainly over time. Kraepelin himself is a key figure in the conceptual genesis of schizophrenia, developing ideas from Ewald Hecker (1843–1909) and Karl Ludwig Kahlbaum (1829–1899), with his own ideas being taken forward by Bleuler and Schneider [20], and the Neo-Kraepelinians of the DSM (Frances, foreword). One of my own concerns as a psychiatrist, and one addressed by Falkai (Chap. 23), is that with DSM and Schneiderian schizophrenia the constructs of Kraepelin (who emphasised cognitive function) and Bleuler have been replaced by one which is heavily determined by the presence of positive symptoms, such as hallucination and delusions, precisely the areas of the clinical presentation we can generally treat well since the advent of anti-psychotics. This allows psychiatrists to both think they are being helpful but also perhaps lead us to neglect the impairment caused by negative and cognitive symptoms, which remain hard to treat. As with Falkai, I hope this will be an area of increasing research going forward as we close the long twentieth century and keep a Kraepelinian dementia praecox in our minds.

Concluding Thoughts

In this brief afterword, I have focussed on themes in the history and philosophy of psychiatry, psychiatric research methods and schizophrenia. Here, there is a strong legacy for psychiatry from Kraepelin's work—his scientific rigour, his use of multiple research methods and his wish to reconnect psychiatry with medicine. But his legacy is by no means wholly positive, and many key contributions to the volume address this in detail. Arguably, Kraepelin left us a concept of serious mental illness that can be viewed as pessimistic and can lead to therapeutic nihilism. Although Kraepelin himself is more nuanced in his writing, Kraepelinian dementia praecox is seen for many clinicians to suggest that schizophrenia is a progressive, degenerative illness, with a limited prospect for recovery and a fulfilling life. Only relatively recently, with more optimistic models of service delivery and community care, and the role of patient advocacy and coproduction, has this partially shifted. One hopes that with research and novel treatments addressing cognitive and negative symptoms, this can be improved further.

Finally, the most distressing element of Kraepelin's legacy is discussed by Turda (Chap. 4) and other contributors. Kraepelin endorsed eugenics and racial hygiene, as a form of public mental health and preventative psychiatry. His support of these ideas, given his academic status, generated an intellectual legacy that may have eased the creation and acceptance of the Nazi T4 euthanasia programme, implemented in part by his own students, and the subsequent extermination of those with mental illness in the Holocaust. With a rise of Far Right and Populism again across the world, clinicians and researchers need to be aware of how science can be used as a tool against the most vulnerable in society and globally, and to guard against that, and to remember our first duty as doctors is to help the suffering individual and as citizens, to improve society. Raymond Williams would endorse Ikkos and colleagues (Chap. 27) in a striving for a (micro) utopia amongst the pessimism: 'To be truly radical is to make hope possible rather than despair convincing'. [21, pg. 118].

References

1. Shorter E. A history of psychiatry: from the era of the asylum to the age of Prozac. New York: John Wiley & Sons; 1997.
2. Engstrom EJ. Clinical psychiatry in imperial Germany: a history of psychiatric practice. Ithaca (NY) and London: Cornell University Press; 2003.
3. Jaspers K. Philosophical autobiography. In: Schilpp PA, editor. The philosophy of Karl Jaspers. La Salle (IL): Open Court Publishing Co.; 1957.
4. Fulford KWM. Commentary. Adv Psychiatr Treat. 2002;8(5):359–63. https://doi.org/10.1192/apt.8.5.359.
5. Fulford KW, Stanghellini G, Broome M. What can philosophy do for psychiatry? World Psychiatry. 2004;3(3):130.
6. Broome MR. Jaspers and neuroscience. In: One century of Karl Jaspers' general psychopathology; 2013. p. 121–32.
7. Halligan PW, David AS. Cognitive neuropsychiatry: towards a scientific psychopathology. Nat Rev Neurosci. 2001;2(3):209–15.
8. Broome MR, Bortolotti L, editors. Psychiatry as cognitive neuroscience: an overview. In: Broome M, Bortolotti L, editors. Psychiatry as cognitive neuroscience: philosophical perspectives, International Perspectives in Philosophy & Psychiatry. 2009; online edn, Oxford: Oxford Academic; 2013. https://doi.org/10.1093/med/9780199238033.003.0001, accessed 28 Aug 2025.
9. Dennett DC. Darwin's dangerous idea: evolution and the meanings of life. New York: Simon & Schuster; 1995.
10. Broome MR. Taxonomy and ontology in psychiatry: a survey of recent literature. Philos Psychiatry Psychol. 2006;13(4):303–19.
11. Jefferson A. Are mental disorders brain disorders? Routledge; 2022.
12. Jefferson A. Are mental disorders brain disorders?–a precis. Philos Psychol. 2024;37(3):552–7.
13. Broome MR. In: Jefferson A, editor. The complexity of brain disorders and the worldliness of mental disorders: are mental disorders brain disorders? Oxford: Routledge; 2022. 108 pp., £ 48.99, ISBN: 9780367421380.
14. De Haan S. An enactive approach to psychiatry. Philos Psychiatry Psychol. 2020;27(1):3–25.
15. Craddock N, Owen MJ. The beginning of the end for the Kraepelinian dichotomy. Br J Psychiatry. 2005;186(5):364–6.
16. Yung AR, McGorry PD. The prodromal phase of first-episode psychosis: past and current conceptualizations. Schizophr Bull. 1996;22(2):353–70.
17. McGorry PD, Hickie IB, Yung AR, Pantelis C, Jackson HJ. Clinical staging of psychiatric disorders: a heuristic framework for choosing earlier, safer and more effective interventions. Aust N Z J Psychiatry. 2006;40(8):616–22.
18. Van Os J, Linscott RJ, Myin-Germeys I, Delespaul P, Krabbendam LJ. A systematic review and meta-analysis of the psychosis continuum: evidence for a psychosis proneness–persistence–impairment model of psychotic disorder. Psychol Med. 2009;39(2):179–95.

© The Editor(s) (if applicable) and The Author(s) 2026
G. Ikkos, T. Becker (eds.), *Psychiatry after Kraepelin*,
https://doi.org/10.1007/978-3-032-09475-9

19. Burger T. Max Weber's theory of concept formation: history, laws, and ideal types. Durham, NC: Duke University Press; 1976.
20. Hoenig J. The Concept of Schizophrenia Kraepelin–Bleuler–Schneider. Br J Psychiatry. 1983;142(6):547–56.
21. Williams R. Resources of hope: culture, democracy, socialism. London: Verso; 1989.

Index

© The Editor(s) (if applicable) and The Author(s) 2026
G. Ikkos, T. Becker (eds.), *Psychiatry after Kraepelin*,
https://doi.org/10.1007/978-3-032-09475-9

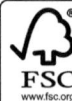

MIX

Papier aus verantwortungsvollen Quellen

Paper from responsible sources

FSC® C105338

If you have any concerns about our products,
you can contact us on
ProductSafety@springernature.com

In case Publisher is established outside the EU,
the EU authorized representative is:
**Springer Nature Customer Service Center GmbH
Europaplatz 3, 69115 Heidelberg, Germany**

Printed by Libri Plureos GmbH
in Hamburg, Germany

V